CURRENT

Diagnosis & Treatment in
Vascular Surgery

a **LANGE** medical book

CURRENT

Diagnosis & Treatment in
Vascular Surgery

First Edition

Edited by

Richard H. Dean, MD
Professor of Surgery
Director, Division of Surgical Sciences
Bowman Gray School of Medicine of
Wake Forest University
Winston-Salem

James S.T. Yao, MD, PhD
Magerstadt Professor of Surgery
Division of Vascular Surgery
Northwestern University
School of Medicine
Chicago

David C. Brewster, MD
Clinical Professor of Surgery
Harvard Medical School
Massachusetts General Hospital
Boston

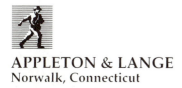

APPLETON & LANGE
Norwalk, Connecticut

Copyright ©1995 by Appleton & Lange
A Simon & Schuster Company

95 96 97 98 / 10 9 8 7 6 5 4 3 2 1

Prentice Hall International (UK) Limited, *London*
Prentice Hall of Australia Pty. Limited, *Sydney*
Prentice Hall Canada, Inc., *Toronto*
Prentice Hall Hispanoamericana, S.A., *Mexico*
Prentice Hall of India Private Limited, *New Delhi*
Prentice Hall of Japan, Inc., *Tokyo*
Simon & Schuster Asia Pte. Ltd., *Singapore*
Editora Prentice Hall do Brasil Ltda., *Rio de Janeiro*
Prentice Hall, *Englewood Cliffs*, *New Jersey*

ISBN: 0-8385-1351-4
ISSN: 1080-5125

ISBN: 0-8385-1351-4

90000

9 780838 513514

Acquisitions Editor: Shelley Reinhardt
Production Editor: Todd Miller
Cover Design: Elizabeth Schmitz

PRINTED IN THE UNITED STATES OF AMERICA

Table of Contents

Authors

John G. Adams, Jr., MD
Resident, Department of Vascular Surgery, University of Missouri at Columbia School of Medicine.

Dennis F. Bandyk, MD
Professor of Surgery, University of South Florida College of Medicine, Tampa.

Marshall E. Benjamin, MD
Research Fellow in Vascular Surgery, Division of Surgical Sciences, Bowman Gray School of Medicine of Wake Forest University, Winston-Salem.

John J. Bergan, MD
Clinical Professor of Surgery, University of California, San Diego School of Medicine, La Jolla.

Ramon Berguer, MD, PhD
Professor of Surgery, Wayne State University School of Medicine; and Chief, Section of Vascular Surgery, Harper Hospital, Detroit.

F. William Blaisdell, MD
Professor and Chairman, Department of Surgery, University of California, Davis School of Medicine, Sacramento.

John Blebea, MD
Assistant Professor of Surgery, University of Cincinnati School of Medicine; and Chief, Section of Vascular Surgery, Cincinnati Veterans Affairs Medical Center, Cincinnati.

David C. Brewster, MD
Clinical Professor of Surgery, Harvard Medical School; and Massachusetts General Hospital, Boston.

Arun Chervu, MD
Assistant Professor, Section of Vascular Surgery, Department of Surgery, The University of Texas Southwestern Medical Center at Dallas; Staff Surgeon, Department of Surgery, University of Texas Southwestern Medical School Affiliated Hospitals.

G. Patrick Clagett, MD
Professor and Head, Section of Vascular Surgery, Department of Surgery, The University of Texas Southwestern Medical Center at Dallas; Staff Surgeon, Department of Surgery, University of Southwestern Medical School Affiliated Hospitals.

Michael A. Cooper, MD
Assistant Clinical Professor, Department of Surgery, University of Colorado Health Sciences Center, Denver; Department of Surgery, Rose Medical Center, Denver.

Joseph S. Coselli, MD
Associate Professor of Surgery, Baylor College of Medicine, Houston, Texas.

Jack L. Cronenwett, MD
Professor of Surgery, Dartmouth Medical School, Hanover, New Hampshire; and Chief, Section of Vascular Surgery, Dartmouth-Hitchcock Medical Center, Lebanon, New Hampshire.

Bruce S. Cutler, MD
Professor of Surgery and Chairman, Division of Vascular Surgery, University of Massachusetts Medical School, Worcester.

Richard H. Dean, MD
Professor and Director, Division of Surgical Sciences, Bowman Gray School of Medicine of Wake Forest University, Winston-Salem.

David H. Deaton, MD
Assistant Clinical Professor of Surgery, University of Pennsylvania School of Medicine, Philadelphia; and Attending Surgeon, Jeanes Hospital, Philadelphia.

Ralph G. DePalma, MD, FACS
Professor of Surgery and Associate Dean, Department of Surgery, University of Nevada, School of Medicine, Reno

Glenn E. Esses, MD
Fellow, Department of Surgery, University of South Florida College of Medicine, Tampa.

Richard L. Feinberg, MD
Assistant Clinical Professor of Surgery, Division of Vascular Surgery, George Washington University School of Medicine, Washington, DC.

Stanley B. Fuller, MD
Bradshaw Fellow in Surgical Research, Bowman Gray School of Medicine of Wake Forest University, Winston-Salem.

Peter Gloviczki, MD
Professor of Surgery, Mayo Medical School, Rochester, Minnesota; and Consultant, Division of Vascular Surgery, Mayo Clinic and Foundation, Rochester, Minnesota.

Richard M. Green, MD
Associate Professor of Surgery; and Chief, Section of Vascular Surgery, University of Rochester School of Medicine, Rochester, New York.

Kimberley J. Hansen, MD
Associate Professor of Surgery, Department of General Surgery, Bowman Gray School of Medicine of Wake Forest University, Winston-Salem.

Robert W. Hobson II, MD
Professor of Surgery and Physiology and Chief, Section of Vascular Surgery, University of Medicine of New Jersey, New Jersey Medical School, Newark.

Douglas B. Hood, MD
Fellow, Department of Surgery, University of Southern California School of Medicine, Los Angeles.

George Johnson, Jr., MD
Roscoe B.G. Cowper Distinguished Professor of Surgery, University of North Carolina School of Medicine, Chapel Hill.

Richard F. Kempczinski, MD
Professor of Surgery and Chief of Vascular Surgery, University of Cincinnati Medical Center, Cincinnati.

Scott A. LeMaire, MD
Resident in Surgery, Baylor College of Medicine, Houston, Texas.

Frank W. LoGerfo, MD
Professor of Surgery, Harvard Medical School; and Chief, Division of Vascular Surgery, New England Deaconess Hospital, Boston.

William A. Marston, MD
Vascular Fellow, University of North Carolina Hospitals, Chapel Hill.

Richard L. McCann, MD
Professor of Surgery, Duke University School of Medicine, Durham.

Wesley S. Moore, MD
Professor of Surgery, University of California, Los Angeles, School of Medicine; and Chief, Section of Vascular Surgery, University of California, Los Angeles Medical Center.

R. Donald Patman, MD
Clinical Assistant Professor of Surgery, University of Texas Southwestern Medical School, Dallas; Attending Surgeon, Baylor University Medical Center, Dallas.

William C. Pevec, MD
Assistant Professor of Vascular Surgery, University of California, Davis School of Medicine, Sacramento.

Robert Y. Rhee, MD
Fellow, Division of Vascular Surgery, Mayo Clinic and Foundation, Rochester, Minnesota.

David Robaczewski, MD
Bradshaw Fellow in Surgical Research, Department of General Surgery, Bowman Gray School of Medicine of Wake Forest University, Winston-Salem.

William D. Routh, MD
Assistant Professor of Radiology and Section Head, Cardiovascular and Interventional Radiology, Bowman Gray School of Medicine of Wake Forest University, Winston-Salem.

Lawrence N. Sampson, MD
Vascular Surgery Fellow, Section of Vascular Surgery, Dartmouth-Hitchcock Medical Center, Lebanon.

Richard J. Sanders, MD
Clinical Professor of Surgery, University of Colorado Health Sciences Center, Denver; and Department of Surgery, Rose Medical Center, Denver.

Mark C. Sebastian, MD
Fellow, Surgical Critical Care, Duke University Medical Center, Durham, North Carolina.

William P. Shutze, MD
Associate Attending in Vascular Surgery, Baylor University Medical Center, Dallas, Texas.

Donald Silver, MD
W. Alton Jones Distinguished Professor and Chairman, Department of Surgery, University of Missouri at Columbia School of Medicine.

James C. Stanley, MD
Professor of Surgery and Head, Section of Vascular Surgery, University of Michigan School of Medicine, Ann Arbor.

William D. Suggs, MD
Assistant Professor of Surgery, Albert Einstein College of Medicine, New York; Division of Vascular Surgery, Montefiore Medical Center, New York.

Hugh H. Trout III, MD, FACS
Clinical Professor of Surgery, George Washington University School of Medicine, Washington, DC.

Frank J. Veith, MD
Professor of Surgery, Albert Einstein College of Medicine, New York; and Chief, Vascular Surgical Services, Montefiore Medical Center, New York.

Fred A. Weaver, MD
Associate Professor of Surgery, University of Southern California School of Medicine, Los Angeles.

Kurt R. Wengerter, MD, RVT, FACS
Assistant Professor of Surgery, Albert Einstein College of Medicine, New York; and Chief of Vascular Surgery, Weiler Hospital, New York.

Rodney A. White, MD
Professor of Surgery, University of California, Los Angeles, School of Medicine; Harbor-UCLA Medical Center, Torrance.

James S.T. Yao, MD, PhD
Magerstadt Professor of Surgery, Division of Vascular Surgery, Northwestern University School of Medicine, Chicago.

Albert E. Yellin, MD, FACS
Professor of Surgery and Chief, Division of Vascular Surgery, University of Southern California School of Medicine, Los Angeles.

Preface

Current Diagnosis and Treatment in Vascular Surgery provides a ready reference for the evaluation and management of vascular diseases. It is designed with the same format as other books in the Lange *Current* series and focuses on the most pertinent aspects of clinical presentation, diagnostic study, and therapeutic options. Other aspects of each disease, such as epidemiology and pathology, are presented only to the extent that they contribute to the book's purpose and overview of patient care. The book includes discussions of clinically important information regarding diseases of the arterial tree, venous system, and the lymphatic system. Each chapter contains references to the relevant scientific literature should the reader desire more extensive information on any aspect of the chapter.

OUTSTANDING FEATURES

- Authors are recognized authorities in their respective fields.
- Comprehensive coverage of vascular diseases.
- Current knowledge of presentation, diagnosis, and management of vascular diseases emphasized.
- Strong art program illustrating surgical and anatomic concepts.

INTENDED AUDIENCE

Health professionals not practicing vascular surgery and medical students will find this text a useful and complete introductory reference to vascular diseases. Salient points provided in each chapter are taught and practiced at major teaching medical centers. Likewise, house officers not pursuing a career in the management of vascular disease will find this text to be a useful reference; it will provide a clinically useful discussion of the diseases they might encounter during their postgraduate education. Finally, practicing physicians, who might be called upon to evaluate and initiate treatment of vascular disease, will find that this book serves as a reference for review and will aid in updating knowledge on the current diagnostic evaluation and management strategies.

ORGANIZATION

The organization of this book follows traditional lines and is arranged into arterial, venous, and lymphatic disease segments. The early chapters are devoted to general topics for the evaluation of the vascular patient. The first chapter appropriately concentrates on the medical history and physical extremities. Subsequent chapters assess the noninvasive diagnostic laboratory studies, angiographic, and other radiologic methods for assessment of vascular disease. Preoperative and postoperative care, clotting abnormalities, and renal dysfunction are afforded individual chapters, underscoring their importance in the management of patients with vascular disease. Subsequent chapters are generally arranged in the order in which blood flows from the heart—specifically, brachiocephalic disease and carotid artery disease followed by thoracic and abdominal aortic disease, visceral and renal disease, and finally, lower extremity occlusive and aneurysmal disease. Other arterial and vascular syndromes that are not occlusive or aneurysmal, such as the vasospastic disorders and thoracic outlet syndromes, are discussed in separate chapters. Evaluation and management of acute and chronic venous disease as well as venous thrombosis and pulmonary embolism are provided in individual chapters reflecting their clinical importance. Finally, an overview of lymphatic disease and management of vascular trauma are included to cover the breadth of vascular disease that the nonvascular surgeon might be called upon to treat.

ACKNOWLEDGMENTS

The editors and respective contributors wish to express their deep gratitude to their secretaries and editorial assistants for their hard work in the creation of this book. The editors provide a special expression of thanks to Jennifer McConnon for her tireless work in formatting the disparate chapters into a uniform presentation consistent with the spirit of the Lange series. Finally, we express our gratitude in advance to any and all readers who, having read and evaluated this text, will provide their comments or criticisms for guidance in preparation of future editions.

March 1995   Richard H. Dean, MD
                                                       James S.T. Yao, MD, PhD
                                                       David C. Brewster, MD

Examination of the Patient with Vascular Disease

1

Marshall E. Benjamin, MD, & Richard H. Dean, MD

As with most disciplines in medicine, the substance of the clinical diagnosis for the patient with vascular disease begins with a thorough history and physical examination. In fact, most clinicians should be able to predict the status of perfusion to the lower extremities simply by obtaining a careful history. Physical findings can then add certainty to the diagnosis. Combining a complete history, physical findings, and a basic knowledge of the disease process being considered, the diagnosis is usually straightforward. When the history and physical examination do not yield sufficient information to firmly establish a diagnosis, noninvasive testing in the clinical vascular laboratory can assist in making an accurate diagnosis.

THE HISTORY

In most cases, the specific diagnosis of a patient with vascular disease can be inferred from a careful, well-directed history. The skillful examiner listens carefully to the patient's account of symptoms and then asks directed questions to clarify or bring out additional information. The following are 5 major areas that are usually the most productive:

- Essential negatives that may eliminate other diagnoses.
- Knowledge of circumstances that aggravate or alleviate the problem.
- Time relationships of the symptom to other medical events.
- Whether the symptom is intermittent or constant.
- The duration of the process as well as the history of prior events or drug use that might have significance as to the onset of the symptom.

For example, although a patient may casually complain of an aching pain in the calf, questions that evoke information that this pain is crampy in nature, that it occurs only with vigorous ambulation, and that it is vividly reproducible after walking for 1 block may provide clues differentiating a vascular cause from a neurogenic one. Patients are frequently referred with a diagnosis already established. A review of their his-

tory often uncovers details that were unappreciated by the previous examiner.

In addition, information should be sought in the patient history concerning risk factors for vascular disease, specifically diabetes mellitus, hypertension, hyperlipidemia, and smoking. Patients who smoke heavily have a more rapid progression of disease and a worse prognosis. Those who continue to smoke after reconstructive surgery are more likely to suffer failure of their bypass. Similarly, the natural history of atherosclerotic disease is often accelerated in patients with diabetes. Information regarding prior vascular reconstructions and associated vascular and other medical problems is also critical.

Furthermore, to obtain a complete history, specific vascular diseases require specific questions. For instance, when evaluating a patient for chronic or acute arterial occlusion, it is important to ask how far or how long the patient can walk before the onset of lower extremity muscular pain (intermittent claudication). However, when evaluating a patient for gastrointestinal ischemia, questions should focus on weight loss and eating habits.

Another example of a specific question for a specific disease is in the case of aneurysms. Because first-degree relatives and siblings of a patient with aneurysm are at high risk for developing an aneurysm, it is essential to gather a family history pertaining to this condition. Therefore, the clinician must be knowledgeable about the appropriate questions to ask regarding the various vascular diseases.

THE PHYSICAL EXAMINATION

Although a complete physical examination is always performed, the astute clinician often tailors the examination according to the information gained in the history. Application of the basic principles of inspection and palpation, with specific attention to the pulse examination, can provide a wealth of information. A few extra minutes spent on the abdominal examination of the patient with a relatively benign-sounding complaint of postprandial abdominal pain may reveal a scaphoid abdomen with an epigastric bruit and signs of aortoiliac occlusive disease. These findings in com-

1

bination with an associated history of significant weight loss strongly suggest a diagnosis of chronic mesenteric ischemia from the history and physical examination alone.

Inspection

The limb with chronic arterial ischemia frequently is cool to the touch and displays all the typical signs of poor nutrition, including decreased hair growth and thin, shiny skin. The nails frequently are thickened or claw-shaped. There may be signs of muscle wasting from longstanding ischemia, particularly marked in the posterior compartment. A simple bedside test (Buerger's test) can provide a reflection of the level of distal perfusion. The skin on a severely ischemic limb shows pallor when elevated, and an intense red color (dependent rubor) will develop after being dependent for several minutes.

The lower extremity should be inspected carefully for the presence of cracks, gangrene, pregangrenous changes, and ulcers. This is especially critical in the diabetic population in whom neuropathy may prevent symptoms even when a critical level of ischemia may be present. Neurotrophic ulcers occur at sites of pressure, most commonly on the plantar surface of the foot, over the first metatarsophalangeal joint. Ulceration from an ischemic cause is generally located laterally or distally and may also be over pressure points (Fig 1–1). These ulcers are painful and bleed little. They frequently have a "punched out" appearance due to the lack of epithelial ingrowth from the periphery. In contrast, ulcers resulting from chronic venous insufficiency are usually located above the medial malleolus, with irregular borders; they are typically painless (Fig 1–2). Table 1–1 describes some of the important differences among ulcers caused by ischemia, trophic ulcers, and venous insufficiency.

Gangrene is usually easily recognized and is illustrated by a typical patient shown in Figure 1–3. The dead tissue is insensate, although the tissue just proximal is ischemic and may be painful. Where the tissue is soft and edematous and may have a foul-smelling drainage, the cause is usually infectious (wet gangrene). In contrast, the tissue of dry gangrene is hard and withered and has no infectious component.

Palpation

Skin temperature and capillary refill can be quickly assessed at the bedside. When compared with the contralateral limb, the ischemic limb may feel cool. However, atherosclerotic disease is generally bilateral, so this may be of little help. In the supine patient, after several seconds of light pressure on the nailbed or tip of the toe, normal color should return almost immediately (capillary refill test). A delay in return is generally a crude reflection of some element of distal ischemia.

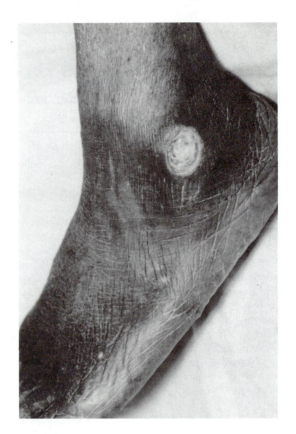

Figure 1–1. Typical appearance of ulceration from arterial insufficiency.

Pulses

Examination of the pulses is probably the most critical element of the vascular examination in patients with lower extremity arterial occlusive disease. The aortic, femoral, popliteal, dorsalis pedis, and posterior tibial pulses all should be assessed. Although there are numerous ways to record the pulse strength, reporting them as aneurysmal, normal, weak, or absent is preferred. In general, if a patient has normal palpable dorsal pedal and posterior tibial pulses, the perfusion to this level suggests normal axial patency. Patients with intermittent claudication typically have superficial femoral artery disease and will therefore have a palpable pulse at the groin, but absent pulses beyond this point. Diabetic patients more commonly have infrapopliteal disease and thus may have palpable pulses at the femoral and popliteal location, but absent distal pulses.

To provide some objective measurement of the level of perfusion when pulses are not palpable, the ankle-brachial ratio is calculated. Normally, the systolic blood pressure at the ankle level is slightly higher than that recorded at the brachial artery, yielding an ankle-brachial index (ABI) of more than 1.0. Ratios between 1.0 and 0.7 usually correlate with a lack of

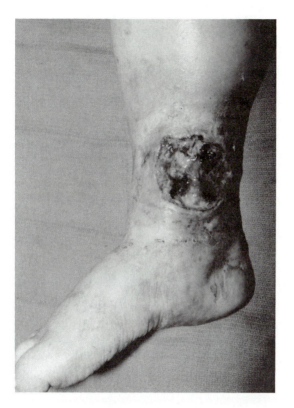

Figure 1–2. Typical appearance of a venous stasis ulcer and surrounding skin changes in a patient with chronic venous insufficiency.

ally associated with limb-threatening ischemia. This will be discussed in greater detail Chapter 2.

Occasionally, patients complain of classic ischemic symptoms during walking or exercising, but have normal palpable pulses at rest. In this setting, a vascular cause may still exist, but the pressure drop across the stenotic lesion only becomes critical with the distal vasodilation caused by walking. If the patient's symptoms are truly a result of arterial insufficiency, the pulse (and blood pressure at this level) will have decreased or disappeared after exercise. Therefore, the presence of normal pulses after exercise strongly suggests a nonarterial cause.

Auscultation with the bell of a stethoscope over a diseased arterial segment may reveal the presence of a bruit, correlating with the presence of turbulent flow. A soft midsystolic bruit is usually associated with a relatively minor lesion that does not significantly reduce flow or pressure. A loud diastolic component suggests a stenosis severe enough to reduce flow and produce a pressure drop. This can be misleading because highly stenotic lesions often have no bruit. In addition, palpation of the arteries occasionally reveal a thrill, suggestive of an arteriovenous fistula at that location.

The cause of acute arterial occlusion is usually a result of acute arterial thrombosis or embolism. Clues obtained during the physical examination can aid in localizing the diseased region. The most common site of acute thrombosis in the lower limb is at the adductor canal where the distal superficial femoral artery passes through the adductor magnus tendon. Typically, the patient has a normal femoral pulse, but an absent popliteal pulse.

When the cause of arterial occlusion is embolic, the embolus tends to migrate until it becomes lodged at a branch point. Larger emboli (*macroemboli*) usually originate from the heart and may settle at the aortic bifurcation, producing absent femoral pulses. Similarly, the patient with embolic occlusion of an iliac or femoral artery has an absent groin pulse on the involved side. Smaller emboli (*microemboli*) tend to

symptoms. Claudication is associated with an ABI of 0.5–0.7, and patients with rest pain, ulcer, or gangrene generally have ABIs of 0.3 or less. An absolute pressure of lower than 40 mmHg at the ankle level is usu-

Table 1–1. Physical findings of ulcers of the lower extremities.

	Chronic Venous Insufficiency	Arterial Insufficiency	Trophic Ulcer
Location	Distally, above medial malleolus	Toes, lateral malleolus, pressure points	Pressure points, areas of decreased sensation, demonstrable neuropathy
Skin around ulcer	Pigmented, sometimes fibrotic	Shiny, atrophic skin	Callused, demonstrable neuropathy
Pain	Not severe, relieved with elevation	Severe, relieved by dependency	None, ulcer may go unnoticed
Associated gangrene	Absent	May be present	Usually absent
Bleeding from ulcer	Venous ooze	Little or none	May be brick red
Associated signs	Edema, pigmentation, possible cyanosis if foot is dependent	Decreased pulses, pallor on elevation, dependent rubor	Decreased sensation, absent ankle reflexes

(From Pousti TJ, Wilson SE, Williams PA: Clinical examination of the vascular patient. In: *Vascular Surgery: Principles and Practice*. Veith FJ et al [editors]. McGraw-Hill, 1994:78.)

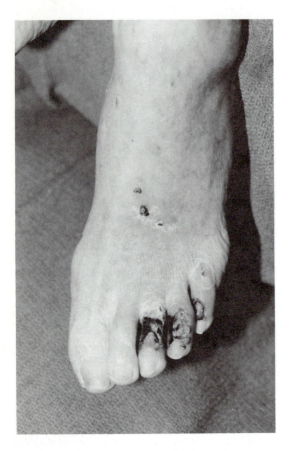

Figure 1–3. Typical appearance of digital (dry) gangrene from arterial insufficiency.

migrate to the most distal aspect of the arterial tree, that is, the digital arteries (Fig 1–4). These emboli commonly originate from an atherosclerotic or aneurysmal aorta, and examination frequently reveals normal pulses throughout.

IMAGING STUDIES

When the history and physical examination cannot provide enough information, imaging studies are extremely helpful. For example, because most aneurysms are asymptomatic, imaging studies such as computed tomography (CT) and magnetic resonance imaging (MRI), ultrasonography, and abdominal x-ray are helpful tools.

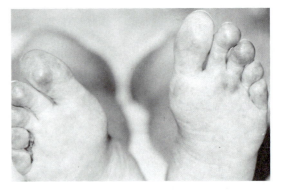

Figure 1–4. Atheroembolism seen in a patient with extensive atherosclerotic disease of the distal aorta.

REFERENCES

Dilley RB: The history and physical examination in vascular disease. In: *Vascular Diagnosis.* Bernstein EF (editor). Mosby-Yearbook, 1993:7.

Joyce JW: Examination of the patient with vascular disease. In: *Vascular Medicine.* Loscalzo J et al (editors). Little, Brown & Company, 1992:401.

Pousti TJ, Wilson SE, Williams RA: Clinical examination of the vascular patient. In: *Vascular Surgery: Principles and Practice.* Veith FJ et al (editors). McGraw-Hill, 1994:74.

Young JR: Clinical Clues to Peripheral Vascular Disease. In: *Peripheral Vascular Diseases.* Young JR et al (editors). Mosby-Yearbook, 1991:3.

Noninvasive Studies of Vascular Disease

2

Glenn E. Esses, MD, & Dennis F. Bandyk, MD

Diagnostics based on ultrasonography and plethysmography have become an integral part of the evaluation and care of patients with vascular disease. Clinicians must be familiar with the spectrum of testing modalities available, including their capabilities and limitations, for appropriate application. The noninvasive vascular laboratory serves as an adjunct to clinical assessment and verifies the presence of disease as well as its location, extent, and severity (Table 2–1). In many patients, simple instruments, such as the hand-held, continuous-wave Doppler device, are sufficient to obtain unique physiologic information and confirm a clinical diagnosis, provide the basis for initial treatment, or indicate the need for other vascular imaging (arteriography, computed tomography [CT]) studies. With duplex ultrasonography, which is a more complex and expensive instrument than continuous-wave ultrasound, detailed physiologic and anatomic information of the vascular tree can be obtained. Scanning often provides sufficient information to predict which patients are candidates for endovascular angioplasty rather than surgical reconstruction. Noninvasive vascular testing is also an important modality for screening high-risk patient populations for advanced atherosclerotic (critical internal carotid artery stenosis), aneurysmal (abdominal aortic aneurysm), or life-threatening venous (lower limb deep venous thrombosis) disease.

Peripheral Arterial Testing

The symptoms and signs of arterial disease are the result of lesions that distort normal pressure and flow and impair blood flow at rest or under conditions of increased metabolic demand (exercise, hyperemia). Thus, physiologic measurements (pressure, blood flow velocity, and volume flow) are necessary for diagnosing occlusive disease, for grading its severity, and for confirming improvement following intervention. The extent of vascular testing should be individualized and dictated by presenting symptomatology, but all patients should have limb blood pressure measured at one or more levels, in combination with Doppler or plethysmographic waveform analysis.

A. Indirect Measurement of Blood Pressure: The most versatile method of peripheral blood pressure measurement is by the Doppler-derived pneumatic cuff occlusion technique. A continuous-wave hand-held Doppler device monitors blood flow with cuff inflation and deflation because Korotkoff sounds cannot be reliably auscultated in distal upper and lower extremity vessels. An appropriate-sized pneumatic cuff is wrapped around the limb and a Doppler probe positioned over a distal artery (radial/brachial in upper extremity; posterior tibial/dorsalis pedis in lower extremity). Cuff size in proportion to limb girth is important for precise and reproducible readings. If the cuff is too narrow, the blood pressure reading will be erroneously high, and if the cuff is too wide, the reading may be falsely low. Positioning pneumatic cuffs at high-thigh and above-knee sites permits assessment for aortoiliac disease and a calculation of pressure gradient across the superficial femoral artery. Systolic pressure is determined by listening to the popliteal artery Doppler flow signal. Similarly, the clinician can obtain calf and ankle pressures by means of cuffs at these locations while listening to the dorsalis pedis (DP) or posterior tibial (PT) signals at the ankle. Blood pressure measurements should be obtained in upper and lower extremities when evaluating peripheral arterial occlusive disease. An ankle/brachial systolic pressure index (ABI) is calculated by dividing the higher DP or PT pressures by the higher of the 2 arm systolic pressures.

Table 2–2 lists the interpretation criteria of Doppler-derived pressures in the limbs. Typical ABIs recorded in patients with vascular claudication are 0.5–0.9, whereas more severe symptoms (ischemic rest pain) or nonhealing leg/foot ulcer typically have levels of less than 0.5. An absolute ankle pressure of 40 mmHg or less indicates critical limb ischemia, and, in the presence of tissue loss, primary healing of ulcer or amputations is unlikely. Artery wall incompressibility is an important limitation to this method, occurring in 5–10% of diabetic patients.

Calcific disease of the tibial arteries can prevent cuff occlusion from occurring, and erroneously high systolic pressure readings will be obtained. The inclusion of Doppler waveform analysis in the measurement prevents an incorrect interpretation of the falsely elevated ABIs. The normal peripheral arterial flow is characterized by a triphasic audible Doppler signal (Fig 2–1). Distal to an obstruction, the Doppler flow

Table 2–1. Clinical applications of noninvasive vascular testing.

Disease Category	Diagnosis	Instrumentation
Peripheral arterial	Identify, localize, and grade severity of obstructive lesions Determine adequacy of tissue nutrition	Doppler-derived pressures, pulse volume recorder, color duplex ultrasonography Transcutaneous oximetry (TcPO₂)
Abdominal visceral	Locate and measure aneurysms Identify and grade renal/mesenteric obstructive lesions	Ultrasonography, CT, MRI Duplex ultrasonography; color duplex ultrasonography
Cerebrovascular	Identify, localize, and grade obstructive extracranial lesions Assess intracerebral collateral circulation Detect presence of intracerebral vasospasm	Duplex ultrasonography Color duplex imaging Transcranial Doppler, oculopneumoplethysmography Transcranial Doppler
Venous	Detect, localize, and characterize venous thrombosis Identify sites of valvular reflux Evaluate severity of venous hypertension	Duplex ultrasonography Impedance plethysmography Duplex ultrasonography Photoplethysmography Air plethysmography

signal has a biphasic configuration with a less rapid acceleration during systole and a more rounded peak. Under conditions of severe ischemia, the Doppler signal may be absent or demonstrate a monophasic flow pattern with minimal pulsatility.

Blood pressure measurements, particularly digital pressure, can be obtained using plethysmographic instruments to monitor blood flow. Measurement of toe pressure is recommended in patients with incompressible tibial vessels, because their digit arteries remain relatively spared of calcific changes. Photoplethysmography is more reliable than Doppler-derived signals in the measurement of digital systolic pressure. A photoelectric cell consisting of a light-emitting diode is taped to the end of the digit, and a photosensor transduces changes in dermal arterial flow. With inflation of a toe cuff to above regional blood pressure followed by slow (3–4 mmHg/sec) deflation, the plethysmographic waveforms reappear when the systolic toe pressure is reached. The technique is useful for evaluating hand ischemia, vasospastic disorders, and impotence (penile pressure).

B. Treadmill Testing: Treadmill testing (walking at 2 mph on a 12% grade) is most helpful in the evaluation of patients with atypical complaints of claudication to exclude a vascular basis for their symptoms or to document the severity of intermittent claudication. Such stress testing can "unmask" arterial occlusive disease in patients with classic symptoms but relatively normal ABIs. The patient is instructed to walk for 5 minutes or until the symptoms forced the patient to stop (Fig 2–2). The location and character of the patient's symptoms, measurements of absolute ankle

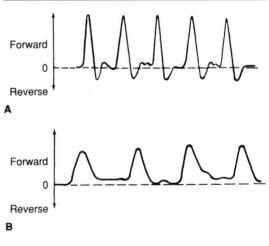

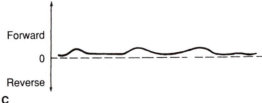

Figure 2–1. Normal and abnormal Doppler velocity waveforms. **A:** The velocity waveform of normal peripheral artery flow is triphasic, but becomes biphasic **B:** and then monophasic **C:** with increasing proximal occlusive disease.

Table 2–2. Interpretation of systolic pressures in the limbs.

Measurement Site	Range of Values
Ankle pressure	Normal: >brachial pressure
Ankle pressure (ABI)	Normal: 1.0–1.2; hemodynamically significant <0.95
Ankle pressure after exercise	Less than 20% of baseline
Proximal thigh pressure	Normal: 30–40 mmHg higher than brachial pressure
Segmental pressures	Normal: <20 mmHg difference between 2 levels in limb
Toe pressure	Normal: 80–90% of brachial pressure

ABI, ankle/brachial systolic pressure index.

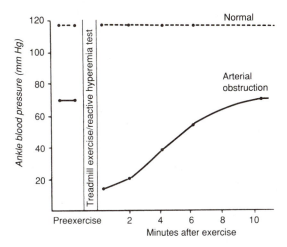

Figure 2–2. Ankle pressure changes with exercise testing in normal limbs and limbs with arterial occlusive disease.

pressure reduction after exercise, and the time required to return to basal levels are important diagnostic features of stress testing. To substantiate a diagnosis of vascular claudication, the ankle pressure should fall to lower than 50 mmHg. A return to baseline values more than 5 minutes indicates multilevel disease or poor collateral development. Table 2–3 lists the clinical categories of chronic limb ischemia based on pressure and pulse waveform criteria.

C. Pulse Volume Recordings: Air plethysmography can be used to record segmental limb blood pressure and provide waveform analysis of volume changes with arterial pulse. Because the quantity of muscle, bone, fat, skin, and venous blood remains relatively constant from second to second, volumes changes of the resting limb reflect the arterial flow. The technique is an indirect measure of blood flow and changes in the waveform amplitude provides an index of local tissue perfusion. Pulse volume recordings (PVRs) require careful application of air-filled cuffs around the extremity at segmental levels (high thigh, above knee, below knee, ankle, transmetatarsal, and

the first toe) and sequential inflation of the cuffs to a standardized pressure, typically 65 mmHg. The instrument is calibrated so that a 1-mmHg pressure change in the cuff provides a 20-mm chart deflection. Criteria for classification of disease severity into 5 categories have been established as well as those for healing foot lesions and amputations (Table 2–4).

PVRs provide information regarding the location and severity of peripheral occlusive disease. Instrument and interpretation errors are uncommon with PVR, and minimal technical expertise is required for accurate patient testing. Digital plethysmography in combination with pressure measurements is particularly useful for differentiating vasospastic disease from occlusive disease in patients with Raynaud's syndrome. Because PVRs provide indirect hemodynamic testing like the Doppler-derived pressure measurements, the precise anatomic localization of occlusive lesions is not possible nor can high-grade stenosis be distinguished from total occlusion of the artery.

D. Measurement of Skin Perfusion: Measurement of the quantity of oxygen available for diffusion to the skin can guide clinical decision regarding healing potential of ulcer, selection of amputation sites, and evaluation of tissue viability (eg, musculocutaneous flaps, tissue transfers). Table 2–5 lists instruments that assess skin perfusion. Measurement of transcutaneous partial tension of oxygen ($TcPO_2$) is the most widely used technique and detects the level of oxygen that has diffused through the stratum corneum. The $TcPO_2$ electrode is placed on the chest or upper arm as a control, and from any region of interest, usually the upper or lower calf or dorsum of the foot. Heating the sensing probe to 43–45°C facilitates oxygen diffusion and vasodilatation. Normal subjects have no gradient in $TcPO_2$ from proximal to distal lower extremity, and values average about 60 mmHg (90% of the chest value). Claudicants demonstrate significant differences between resting values at thigh and foot values. Exercise testing further accentuates this difference. Limbs with critical limb ischemia have values of less than 40 mmHg. Wound healing can be anticipated if the $TcPO_2$ in the region is greater than 24

Table 2–3. Lower-limb ischemia based on pressure and waveform criteria.

Clinical Features	ABI	TP	Treadmill Test/PVR
Asymptomatic	≥1.0	80% of brachial pressure	Normal treadmill test
Mild claudication	>0.8	>60 mmHg	Completes treadmill exercise, AP after exercise <50 mmHg
Moderate to severe claudication	0.4–0.8	>40 mmHg	Cannot complete treadmill exercise and AP after exercise <50 mmHg
Ischemic rest pain	<0.4	<30 mmHg	Flat or minimal pulsatility of metatarsal PVR
Tissue loss	<0.5	<40 mmHg	Ankle metatarsal PVR flat, barely pulsatile
Threatened limb	<0.15		Inaudible Doppler arterial signal, but audible signals at ankle; mild sensory and motor deficit
Irreversible ischemia	0.0		Inaudible Doppler arterial and venous signals at ankle; anesthestic, paralyzed limb

ABI, ankle/brachial index; TP, toe pressure; PVR, pulse volume recording; AP, ankle pressure.

Table 2–4. Pulse volume recording categories.

	Chart Deflection (mm)	
Category*	Thigh/Ankle	Calf
Normal	>15	>20
Mild	>15	>20
Moderate	5–15	5–20
Severe	<5	<5
Critical	Flat	Flat

*Severity of ischemia.

Table 2–6. Duplex criteria for lower limb arterial occlusive disease.

	Duplex-Derived Velocity Spectra	
% Stenosis*	Peak Systolic Velocity	Velocity Ratio†
Normal	<150 cm/sec	<1.5
30–49	150–200 cm/sec	1.5–2.0
50–75	200–400 cm/sec	2.0–4.0
>75	>40 cm/sec	>4.0
Occlusion analysis	No flow by color Doppler/pulsed Doppler spectral	

* Diameter reduction.
† V_1 is peak systolic velocity at the level of the stenosis; V_2 is peak systolic velocity of normal-caliber graft within 2 diameters length distance from the stenosis.

mmHg, particularly when the value increases when the patient breathes supplemental oxygen.

E. Duplex Ultrasonography: Duplex scanning, which combines high-resolution, real-time B-mode imaging with pulsed-wave Doppler spectral analysis, should be used to address specific queries concerning disease morphology (stenosis, occlusion, or aneurysm), to measure vessel diameter, to grade stenosis severity, or to determine length of vessel occlusion based on visualization of exit and re-entry collateral vessels. With color Doppler technology, the arterial tree can be mapped in a manner analogous to that of arteriography in body regions accessible to interrogation by ultrasonic energy. Color flow imaging facilitates localization of stenosis, aneurysmal dilatation, or occlusion. Compared with arteriography, diagnostic accuracy is more than 80% successful in detection of more than 50% diameter reduction of arterial stenosis or occlusion (Table 2–6).

Accepted clinical applications of duplex ultrasonography include the evaluation of symptomatic patients with abnormal ABIs to ascertain intervention options (angioplasty versus direct surgery), exclude occult aortoiliac disease in patients with femoral pulses in whom a distal bypass is contemplated, evaluate specific diseased arterial segments whose hemodynamic significance is not clear following angiographic visualization, and surveillance of infrainguinal vein bypasses for myointimal hyperplasia.

In general, patients with multilevel disease and severe ischemia are best evaluated with arteriography because diagnostic accuracy of duplex scanning in grading secondary and tertiary occlusive lesions is poorer than with arteriography. Patients with mild to moderate symptoms of claudication do not require duplex scanning for disease characterization unless consideration of percutaneous transluminal angioplasty is judged necessary.

Duplex scanning is an important modality in the surveillance of an arterial disease (bypass graft patency, abdominal and peripheral aneurysm). The rationale for this application is that intervention can be safely delayed until the arterial lesion is severe enough that symptoms or its natural progression pose a risk to the patient. The development of lesions, which may precipitate graft failure, can be identified and repaired before thrombosis occurs, resulting in improved graft patency and limb salvage. At present, high-grade (>75% diameter reduction) stenotic lesions should be corrected. Aneurysm enlargement can be accurately determined by serial scans. Intervention is based on the size of the aneurysm and, for peripheral arteries crossing joints or arterial anastomotic sites, when mural thrombus is identified.

An important limitation of duplex ultrasonography is the high level of technical expertise required to obtain interpretable studies. The instrumentation is considered essential in the areas of cerebrovascular, venous, and abdominal visceral testing. High-quality testing can be anticipated at accredited vascular laboratories staffed by persons with skills and experience sufficient for accurate scanning of the peripheral arterial system.

F. Magnetic Resonance Angiography (MRA): MRA is a relatively new technique, which can be used to construct 3-dimensional images of the arterial tree. The technique is not available in vascular laboratories, and clinical applications are in an evolutionary phase of development. With refinements in software, it has been possible to identify lower limb vessels that were not well visualized with conventional or digital subtraction angiography. In centers with MRA expertise, surgical bypass based on this imaging technique alone has proved to be safe and effective, indicating that diagnostic arteriography may be replaced with this technique in most patients.

Instrument availability and prolonged scanning times limit clinical use, as do artifacts produced by

Table 2–5. Skin perfusion tests.

Epicutaneous xenon-133 clearance
Laser Doppler flux
Photoplethysmography
Skin arterial blood pressure
Skin thermometry
Thermal clearance
Thermal conductance
Transcutaneous partial tension of oxygen ($TcPO_2$)
Venous occlusion plethysmography

tissue motion, highly disturbed flow, and vessel tortuosity. The intensity of the magnetic fields and procedure times required for arterial imaging limit its use to cooperative, stable patients without implanted metallic devices (pacemakers, cerebral aneurysm clips).

Cerebrovascular Testing

A. Duplex Scanning: Duplex ultrasonography is essential instrumentation for evaluation of the extracranial carotid and vertebral arteries for occlusive or aneurysmal lesions. Patients with appropriate indications for testing include those with suspected cerebrovascular ischemia (hemispheric or nonhemispheric stroke syndromes), transient ischemia attack (TIA), amaurosis fugax, and a high risk for stroke based on history and physical examination (ie, cervical bruit). Testing is also performed for surveillance of known disease or after carotid endarterectomy. The principal component of the examination is to assess anatomy and flow hemodynamics to locate and grade disease severity. The degree of stenosis is assessed by quantitative pulsed-wave Doppler spectral analysis (Table 2–7), whereas atherosclerotic lesion features (ulceration, calcification, acoustic heterogenicity, intraplaque hemorrhage) are determined by real-time B-mode imaging.

A complete extracranial duplex examination requires bilateral, sagittal, and transverse imaging along the course of the common, external, and internal carotid arteries and, to the extent possible, the origin and course of the vertebral arteries. Areas of stenosis are categorized using velocity spectra criteria recorded proximal to and at the point of maximum stenosis. Use of a Doppler angle of insonation of less than 65 degrees is essential whenever color Doppler imaging and spectral analysis are performed. Compared with arteriography, the accuracy of duplex scanning exceeds 90% for all categories of disease. Lesions not amenable to surgical repair (eg, total internal carotid artery [ICA] occlusion) can be identified with a positive predictive value of 95–98%. Disease classification facilitates patient care because thromboemboli typically originate from complex lesions (heterogenous plaque, irregular surface, intraplaque hemorrhage)

with significant (50% diameter reduction) stenosis, whereas smooth homogenous plaques with less than 50% diameter reduction are less likely to be associated with cerebrovascular ischemia syndromes. Subclavian steal syndrome can be identified by a retrograde flow in the vertebral artery ipsilateral to a subclavian artery stenosis.

Duplex scanning cannot reliably identify proximal lesions of the common carotid artery or distal lesions in the ICA, especially in the cavernous portion of the ICA. Because most carotid occlusive disease is confined to the area of the carotid bifurcation, this does not usually present a problem. However, patients with suspected proximal common carotid artery disease or very distal ICA disease should undergo some additional study (MRA, transcranial Doppler, arteriography) to define these areas.

B. Transcranial Doppler (TCD) Ultrasonography: Transcranial Doppler uses a low-frequency (2 MHz), high-intensity, pulsed-wave Doppler probe to evaluate intracerebral vessels. Ultrasound waves do not penetrate bone easily. Therefore, 3 separate "windows" in the skull have been identified with relatively thin bone where ultrasound may be used: the transtemporal, transorbital, and posterior through the foramen magnum. The first 2 windows may be used to assess the intracerebral portions of the ICA, the middle cerebral artery (MCA), the anterior cerebral artery (ACA), and the anterior communicating artery (AcoA). The posterior approach may be used to assess the intracranial portions of the vertebral arteries (VA), the basilar artery, and the posterior communicating artery.

Current applications for TCD include (1) assessment of cerebral vasospasm, particularly after subarachnoid hemorrhage, (2) detection of intracranial arterial stenoses, (3) evaluation of the collateral circulation patterns in patients with known severe extracranial disease, and (4) diagnosis of brain death. Clinical uses are firmly established in neurology and neurosurgery, but the role of TCD in vascular surgery remains an active area of research. Limitations of TCD examinations include a high degree of operator dependence, the inability to find a window in about 10–15% of patients studied, and the use of velocity data alone

Table 2–7. Categories of internal carotid artery disease.

Duplex Category	Angiographic Criteria	Velocity Spectra Characteristics
A,B	Normal, 0–15% DR	ICA systolic peak flow velocity <100 cm/sec; no spectral broadening or only in deceleration phase of systole
C	16–49% DR	ICA systolic peak flow velocity >100 cm/sec but <125 cm/sec; spectral broadening throughout systole
D	50–75% DR	ICA systolic peak flow velocity >125 cm/sec; spectral broadening throughout systole and during diastole
D+	76–99% DR	ICA diastolic peak flow velocity >125 cm/sec; spectral broadening throughout pulse cycle
E	Occlusion	No ICA signal, flow to zero during diastole in common carotid artery

DR, diameter reduction; ICA, internal carotid artery.

to reflect blood flow in the highly vasoactive cerebral vasculature.

C. MRA Cerebral Angiography: MRA of the extracranial and intracranial circulation can provide both anatomic and physiologic data. The combination of MRA and duplex scanning of the extracranial carotid arteries is particularly useful in the patient with carotid occlusive disease who is being considered for carotid endarterectomy. Tandem lesions (areas of atherosclerotic occlusive disease in the distal ICA inaccessible to the duplex scanner) can be identified, and the intracerebral collateral patterns can be assessed. This combination of tests may supplant cerebral arteriography in selected patients.

Abdominal Visceral Vascular Testing

A. Renal Duplex Ultrasonography: Indications for the use of duplex scanning to evaluate for renal artery stenosis include the presence of hypertension (HTN) and ischemic nephropathy. Because HTN affects about 60 million people in the USA, a smaller subset of patients, including those who develop HTN before age 30 or after 50 years, those with abrupt onset of HTN, malignant HTN, or HTN requiring 3 or more drugs for control, and those with deteriorating renal function on angiotensin-converting enzyme inhibitors, have been candidates for screening for renovascular HTN. Using the latter criteria, investigators have identified a higher percentage of patients screened with renovascular HTN. Unfortunately, no reliable clinical criteria set apart patients with renovascular HTN from those with HTN from other causes, including essential HTN. Similarly, renal artery occlusive disease accounts for only a minority of patients who suffer from progressive failure of renal function.

The identification of renal artery stenosis is based on velocity recordings in the aorta compared with those found in the renal arteries. Spectral criteria alone have not been found to be as useful as velocity recordings, although peak systolic velocities greater than 180 cm/sec indicate a stenosis. Table 2–8 lists the criteria for identifying renal artery stenosis. Limitations of this method are operator dependence and the inability to perform the examination in 10–15% of patients based on obesity, bowel gas, or recent abdominal surgery.

Chronic mesenteric occlusive disease of the celiac and superior mesenteric arteries is a rare disorder. Duplex scanning has been used to evaluate these arteries, as well as other intra-abdominal arteries. However, the discussion of the specific diagnostic criteria for each of these is beyond the scope of this text. Limitations to duplex scanning of these vessels are similar to those for the renal arteries.

B. Aneurysmal Imaging: Color Doppler flow imaging can detect aneurysms involving the abdominal aorta, iliac segments, or extremity vessels. External diameter, length, presence of mural thrombus, and anatomic relations to adjacent structures (renal arteries, ureters, duodenum) are possible to measure with a high degree of accuracy. The precision and reproducibility of measurements are sufficient for detection of aneurysm enlargement in surveillance applications. In selected patients, a high-quality duplex study can replace arteriography in assessing concomitant occlusive (renal, mesenteric, or iliac) disease and cholelithiasis and in seeking sites for safe vascular clamp placement. Vascular imaging of aneurysms for diagnosis or surveillance may require use of several diagnostic modalities (chest radiograph, CT, magnetic resonance imaging [MRI]), depending on the location. Thoracic and abdominal aortic aneurysms can be identified by conventional radiography, but CT scanning is recommended to accurately measure size and extent and provide anatomic information important for surgical repair.

B-mode ultrasonography is the recommended method for screening/surveillance of abdominal, femoral, and popliteal aneurysms. The features of low cost, lack of ionizing radiation, and reproducibility make this method particularly useful for detection of enlargement or of rapid (>0.6 cm/6 months) growth rates. Disadvantages include the lack of precise anatomic data regarding the renal vessels, the adjacent bowel, and the iliac arteries that are helpful in planning the operative repair of an abdominal aortic aneurysm. Most surgeons obtain a CT scan or MRI prior to planned surgical or endovascular repair. In hemodynamically stable patients with equivocal symptoms of rupture of abdominal aortic aneurysm, CT can identify loss of aneurysmal wall integrity or other conditions (renal or biliary colic) that can mimic this vascular emergency. MRI provides similar anatomic information as CT, but it is not routinely obtained because of its higher cost. MRA should be considered in patients who are candidates for aneurysm repair but at high risk for complications with conventional arteriography such as contrast-induced renal failure (in patients with chronic renal insufficiency or type I diabetes mellitus). Current limitations in image acquisition and software preclude abdominal and pelvic arterial imaging with the degree of resolution achieved by conventional arteriography.

Table 2–8. Renal duplex diagnostic criteria.

Criteria	Normal	<60%	>60%	Occluded
Renal/aortic ratio	<3.5	<3.5	>3.5	N/A
Velocity	<180 cm/sec	>180 cm/sec	>180 cm/sec	No flow, kidney <9 cm/sec; parenchyma <10 cm/sec

Peripheral Venous Testing

A. Deep Venous Thrombosis: Duplex imaging has replaced the previous gold standard of ascending phlebography as well as physiologic testing methods (impedance plethysmography, continuous-wave Doppler imaging) for the diagnosis of deep venous thrombosis (DVT). Numerous clinical trials have documented sensitivity and specificity rates of greater than 90% for venous duplex imaging compared with phlebography for the diagnosis of calf, popliteal, and superficial femoral DVT. Superficial and deep veins of the extremity are imaged transversely, and gentle external compression is performed to coapt the vein walls.

A normal vein will collapse with probe pressure and will dilate in response to a Valsalva maneuver. Veins with acute thrombus are enlarged because of increased venous pressure and are noncompressible (Table 2–9). Pulsed-wave Doppler interrogation of venous flow characteristics is also an integral part of the examination. A normal vein at or proximal to the popliteal level will demonstrate 3 hemodynamic features: (1) respiratory variation in flow, (2) no evidence of reflux flow on Valsalva's maneuver or proximal limb compression, and (3) augmentation of flow with distal limb compression. An occluded vein demonstrates no flow, and veins proximal to occlusion have continuous flow and minimal or no augmentation of flow with distal limb compression. Venous segments with nonocclusive thrombus may have minimal Doppler flow abnormalities. However, with transverse probe pressure, the vein wall will not completely coapt.

Indications for testing include suspected DVT or pulmonary embolus. In making the diagnosis of DVT in symptomatic patients, compression ultrasonography is preferable to hemodynamic testing methods (impedance plethysmography, bidirectional Doppler examination). The positive predictive values were 94% and 83%, respectively. Testing is also appropriate for surveillance of high-risk patients after orthopedic, neurosurgical, or general vascular surgical procedures and during recovery after DVT for assessment of venous system patency and the need for elastic stockings. Venous duplex scanning has the advantages of portability and repeatability, but testing depends on operator skill and identification of iliac vein thrombus must be made on color Doppler flow characteristics alone, because the iliac veins and inferior vena cava cannot be adequately compressed.

B. Evaluation of Venous Valvular Function: Peripheral superficial and deep veins have valves that direct blood flow from distal to proximal and from superficial to deep. Abnormalities of valvular function can exist in the deep venous system, the superficial (greater and lesser saphenous) venous system, and the communicating (perforator) venous system. Duplex scanning can evaluate each of the venous systems and determine their functions. By identifying areas of valvular reflux with compression and Valsalva's maneuvers, a rational treatment strategy for chronic venous insufficiency can be developed. In accessible veins such as the femoral, popliteal, and PT veins, a bidirectional Doppler device is useful for confirming patency and directional flow. Reversal of flow with limb compression proximal to the recording site occurs when the valves are incompetent.

C. Plethysmography: Photoplethysmography (PPG) is used to evaluate the presence and severity of venous hypertension. Venous hypertension may be the result of venous outflow obstruction, venous valvular reflux, or more commonly a combination of both. PPG measures the rate of venous capillary refill of the skin following emptying after exercise. The probe is fixed to the medial calf 8–10 cm above the medial malleolus. Five calf compressions (heel raises with the patient seated and the feet resting on the floor) are performed with the patient non-weight-bearing. The venous refilling time (RT) is the time it takes for the calf veins to refill and should be more than 20 seconds. In patients with severe venous hypertension, the calf veins may refill as quickly as 7–10 seconds. The testing may then be performed with an occlusive superficial tourniquet (see Chapter 32). If the venous RT normalizes, the reflux is present in the superficial veins (being compressed); if the RT remains abnormal, the valvular incompetence is in the deep venous system.

Air plethysmography (APG) has emerged as the best noninvasive test to estimate invasive measurements of ambulatory venous pressure. The test is used primarily to grade the severity of venous hypertension in patients with chronic venous insufficiency and assess those who may be candidates for reconstructive surgery of the deep veins. An air-filled chamber placed around the lower leg can quantify the volume of the leg. Various maneuvers including leg elevation, leg dependency, and calf muscle contraction are used to evaluate the functional volume changes in the leg. The volume changes and the time it takes to achieve them

Table 2–9. Duplex criteria for venous thrombosis.

Normal	No thrombus visualized; flow spontaneous and phasic or easily augmented; veins easily compressed by probe pressure. Color flow image demonstrates flow within entire vein lumen.
Positive	Flow nonphasic with respiration or absent with augmentation; vein compressibility absent or incomplete. Luminal thrombus, depending on its echogenicity, may or may not be visualized; color flow imaging demonstrates no flow in lumen and presence of collateral vein development (increased flow in superficial veins).
Equivocal	No thrombus visualized, but venous flow patterns abnormal. Color flow image demonstrates irregularities in vessel lumen without consistent areas of no flow (findings of small, nonocclusive thrombi).

form the basis for quantifying the severity of venous hypertension. Good correlation has been demonstrated between both APG-derived values, ambulatory venous pressure measurements, and the clinical presence of venous ulceration in legs being studied.

Surveillance Studies

Duplex scanning is the preferred method for surveillance of high-risk patients for DVT or ICA disease progression and for monitoring the functional patency of infrainguinal bypass grafts. Follow-up after arterial surgery involves imaging the reconstruction/bypass graft to detect high-grade stenosis, which could lead to thrombosis or thromboemboli. A localized increase in peak systolic velocity of greater than 100% identified lesions of 50% or more reduction in diameter. When the lesions progress to more than 70%, peak systolic velocities are generally greater than 300 cm/sec. In vein bypass grafts, flow velocity remote from the stenosis falls to low (<40 cm/sec) levels, that is, the low-flow state.

After carotid endarterectomy or percutaneous transluminal angioplasty duplex scanning provides objective information regarding the hemodynamics of the repair. A normal duplex scan predicts a durable result, whereas velocity spectra of a 50% or greater stenosis within the reconstruction increase the likelihood of clinical failure. Most patients with abnormal surveillance studies do not require operation, but should be followed-up at 3–6-month intervals to detect progression to high-grade stenosis, a lesion that threatens the patency of the arterial repair/bypass.

REFERENCES

Bandyk DF: Noninvasive vascular laboratory in clinical practice. Echocardiography 1992;9:525.

Belcaro G et al: Noninvasive tests in venous insufficiency. J Cardiovasc Surg 1993;34:3.

Carpenter JP et al: Magnetic resonance angiography of peripheral runoff vessels. J Vasc Surg 1992;16:807.

Cossman DV et al: Comparison of contrast arteriography to arterial mapping with color-flow duplex imaging in the lower extremities. J Vasc Surg 1989;10:522.

Edwards JM et al: The role of duplex scanning in the selection of patients for transluminal angioplasty. J Vasc Surg 1991;13:69.

Franzeck UK et al: Transcutaneous PO_2 measurements in health and peripheral arterial occlusive disease. Surgery 1982;91:156.

Heijboer H et al: A comparison of real-time compression ultrasonography with impedance plethysmography for the diagnosis of deep-vein thrombosis in symptomatic outpatients. N Engl J Med 1993;329:1365.

Kirkendall WM et al: Recommendations for human blood pressure determination by sphygmomanometers. Circulation 1980;62(5):1146.

Kohler TR et al: Duplex scanning for diagnosis of aortoiliac and femoropopliteal disease: A prospective study. Circulation 1987;76:1074.

Malone JM et al: Prospective comparison of noninvasive techniques for amputation level selection. Am J Surg 1987;154:179.

Yao JT: Haemodynamic studies in peripheral arterial disease. Br J Surg 1970;57:761.

Contrast Angiography

3

William D. Routh, MD

Conventional and digital radiographic blood vessel imaging after injection of iodinated contrast material continues to play an essential role in the planning and performance of surgical and endovascular interventional therapies. However, technologic advances in noninvasive vascular imaging have substantially decreased reliance on contrast angiography as a diagnostic tool. Optimal use of diagnostic angiography in patients with vascular disease requires that their physicians (1) have a thorough knowledge of the indications for, risks of, and alternatives to angiography, (2) recognize modifiable factors that contribute to risk, and (3) properly recognize and institute treatment for complications. A general understanding of the technical and procedural aspects of diagnostic angiography and the pitfalls in interpretation of angiographic images is also desirable.

EQUIPMENT

The conventional film-screen angiographic unit consists of a radiographic table with movable top to facilitate proper patient positioning within the x-ray beam (Fig 3–1A). The table is interposed between an x-ray source (located above or below the patient) and a rapid film changer capable of transporting up to 30, 14 × 14-in radiographic films at a maximum rate of either 4 or 6 films per second, depending on design (Fig 3–1E). High-resolution fluoroscopy, essential for preangiographic catheter positioning, is provided by a large field of view (maximum diameter, 40 cm) image intensifier (Fig 3–1C and D). The image intensifier is interfaced with a television system providing a real time video image during fluoroscopy (Fig 3–1G).

The following monitoring and life support equipment should be immediately available during each angiographic procedure:

(1) Continuous ECG monitor with paper strip recorder

(2) Automated external blood pressure monitor

(3) Multichannel intravascular blood pressure monitor and pressure transducers

(4) Pulse oximeter with continuous digital display of oxygen saturation

(5) Approved institutional resuscitation cart and external monitor-defibrillator

Older angiographic units generally use a ceiling-suspended image intensifier exposed by a below-the-table x-ray source, which is separate from that used for angiographic filming. Current state-of-the-art systems incorporate the image intensifier on a rotational stand along with the rapid film changer. The same x-ray source is used for fluoroscopy or angiographic filming, and variable x-ray beam angulation is possible without rotation of the patient (see Fig 3–1).

Catheters

Angiographic catheters are made from polyethylene, polyurethane, nylon, Teflon, and a variety of other polymers that exhibit inherent differences in stiffness, surface friction, and ease of passage over a guidewire. Wire mesh stainless-steel reinforcement, incorporated into the walls of some catheters, imparts improved torque control, which may be desirable during selective vessel catheterization.

Several factors contribute to the selection of an angiographic catheter: caliber, length, tip configuration, and presence (or absence) of side holes. Furthermore, the type of vessel to be injected, the type of angiographic study to be performed, the size of the patient, the pathologic entity being investigated, and the experience of the angiographer determine the type of catheter to be used.

Guidewires

For angiographic procedures performed using the Seldinger technique, guidewires are required for initial catheter insertion. Guidewires are also used for catheter exchange, during selective branch vessel catheterization, for negotiation of tortuous, stenotic, or occluded vessels, and for delivery of a variety of endoluminal devices.

The most commonly used guidewires are composed of a tightly wound stainless-steel coil spring wrapped around a central monofilament stainless-steel core, or mandril. Selection of a guidewire requires specification of a variety of parameters including length, caliber, tip configuration (J versus straight), and tapered versus nontapered core. Teflon coating of guidewires

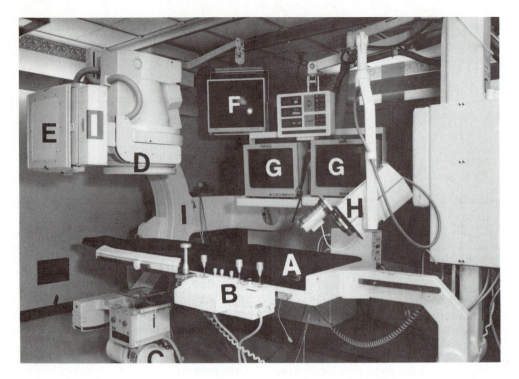

Figure 3–1. Angiographic procedure room. **A:** Ceiling-suspended angiographic table. **B:** Tableside controls. **C:** X-ray tube for fluoroscopy, conventional and digital angiography. **D:** Image intensifier (for generation of fluoroscopic image). **E:** Rapid film changer. **F:** Video monitor for physiologic data. **G:** Video monitors for fluoroscopic images. **H:** contrast injector. **I:** C-arm angiographic support allowing variable angulation for fluoroscopy and angiography.

reduces surface friction and improves the ease of over-the-wire catheter passage.

A variety of new customized guidewires exhibiting improved steerability, added kink resistance, and low-friction hydrophilic surface coatings are currently available. These design modifications can greatly facilitate difficult selective branch vessel catheter positioning or negotiation of severely diseased or tortuous vessels.

CONTRAST MATERIAL

Iodinated contrast agents currently used for angiography can be categorized according to their osmolality. High-osmolality agents are ionic; low-osmolality agents may be either ionic or nonionic.

High Osmolality: Ionic Contrast

Ionic contrast agents currently used in the USA are sodium or meglumine salts of the triiodinated benzoic acid derivatives, diatrizoate and iothalamate. The ratio of iodine atoms to osmotic particles is 1:5. The pharmaceutical properties of equivalent cationic preparations of the 2 different anions are similar.

Preparations are marketed with differences in percentage of weight per volume of iodine, relative iodine concentration, and relative ratio of sodium to meglumine. For equal iodine concentrations, the viscosity of the meglumine preparations exceeds that of sodium preparations. Osmolalities of the 60% and 76% weight per volume preparations most frequently used in angiography range from 1400 to 2000 mOsm per kilogram (mOsm/kg).

Low Osmolality: Nonionic Contrast

Low-osmolality contrast agents consist of a triiodinated multisubstituted benzene ring that is nonionic. The ratio of iodine atoms to osmotically active particles is therefore increased to 3:1. Since the radiographic density of contrast is directly related to its iodine concentration, a given contrast density is achieved at a much lower contrast osmolality than would be necessary with standard ionic contrast.

The 2 nonionic agents most frequently used in angiography are iohexol and iopamidol. At the concentrations typically used, osmolalities range from 616 to 862 mOsm/kg, about 50% of that of ionic agents with equivalent iodine content. This reduced osmolality likely accounts for the substantial reduction in pain and other adverse effects observed during angiography.

Low Osmolality: Ionic Contrast

The prototype low-osmolality ionic agent combines the anion of ioxaglic acid, a triiodobenzoic acid dimer containing 6 iodine atoms, with meglumine sodium. Since each molecule dissociates in solution into 2 osmotically active particles, the ratio of iodine atoms to osmotic particles is 3:1, the same as that of nonionic agents. The commercially available preparation used for angiography is Hexabrix (Mallinkcrodt, St. Louis, MO), which has an osmolality of 600 mOsm/kg and causes much less pain than conventional ionic agents for extremity angiography.

PATIENT PREPARATION FOR ANGIOGRAPHY

Preangiographic Evaluation

Consultation between the referring physician and the angiographer, review of the medical record and previous imaging studies, and a patient interview all are essential for clarifying the indications for angiography, the type of examination to be performed, and the possible factors increasing the risk of the study. Pertinent preangiographic physical findings including patient weight, blood pressure, peripheral pulses, presence of arterial bruits, and signs of tissue ischemia should be noted. A minimal laboratory evaluation prior to diagnostic angiography usually includes blood urea nitrogen, serum creatinine, prothrombin time, partial thromboplastin time, hematocrit, and platelet count.

Preangiographic orders include modification of diet, puncture site preparation, and intravenous hydration. Special considerations may include modification of anticoagulant or antidiabetic medications, preprocedure correction of coagulation defects, or premedication in patients considered at high risk for pseudoallergic contrast reaction. Preprocedure sedative and analgesic medications are not generally given prior to patient transport to the angiographic suite.

THE ANGIOGRAPHIC PROCEDURE

The patient is positioned on the angiographic table to optimize operator access to the catheter entry site and to allow full fluoroscopic and angiographic coverage of the anatomic areas to be evaluated. Constant ECG, automated external blood pressure, and pulse oximetry monitoring are instituted. Premedication with an intravenous sedative/analgesic combination is administered in incremental doses to allay anxiety and reduce discomfort while avoiding depression of protective reflexes. A combination of a benzodiazepine (midazolam hydrochloride, diazepam) and a narcotic analgesic (fentanyl citrate, morphine sulfate) is commonly used.

Femoral Artery Cannulation

Most diagnostic arteriography is currently performed via the common femoral artery using the needle-guidewire-catheter replacement technique perfected by Seldinger in the early 1950s. This usually allows selective catheterization of any of the major branches of the thoracic or abdominal aorta from a single arterial access site. The catheter skin entry site is best determined fluoroscopically. An infrainguinal arterial entry over the femoral head allows for effective compression of the artery against the underlying bone after catheter removal, reducing the risk of puncture site hemorrhage. After infiltration of the skin and perivascular tissues with a local anesthetic, the common femoral artery is entered with a beveled, styletted cannula. A guidewire is advanced through the cannula, which is then replaced over the wire with an appropriate catheter. Catheter exchanges may be performed over a guidewire of sufficient length to safely maintain arterial access. Use of a hemostatic introducer sheath may be desirable to minimize puncture site trauma if multiple catheter exchanges are anticipated.

Brachial Artery Cannulation

Catheter access may be obtained from the upper extremity when the transfemoral route is not feasible. This is most frequently due to the existence of severe aortoiliac occlusive disease. Cannulation of the brachial artery may entail less risk than entry at the axillary level. Debate continues regarding optimal site of brachial entry (proximal, middle, or distal).

For catheterization of the abdominal aorta or more distal vessels, the left brachial approach is preferred. Catheter passage into the descending aorta may be more difficult in elderly or hypertensive patients because of elongation and ectasia of the aortic arch, creating an unfavorable angle between the left subclavian artery and the descending aorta. Right brachial access may be selected when catheterization of the ascending aorta is required or when there is occlusive disease central to the left brachial artery. The relative risk of central nervous system complications is higher for right brachial than for left brachial access.

Translumbar Aortic Cannulation

Direct aortic cannulation from the translumbar approach may be required for performance of aortography when neither femoral nor brachial access is feasible. An example would be the patient with coexisting severe aortoiliac and brachiocephalic occlusive disease. Since the abdominal aorta is typically more diseased in its infrarenal segment, a "high" translumbar approach is generally preferred. A skin entry site is selected 8–10 cm to the left of the midline and caudal to the posterior 12th rib. A 16-gauge trocar sheath cannula is advanced under fluoroscopic guidance to contact the left lateral aspect of the 12th thoracic vertebral body. The cannula is then redirected slightly more ventrally and advanced just past the left anterolateral margin of the vertebral body to enter the aorta. The central stylet is replaced with a guidewire that is directed cephalad into the descending aorta. The outer sheath is then advanced into the descending aorta, and the guidewire and stiffening cannula are removed.

Depending on the initial abdominal aortographic findings, it may be desirable to redirect the tip of the translumbar sheath into an infrarenal position to optimize contrast opacification of the lower-extremity vessels. This is usually accomplished by retraction of the sheath until its tip is near the aortic entry site, manipulation of a guidewire through the sheath into the infrarenal aorta, and readvancement of the sheath.

Aortofemoral Graft Cannulation

In patients who have patent aortofemoral grafts with well-healed noninfected incisions, angiographic access from the groin by direct graft puncture generally carries less risk than transbrachial access. Administration of prophylactic antibiotics may be warranted to further reduce the small risk of graft infection, although the efficacy of this therapy has not been scientifically established. Single wall entry with a beveled cannula into the graft central to its femoral anastomosis allows guidewire access into the aorta. Slight overdilatation of the puncture site or use of an introducer sheath may be required for catheter insertion through the graft and fibrotic perigraft tissue. Catheter breakage has been reported when removal is attempted through a prosthetic graft. The risk of breakage may be reduced by catheter retraction over a guidewire or by initial catheter introduction through a sheath.

Angiographic Filming

For conventional angiography, a preliminary "scout" radiograph is obtained to ensure correct patient position and radiographic technique prior to contrast injection. X-ray beam energy and intensity are adjusted to optimize image density and detection of iodinated contrast.

Manual injection of contrast may suffice for evaluation of small, slow-flow vessels during digital subtraction angiography. However, optimal vessel opacification during film-screen angiography usually requires use of an automated mechanical contrast injector. For each angiographic run, contrast injection rate, total volume, and time interval between onset of injection and filming are programmed. These injection parameters are chosen according to the vessel size and flow rate, as judged by a manual injection of contrast viewed fluoroscopically. Filming rate (number of films/sec) and duration of filming are also selected to maximize the angiographic yield from each contrast injection while minimizing patient exposure and film waste.

Conventional angiographic films and laser-imaged photographic copies of digital angiograms are developed and fixed in an automated film processor and displayed for review on fluorescent-lighted illuminators.

These facilities should be in close proximity to the angiographic procedure room to allow for preliminary review of films by the angiographer prior to catheter removal, ensuring the performance of a complete and diagnostic examination.

Angiographic Artifacts & Interpretive Pitfalls

Overlapping opacified vessels, disease near vessel bifurcations, and superimposed skeletal structures may hinder angiographic interpretation. Additional angulated views or angiographic subtraction may then be helpful. When possible, external radiopaque hardware and monitoring devices should be repositioned out of the angiographic field of view. Contrast within the urinary bladder or spilled over the area of interest may also obscure vascular pathology.

Patient motion during the angiographic series degrades image sharpness. Additional patient sedation or use of external restraints may be necessary to reduce motion. For extremity angiography, limb motion may be a consequence of pain experienced during the contrast injection. Use of low-osmolality contrast may then be beneficial. Reduction in film exposure time, when technically feasible, reduces the reduction in image sharpness created by patient motion.

Postangiographic Care

After review of the angiographic films, the catheter is removed and the puncture site is manually compressed to achieve hemostasis. Patients are restricted to bedrest for 6–8 hours with frequent nursing assessment of heart rate, blood pressure, status of extremity circulation, and signs of puncture site hemorrhage. After brachial artery catheter removal, frequent assessment of upper-extremity neurologic status is also necessary to detect early signs of nerve injury.

PHARMACOLOGIC AGENTS USED DURING ANGIOGRAPHY

Pharmacologic agents may be used during angiography to enhance diagnostic yield or reduce risk.

Vasodilators

Tolazoline hydrochloride (Priscoline, Ciba Pharmaceuticals, Edison, NJ) acts directly on vascular smooth muscle. Its vasodilatory effect can improve contrast opacification of peripheral vessels during selective extremity angiography, accentuate portal and mesenteric venous opacification during arterial portography, alleviate catheter-guidewire-induced vasospasm, and aid in direct hemodynamic assessment of arterial stenoses. A typical adult dose of 25 mg diluted in 5–10 mL of sterile saline is injected intra-arterially with maximal vasodilatation occurring 20–30 seconds postinjection.

Intra-arterial nitroglycerin given in 100–200-μ increments can also be used to enhance opacification of extremity arteries and to counteract catheter-guidewire-induced vasospasm. Because of its rapid clearance, repeated doses may frequently be necessary.

Papaverine hydrochloride is another direct vascular smooth muscle relaxant with vasodilator effects that have been primarily used by angiographers in the evaluation and treatment of nonocclusive mesenteric ischemia. In such cases, if angiographic improvement in the severity of splanchnic vasoconstriction can be demonstrated following a selective 20–30-min infusion of papaverine into the superior mesenteric artery at a rate of 3 mg per minute, then continued infusion at 30–60 mg per hour may help to preserve intestinal viability. This therapy does not obviate the need for surgical therapy in patients with clinical signs of bowel infarction.

Calcium channel blockers are frequently used to prevent arterial spasm during angiography, angioplasty, and other catheter interventions. Nifedipine, given in 10-mg dose increments, exerts an effect 10–15 minutes following sublingual administration.

Systemic hypotension, which can result from use of the forementioned vasodilators, usually responds rapidly to infusion of intravenous fluids and leg elevation. Caution must be observed if pretreatment blood pressure is marginally low. The reflex tachycardia seen with some vasodilators may be harmful in patients with ischemic heart disease.

Anticoagulants

Heparin is routinely added to solutions used for catheter flushing during angiography to prevent catheter thrombosis or embolism. The small doses administered for this purpose usually have no significant systemic anticoagulant effect. There is some evidence to support giving a 50–100-U-per-kg bolus dose during angiography as additional protection against catheter-related thromboembolism. A bolus dose of heparin (typically 5000 U) is routinely given prior to balloon angioplasty and endovascular stent placement, and continued intravenous infusion may be indicated following the procedure, depending on the size and flow rate of the treated artery and the adequacy of the result. Rapid automated determination of activated clotting time allows for quick assessment of the adequacy of the heparin effect and helps to determine the need for heparin reversal prior to catheter removal.

TYPES OF DIAGNOSTIC ANGIOGRAPHY

Aortography

A. Aortic Aneurysm: The existence, size, and location of aortic aneurysms can generally be determined by noninvasive imaging studies such as ultrasonography, computed tomography (CT), and magnetic resonance imaging (MRI). Aortography may be indicated as an additional preoperative study to clarify the extent of the aneurysm, its relation to major aortic branches, and the presence and severity of branch vessel aneurysmal or occlusive disease.

Contrast injection rates and filming sequences may need to be modified because of the large capacity and slow-flow characteristics of the aneurysmal aortic segment. Additional oblique or lateral views may be required for full delineation of branch vessel origins.

B. Aortic Dissection: Aortic dissection may be specifically diagnosed by a variety of imaging modalities such as CT, MRI, and transesophageal echocardiography. Diagnostic angiography may be indicated for confirmation of diagnosis, delineation of the extent of dissection and sites of intimal disruption, and assessment of branch vessel involvement. Optimally, catheter access is obtained from the femoral approach into the true lumen of the aorta with overlapping angiographic views extending from the aortic root to beyond the distal extent of the dissection. Femoral pulse deficits due to iliac dissection may necessitate transbrachial aortography.

C. Chronic Aortic Occlusive Disease: In the symptomatic patient who is a candidate for revascularization, preoperative anatomy of the abdominal aorta, pelvic arteries, and distal run-off vessels is required. Oblique or lateral aortic views may be necessary for delineation of coexistent renal or visceral occlusive disease. Transfemoral catheter introduction into the aorta may not be feasible, thus necessitating either transbrachial or translumbar entry.

D. Miscellaneous: Emergency aortography remains the diagnostic procedure of choice in most patients with suspected acute thoracic aortic trauma. Digital subtraction aortography greatly reduces examination time without significant compromise of diagnostic resolution. More than one angiographic projection is required to exclude significant aortic injury, and the aorta must be evaluated from the aortic valve to at least the level of the diaphragm. If clinical findings, plain film findings, or abnormalities seen on the initial aortograms suggest brachiocephalic vessel injury, additional selective angiograms are obtained.

Aortography is also routinely performed for evaluation of the aorta and its branches prior to selective branch vessel angiography and for evaluation of aortitis or congenital abnormalities of the aorta.

Abdominal Visceral Angiography

A. Visceral Ischemia: Chronic mesenteric ischemia, manifested clinically by postprandial abdominal pain and weight loss, is evaluated primarily with aortography in frontal and lateral projections to assess for evidence of proximal visceral occlusive disease. Selective visceral angiography may be performed to better define visceral collateral pathways.

Suspected acute intestinal ischemia is evaluated emergently with aortography to exclude proximal superior mesenteric artery (SMA) thrombosis. If the proximal SMA is patent, selective mesenteric angiography is performed to search for more distal occlusions that are usually embolic in nature. In the absence of these findings, the existence of diffuse mesenteric vasoconstriction may be an indication of nonocclusive mesenteric ischemia. In such cases, extensive reflux of contrast into the aorta during selective SMA injection is further evidence of reduced mesenteric perfusion. If repeat SMA angiography following selective intra-arterial vasodilator injection shows substantial reversal of the vasoconstriction, the patient may benefit from continued papaverine infusion (see discussion under Pharmacologic Agents Used During Angiography).

Acute mesenteric ischemia is occasionally the result of mesenteric venous thrombosis, which may be manifested on late-phase SMA angiography as mesenteric venous occlusion with or without a lucent intraluminal filling defect. A prominent, thickened intestinal mucosal blush may also be noted. Dilation of peripheral mesenteric venous tributaries or abnormal venous collaterals may be seen.

B. Miscellaneous: Additional primary visceral vascular abnormalities that may be evaluated by selective angiography are visceral artery aneurysms, vascular malformations, and vasculitis.

Portal Hypertension

Selective visceral angiography is indicated in patients with portal hypertension and gastroesophageal varices who are candidates for a portosystemic shunt procedure. Superior mesenteric angiography with delayed filming following selective injection of tolazoline (arterial portography) usually depicts mesenteric and portal venous anatomy and defines portosystemic collaterals. Splenic vein anatomy is assessed with selective splenic angiography and delayed filming. Selective hepatic angiography may detect the arterial changes of cirrhosis or evidence of an unsuspected hepatocellular carcinoma. Systemic venous catheterization is usually also performed for hepatic venography, left renal venography, and hemodynamic assessment, including free and wedged hepatic vein pressures and a pull-back gradient from the right atrium to the infrahepatic inferior vena cava.

Visceral angiographic evaluation may be indicated postoperatively in patients with suspected portosystemic shunt malfunction.

Renal Angiography

For evaluation of suspected renal artery occlusive disease, an initial abdominal aortogram is obtained to determine the number, location, and patency of renal arteries. Selective renal angiography also is generally indicated when significant disease of the proximal renal arteries is absent. This is typically the case with fibromuscular disease. Selective angiography gives more detailed assessment and better delineates intrarenal involvement than does aortography.

In patients with atherosclerotic renal artery stenosis,

which more typically involves the proximal renal arteries and their origins, selective angiography is reserved for assessment of lesions of uncertain hemodynamic significance or for more detailed evaluation of intrarenal pathology. Otherwise, to minimize risk, catheterization of renal arteries exhibiting significant stenotic disease is generally deferred unless balloon angioplasty is being performed.

Less common indications for selective renal angiography are suspected blunt or penetrating renal artery trauma, embolus, dissection, aneurysm, vascular malformation, and vasculitis.

Pelvic Angiography

Angiographic evaluation of the pelvic vessels is routinely performed in patients with aortoiliac occlusive disease, abdominal aortic aneurysm, and known or suspected iliac artery aneurysm. In these cases, the evaluation is often part of a more complete angiographic evaluation of the aorta and peripheral vessels.

Pelvic angiography may be performed for evaluation and transcatheter therapy of retroperitoneal hemorrhage due to pelvic trauma, tumor, obstetric complication, or other causes. Pelvic arteriovenous fistulas, vascular malformations, and male impotence due to arterial occlusive disease are also indications for pelvic angiography.

Lower-Extremity Angiography

Bilateral lower-extremity angiography (femoral run-off angiography) is routinely performed in patients with chronic symptomatic arterial occlusive disease prior to surgical or endovascular therapy. To confirm existence of hemodynamically significant occlusive disease and to predict the anatomic levels of involvement, one or more of the following noninvasive evaluation methods is generally obtained prior to angiography: ankle-brachial index, pulse volume recording, Doppler waveform analysis, and duplex ultrasonography.

Complete angiographic evaluation consists of abdominal aortography followed by angiography of the pelvic and distal run-off vessels down to the pedal arches of both feet. A variety of techniques exist for evaluation of the extremity run-off vessels. Conventional or digital angiograms can be performed during an extended contrast injection into the distal aorta with incremental stepping of the angiographic table timed appropriately to image contrast-filled arteries at each step. Alternatively, both legs can be filmed during an aortic injection using 14×51-in film cassettes in a long-leg (BCM) film changer (BC Medical Ltd. St. Hubert, Quebec, Canada) (Fig 3–2). Timing of film exposure is generally less critical for this technique than for the stepped run-off technique. With either system, supplemental digital subtraction images may be desirable to better delineate distal vessels. Also, additional oblique angulated views may be necessary to fully define lesions near arterial bifurcations.

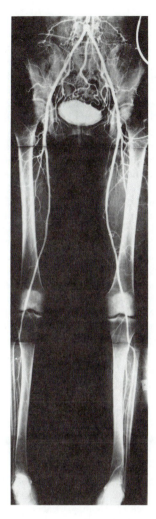

Figure 3–2. Bilateral lower-extremity run-off arteriogram performed with a long-leg cassette changer displays arterial anatomy from the lower abdomen to the feet. Stenosis of the distal aorta is noted with enlarged lumbar arteries and rectal branches of the inferior mesenteric artery providing collateral flow distally.

Full angiographic visualization of run-off vessels can be a technical challenge in patients with multisegmental occlusive disease, severe infrapopliteal disease, or peripheral vasoconstriction. Reactive hyperemia created by suprasystolic inflation of calf vein blood pressure cuffs for about 5 minutes immediately prior to contrast injection can substantially improve opacification of distal vessels.

Other techniques that may improve distal vessel opacification are more selective catheter positioning into the external iliac artery, selective injection of vasodilators, systemic vasodilators (topical nitroglycerin, subinguinal nifedipine), or balloon occlusion angiography. With any of these manipulations, digital subtraction angiography generally improves contrast

detection compared with that achieved with conventional angiography.

The presence and size of femoral and popliteal aneurysms can be readily defined with duplex ultrasonography. Angiography is indicated prior to surgery to assess the status of inflow and distal vessels. Because of the frequent bilaterality of these lesions and the frequent coexistence of aortic aneurysmal disease, abdominal aortography and bilateral lower-extremity angiography should be performed.

In patients with failed lower-extremity bypass grafts, angiography may be performed to assess inflow and run-off vessels prior to surgery or to serve as an initial step in local transcatheter delivery of a thrombolytic agent into the clotted graft. Angiography may be warranted prior to surgery in patients with patent grafts in whom routine surveillance studies such as duplex ultrasonography suggest developing graft or anastomotic abnormalities.

Lower-extremity angiography may also be performed in patients with acute limb ischemia due to arterial thrombosis or embolism and in patients with suspected arterial injury due to blunt or penetrating trauma.

Upper-Extremity Angiography

Symptomatic hand or upper-extremity ischemia may be due to proximal occlusive disease (atherosclerosis, thoracic outlet syndrome, vasculitis), emboli from a cardiac or proximal upper extremity source, or intrinsic small vessel disease (thromboangiitis obliterans, collagen vascular disease, repetitive trauma). Angiography is indicated to aid in diagnosis and to delineate anatomy prior to therapeutic intervention. Complete evaluation generally requires arch aortography followed by selective angiography of the involved extremity down to and including the hand. Selective intra-arterial injection of a vasodilator such as tolazoline or nitroglycerin is usually required to adequately opacify distal vessels in the hand. In patients with small vessel occlusive disease seen angiographically in one hand, examination of the other hand may reveal an unsuspected systemic process. High-resolution digital subtraction angiography is ideal for this evaluation, greatly reducing procedure time and contrast dose. Low-osmolality contrast agents can greatly reduce injection pain.

Upper-extremity angiography is frequently performed for evaluation of malfunctioning dialysis access sites. Optimal site of catheter insertion depends on location and type of access, physical examination, and hemodynamic parameters obtained during dialysis. Prosthetic grafts most commonly malfunction because of venous obstruction at or central to the graft anastomosis and can usually be studied by contrast injection into the venous end of the graft. Lesions detected may be amenable to angioplasty through this same access site. Patients with malfunctioning distal forearm arteriovenous fistulas (Brescia-Cimino fistulas) may exhibit stenosis of the fistula, the feeding artery, or the draining vein. Contrast injection into the vein with external compression central to the injection site may reflux sufficient contrast retrogradely through the fistula to allow evaluation of artery and vein. Alternatively, retrograde brachial artery or transfemoral catheterization may be necessary for complete assessment.

Brachiocephalic & Cerebral Angiography

Carotid angiography is most frequently performed in patients who are candidates for surgical therapy of extracranial carotid occlusive disease. These may include symptomatic patients with hemispheric transient ischemic attacks or amaurosis fugax, some patients with completed stroke, and some asymptomatic patients with evidence of severe stenosis or ulcerated plaque detected by noninvasive imaging studies.

Optimally, a left anterior oblique arch aortogram is initially performed to assess the origins of the major brachiocephalic vessels, followed by bilateral selective common carotid angiography in multiple views to delineate the carotid bifurcations in detail. Frontal and lateral views of the intracranial vasculature are routinely obtained to check for other sites of occlusive disease and to assess the status of collateral cerebral perfusion. The vertebrobasilar circulation is evaluated by selective catheterization of the dominant vertebral artery, or, if not feasible, by ipsilateral proximal subclavian injection and filming of the cervical and intracranial vasculature. The spatial resolution of state-of-the-art digital angiographic systems is such that conventional angiography has largely been replaced for this evaluation. Contrast load and procedure time may be further shortened by use of simultaneous biplane imaging.

Angiographic evaluation of the aortic arch and its branches may also be indicated in patients with symptoms of posterior circulation ischemia and those with suspected subclavian steal who are candidates for surgical revascularization.

Carotid, vertebral, and cerebral angiography is also used in the evaluation of suspected arterial trauma, dissection, vascular malformations, and intracranial aneurysms.

Venography

A. Lower Extremity: Duplex ultrasonography has gained acceptance for the initial imaging evaluation of suspected lower-extremity deep venous thrombosis. Venous noncompressibility is the sine qua non of a positive diagnosis. Supplemental findings include intraluminal echogenicity and altered venous flow. In most cases, the deep venous system of the leg is readily examined from the popliteal to the external iliac level. Efficacy in detection of calf vein thrombus has been questioned, although results from some recent clinical series are promising.

Contrast venography is reserved for cases with inconclusive ultrasound results or for suspected isolated calf vein thrombosis. A diagnostic alternative in patients with suspected calf vein thrombosis and a normal initial ultrasound examination is performance of serial follow-up ultrasound studies, given the relative lack of propensity for calf vein thrombus to cause clinically significant pulmonary embolism unless propagation above the knee occurs.

Contrast venography may also be requested for assessment of incompetent perforating veins prior to varicose vein surgery.

A superficial vein on the dorsum of the foot is cannulated. With the patient positioned in a 45–60-degree reverse Trendelenburg position, contrast is manually injected and overlapping radiographs are obtained to encompass the entire lower extremity. Additional films of the pelvis, obtained as the table is leveled, are necessary to assess the iliac veins. A tourniquet applied at the ankle promotes contrast flow from the superficial venous injection site into the deep veins of the calf. Dilute nonionic contrast is used to reduce the risk of chemical phlebitis or tissue necrosis if contrast extravasates. Deep venous thrombosis is definitively diagnosed upon finding contrast material around a radiolucent intraluminal filling defect. Abrupt termination of an opacified deep vein, nonopacification of a segment of deep vein, and abnormal venous collaterals are indirect but nonspecific signs of deep venous thrombosis. Vessel recanalization and luminal irregularity may be seen as manifestations of chronic thrombosis.

In patients with clinical sequelae of chronic venous stasis (pain, edema, skin pigmentation, ulceration), evaluation for the presence of deep venous valvular incompetence may be indicated. The status of the central-most valves of the major lower-extremity veins (superficial femoral, profunda femoral, and greater saphenous veins) can be directly assessed with descending venography. Contrast is manually injected into the external iliac vein with the patient in a 60-degree reverse Trendelenburg position and performing Valsalva's maneuver. Videofluoroscopy and plain radiographs record the severity and peripheral-most extent of contrast reflux down the leg. Various grading schemes have been proposed and correlated with indications for and efficacy of venous valvular repair. Similar information may be obtainable with duplex ultrasound imaging, which also has the advantage of detecting venous reflux at levels peripheral to a competent central valve.

B. Upper Extremity: Upper-extremity venography is performed for confirmation of clinically suspected venous thrombosis or stenosis and as a preliminary step in catheter-directed local thrombolytic therapy. Contrast injected into a superficial vein in the distal forearm usually opacifies all patent major venous channels central to the elbow. Alternatively, cannulation of a medial antecubital vein optimizes opacification of the axillary and subclavian veins and provides the most direct route for peripheral introduction of a catheter to these sites. Digital acquisition of images greatly expedites the examination, and digital subtraction improves detection of central venous abnormalities, which may otherwise be obscured by superimposition of the spine or mediastinal soft tissues.

When venography is performed via peripheral upper-extremity contrast injection, overestimation of the extent of central venous thrombosis may result from preferential flow through venous collaterals, causing poor opacification of more central veins. For more accurate assessment in such cases, it may be necessary to advance an angiographic catheter centrally to allow contrast injection in close proximity to the site of obstruction.

C. Inferior and Superior Venacavography:
Contrast opacification of the inferior or superior vena cava may be indicated for diagnosis and pretreatment evaluation of obstruction due to thrombosis, tumor ingrowth or compression, postirradiation stricture, or other causes. Inferior venacavography is also routinely performed prior to vena cava filter insertion. Direct catheterization may be performed from the femoral, jugular, or antecubital routes. Simultaneous contrast injection from peripheral sites in both upper extremities may provide sufficient opacification for evaluation of the superior vena cava in some cases.

INTRAOPERATIVE ANGIOGRAPHY

In patients undergoing surgical reconstruction for chronic lower-extremity ischemia, detailed preoperative angiography should generally be sufficient for guidance of the operative repair. Prereconstructive intraoperative angiography may be necessary in patients with acute ischemia or acute arterial trauma in whom detailed preoperative angiography has not been performed.

In patients undergoing infrainguinal bypass grafting, routine intraoperative completion angiography is efficacious in the detection of significant technical flaws including intragraft or graft anastomotic stenosis, graft kinks or twists, and unsuspected distal arterial lesions. Correction or additional bypass of these abnormalities has been shown to contribute favorably to early graft patency.

For intraoperative evaluation of infrainguinal grafts, iodinated contrast is manually injected through a cannula inserted into the native inflow artery or proximal graft during proximal occlusion of arterial flow. A standard 14×16-in radiographic film is exposed at the completion of the injection. Contrast volumes vary with the size and length of graft. Additional films are obtained if necessary for complete graft coverage and evaluation of distal run-off vessels.

Portable C-arm fluoroscopic units can now be equipped with high-resolution digital angiographic systems, allowing rapid serial imaging, video image display, and postacquisition image manipulation. Selected images may be copied onto photographic film for long-term storage. The enhanced contrast resolution of digital angiography and capability of subtraction acquisition with immediate video review of images may be advantageous compared with conventional intraoperative angiography. The main disadvantage of these portable digital systems is limited anatomic coverage—usually a maximum 9-in diameter round field of view.

COMPLICATIONS OF ANGIOGRAPHY

Adverse Reactions to Contrast

Adverse reactions to contrast agents may be categorized as either pseudoallergic or chemotoxic (Table 3–1). Pseudoallergic or anaphylactoid reactions, which include urticaria, bronchospasm, laryngeal edema, hypotension, and cardiac arrest, closely resemble true allergic reactions but are not thought to be antigen-antibody mediated. No specific etiologic mechanism has been uniformly accepted. Theories include direct contrast-induced release of histamine and other mediators from mast cells, complement activation, and direct central nervous system effects. Pseudoallergic reactions typically occur independent of dose.

Chemotoxic reactions represent direct effects of contrast on the injected vessel or perfused organ. These reactions depend on contrast dose, concentration, formulation, and site and rate of injection. Examples are pain during arterial injection, systemic vasodilatation, pulmonary hypertension, and renal tubular toxicity.

The overall incidence of acute adverse reactions to conventional ionic contrast agents is 5–8%. One to 2% of patients experience moderate reactions requiring therapy. Severe life-threatening reactions occur in 0.05–0.10% of patients. Reported incidence of mortality has ranged between 1 in 10,000 and 1 in 169,000 patients exposed to contrast agents. The overall risk of adverse reactions to low-osmolality contrast agents appears to be substantially lower than that for conventional agents. Although laboratory studies suggest that nephrotoxic effects are reduced by the use of low-osmolality agents, this has not been definitively proved in clinical studies.

Factors that may be associated with increased risk of contrast toxicity are previous contrast reaction, diabetes mellitus, elevated serum creatinine, advanced age, severe cardiopulmonary disease, history of severe allergy, and asthma.

The risk of pseudoallergic reactions may be reduced by pretreatment with corticosteroids and antihistamines. Since a previous major adverse reaction to contrast carries a substantial risk of repeat reaction (20–33% with ionic agents), such patients should be

Table 3–1. Guide for the treatment of acute reactions to contrast media.

Signs and Symptom	Treatment	Treatment Dose/Route of Administration		Treatment Interval	Treatment Precautions
		Adults	Children		
Nausea/vomiting					
Transient	Supportive				Observe patient
Severe, protracted	Prochlorperazine injectable (Compazine)	5–10 mg/intramuscular, IV	>2 years old: 0.13 mg/kg/intramuscular <2 years old: not recommended	Every 3–4 hr	IV—administer slowly; drowsiness
Urticaria					
Scattered, transient	Supportive				Observe patient
Scattered, protracted	Diphenhydramine injectable (Benadryl)	25–50 mg/IV, intramuscular	1.25 mg/kg/IV, intramuscular	Every 2–3 hr	Drowsiness
Profound	Cimetidine injectable (Tagamet) *or*	300 mg (diluted—10 mL)/IV	5–10 mg/kg (diluted)/IV	Every 6–8 hr	Administer slowly; drowsiness
	Ranitidine injectable (Zantac)	50 mg (diluted—10 mL)/IV	Use not established	Every 6–8 hr	Administer slowly
Bronchospasm					
Mild-moderate	Oxygen	3 L/min	3 L/min		
	Subcutaneous epinephrine 1:1000	0.1–0.2 mg (0.1–0.2 mL)/subcutaneous	0.01–0.02 mg/kg to 0.2 mg maximum subcutaneously	Every 10–15 min	Noncardioselective β-blockers
Accelerating, severe	IV epinephrine 1:10,000	0.1 mg (1 mL)/IV	0.01 mg/kg to 0.1 mg maximum/IV	Every 2–3 min	Administer slowly; β-blockers (especially noncardioselect)
Wheezing-protracted, isolated	Metaproterenol (Alupent) *or* Terbutaline (Brethaire) *or* Albuterol (Proventil)	Two deep inhalations (all)/metered dose inhaler	If possible: one to two deep inhalations (all)/metered dose inhaler	Every 4–6 hr	Proper inhalation technique (use of insert)
Hypotension					
Normal sinus rhythm, tachycardia	IV fluids (eg, normal saline, Ringer's solution)	1–2 L/IV (rapid)	10–20 mL/kg/IV (rapid)	As per blood pressure, urine output	Fluid overload
Bradycardia	IV fluids (eg, normal saline, Ringer's solution) *plus*	1–2 L/IV (rapid)	10–20 mL/kg/IV (rapid)	As per blood pressure, urine output	Fluid overload
	Atropine injectable	1 mg/IV (push)	0.02 mg/kg to 0.60 mg (maximum)/IV	Every 3–5 min to total 3 mg for adults or 2 mg for children	Monitor pulse rate
Seizures/convulsions					
Isolated	See hypotension				
Multiple, continuous	Diazepam injectable (Valium)	5–10 mg/IV	0.2–0.5 mg/kg/IV	Every 20 min	Respiratory depression

From Bush WH, Swanson DP: Acute reactions to intravascular contrast media: Types, risk factors, recognition, and specific treatment. AJR 1991;157:1153.

premedicated. A variety of regimens using prednisone, 50 mg, or prednisolone, 32 mg, in combination with H_1 or H_2 blockers have been advocated. To be efficacious, the regimen must include at least 2 doses of corticosteroids, one given 1–2 hours and one at least 12 hours prior to contrast injection. Nephrotoxic effects may be minimized by careful attention to patient selection, preprocedure hydration, and contrast dose. Use of low-osmolality agents should be considered in patients deemed at increased risk of adverse reactions. Otherwise, the substantially higher cost of low-osmolality contrast agents may be an impediment to their universal use for angiography.

Arterial Catheterization

Angiographic complications directly related to arterial catheterization may occur at or distant from the puncture site. Local puncture site complications include hematoma, pseudoaneurysm, arteriovenous fistula, and arterial thrombosis. Doppler ultrasonography may be extremely helpful in assessment, allowing detection and characterization of pseudoaneurysms and arteriovenous fistulas. Some patients with pseudoaneurysms may be candidates for nonsurgical treatment by direct ultrasound-monitored vessel compression. Otherwise, any of these local complications may require surgical intervention.

Transbrachial angiography carries the added risk of nerve compression injury owing to local bleeding within the contained medial brachial fascial compartment. Nerve injury, which may manifest as pain or sensory or motor deficit, most frequently involves the median nerve initially but subsequently may extend to the radial or ulnar nerve. Early surgical exploration is mandatory, especially if motor deficits are detected, to prevent permanent neurologic sequelae.

Catheter guidewire complications may occur distant from the puncture site, including vessel perforation, dissection, contrast extravasation, embolism, or catheter breakage.

The overall incidence of complications is lowest for transfemoral, highest for transaxillary/transbrachial, and intermediate for translumbar arterial access.

Treatment of Adverse Reactions

Optimal management of adverse contrast reactions requires availability and use of proper monitoring and resuscitation equipment, availability and adequacy of intravenous access, training of all personnel in basic cardiac life support (CPR), and familiarity of personnel with the early symptoms and signs of adverse contrast reactions, allowing for early institution of therapy. Additional training in advanced CPR is desirable. Specific treatment measures depend on the type and severity of reaction encountered. Mild reactions such as nausea or mild urticaria may simply be observed and generally resolve without specific therapy. More severe reactions necessitate specific pharmacologic interventions, details of which are included in the accompanying table.

CONVENTIONAL VERSUS DIGITAL ANGIOGRAPHY

For conventional femoral run-off arteriography, some angiographic tables are designed to perform a series of programmable longitudinal translations or steps, allowing filming from the pelvis to the feet during a single-contrast injection. Alternatively, a long-leg cassette film changer (BCM) using 14×51-in film cassettes and requiring a separate ceiling-mounted x-ray source can be used (Fig 3–3). Depending on patient height, film size is usually sufficient to encompass the aortic bifurcation to the toes.

Digital angiographic units may be interfaced with the image intensifier to allow rapid digital image acquisition in a subtracted or nonsubtracted mode. Digital "road mapping" can provide a sustained real-time fluoroscopic image of the opacified vessel lumen to aid in difficult catheter manipulations. Digital fluoroscopy allows for reduction in radiation exposure and improved fluoroscopic image quality. Most digital systems offer a variety of additional postprocessing software algorithms for manipulation of image quality and quantitation of vessel size and stenosis severity.

Digital images may be reviewed on a video monitor or copied onto photographic film by use of a multiformatted laser imaging system. Selected images may be archived onto standard magnetic or digital tape.

The inherent technical differences between conventional film screen angiography and digital angiography are such that each has its strengths and weaknesses. Potential advantages of conventional angiography are greater image sharpness and resolution power (ability to delineate fine anatomic detail) and larger field of view. Also, image degradation by patient motion is less of a problem with conventional angiography than with digital imaging. Although subtraction films may be created from conventional angiograms, this requires additional time and manual processing. Postprocessing manipulation of image quality is generally not possible.

Digital angiographic images can generally be acquired in a subtracted or nonsubtracted format, and additional postacquisition manipulation of image quality is possible. Contrast resolution exceeds that of conventional angiography, allowing for reduction in contrast volume or concentration and improving visualization of faintly opacified vessels. Scout radiographs are largely eliminated and images may be quickly reviewed on a video monitor, resulting in substantial reduction in procedure time. Digital "road mapping" software, which allows real-time 2-dimensional fluoroscopic imaging of vessel luminal geometry, facilitates safe catheter-guidewire advancement through tortuous or diseased vessels. This feature is particularly helpful for guidance of endovascular interventions.

Although current digital systems offer electronic image archival capabilities, limitations of image storage space and retrievability are such that photographic

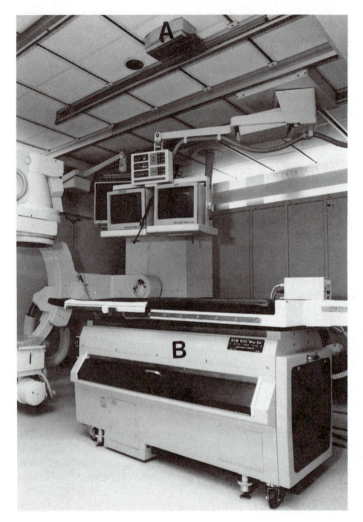

Figure 3–3. Angiographic procedure room equipped for long-leg femoral run-off angiography. *A:* Ceiling-mounted x-ray source. *B:* Long-leg cassette changer.

copies of selected images are usually saved. Even so, overall photographic film costs may be substantially reduced by use of digital angiography.

Compared with conventional angiography, digital angiography suffers from a generally smaller field of view, and digital subtraction images may be severely degraded by motion. Motion of the patient or cardiac, respiratory, or peristaltic bowel motion all may degrade image quality.

Considering the previously mentioned considerations, conventional angiography continues to be preferable for detailed evaluation of pulmonary or visceral arteries, in which small-vessel detail must be preserved in the face of inherent anatomic motion. Conventional angiography may also be preferable for aortography if resolution of peripheral branch vessels such as intrarenal arteries is desirable and selective

catheterization is not feasible. Otherwise aortography, selective extremity angiography, brachiocephalic and cerebral angiography, central venous and upper-extremity venography, and dialysis access angiography can usually be satisfactorily performed with digital angiography.

Bilateral lower-extremity (femoral run-off) angiography, which has traditionally been performed with conventional stepped or long-leg technology, can now be performed with multiple separate digital subtraction angiographic runs or by newer systems that allow for stepped nonsubtracted digital or digital subtraction acquisition.

See Chapter 4 for a discussion of other imaging modalities that are being used for vascular diagnosis, either as initial screening studies or as alternatives to contrast angiography.

REFERENCES

Bush WH, Swanson DP: Acute reactions to intravascular contrast media: Types, risk factors, recognition, and specific treatment. AJR 1991;157:1153.

Dyer R (editor): *Handbook of Basic Vascular and Interventional Radiology.* Churchill Livingstone, 1993.

Fellmeth BD et al: Postangiographic femoral artery injuries: Nonsurgical repair with US-guided compression. Radiology 1991;178:671.

Mills JL, Fujitani RM, Taylor SM: Contribution of routine intraoperative completion arteriography to early infrainguinal bypass patency. Am J Surg 1992;164:506.

Swanson DP, Chilton HM, Thrall JH: *Pharmaceuticals in Medical Imaging.* Macmillan, 1990.

Interventional Endovascular Techniques

Rodney A. White, MD

A brief overview of the causes and distribution of atherosclerotic lesions is relevant to a discussion of the development and application of endovascular imaging and therapeutic techniques. Atherosclerosis is primarily an intimal disease with secondary changes occurring subsequently in the media of the artery. Many believe that the atherosclerotic process begins in childhood with the development of flat, lipid-rich intimal lesions. Histologically, the initial lesions in the thickened intima resemble the structure of the media. Progressive thickening of a simple lesion by continued proliferation of smooth muscle cells and production of extracellular matrix lead to stenotic or occlusive fibrous plaques. Early simple plaques progress to complex lesions with the accumulation of cellular debris, hemorrhage, and calcification of nonviable components.

ATHEROSCLEROTIC LESIONS

About 70% of both coronary and peripheral lesions develop with an eccentric position in the vessel so that the residual lumen is usually off-center in relation to the outside walls of the artery (Fig 4–1). The distribution of atherosclerosis is integral to the development, application, and success of various interventional methods. Atherosclerotic lesions are frequently short localized segments with softer clot and organized material filling the lumen proximal to the lesion up to the site of the next patent branch carrying collateral flow distally. The significant component of soft material enables successful passage of wires across many long occlusions. For the same reason, the length of many occlusions can be shortened or almost completely cleared by thrombolytic therapy. Following thrombectomy with a balloon catheter or thrombolytic therapy, localized atherosclerotic lesions can subsequently be treated by means of various interventional methods. The success rates of current devices are best in short fibrous lesions, whereas failures are related to inade-

quate guidance and debulking of lesions in vessels that are occluded by longer segments of fibrotic or calcified material.

ENDOVASCULAR THERAPY

The distribution of atherosclerotic lesions plays an important role in most interventional vascular procedures. Conventional vascular reconstructions bypass heavily diseased arteries and long occlusions by connecting relatively normal areas proximal and distal to the lesions. Balloon angioplasty increases the size of the artery lumen by producing a fracture of an atherosclerotic lesion and by displacing the plaque. Eccentric positioning of the atherosclerotic lesions within the artery wall predisposes to controlled fracture of the thinner portion of the plaque to create a neolumen. In a similar fashion, surgical endarterectomy relies on the eccentric (usually posterior) localized nature of lesions so that complete removal can be accomplished through a transmural incision leaving a smooth transition to the adjacent luminal surface.

Candidates for endovascular therapy present with a spectrum of symptoms, although most of the lesions amenable to this form of therapy are isolated, relatively short lesions. For this reason, most patients who have been treated with endovascular therapy are those with less severe disease (eg, claudication of the lower extremities), since most endovascular modalities are less successful for treating severe ischemia. With advancing technology, treatment of more diffuse and complex lesions is being investigated with the eventual potential for effectively treating a broad group of pathologies. Throughout this chapter, the usefulness of and potential for treating disease of various forms and severity will be addressed as each method is described.

DIAGNOSTIC EVALUATIONS

Physical Examination

Diagnostic evaluation of patients amenable to endovascular therapy is essentially the same as routine evaluation of patients with peripheral vascular disease.

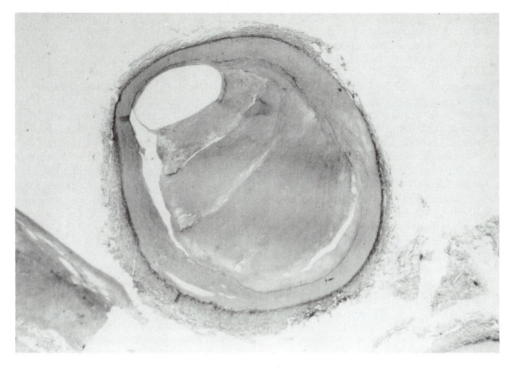

Figure 4–1. Histologic section of a typical atherosclerotic artery with a posteriorly located eccentric plaque. As the vessel narrowing progresses, the lumen becomes smaller and the eccentricity is further accentuated.

Physical findings such as asymmetric extremities, fragile skin, hair loss, and xanthomas are suggestive of vascular disease. Careful palpation, auscultation, Doppler segmental pressure measurement of pulses, and pulse-volume recording can indicate the severity and distribution of vascular lesions.

Vascular Imaging Techniques

Vascular imaging modalities are evolving rapidly and have a significant influence on the patient's choice for endovascular procedures. Real-time imaging of complex structures is improving with enhanced resolution and 3-dimensional reconstruction, making the images easily interpretable and useful for most physicians. Catheter-based imaging technologies are applicable only when intravascular puncture is indicated. Vascular access may be accomplished either at the time of a diagnostic percutaneous procedure or at surgery. Although the images acquired by intraluminal methods are of particularly good quality, the nature of the technology restricts the diagnostic potential to invasive procedures such as peripheral or coronary angiography.

In current practice, the expense of these procedures devices limits their availability. This factor is accentuated by the difficulty in obtaining reimbursement for use of catheter-based techniques solely for diagnostic purposes. Widespread use will probably not occur until the catheter-based imaging methods are combined with therapeutic interventional devices so that more cost-effective therapeutic applications can be established using these modalities.

Angiography

Contrast angiography is the most accurate method of diagnosing arterial and venous disease, although Doppler and ultrasound imaging techniques, as well as intravenous angiography, are used increasingly for noninvasive diagnosis of vascular lesions. Treadmill exercise combined with electrogram (ECG) monitoring quantitates ischemic symptoms and is particularly useful for screening patients with peripheral vascular disease for concomitant coronary artery lesions correctable by surgery.

Angiography is the "gold standard" for imaging the distribution and severity of vascular lesions. Uniplanar angiography can be accurate in defining vessel luminal dimensions and cross-sectional area if the luminal profile is circular, as in most normal and mildly diseased arteries. The method is also useful to demonstrate the distribution and continuity of patent vessels.

In severe disease, **arteriography** yields limited information regarding the morphology and extent of lesions in the arterial wall, aside from demonstrating visible calcification and topography of the luminal surface. Clinically significant atherosclerosis is usually eccentrically positioned in the arterial lumen, and the lumen may be either circular or elliptical. In instances in which the lumen is elliptical, biplanar angiograms are required to define the luminal cross-sectional area and calculate percentage of area stenosis. Where the lumen is not circular, the accuracy of estimated areas can be limited.

The quality of equipment available for radiologic imaging during vascular procedures varies from traditional C-arm fluoroscopes to sophisticated high-resolution intensifiers and TV monitoring systems contained in mobile units suspended from the ceiling. Some cinefluoroscopy systems lack good spatial and contrast resolution and may require serial examinations to visualize the entire field of interest. The most desirable cinefluoroscopy units permit panning the entire length of the patient to monitor the progression of contrast agents. Carbon fiber tables expedite rapid examinations by eliminating artifacts produced by metal support structures. Digital subtraction techniques have increased contrast sensitivity, allowing detection of low levels of iodinated contrast. Many digital units have freeze-frame and "road-mapping" features that permit superimposition of a subtracted contrast image of the stenotic or occluded vessel on a live fluoroscopic image. The real-time image of the manipulation of guidewires or angioplasty instruments can then be viewed overlying the retained angiographic road map of the lesion, enhancing the safety and accuracy of the intervention by constant visual guidance.

A. Computed Tomography: Conventional transmission computed tomography (CT) was developed in 1972 and represented the first association of an x-ray imaging technique with computed image acquisition and processing. This was a landmark innovation, with extraordinary quality images providing clinicians with clear, accurate anatomic information. The initial application of CT to cardiovascular disease centered around examination of large vessels (aorta and branches) and associated diseases including aneurysms, thrombosis, and tumors. There was limited application of CT to the heart and great vessels because of its relatively slow image acquisition time with respect to the cardiac cycle. Attempts at ECG gating of CT scans were not clinically successful.

To overcome these limitations, high-speed CT was developed in the late 1970s, but resulted in an expensive, cumbersome device that was used principally as a research tool. Ultrafast CT solves many of the problems in imaging of the cardiovascular system because of its ability to acquire a multilevel sequence of scans in a fraction of a second (about 200 msec for a multilevel scan of an 8-cm longitudinal segment of the heart). Various scanning protocols are used for cardiovascular studies. Flow mode imaging requires a peripheral intravenous contrast bolus, and ECG triggered scans are obtained at a selected percentage of the cardiac cycle. This mode is used to demonstrate cardiovascular anatomy, and analysis of the iodine time-density curves that are produced permits calculation of cardiac output, intracardiac shunt volume, and

regional flow. A cine-CT loop is available for evaluation of myocardial wall and valvular motion as well as calculation of ejection fractions.

Perhaps the most exciting and important new application of ultrafast CT scanning is the assessment of coronary artery bypass graft patency and degree of native coronary artery calcification. Ultrafast CT has been used to detect and quantify coronary artery calcification, which indicates the presence and severity of atherosclerosis. The capability of ultrafast CT to predict coronary artery disease in patients with significant disease—and its high negative predictive value for disease absence—has been shown to be better than other noninvasive diagnostic tecniques including fluoroscopy, exercise testing, and exercise thallium myocardial perfusion scintigraphy.

The usefulness of ultrafast CT in peripheral endovascular interventions is to help determine the size, extent, and character of lesions and to help determine the candidacy for endovascular treatment. CT is also useful for screening of patients for associated cardiovascular risk, as described in the preceding discussion, and is helpful for noninvasive assessment of interventions at various follow-up intervals. This technology has been most helpful in determining the morphology and distribution of lesions in larger arteries, although adaptability to smaller vessels is improving. New computed 3-dimensional spiral CT imaging methods are dramatically improving the usefulness of CT for interpreting the distribution of disease and for assessing appropriate therapy (Fig 4–2).

B. Magnetic Resonance Imaging: Magnetic resonance imaging (MRI) has also recently developed as an important method of noninvasive screening of patients for endovascular therapy and for following up patients at various intervals after the procedure. A brief discussion of this technology follows to provide a complete perspective of the potential of this method in endoluminal therapy.

The **principle of flow void,** in which rapidly moving protons fail to elicit a perceptible signal, forms the basis for imaging blood vessels using MRI methods, called **magnetic resonance angiography** (MRA). Although the detection of flowing blood using MRA is far more complicated than the simplistic concept of flow void might suggest, the technique essentially produces a luminogram of the vessel. More sophisticated techniques have evolved over the past few years for the evaluation of medium-sized vessels such as the carotid, renal, and femoral arteries. Most of these methods are based on **gradient-echo** (GRE) pulse sequences, which produce bright blood images from 2- or 3-dimensional data sets. Postprocessing of the information into angiographic display format enables the viewer to evaluate the vessels from various optimal viewing angles.

MRI has been shown to be an excellent diagnostic tool for vascular pathology within the mediastinum. Information regarding luminal dimensions, vessel

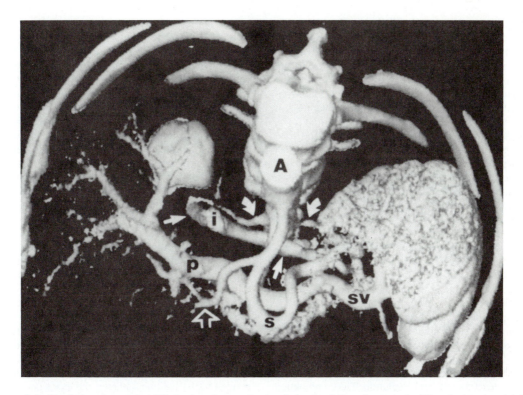

Figure 4–2. Shaded-surface spiral CT display of normal splanchnic circulation shows aorta (A), splenic artery (s), hepatic artery (*open arrow*), splenic vein (sv), and portal vein (p). Renal arteries with stenosis of left renal artery origin (*curved arrows*) and renal veins (*straight arrows*) entering inferior vena cava (i) are also demonstrated. Because cephalad aspect of CT angiogram is obtained 30 seconds before caudal aspect, spatial variations in contrast material appear in spleen. (Reproduced, with permission, from Rubin GD et al: Three-dimensional spiral computed tomographic angiography: An alternative imaging modality for the abdominal aorta and its branches. J Vasc Surg 1993;18:656.)

wall, relation of pathology to the arch vessels and para-aortic structures can be obtained without the use of contrast media. Both CT scanning and MRI are effective in diagnosing aortic dissection, but MRI is more sensitive in demonstrating the dissection entry site and end point. Intimal flaps are seen as linear structures of intermediate signal density, with blood flowing in the adjacent lumens appearing as flow void or anomalous intraluminal flow signal. MRI is also well suited to the evaluation of aortic aneurysmal disease, with demonstration of the outer dimensions of the aorta, presence of mural thrombus, size of the residual lumen, and relation of the aneurysm to major branch vessels.

C. Magnetic Resonance Angiography: There has been recent extensive investigation of MRA in evaluating cerebrovascular disease, particularly the extracranial carotid circulation. High-intensity signal "bright blood" projections of the carotid bifurcation can be generated from the 2- and 3-dimensional acquisitions similar in appearance to contrast angiograms. The accuracy of MRA has been the subject of extensive investigation, with the current consensus cautiously adopting carotid MRA primarily as an un-

proven research tool, accepting that it may overestimate the degree of stenosis or atheroma in some cases, particularly in tortuous vessels.

The effectiveness of MRA in evaluating intracranial vessels is a matter of ongoing research, using complex computer-generated reconstructions as the display mode. Images of major intracranial vessels are generated by means of a computer algorithm called **maximum intensity projection** (MIP), which connects the high-intensity elements of the vessels in 3 dimensions. The resulting series of projections can be viewed from various user-defined angles by rotating the image.

MRA has been used to image virtually all other major circulations (eg, abdominal, peripheral limb, venous), but appears to offer little advantage over other established methods in these areas. It is commonly used as an adjunct to ultrasound imaging in the assessment of patients who are not suitable for radiologic contrast infusion due to renal failure or history of major allergic reactions. Continued development of data acquisition and dynamic 3-dimensional display techniques may improve the resolution of smaller vessel examinations.

D. Transcutaneous Ultrasound Imaging: Transcutaneous ultrasonography plays an important role in imaging lesions. Like CT and MRI, transcutaneous ultrasonography is useful for selecting patients for endovascular therapy and assessing the long-term function of therapy. Research is being conducted for the use of external ultrasound imaging during procedures.

Using ultrasound technique to diagnose and treat patients with cardiovascular disease is one of the most notable medical successes of the past 2 decades. Transcutaneous ultrasonography can image arteries in a tomographic (perpendicular to the long axis) or coronal projection (parallel with the long axis). It is limited by the intervening skin and soft tissue that attenuates the signal and decreases signal penetration. The use of lower frequency transducers (>10 MHz) allows definition of deeper structures but sacrifices 2-point resolution.

An extremely safe technique, ultrasound imaging has become an integral component of modern cardiac and peripheral vascular centers. Initially developed in the late 1950s to examine the fetus in pregnancy, ultrasonography rapidly found use in many specialties with the introduction of more sophisticated techniques including M- and B-mode imaging and improvements in transducer designs and resolution. The combination of B-mode imaging with Doppler-derived waveform analysis (duplex scanning) allowed combined morphologic and hemodynamic assessment of vascular disease. Refinements in transducer configurations, such as linear sequenced and phased arrays, mechanical sector scanners, and variable frequency devices produced a powerful noninvasive technique for investigation of cardiovascular diseases. Color Doppler imaging, which can be performed in real time, has added greatly to the capability of vascular ultrasound imaging by rapidly examining each volume element of the display (voxel) for the presence, direction, and velocity of blood flow.

E. Duplex Ultrasonography: Duplex ultrasound scanning has become the most commonly used method for evaluation of peripheral arterial and venous diseases. It is considered the standard method for primary evaluation of carotid arteries in patients with carotid bifurcation disease, with concomitant examination of the aortic arch branches and vertebral vessels becoming routine. Previously inaccessible circulations, such as the intracranial vessels, can now be imaged with remarkable clarity, and when combined with MRA, a completely noninvasive assessment of cerebral circulation is possible. The accuracy and reliability of these new imaging techniques have not been extensively established, but the prospect of high-resolution, noninvasive imaging of the most inaccessible vessels is exciting.

Duplex scanning is also accepted as the standard method for evaluation of lower-extremity arterial disease, with better correlation than segmental pressure measurements for selecting patients for the possibility of interventional catheter-based procedures. Color Doppler imaging is frequently used to screen patients with claudication, limiting angiography to only those who would benefit from an endovascular or surgical intervention. Duplex scanning is used to evaluate traumatic injuries in the operating room as completion assessment after arterial reconstruction and postoperatively to monitor recurrent or progressive lesions. Although providing valuable morphologic data, angiography does not yield precise information regarding residual flow abnormality or pressure gradient at the site of balloon angioplasty. A more sensitive assessment of angioplasty can be made with duplex scanning, with identification of functional stenosis or normalization of flow hemodynamics being predictive of long-term failure or success, respectively. Renal, celiac, and mesenteric arteries, pancreatic and renal transplant lesions, tumor vascularity, and renal parenchymal lesions are routinely studied with duplex equipment.

Ultrasound-directed balloon angioplasty is an innovative technique that enables the operator to guide and evaluate the progress of the procedure without using radiographic imaging. Using piezoelectric material bonded to the balloon catheter, the exact position of the balloon can be identified on a duplex image of the arterial segment being treated. This technique records physiologic and anatomic data in real time so that the progress of the angioplasty can be continuously monitored.

F. Intravascular Ultrasound Imaging: Intravascular or intraluminal ultrasound (IVUS) is an imaging modality that enables transmural visualization of blood vessels by an ultrasound transducer (10–30 MHz) placed at the tip of a catheter that is introduced into the vascular system either percutaneously or through an arteriotomy or venotomy. Imaging of the vessel lumen and wall is performed in a tomographic fashion by advancing the tip of the catheter to the areas of interest. A computed processing system displays real-time images of the vessels. Luminal dimensions obtained using IVUS catheters have been shown to correlate significantly with values measured from corresponding histologic specimens and vessel angiograms both in vitro and in vivo. The devices have also been used to identify intimal flaps and dissections and to differentiate normal artery from plaque. In addition, computed longitudinal reconstruction of serial ultrasound images along the vessel yields a 3-dimensional view of the vessel anatomy. This technology has significant potential in future diagnostic and interventional procedures.

Intravascular ultrasound evaluations are adding a new perspective to current vascular diagnostic modalities. The benefit is apparent in 2 respects: (1) by defining the distribution of disease within the arterial lumen by visualizing transmural anatomy of the vessel and (2) by providing control cross-section information regarding vessel luminal and wall morphology before and after interventions. This is of particular importance in addressing the phenomenon involved in angioplasty recurrence (**restenosis**), in which adequate controls are not currently available.

Tobis and colleagues (1990) compared the sensitivity of IVUS with that of coronary angiography for diagnosing coronary atherosclerosis. In segments of arteries determined to be normal angiographically, calculations of cross-sectional area by both methods was essentially the same. In contrast, IVUS revealed a substantial amount of atheroma within the wall in either a concentric or smooth eccentric distribution involving about 40% of the available area bounded by the vessel wall media. This demonstrates that angiography underestimates the extent of disease in coronary arteries compared with that which occurs intravascular ultrasound. Nissen and colleagues (1990) also confirmed a significant difference between IVUS and cine-CT in measurements of coronary dimensions and degree of stenosis, particularly at sites of lesion eccentricity.

Comparison of IVUS and angiography images of coronary balloon angioplasties demonstrates that IVUS is more sensitive in defining the extent of atherosclerosis and calcification. Tears and dissections occurred in 80% of vessels, and the mean cross-sectional lumen area postdilatation measured by ultrasound correlated poorly with the value calculated by angiography. The inaccuracy of determination of luminal area using cineangiography discourages the use of this method as the standard for evaluating lesion recurrence. The investigators also reported that IVUS documented that the mean residual atheroma area at the site of prior dilatation was 73% of the available arterial cross-sectional area of the artery. They postulated that this finding may explain the high incidence of restenosis after percutaneous transluminal coronary angioplasty. These data highlight the inability of conventional cineangiography systems to provide adequately sensitive data regarding the distribution and consistency of lesions and illustrate the outcome of current methods. It is questionable whether angiography should still be used as the gold standard for quantitating restenosis, particularly since IVUS offers a more precise alternative and can evaluate the distribution of disease in the vessel wall.

Preliminary investigators have confirmed the usefulness of angioscopy and IVUS in identifying the distribution and cross-sectional analysis of plaque morphology before and after atherectomy. These data will be useful in quantitating the amount of plaque removed and in redefining the recurrence of lesions based on these observations (Fig 4–3).

IVUS has recently been used to help define the mor-phology of lesions in the arterial wall during catheter-based interventions such as stent repairs of aortic dissections. The use of IVUS real-time imaging during endovascular procedures is appealing from several perspectives. IVUS provides improved precision for quantitating disease, choosing appropriate interventional methods, and assessing the outcome of an intervention. Its role in enhancing the interpretation of preoperative angiographic and CT imaging studies is exemplied in Figure 4–4.

G. Angioscopy: Angioscopy, the endoscopic examination of the luminal anatomy of blood vessels, is useful in determining the diagnosis and cause of vascular diseases, in evaluating the technical accuracy of vascular reconstructions, and in visualizing intraluminal instrumentation. Newly developed angioscopes (0.5–3.3 mm in diameter) have improved fiberoptic systems and light sources, enabling high-resolution imaging if blood can be adequately cleared from the vessel lumen (Fig 4–5).

Several investigators have reported that angioscopy reveals clinically important information that is not apparent by extraluminal inspection, probing, or angiography in 20–30% of vascular procedures. The angioscopic findings have altered the surgical therapy in a significant number of patients. Angioscopic examination of vessels after thrombectomy not only identifies critical stenoses but also demonstrates residual thrombus missed by angiography.

Angioscopy provides repeatable 3-dimensional intraluminal views of treated vessels before blood flow is restored. The procedure also helps limit the need for contrast dye and exposure to ionizing radiation. Potential complications of angioscopy include fluid overload from excessive administration of irrigation and direct intimal damage. Fluid overload can be averted by occluding both the vessel being inspected and its collateral branches or by performing the procedures with a tourniquet on the extremity. Inspection of vessels that approximate or are smaller than the diameter of the angioscope can produce spasm and possible thrombosis. The clarity of angioscopic images is usually excellent, but adequate clearing of blood flow from collateral and distal vessels by fluid infusion and centering of the device for good examination require an initial learning curve. These factors frequently limit visualization.

During angioplasty procedures, experience has shown that the most valuable applications of angioscopy may be in pre- and postprocedural assessment of arterial morphology rather than in direct monitoring of the angioplasty. Of special benefit is the ability to immediately examine the vessel for complications and to gain a graphic 3-dimensional representation of the vessel lumen and adequacy of recanalization. A limiting factor with angioscopy is that evaluation of wall thickness or concentricity of lesions is not possible.

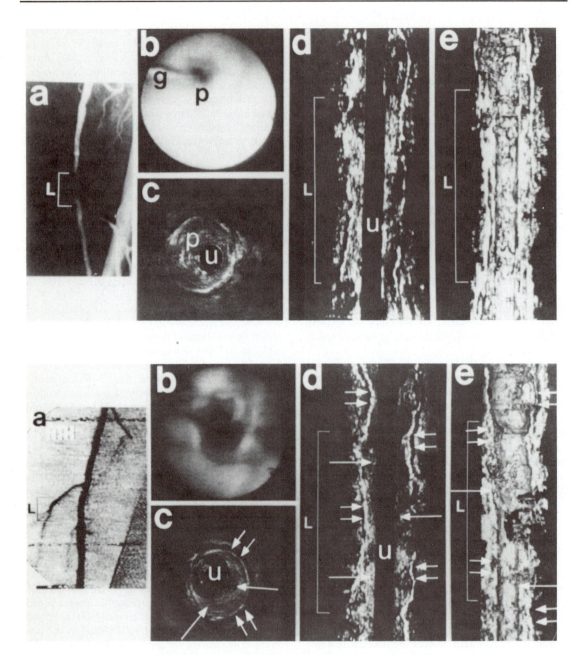

Figure 4–3. Comparison of angiography *a:* angioscopy *b:* and intravascular ultrasound cross-section *c:* longitudinal *d:* and surface-rendered 3-dimensional reconstruction *e:* before (***top***) and after (***bottom***) recanalization of an occluded segment (L) of the superficial femoral artery using an Auth rotablater. Before the intervention, the lesion completely occludes the vessel lumen with plaque (P) directly abutting the guidewire (g)) on the angioscopy image and the ultrasound catheter (u) on the intravascular ultrasound images. Following the intervention, the angiogram of the lesion suggests that the plaque was completely removed when compared with the appearance of adjacent normal artery. Although angioscopy shows a significantly larger lumen following atherectomy, the intravascular ultrasound images demonstrate that most of the lumen inside the media of the artery (*double arrows*) has significant residual plaque (*single arrows*) occupying greater than 60% of the luminal volume of the vessel (Reproduced, with permission, from Cavaye DM et al. Three-dimensional ultrasound imaging. In: *An Atlas and Text of Arterial Imaging: Modern and Developing Technology.* Cavaye DM, White RA [editors]. Chapman & Hall, 1993:138.)

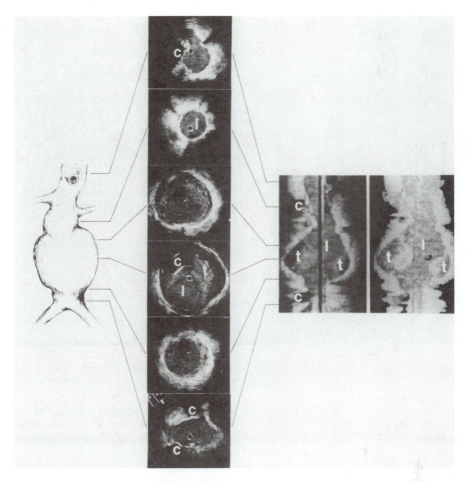

Figure 4–4. Selected cross-sectional images of the aorta and aneurysm at various levels (***center***) compared with a schematic diagram of the lesion (***left***) and the longitudinal gray scale and 3-dimensional intravascular ultrasound images (***right***) of the aneurysm. Note the evidence of thrombus (t) and calcification (c) at several levels throughout the length of the vessel. (l, lumen; reproduced, with permission, from White RA et al: Innovations in vascular imaging: Angiography, 3D CT, and 2D and 3D intravascular ultrasound of an abdominal aortic aneurysm. Ann Vasc Surg 1994;8:285-89.)

ENDOVASCULAR TREATMENT TECHNIQUES

Balloon Angioplasty (BA)

Transluminal dilatation of stenotic atherosclerotic arterial lesions was initially advocated by Dotter in 1964. Dilatation was performed using successively larger coaxial polyethylene catheters (a 12F catheter over an 8F catheter). Staple later used tapered-tip 5–12F catheters with similar effect. The taper configuration reduced trauma to the arterial wall, which had been a common occurrence with Dotter's blunt-nosed catheters.

Dotter subsequently postulated that balloon dilatation of an atherosclerotic lesion might effectively enlarge the lumen. In 1965, he successfully dilated a stenosed iliac artery using a Fogarty balloon embolectomy catheter. The concept of balloon dilatation was advanced by Gruntzig and Hopff in a 1974 report of the use of a double lumen polyvinyl balloon catheter. Design and construction of angioplasty balloons have advanced, particularly with the development of stronger noncompliant, nonelastomeric balloons that can withstand high inflation pressures without distortion of shape or overstretching of diameter. Early polyvinyl chloride balloons stretched easily with moderate pressure, whereas the later expandable polymer balloons are stronger and provide forceful radial dilatation of lesions. Increased catheter flexibility and decreased catheter diameters have improved the maneuverability of the devices and the ability to cross tight stenotic regions of stenosis, including those in small tortuous arteries of the coronary circulation and the lower leg.

The following characteristics must be considered in the choice of a balloon catheter for a particular patient:

- Balloon diameter
- Balloon length

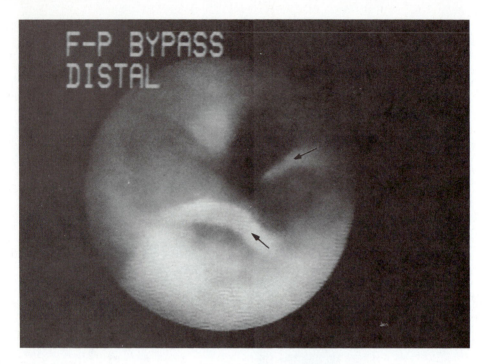

Figure 4–5. Angioscopic view of an intimal flap (*arrows*) beyond the distal anastomosis of a femoropopliteal bypass graft.

- Catheter diameter
- Catheter length
- Catheter flexibility
- Profile and diameter of the catheter tip and the deflated balloon

Recent high-pressure balloons may allow inflation to pressures of 12–15 atmospheres without increase in diameter. This means that a greater dilating force is achieved without overexpansion; this characteristic may be particularly favorable in densely fibrotic atherosclerotic stenoses.

Following placement of the balloon at the site of an atherosclerotic narrowing, the weakest point in the plaque is fractured by expansion of the balloon (Fig 4–6). BA is especially effective for localized, short stenotic lesions (or short-length occlusions) of the iliac arteries, with good rates of initial recanalization (>90%) and long-term patency. Cumulative patency rates of about 60–70% at the 4-year interval have been reported. A retrograde femoral approach is usually used, and frequently bilateral iliac angioplasty may be performed through one femoral access site. Measurement of pressure gradients are helpful in determining the success of a BA procedure. Pressure gradients across a lesion may be measured simultaneously with dual catheters or separately by measuring the pressure as the catheter is passed through the stenosis.

The results of percutaneous BA of infrainguinal arterial disease are not as good as for aortoiliac disease. Several generalizations regarding the usefulness of in-

frainguinal BA can be made following a survey of current literature. In a prospective randomized study of BA and surgery, the initial technical failure rate of BA was higher, whereas the results between successful BAs and surgery were similar up to 3 years. These results are different from those of other series, which report BA patency rates as being lower than with surgery. This is probably because patients in the randomized study had less advanced disease, since an entry criterion for this study was that both groups be amenable to BA.

Factors that predict success of BA of infrainguinal lesions are claudication as the presenting symptom rather than limb salvage, short stenoses, and good runoff of the distal arterial bed. An increased risk in patients with diabetes has been suggested, but this has not been substantiated in patients with short lesions and claudication.

Complication rates for infrainguinal BA range from 8% to 20%, depending on the criterion chosen and the severity of the ischemia. About 10% of claudicators with BA failures are clinically worse with coincident reduction in ankle-brachial indices (ABI). Particularly poor results are reported for BA in patients with limb threat. The only suitable approach for femoropopliteal or tibial angioplasty in severe limb ischemia is to use the technique in a limited and highly selected group of isolated short lesions.

Success rates of BA have been questioned from several perspectives. Even in carefully selected patients in whom BA effectively treated limb threat with salvage

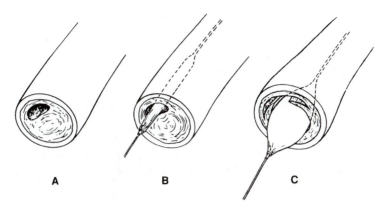

Figure 4–6. Schematic drawing of the mechanism of balloon dilatation of an arterial stenosis. **A:** Eccentric arterial stenosis. **B:** Angioplasty balloon positioned within the atherosclerotic narrowing. **C:** The weakest point in the plaque is fractured by expansion of the balloon. (Reproduced, with permission, from White RA, White GH: Balloon angioplasty. In: *A Color Atlas of Endovascular Surgery.* White RA, White GH [editors]. Chapman & Hall, 1993:24.)

rates comparable to reconstructive surgery, BA patients required a significantly greater number of subsequent procedures compared with that of a surgery group. An additional study reporting a 24-fold increase in BA and 2-fold increase in bypass surgery over a 10-year period from 1979 to 1989 in Maryland hospitals with no change in the incidence of lower extremity amputation rate questions the liberal use of BA for the treatment of lower-extremity vascular disease.

Additional data have evaluated the long-term usefulness of BA in those with claudication—the group identified to be the best candidates for BA and the patients who obtain immediate hemodynamic improvement determined by ABI. In 36 patients randomized to BA or exercise for treatment of intermittent claudication, BA treatment produced significant mean ABI increases of 0.21 at 3 months, which was maintained at 6 and 9 months. The mean claudication distance increased only at 3 months, and the mean maximal walking distance improved slightly at 3 months and deteriorated progressively thereafter. The exercise patients had no increase in mean ABI at any interval, but the mean claudication distance and maximal walking distance improved progressively at each interval up to 15 months. It was concluded that supervised graduated exercise therapy may produce a better long-term improvement in symptomatic patients with mild or moderate claudication by improving mean claudicating and maximal walking distances in patients suitable for BA.

BA can also be used to treat disease in the branches of the abdominal aorta, particularly the renal and mesenteric arteries. Renovascular disease is found to be the cause of hypertension in about 5% of hypertensive patients and may often be amenable to dilatation, especially if there is a short, focal stenosis of the renal artery that does not involve the ostium. Lesions of the orifice of the renal artery formed by an extension of aortic plaque are less favorable and more difficult to treat successfully, as are totally occlusive lesions of the renal artery.

Lasers

For less than a decade, lasers have been investigated as a method of recanalizing and debulking atherosclerotic occlusions. These devices, more than any other device, have undergone rapid development and application. Controversy concerning the use of lasers as angioplasty devices highlights the problems and discussions relevant to the use of all endovascular surgical instruments.

The initial laser devices used available energy sources such as the continuous wave argon and Nd:YAG lasers. Preliminary attempts to recanalize lesions using fiberoptic delivery from these continuous-wave thermal sources produced a high incidence of vessel perforation and thermal damage. To capture the thermal energy and attempt to help prevent perforations, ovoid metal tips were placed on the ends of the fibers. Although there were enthusiastic preliminary reports based on treatment of stenotic lesions and short occlusions using the laser thermal devices plus BA compared with patency for BA alone, application of this technology to longer lesions that conformed to surgical indications for therapy have higher complication and failure rates. Even when obstructions are successfully recanalized, the long-term patency is disappointing. Newer devices include a hybrid concept with partial emission of laser energy combined with the thermal effect, pulsed high-energy laser devices for precise ablation of tissue, and guided laser angioplasty systems. At this time, the current role of laser devices is undetermined and is dependent on whether future technology can eliminate some of the present limitations.

The most common complication of laser angioplasty is vessel wall dissection or **perforation.** Regardless of the device, if the probes are used in lesions where a guidewire cannot be initially passed, perforations are a common limiting factor. Laser angioplasty highlights the problems regarding guidance of endovascular devices, since most atherosclerotic lesions are positioned eccentrically within the vessel lumen and failures including perforations, dissections, and short-term reocclusions are due to inaccurate guiding and debulking of lesions.

An additional complication of laser angioplasty, which is related to imprecise delivery of energy to normal or minimal diseased artery, is the development of lesions in previously unaffected sites adjacent to the treated segment. The most evident presentation of this complication is apparent when patients who were previously treated for short stenoses or occlusions return with long segments of reoccluded vessels. This limitation emphasizes the importance of treating only well-defined lesions that can be precisely ablated with current devices. It also emphasizes that treatment of minimal disease, such as claudication, should be reserved for interventionalists who have technical excellence, vast experience, and optimal systems available to treat these lesions.

The benefit promised by laser technology is the ability to recanalize arterial lesions that would otherwise require a surgical procedure to reconstruct the segment. Patency of vessels treated by laser angioplasty at 12 months' follow-up appears to be comparable to percutaneous transluminal angioplasty for similar lesions, but inferior to surgery for occlusions over 3 cm long. Although the method is applicable to iliac, superficial femoral, and popliteal arteries, current results are not optimal because (1) current devices make only small channel, which must be enlarged by subsequent balloon dilatation; (2) it cannot precisely deliver the energy at the lesion; and (3) there is a significant incidence of perforation of the vessel wall and early thrombosis.

Although clear indications for laser angioplasty are still undefined, pilot studies show possible benefit for a limited number of patients (1) who have arterial stenoses and short occlusions, (2) who have iliac artery lesions, (3) who have polytetrafluorethylene graft occlusions due to anastomotic intimal hyperplasia, and (4) who are not good surgical candidates because of being high risk or who have experienced failures with conventional therapy.

The major advantage of laser energy is that it can provide precise, high-energy ablation of tissue through miniaturized endoluminal delivery systems that require only minimal intervention to recanalize occluded arteries and to debulk lesions. It is important to recognize that the current laser devices establish feasibility only for the future application of advanced systems to angioplasty. For example, the "hot-tip" devices are not a guided laser energy source but a laser-powered thermal probe. Newer prototype instruments, the most promising of which emit free laser energy, demonstrate the feasibility of the evolution of this technology.

Atherectomy Devices

Atherectomy devices are designed to remove atherosclerotic plaque from the vessel by cutting, drilling, or pulverizing atheroma. This technique produces a luminal surface different from that of BA or open surgical endarterectomy. Some currently available atherectomy devices have mechanisms for extraction of the fragments of ablated plaque, whereas others reduce the plaque to microparticles that are circulated within the bloodstream and removed by the lungs and reticuloendothelial organs. Atherectomy catheters may be used percutaneously through an arterial sheath, introduced through an incision, or used as part of a conventional vascular operation. Larger catheter sizes are more suited to intraoperative application.

Atherectomy may be used as sole therapy or in conjunction with balloon dilatation. Most current atherectomy devices are suitable for stenotic lesions only and are inserted over a guidewire. If the stenotic arterial lumen is not sufficiently enlarged after a successful atherectomy procedure, adjunctive balloon dilatation is often performed. As a corollary, angioplasty device complications (particularly dissection or acute occlusion) or inadequate recanalization may be improved by subsequent passage of an atherectomy catheter.

Precise indications for atherectomy have not been defined, and its true role in the management of vascular disease will be determined by further technologic developments of the instrumentation and extensive clinical experience. Although initial successes have been achieved with several devices, restenosis has been a problem in some initial clinical studies, particularly when an inadequate amount of plaque was removed. Preliminary data suggest that precise control of the level of removal of the lesion within the arterial wall dramatically improves patency on follow-up as well as hemodynamic results. If this finding is substantiated, development of this principle could dramatically improve the results of endovascular recanalizations.

A. Simpson Atherectomy Device: The Simpson atherectomy catheter consists of a catheter with a distal cutting blade and its housing chamber, including an attached positioning balloon. The proximal aspect of the catheter is coupled to a hand-held motor unit and has 2 ports—one for fluid flush and one for balloon inflation. A lever on the motor drive unit is used to advance the rotating cutting blade down the distal chamber. The nonelastic balloon pushes the cutaway against the plaque. The tubular cutter shaves a section of plaque and impacts it in the distal chamber.

Simpson catheters for use in the peripheral vascular system range in diameter from 7F to 11F and have windows of 15 mm and 20 mm length. Excised atheromatous material is pushed by the blade into the distal containing section of the chamber so that it may be extracted by removing the catheter. Early designs of the device had a small chamber that filled after only 5 or 6 blade passes; the more recent design has a larger chamber that will accommodate material from 20 to 25 cuts. Atherectomy devices designed for coronary artery use are narrower (4.6–7F) and more flexible, with window opening length of 10 mm. The housing moves over a guidewire through a central lumen.

Simpson atherectomy catheter may be indicated for management of complications of BA, particularly dissection, intimal flap, inadequate recanalization, and early restenosis. Restenosis tends to occur rapidly if insufficient material is removed from the treated artery. If the residual lumen after treatment has less than 20% stenosis, the incidence of recurrent stenosis is reduced.

B. Kensey Atherectomy Catheter: The Kensey atherectomy catheter uses a different mechanism of action to debulk atheromatous plaque. A rotating cam tip, not a cutting blade, acts by pulverizing firm or fibrous atheromatous tissue into microparticles. The cam tip is rotated by a central drive shaft housed within a flexible polyurethrane catheter. An external electric motor drive unit rotates the tip at speeds of up to 200,000 rpm, but rates of less than half this speed are recommended. A coaxial lumen within the catheter is used for infusion of fluid. Fluid ejected from the rotating tip generates a radial jet that creates a vortex effect within the vessel, enhancing the emulsification of dislodged atherosclerotic debris. The fluid also serves to cool and lubricate the rotating cam. Elastic tissue of the normal arterial wall is pushed aside and not damaged, whereas firm or fibrous atheroma is sculpted by the rotating tip and the fluid jet. There is no mechanism for removal of fluid or microparticles from the vessel. Access may be by percutaneous sheath or intraoperative cutdown to the vessel. The fluid injected through the catheter often consists of a mixture of fluoroscopic contrast, heparin, dextran, and thrombolytic agent. The fluid is usually injected at a rate of about 30 mL/min.

The catheter is typically advanced in a to-and-fro fashion with gentle and gradual progress down the vessel. A guidewire is not required, and the system is considered suitable for treatment of total occlusive lesions as well as arterial stenosis. Initial experiences were complicated by a fairly high rate of vessel perforation, since the catheter tends to follow the plane of least resistance, which oftens takes it into the arterial wall. Modifications of the instrument and experience with the techniques have considerably reduced the incidence of this complication.

C. Auth Rotablater: The Auth rotablater consists of a rotating shaft that is used to drill out a core down the vessel lumen. In this case, the tip is a burr with its leading surface covered by metal-impregnated diamond chips. A flexible mechanical drive shaft attached to the metal burr tip is housed within a Teflon sheath within the atherectomy catheter. The whole system is designed to be fed down the artery over a guidewire and is essentially suitable for treatment of stenotic lesions alone. For total occlusions, a guidewire must first be passed through the lesion. The drive shaft is controlled by a turbine that is housed in plastic casing attached to the proximal end of the catheter.

Compressed air powers the turbine with rotation speeds greater than 100,000 rpm; the speed of rotation is determined by the air pressure. The system also contains an irrigation port for infusion of fluid. The burrs are available in various sizes from 0.7 to 6 mm in diameter. The small-size tips are suitable for tibial and coronary arteries, and the larger sizes are designed for the peripheral vascular system, particularly the superficial femoral and popliteal arteries. The multiple diamond chips on the tip function as microknives that fracture and fragment atheromatous plaque. A control knob on the motor drive casing allows the surgeon to advance or retract the burr tip over a guidewire. The drive shaft has a disengagement mechanism that prevents the artery from wrapping around the rotating burr or catheter at low torque. Animal experiments using labeled particles of atheroma have demonstrated that these particles are generally less than 1 μ, pass through the small vessels of the leg and accumulate in the lung, liver, and reticuloendothelial system.

Preliminary investigations have confirmed the usefulness of angioscopy and IVUS in identifying the distribution and cross-sectional analysis of plaque morphology before and after atherectomy. This data will be useful in quantitating the amount of plaque removed and in redefining the recurrence of lesions based on these observations (see Fig 4–3).

D. Transluminal Extraction Catheter: The transluminal extraction atherectomy catheter (TEC) developed by Interventional Technologies also uses a rotating burr tip technique. In TEC, he tip has 2 sharp blades that are used to cut plaque, and the internal lumen of the hollow-tubed catheter is connected to suction to allow extraction of the fragmented particles. The procedure is performed over a guidewire and is suitable for stenotic lesions only. Preliminary studies using TEC have been promising and ultimate usefulness awaits further evaluation.

Complications–Complications of transluminal atherectomy are similar to those of other interventional techniques within the peripheral vascular system. The incidences of complications should be less than 10%, with thrombosis and embolization being the most important. In experienced hands, less than 5% of patients suffer complications; the long-term systemic effects of microembolization have not been fully determined. Hemoglobinuria and hemolysis have been recorded on several occasions. Microembolization to distal tissues in the leg has not been a serious clinical problem even though many particles must be embolized to the distal arterial beds.

INTRAVASCULAR STENTS

Vascular stents or intraluminal splints were first investigated by Dotter in 1969 using nonexpanding stainless-steel coils placed in dog femoral arteries. His work prompted studies by other investigators using a variety of stent designs. Early prototypes suffered from limitations including bulky configurations, unpredictable expansion of the stent, migration, abrupt thrombosis, and gradual restenosis from intimal hyperplasia.

There are 3 basic designs: stainless-steel spring-loaded stents, thermally expanded memory metal stents, and balloon-expandable stents. The latter type is used most frequently because it is the only device approved in the USA for insertion at the time of concomitant BA. In animal studies, intra-arterial stents can prevent elastic recoil of the vessel wall and maintain luminal diameter by plaque compression following angioplasty. Although stents do become incorporated in the vessel wall and are covered by endothelium, preliminary histologic studies performed 12 months after placement reveal that the stented segments show thinning of the media and neointimal proliferation over the stent.

Stents are most beneficial clinically in large-diameter high-flow vessels. Stenting of lesions in iliac arteries and veins and superior vena caval stenoses have been particularly useful. There has also been impressive initial data of procedures using stents to treat aortoiliac stenoses that remain following thrombolytic therapy recanalizations of aortic occlusions (Fig 4–7).

The use of stents in medium-caliber vessels of lower velocity such as the femoral and popliteal arteries are unknown and will be determined by the results of ongoing clinical trials. The usefulness of stents may be to treat acute reclosure of angioplasties from residual thrombotic material, flaps, or dissections or from recoil of the vessel wall. Preliminary clinical evaluation of these devices has demonstrated a benefit in salvaging patients who have abrupt closure of coronary BAs by restoring patency and preventing myocardial infarctions. Prevention of restenosis by stent therapy remains to be demonstrated; thus, use of stents for this indication remains controversial particularly regarding the risks of chronic thrombosis, dislodgment and migration, or embolization. As in other areas of endovascular therapy, intravascular ultrasonography is enhancing the precision of stent therapy and appears to reduce the long-term complications of restenosis and thrombosis by improving the accuracy of deployment.

OTHER ENDOVASCULAR ANGIOPLASTY DEVICES

After preliminary reports of success of laser thermal devices, several nonlaser thermal angioplasty systems were developed. These include radiofrequency and ultrasonic, electric, and catalytic thermal ablation de-

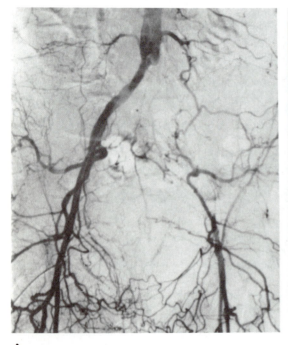
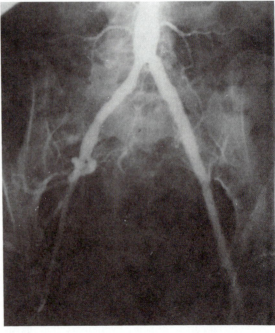

A   B

Figure 4–7. A 73-year-old woman with incapacitating left thigh claudication. **A:** Arteriogram demonstrates occlusion of the left common and external iliac arteries. **B:** Follow-up arteriogram 1 year after thrombolysis and placement of stents in the left iliac system. (Reproduced, with permission, from Wolf YG et al: Initial experience with the Palmaz Stent for aortoiliac stenoses. Ann Vasc Surg 1993;7:254.)

vices, which may be alternatives to the laser thermal devices if thermal ablation remains a viable modality.

Ultrasonic ablation of atherosclerotic plaques has been evaluated as a method to remove abnormal tissue while preserving normal arterial wall. Pulsed and continuous energy have been delivered to plaques by wire probes with histologic evidence of tissue ablation, which conforms to the shape of the probes tips. Other intriguing methods of plaque dissolution have been identified such as the pulsatile, high-velocity water jet. Additional modalities are certain to develop as angioplasty continues to evolve.

INTRALUMINAL VASCULAR PROSTHESES

A new and exciting aspect of endovascular therapy entails the insertion and delivery of vascular bypass graft using catheter-based methods. Conventional surgical bypass procedures use commercially available synthetic Dacron or Teflon tubes or autologous veins to reconstruct aneurysmal or narrowed segment of vessels. Although conventional bypass opertions are highly successful, they require major surgical procedures, which have significant morbidity and mortality.

Preliminary and experimental laboratory and clinical studies have demonstrated the feasibility of successfully placing intraluminal vascular prosthesis in normal and diseased arteries such as aneurysmal arteries, traumatic injuries, and atherosclerotic occlusions. Figure 4–8 is a schematic drawing of endovascular grafts placed inside an abdominal aortic aneurysm with the prosthesis being fixed to the aortic wall with intravascular stents on either side of the aneurysm. Although many variations of devices and graft/stent prostheses are being tested to evaluate this technology, early clinical reports of success at 1–3-year follow-up

periods are promising. Future developments and evaluations may substantiate the improved therapy and cost-efficiency of these catheter-based methods, dramatically influencing the evolution of vascular surgical reconstructive procedures.

THE FIBRINOLYTIC SYSTEM

The fibrinolytic system, which is responsible for clot lysis, is activated when plasminogen is converted to plasmin by mediators such as tissue plasminogen activator (tPA). Fibrinolysis can also be initiated by exogenous activators such as **urokinase** (UK) and **streptokinase** (SK). Plasmin degrades fibrin and fibrinogen into fragments, some of which have antithrombotic activity. The fibrinolytic system is most effective on fresh thrombus, but has also been shown to be effective in more organized thromboses.

Plasminogen and plasmin exist in free circulating and thrombus-bound forms. To protect against the development of a generalized fibrinolytic state, the plasma contains antiplasmins: α_2-antiplasmin, which instantly neutralizes free plasmin; α_2-microglobulin, a slower, more stable inhibitor of plasmin; α_1-antitrypsin; antithrombin 3; and C1 inactivator. Plasmin bound within thrombus is protected from neutralization by the antiplasmins and therefore is free to degrade fibrin. Thus, the interaction between plasmin and antiplasmin provides a system of selective fibrinolysis.

Tillett and Garner reported the exogenous thrombolytic activity of streptococcal extract in 1933. Later, the lytic agent streptokinase (SK) was isolated from

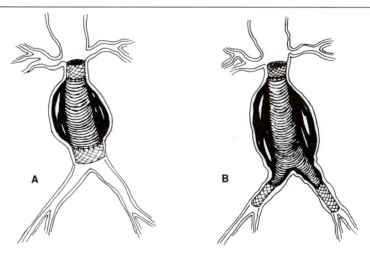

Figure 4–8. Schematic drawing of intraluminal prosthesis deployed in an abdominal aortic aneurysm in tubular **(A)** and bifurcated **(B)** graft configurations. Fixation of the ends of the prostheses is by intravascular metal stents.

β-hemolytic streptococci. SK is a purified preparation of a bacterial protein elaborated by group C, β-hemolytic streptococci. It is supplied as a water-soluble, white lyophilized powder. SK has 2 peaks of activity: one at 16 minutes and the other at 83 minutes. SK combines with plasminogen to form SK-plasminogen. This complex then unites with another plasminogen molecule to form plasmin. Since each molecule of SK utilizes 2 molecules of plasminogen to generate a molecule of plasmin, it is less efficient and also causes greater plasminogen depletion than UK. Because SK-plasminogen is a more potent activator than UK, fibrinogen degradation is also greater than during SK administration.

Streptococcal antibodies produced during a prior bacterial infection directly inactivate the agent by forming an irreversible complex. Therefore, all the antibody sites must be saturated by an initial loading dose of SK before a subsequent dose can be active systemically. A standardized loading dose of 250,000 U of SK has been found to neutralize antibodies in 90% of the American population. As a foreign protein, SK causes a pyretic reaction in 5–10% of patients. Anaphylaxis and serum sickness have been reported, but serious reactions are rare.

UK is an enzyme produced by the kidney and found in the urine. When isolated from human urine in 1946, it showed thrombolytic activity. The 2 forms of UK differ in molecular weight but have a similar clinical effect. Abbokinase (injectable UK) is a thrombolytic agent obtained from human kidney cells by tissue culture techniques and is primarily the low molecular weight form. UK differs significantly from SK in several aspects. First, UK has no antibodies to cause inactivation, so that no loading dose is necessary. In addition, UK is a direct plasminogen activator. All plasminogen activated by UK is converted to plasmin. UK is nonantigenic and does not induce an allergic response. Its half-life is relatively short, averaging 14 minutes.

Thrombolytic therapy was first used systemically in the mid-1950s for thromboembolic peripheral arterial occlusions. Although complete or partial thrombolysis was achieved in 20–50% of patients, the high incidence of hemorrhagic complications led investigators to explore methods to perform selective local treatment. Local intra-arterial infusion of SK was reported early as 1963 by McNico and associates. In 1974, Dotter and colleagues described the angiographic technique for intra-arterial infusion of thrombolytic agent (SK) in the treatment of arterial thromboembolic disease. Although their success was not as impressive as that of later reports, it represented the beginning of a new therapeutic modality.

In 1981, Katzen and van Breda reported an exceptionally high rate of success of intra-arterial administration of thrombolytic therapy in a small series (11 of 12 patients) of acute or recent arterial thromboembolic occlusions. They infused SK at a rate of 5000 U per hour intra-arterially at the site of occlusion. Although UK was occasionally used as an alternative to SK, it was not used intra-arterially until 1985, when McNamara and Fischer reported their experiences in a series of 85 patients.

In most reports, UK is considered safer and more effective than SK and is now the preferred thrombolytic agent by many physicians. The most popular method of administration consists of initial continuous intrathrombus infusion of 4000 U/min with serial advance of the catheter into any remaining occluded segment at 1–2-hour intervals until antegrade flow is accomplished. Following restoration of flow, the catheter tip is repositioned proximal to any residual clot, and the dose is decreased to 1000 U/min and continued for an additional 8–12 hours before reexamination. The infusion is continued until complete clot lysis has been accomplished, unless complications or the patient's degree of ischemia requires cessation and operative intervention. Heparinization (about 1000 U/hr) is maintained during UK infusion to prevent thrombus development along the delivery catheter.

Recombinant human tissue plasminogen activator (rtPA) is being evaluated for local thrombolysis in peripheral arterial or bypass graft occlusions. This tPA, produced by recombinant DNA technology, is an enzyme that has the property of fibrin-enhanced conversion of plasminogen to plasmin. It produces limited conversion of plasminogen in the absence of fibrin. When introduced into the systemic circulation at pharmacologic concentration, rtPA binds to fibrin in a thrombus and converts the entrapped plasminogen to plasmin. This initiates local fibrinolysis but also has some limited systemic proteolysis.

Prourokinase (Pro-UK), a single-chain, zymogen form of UK, also known as **kidney plasminogen activator,** is naturally present in the body in the same concentration as native tPA. Pro-UK has a longer half-life and higher enzyme activity then tPA; thus, smaller doses are required. The effectiveness of Pro-UK in humans is under investigation.

The complications of thrombolytic therapy include allergic reactions to SK, localized bleeding and bruising, systemic fibrinolysis causing diffuse hemorrhage, gastrointestinal hemorrhage or cerebral bleeding, and embolization of dislodged clot to distal arteries.

THROMBOLYTIC THERAPY

Thrombolytic therapy involves the use of medications to lyse thrombus in the arterial or venous system. These medications have an expanding role in the treatment of vascular diseases. In particular, thrombolysis is being used widely in combination with other interventional methods to dissolve thrombus and define the extent of lesions as well as to clear thrombus from vessels inaccessible to other methods.

Perioperative Evaluation & Management of Cardiac Disease

5

Bruce S. Cutler, MD

Thanks to a number of recent innovations in the evaluation and treatment of both coronary and peripheral vascular disease, a wide variety of management strategies are available to minimize the risk of cardiac complications after vascular surgical procedures. This chapter reviews some of the current methods used to detect coronary artery disease (CAD), to classify cardiac risk preoperatively, and to prevent myocardial ischemia during and after operation.

CORONARY ARTERY DISEASE

General Considerations

The prevalence and severity of CAD in vascular patients have been estimated from studies in which all patients underwent coronary angiography before vascular surgery. Myocardial infarctions account for 56–69% of the mortality following peripheral vascular operations, reflecting the common association of coronary and peripheral vascular disease. The collective results from 5 studies of a total of 1545 patients showed that 77% had greater than 70% stenosis of at least 1 coronary artery and 44% had significant narrowing of all 3 vessels. These studies also found that 40% of patients with no history of previous myocardial infarction or angina had at least single vessel disease. Of the asymptomatic patients, 29% had advanced involvement of all 3 vessels or the left main coronary artery.

The high incidence of asymptomatic CAD is important because the risk of cardiac events correlates with the severity of the CAD and is independent of symptoms. Consequently, all vascular patients, even those who have no symptoms of CAD, should be considered to be at risk for a perioperative cardiac complication.

Myocardial Ischemia

Myocardial ischemia occurs when there is an imbalance between myocardial oxygen requirements and the supply of oxygen. Any factor that causes a critical reduction in the supply of oxygen or increases the heart's need for oxygen in the presence of restricted coronary blood flow may precipitate myocardial ischemia. The heart is more efficient than any other organ in extracting oxygen from the circulation, removing 65% of the oxygen from coronary blood. In fact, oxygen extraction is near maximum, even under resting conditions. Consequently, when the demand for oxygen increases, as with exercise or the stress of a surgical procedure, the increased demand is primarily met by reflex coronary vasodilatation and an increase in coronary blood flow. Autoregulation of coronary blood flow is severely limited by CAD or vasospasm.

Most of the coronary blood flow occurs during ventricular diastole, when the pressure gradient across the coronary vascular bed is at a maximum. The coronary perfusion gradient is the difference between systemic arterial diastolic pressure and left ventricular end-diastolic pressure (LVEDP). Consequently, factors such as systemic hypotension and elevated LVEDP from left ventricular (LV) failure decrease the perfusion gradient and reduce coronary blood flow. Tachycardia is particularly detrimental because the elevated heart rate causes an increase in myocardial oxygen demand at the same time that the duration of LV diastole is reduced, which in turn decreases the time for coronary perfusion. It is not surprising that tachycardia is a common cause of myocardial ischemia in the presence of CAD. LV failure also has a deleterious effect on both sides of the myocardial oxygen balance. The increased wall tension from ventricular dilatation increases oxygen demand and at the same time the elevated LVEDP decreases the coronary perfusion gradient.

Coronary vasospasm is an important cause of myocardial ischemia, which may occur in conjunction with coronary occlusive lesions and further impair coronary blood flow. To avoid coronary vasoconstriction, nitrates and calcium channel blockers should be continued perioperatively in patients with known CAD. Since patients with CAD have a limited ability to increase coronary blood flow in response to oxygen demand, it is especially important that the oxygen carrying capacity of the blood be at a maximum. In the presence of CAD, even mild anemia or oxygen desaturation may contribute to myocardial ischemia. Unfortunately, many of the factors just mentioned may occur concurrently during and immediately after a vascular operation to produce myocardial ischemia.

CARDIAC RISK ASSESSMENT

Cardiac risk assessment in vascular patients relies on an estimation of the severity of CAD as determined by evaluation of symptoms, review of risk factors, and application of tests that have been shown to bear a relationship to the degree of coronary occlusive disease. The fact that many vascular patients with known severe CAD survive major vascular operations does not diminish the value of preoperative risk assessment. Rather, it means that other important factors, in addition to the underlying anatomic extent of CAD, determine whether a patient may have a cardiac complication.

Symptoms & Risk Factors

Continuous ECG (Holter) monitoring of patients with known CAD has indicated that 70–90% of episodes of myocardial ischemia are clinically silent, that is, unaccompanied by chest pain. It is not known why many episodes of ischemia are asymptomatic, but the incidence of severe CAD and subsequent mortality from cardiac events appears to be independent of symptoms. In fact, it is possible that patients with silent ischemia may be at an even greater risk than those who experience angina, because they perform higher levels of exercise than those whose activity is limited by angina. The incidence of silent ischemia is highest in diabetics, possibly because of autonomic neuropathy, which interferes with the perception of pain. The fact that most episodes of myocardial ischemia are asymptomatic may explain why multivariant analyses have not found angina to be a useful predictor of perioperative cardiac events.

An operative procedure during convalescence from an acute myocardial infarction increases the risk of reinfarction. Although thrombolytic therapy and early revascularization have improved survival after acute myocardial infarction, the mortality rate for a variety of extra-abdominal vascular operations performed within 6 weeks of an infarction was recently found to be 17% within a group of 30 patients. It is surprising that a non-Q wave or subendocardial infarction has been shown to carry at least the same risk of reinfarction as a transmural event. It is postulated that a subendocardial infarction is surrounded by a zone of ischemia, which is in jeopardy for subsequent damage during the stress of a surgical procedure. In a transmural infarction, the injury is complete without a surrounding vulnerable area. Consequently, patients with a recent subendocardial infarction may have the same or even greater risk of reinfarction from the stress of a major vascular operation as those who have had a transmural event.

Congestive heart failure is the most ominous symptom of CAD. It is the end result of extensive myocardial infarction or fibrosis resulting in severe LV dysfunction. At one extreme are patients who have had a single episode of failure, accompanying a remote my-

ocardial infarction, have returned to a nearly normal level of exercise, and will tolerate a major vascular procedure. At the other extreme are those with recurrent or continuous failure for whom even a limited procedure may carry a mortality rate higher than 50%.

Multivariant analysis of clinical risk factors has identified the following as potentially useful in predicting perioperative cardiac morbidity: 1, myocardial infarction within 6 months; 2, history of congestive heart failure; 3, Q wave on electrocardiogram; 4, angina; 5, diabetes; 6, ventricular arrhythmia; 7, age over 70; 8, emergency operation; and 9, recent cardiovascular accident. Goldman, Detsky, Yeager, Cooperman, and Eagle and colleagues developed risk factor indices in which a weight is assigned to each risk factor, which is then totaled or entered into a formula to determine operative risk. Although the indices undoubtedly have a strong association with underlying CAD, other studies show that they do not reliably predict cardiac complications.

Screening Tests

Since as many as 40% of peripheral vascular patients may have clinically silent CAD, the only means of identifying all patients with hemodynamically significant CAD is to apply an objective screening test to all patients before operation. A number of tests, originally developed to evaluate patients following myocardial infarction have been adapted to detect and quantify CAD in peripheral vascular patients.

A. Electrocardiogram (ECG): It is common practice to perform a resting 12-lead ECG at the time a patient is admitted to the hospital for vascular surgery. Although the ECG is useful in identifying old Q-wave infarctions and arrhythmias, it is of limited value in predicting cardiac complications. The observation that 35% of patients who had a previous cardiac event had a normal resting ECG led to the addition of exercise to improve the sensitivity of the test. Although the development of exercise-induced myocardial ischemia was a useful predictor of cardiac risk, its applicability among vascular patients was limited by the need for treadmill exercise. As many as 50% of vascular patients were unable to achieve the target heart rate necessary for a meaningful test because of claudication, amputation, or β-blocking medication. Consequently, stress testing has been largely replaced by other screening tests that do not require exercise.

B. Radionuclide Ventriculography: This test is a widely used method of evaluating LV function after myocardial infarction. It has been proposed as a method of evaluating cardiac risk in preoperative vascular patients because it does not require exercise and is minimally invasive. However, the test has not proved useful because reduction of LV function is primarily a reflection of previous myocardial infarction or fibrosis, which, in the absence of ischemia, poses relatively little threat of reinfarction. On the other hand, severe impairment of LV function greatly increases the operative risk due to congestive heart failure. Conversely, a normal ejection fraction is no assurance that a patient does not have significant underlying CAD. Therefore, radionuclide ventriculography should be used selectively to evaluate patients suspected of having impaired LV function or to complement the results of another screening test such as dipyridamole-thallium scintigraphy.

C. Electrographic Monitoring: Continuous electrographic monitoring has shown that silent myocardial ischemia occurs frequently throughout the perioperative period, affecting 20% of patients before operation, 25% during operation, and 41% after operation. Multivariant analysis showed that the development of postoperative ischemia increases the risk of an ischemic cardiac event 9.2 times. Unfortunately, these same studies also failed to demonstrate any predictive value for myocardial ischemia occurring in the preoperative period, obviating its use as a screening test.

D. Dipyridamole-Thallium Scintigraphy (DTS): DTS has become the most widely used test to stratify cardiac risk in vascular patients. The vascular surgeon should therefore be familiar with the physiologic mechanism of the test, its clinical usefulness, and its limitations. The intravenous administration of dipyridamole results in maximum dilatation of precapillary resistance arterioles with almost no effect on the major coronary arteries or on systemic vascular resistance. The result is a decrease in coronary resistance equal to that produced by maximum exercise, but without an increase in myocardial oxygen consumption. Total coronary blood flow may increase by as much as 500%, but it is proportionately reduced in areas supplied by stenotic vessels. The net effect is to maximize regional flow abnormalities. Thallium-201 (^{201}T) is used as a marker for viable myocardium and is injected a few minutes after dipyridamole, when coronary vasodilatation is at a maximum. The uptake of ^{201}T is reduced in areas supplied by stenotic vessels, creating a defect detectable by scintigraphy. Scanning is performed in 3 views 15 minutes and 3 hours after injection of ^{201}T. The isotope is promptly absorbed by normal myocardium on the initial scan.

Infarcted or scarred tissue does not absorb ^{201}T and produces a "fixed defect" on the initial scan, which remains unchanged on the delayed image. Ischemic tissue supplied by stenotic or collateral vessels absorbs the isotope more slowly, resulting in delayed uptake or redistribution on the 3-hour scan (Fig 5–1). Ischemic areas and infarcts may be localized to territories supplied by each of the 3 coronary arteries (Fig 5–2). For descriptive purposes, each of the 3 scintigraphic views is divided into 3 segments.

Aminophylline is used to treat side effects of DTS because it antagonizes the vasodilatation produced by dipyridamole. Consequently, xanthine derivatives including aminophylline and caffeine should be withheld for 48 hours before testing. Since dipyridamole

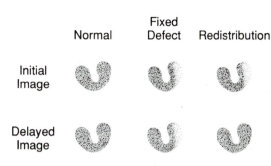

Figure 5–1. Dipyridamole-thallium scintigraphy. Normal, Thallium is promptly absorbed by normal myocardium on the initial scan and remains unchanged on the delayed image. Fixed defect, Infarcted tissue does not absorb thallium on the initial or delayed scans. Redistribution, Ischemic tissue absorbs the isotope more slowly, resulting in delayed uptake on the 3-hour scan.

can also cause bronchospasm, DTS should not be performed on patients who have severe bronchospastic disease. Minor adverse reactions during testing affect 51% of subjects, but fortunately are reversible with intravenous administration of aminophylline. The incidence of life-threatening reactions is 0.3% and of fatal myocardial infarction 0.05%.

In 1985, Boucher and associates published the first report of the use of DTS to predict cardiac complications. In a group of 48 patients scheduled for peripheral vascular surgery, 8 of 16 with redistribution on a preoperative DTS had cardiac events, compared with none in 32 others whose ^{201}T scan was normal or showed only persistent defects. Since this initial study, a number of similar reports have confirmed the validity of the relationship between redistribution and the risk of perioperative cardiac complications. Pooled data from 5 of the largest series involving 759 patients showed that the risk of perioperative events in patients with 2 or more segments of redistribution was 30%, compared with a risk of 1% in those whose scan was normal. The sensitivity of predicting cardiac events was 86%; the specificity was 57%. Despite the relatively high sensitivity of DTS, its clinical usefulness has been questioned because of its limited specificity: As many as 70% of patients with a positive test will not have a cardiac event.

Various measures have been developed to improve the specificity of DTS. A quantitative relationship has been demonstrated between the number of segments of redistribution, the number of coronary territories involved, and the risk of an event. With this approach, the risk of cardiac events is 0 for 1 segment of redistribution, 12% for 2–3 segments, and 36% for 4 or more segments. Furthermore, when redistribution involves the territory of a single coronary artery, the event rate is 13% compared with 43% when all 3 territories are involved. Consequently, the risk of cardiac complications is related not only to redistribution on DTS but

Anterior　　　　　　**LAO/45°**　　　　　　**Left Lateral**

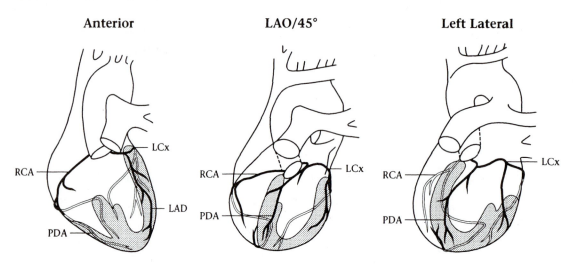

Figure 5–2. Dipyridamole-thallium scan (*shaded area*) corresponding to the territory supplied by each coronary artery in 3 projections: anterior, LAO/45°, and left lateral. LAD, left anterior descending artery; LCx, left circumflex artery; PDA, posterior descending artery; RCA, right coronary artery; LAO, left anterior oblique.

also to the total number of segments involved and to its presence in the distribution of multiple coronary arteries.

Several sources of error can lead to misinterpretation of DTS, the most serious of which is global ischemia. Since DTS relies on the differential uptake of ^{201}T to distinguish areas of ischemia from normal myocardium, uniformly poor ^{201}T uptake may occur because of left main coronary or balanced 3-vessel disease, which may be mistaken for a normal test. LV hypertrophy, soft tissue attenuation from overlying breast tissue and variations in coronary anatomy may yield falsely positive results.

Dipyridamole-thallium scintigraphy has been found to be a better predictor of adverse cardiac events when directly compared with risk factor indices, exercise testing, or radionuclide ventriculography. Consequently, despite the drawback of limited specificity, DTS has become the most widely used screening test for CAD in vascular patients, because of its lack of need for exercise, ability to detect asymptomatic disease, relative safety, wide availability, and general familiarity with interpretation.

E. Dobutamine Stress Echocardiography (DSE): DSE is another test originally developed to provide prognostic information following myocardial infarction, which has been recently adapted to preoperative cardiac risk assessment. The essential premise of echocardiography is that ischemia or infarction results in abnormal mechanical function of a portion of the wall of the LV detectable by ultrasonography. Segmental wall motion abnormalities (SWMA) can be identified as areas of the LV wall that fail to demonstrate a normal increase in thickness during systole (Fig 5–3). Dobutamine is a β_1-receptor agonist that exerts a strong inotropic but weak chronotropic effect on the heart. During DSE, dobutamine is infused at a gradually increasing rate at the same that 2-dimensional echocardiography is used to detect SWMA. Atropine may be used to augment the heart rate response. The test is terminated when an ischemic response is detected or when the target heart rate is achieved.

The predictive value of DSE to assess cardiac risk in vascular patients appears to be similar to that of DTS. In 2 recent prospective studies, DSE was performed before operation without revealing the results of the test to the clinicians. The negative predictive value for each of the 2 studies was 100%. The positive predictive value was 19% and 42%, respectively. Therefore, both DTS and DSE share a very high sensitivity in detecting significant CAD, but both tests suffer from a lack of specificity. Nonetheless, DSE has some potential advantages over other screening methods including DTS. Testing requires only about 20 minutes, compared with 3 or more hours for DTS, and DSE can even be performed at the bedside, if necessary. DSE is cheaper, costing only about one-third as much as DTS. In addition, echocardiography provides an estimate of the ejection fraction and valvular dysfunction not available with DTS. Proponents of DSE feel that the accelerated heart rate produced by the dobutamine infusion is more analogous to the stress of a vascular operation than the vasodilatation produced by DTS. Furthermore, the heart rate that produces SWMA or electrocardiographic ST-segment depression can define an "ischemic threshold" that is potentially useful in preventing or detecting myocardial ischemia both intraoperatively and postoperatively.

Since dobutamine does not cause bronchospasm, it is a potential alternative to DTS in patients with reactive airway disease. However, there are several important drawbacks. DSE may be nondiagnostic in patients who are on β-blocking medications, which may blunt

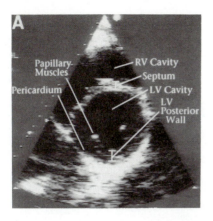
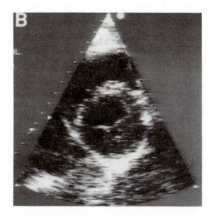
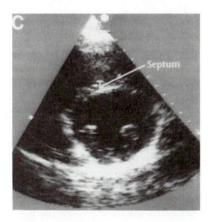
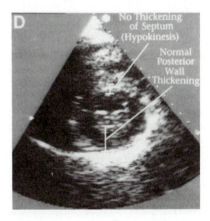

Figure 5–3. Dobutamine stress echocardiogram. **A:** Diastole. **B:** Systole, no SWMA. **C:** Diastole and dobutamine 40 μg/min/kg. **D:** Systole and dobutamine 40 μ/min/kg, absence of normal thickening of septum, which correlated with 90% stenosis of LAD (left anterior descending) artery on coronary angiogram.

the heart rate response. In at least 5% of patients, the echocardiographic image quality is insufficient for accurate analysis. Finally, the test is so new that there is not yet universal agreement on the interpretation of wall motion abnormalities and their significance. Until more experience is gained with this technique, DTS remains the most widely used and the best understood screening test for CAD in vascular patients.

Treatment

A. Preoperative: The goal of the preoperative period is to detect and to quantify the severity of CAD and thereby to estimate the cardiac risk of the proposed operation. The value of the surgeon's and the cardiologist's clinical assessment should not be overshadowed by the results of screening tests, which have come into recent popularity. Preliminary evaluation of cardiac risk should still be based on a clinical history of CAD and the magnitude of the proposed operation, bearing in mind that the risks of infrainguinal operations have recently been shown to equal those of operations on the abdominal aorta. Screening tests such as DTS are of most value in helping quantify the risk in

patients whose CAD is asymptomatic, who have chronic stable angina, or who have suffered a remote myocardial infarction. DTS is of limited value in assessing risk in patients with more severe forms of CAD, in whom it only confirms the presumption that the patient has extensive disease (Table 5–1).

In general, patients with chronic stable angina or an old myocardial infarction who have less than 2 segments of redistribution by scan can undergo major vascular procedures with a 2% risk of cardiac complications. Patients who have more than 2 segments of redistribution, particularly if it involves the territories of multiple coronary arteries, are at increased risk. The risk of the operation may be reduced by modification of the magnitude of the operation or by measures that will improve cardiac tolerance for the procedure. An alternative procedure is most applicable in the treatment of occlusive disease. If the only symptom is claudication, nonoperative treatment is the safest alternative. For limb-threatening ischemia, an angioplasty, atherectomy, or extra-anatomic bypass graft is usually safer than a procedure requiring laparotomy. When a major procedure is unavoidable, such as for treatment

Table 5–1. Evaluation & management of combined coronary & peripheral vascular disease.

Symptoms of CAD	Cardiac Risk	Initial Test	Management Alternatives
Asymptomatic	Variable	DTS	DTS normal: major operation, low-risk DTS abnormal: major operation, accept increased risk; reduced magnitude of operation; or preliminary coronary angiography
Chronic stable angina	Variable	DTS	Same as above
Myocardial infarction >6 mo.	Variable	DTS	Same as above
Subendocardial MI <6 wk	Very high	Coronary angiography	Delay operation or preliminary CABG
Transmural MI <6 wk	High	Coronary angiography	Same as above
Unstable angina	Very high	Coronary angiography	Avoid operation; minimal operation; or major operation and IABP

CAD, coronary artery disease; DTS, dipyridamole-thallium scintigraphy; CABG, coronary artery bypass graft; IABP, Intra-aortic balloon pump; RVG, radionuclide ventriculography; MI, myocardial infarction.

of a large or symptomatic abdominal aortic aneurysm or for ischemic rest pain from infrainguinal occlusive disease, the cardiac risk may be minimized through careful preoperative preparation followed by invasive intraoperative cardiac monitoring or preliminary coronary revascularization.

Several nonrandomized and uncontrolled studies have suggested that coronary artery bypass grafting (CABG) before vascular surgery can reduce the likelihood of myocardial infarction after vascular surgery. The results of such retrospective studies, however, are not directly applicable to patients with symptomatic peripheral vascular disease, who tend to be older with more associated illnesses including diabetes and COPD and who have a mortality rate for aortocoronary surgery as high as 10%. Consequently, the risks of coronary angiography, CABG, and the vascular procedure must be summed up and considered together with the requisite delay in treatment of any life-threatening diagnosis such as abdominal aortic aneurysm, then balanced against the potential for improved perioperative and long-term survival.

When an operation is necessary for patients with more severe symptoms of CAD such as a recent myocardial infarction, unstable angina, or congestive heart failure, coronary angiography should be considered as part of the preoperative assessment (see Table 5–1). Unfortunately, angiography frequently demonstrates severe 3-vessel disease, which is often not treatable by a limited procedure such as angioplasty or atherectomy. About one-third of vascular patients who undergo preoperative coronary angiography have disease that is so diffuse that coronary artery bypass grafting is either not anatomically feasible or could not be expected to improve myocardial perfusion. Of the patients in whom aortocoronary grafting is possible, those with high-grade stenosis of the left main coronary artery or its 3-vessel equivalent are clearly at high risk and should undergo coronary revascularization before vascular surgery. Whether patients without left main coronary occlusive disease will have improved perioperative survival from preliminary coronary

revascularization is uncertain. The decision should be highly individualized and based on age, associated illness, and the patient's willingness to undergo 2 procedures.

Occasionally, a patient with a recent myocardial infarction, unstable angina, or left main CAD requires an urgent procedure for a large or symptomatic abdominal aortic aneurysm. Such a patient may be considered for combined aortocoronary bypass and aneurysm resection. Although mortality rates for elective combined operations have been reported to be as low as 4%, the risk may be as high as 25% in the presence of impaired LV function or left main CAD. When coronary revascularization is not feasible because of diffuse disease or poor LV function, the risk of operation may be reduced by counterpulsation using an intra-aortic balloon pump.

B. Intraoperative: The goal of intraoperative management of patients with CAD is the prevention, detection, and treatment (if necessary) of myocardial ischemia before permanent injury occurs. Prevention begins during the preoperative period. Hypertension should be carefully controlled because of its deleterious effect on the myocardial oxygen balance. Beta- and calcium channel-blocking medications or nitrates should be continued intra- and postoperatively because their withdrawal may cause rebound hypertension, tachycardia, or coronary vasospasm. Anxiety and catecholamine-associated tachycardia should be controlled with preoperative sedative medication.

Optimal hydration is critical to cardiac performance. Many vascular patients are in a state of mild chronic dehydration from diuretic therapy for hypertension. They may also be acutely dehydrated from fasting for diagnostic tests or from contrast-induced diuresis for angiography. Conversely, even mild degrees of congestive heart failure markedly increase myocardial oxygen requirements and the risk of ischemia. The preoperative state of hydration is so important that some institutions have advocated transfer to an intensive care unit the evening before operation to place a flow-directed pulmonary artery catheter for controlled hydration and to develop an LV performance curve by plotting cardiac index against pulmonary capillary wedge pressure (PCWP). Although this approach is probably not necessary for most patients, it is still a useful technique for patients with impaired LV function.

All inhalation anesthetic agents have a negative inotropic effect, a property that may be advantageous in patients with good LV function. Potent inhalation agents produce excellent analgesia for intra-abdominal surgery and controlled myocardial depression, which reduces myocardial oxygen requirements. In contrast, patients with reduced LV function (eg, ejection fraction < 0.35) tolerate inhalation agents poorly. Intravenous narcotics such as fentanyl are often used as an alternative to inhalation anesthetics because they cause less LV depression. However, narcotics alone may not provide adequate analgesia for an intra-abdominal procedure, and supplementation with nitrous oxide may be needed to control hypertension. Spinal and epidural anesthetics do not depress the myocardium directly but may be associated with anxiety and hypertension in the awake patient or bradycardia and hypotension due to peripheral sympathetic block, which can cause an increase in myocardial oxygen consumption.

In prospective studies that have compared epidural with general anesthesia, there was no advantage to either technique in reducing perioperative cardiac complications.

There is no single reliable means of detecting myocardial ischemia in the anesthetized patient. The commonly monitored parameters of heart rate, blood pressure, and PCWP are useful guides to analgesic and fluid requirements, but cannot accurately identify ischemia soon enough to permit prompt treatment.

Transesophageal echocardiography (TEE) has been proposed as a possible method of detecting ischemia intraoperatively. In animal studies, SWMA produced by progressive coronary constriction were shown to precede infarction. Clinical studies, however, found that SWMA occur frequently during vascular operations, particularly when the aorta is cross-clamped. The wall motion abnormalities usually resolved spontaneously and were found to be poorly predictive of postoperative cardiac events. Because of the inconvenience and limited sensitivity of TEE monitoring, it is unlikely to become a widely used method to detect intraoperative ischemia. Continuous-lead ECG monitoring using limb and precordial leads is still the most practical method of detecting intraoperative myocardial ischemia, despite its limited specificity. When new ST-segment depression is temporally associated with physiologic parameters known to cause ischemia such as tachycardia and aortic cross-clamping, it is strong presumptive evidence for ischemia.

Therapy depends on the cause of ischemia. Obviously, causative factors, if they can be identified, should be corrected. For example, hypertension and tachycardia often indicate inadequate analgesia and is treated by reinforcement of anesthesia. On the other hand, ischemic ECG changes accompanied by hypotension may be caused by blood loss, reduction in peripheral resistance from release of the aortic cross-clamp, or ventricular dysfunction.

Initial treatment of hypotension is usually volume expansion, except in the case of ventricular failure, where positive inotropic agents may be necessary to restore systolic pressure and coronary blood flow. An infusion of nitroglycerin is often used prophylactically to produce coronary vasodilatation. Calcium channel-blocking agents such as verapamil or nifedipine may be used to treat coronary spasm not responsive to nitroglycerin. β-Blocking medication, which decreases myocardial oxygen requirements, has been shown to reduce the incidence of myocardial infarction in vascular patients with good LV function. Despite the evidence that silent myocardial ischemia is a fairly frequent occurrence during vascular operations, intraoperative myocardial infarction is unusual, indicating the beneficial effects of attentive hemodynamic monitoring for this group of patients.

C. Postoperative: The risk of myocardial infarction is greatest during recovery from a major vascular operation. More than 80% of infarctions occur during the postoperative period, with the peak incidence being on the third day. The occurrence of infarction several days after operation, when most patients are hemodynamically stable, suggests that infarction may be the consequence of multiple factors including hypercoagulability due to platelet activation, which is at a maximum at this time. Continuous ECG monitoring has shown that 40% of patients develop ischemic changes postoperatively and that there is a strong multivariate correlation with subsequent infarction. Since the ischemia is usually silent and infarction occurs at a time when most patients have left the intensive care unit, many episodes of myocardial ischemia and injury are undetected, unless ECG and creatine phosphokinase enzyme monitoring is extended. As pointed out earlier, even subendocardial infarctions, detectable only by enzyme studies, carry an adverse late prognosis.

Many seemingly minor postoperative problems such as anemia, anxiety, fever, atelectasis, mild oxygen desaturation, and sinus tachycardia have a cumulative deleterious effect on myocardial oxygen needs. Furthermore, elevations in heart rate or blood pressure may not receive the same prompt attention as they might have intraoperatively and therefore may contribute to the incidence of postoperative infarction. Intensive care unit personnel should be aware of the frequency and importance of silent myocardial ischemia so that they can promptly recognize and treat those physiologic alterations that cause ischemia before infarction ensues.

To date, efforts to reduce the cardiac risk of vascular operations have focused primarily on the preoperative and intraoperative periods. However, it is now clear that further improvements in cardiac morbidity

Table 5–2. Screening tests to predict long-term survival following vascular surgery.

Screening Test	Cumulative Survival			
	1 Yr (%)	2 Yr (%)	3 Yr (%)	4 Yr (%)
Radionuclide ventriculography*				
EF > 0.35	90	82	82	—
EF < 0.35	56	56	37	—
Dipyridamole-thallium scintigraphy†				
Normal	97	97	97	97
Redistribution	88	88	88	82
Fixed defects	88	79	69	55
Holter monitor‡				
No ischemia	97	92	—	—
Ischemia	83	63	—	—

EF, ejection fraction.
* Data from Kazmers, Cerqueira, Zierler (1988).
† Data from Cutler, Hendel, Leppo (1992).
‡ Data from Raby et al (1990).

are likely to result from increased attention to myocardial ischemia that occurs during the postoperative period.

Prognosis

Myocardial infarction is the primary cause of death during the first 5 years after a vascular procedure. In a collected series of 3755 aortic aneurysm patients, 53% of the late deaths were cardiac. Unfortunately, the prognosis for long-term survival is often overlooked at the time of the initial assessment of operative risk; nevertheless, useful data are available from the results of many of the tests used to screen for CAD. LV function is directly related to long-term survival; consequently, the tests that measure some aspect of ventricular function are most useful in predicting longevity. For example, patients with an ejection fraction less than 0.35 by radionuclide ventriculography have a 3-year survival rate of only 37% compared with 82% in those whose ejection fraction is greater than 35% (Table 5–2).

The presence of fixed defects on a preoperative DTS have been largely ignored because they are not associated with perioperative cardiac events. However, fixed defects, which indicate infarcted myocardium and reduced LV function, have been shown to have a strong correlation with long-term survival by multivariate analysis (see Table 5–2). Cumulative survival data are not yet available from DSE studies, but a correlation will likely be observed between resting SWMA abnormalities and reduced long-term prognosis.

Prognostic data about long-term survival should be considered together with predicted perioperative risk when making initial treatment decisions. After a successful vascular reconstruction, patients who previously had no symptoms of CAD by virtue of their sedentary lifestyle may increase their level of physical activity to the point where they develop angina. Symptomatic patients may have the severity of their CAD appreciated for the first time as a consequence of their preoperative evaluation or a nonfatal cardiac complication. Because of the prevalence of silent myocardial ischemia, all vascular patients—symptomatic or asymptomatic—are at risk for developing late cardiac morbidity and therefore should be followed with strict control of risk factors, periodic assessment of the progression of their CAD, and, when appropriate, consideration of coronary revascularization to derive the best quality of life and longevity after a major vascular operation.

REFERENCES

Baron JF et al: Combined epidural and general anesthesia versus general anesthesia for abdominal aortic surgery. Anaesthesia 1992;75:611.

Bonchek LI, Olinger GN: Intra-aortic balloon counterpulsation for cardiac support during noncardiac operations. J Thorac Cardiovasc Surg 1979;78:147.

Boucher CA et al: Determination of cardiac risk by dipyridamole-thallium imaging before peripheral vascular surgery. N Engl J Med 1985;312:389.

Calvin JE et al: Cardiac mortality and morbidity after vascular surgery. Can J Surg 1986;29:93.

Carrel T et al: Simultaneous revascularization for critical coronary and peripheral vascular ischemia. Ann Thorac Surg 1991;52:805.

Cooperman M et al: Cardiovascular risk factors in patients with peripheral vascular disease. Surgery 1978;84:505.

Cutler BS: Cardiac complications. In: *Vascular Surgery*, 3rd ed. Rutherford RB (editor). WB Saunders, 1994 (in press).

Cutler BS, Hendel RC, Leppo JA: Dipyridamole-thallium scintigraphy predicts perioperative and long-term survival after major vascular surgery. J Vasc Surg 1992;15:972.

Cutler BS, Wheeler HB, Paraskos JA, Cardullo PA: Applicability and interpretation of electrocardiographic stress testing in patients with peripheral vascular disease. Am J Surg 1981;141:501.

Dawson I, van Bockel JH, Brand R: Late nonfatal and fatal cardiac events after infrainguinal bypass for femoro-popliteal occlusive disease during a thirty-one-year period. J Vasc Surg 1993;18:249.

Detsky AS et al: Predicting cardiac complications in patients undergoing non-cardiac surgery. J Gen Intern Med 1986; 1:211.

Eagle KA et al: Combining clinical and thallium data optimizes preoperative assessment of cardiac risk before major vascular surgery. Ann Intern Med 1989;110:859.

Eagle KA et al: Dipyridamole-thallium scanning in patients undergoing vascular surgery: Optimizing preoperative evaluation of cardiac risk. JAMA 1987;257:2185.

Eichelberger JP et al: Predictive value of dobutamine echocardiography just before noncardiac vascular surgery. Am J Cardiol 1993;72:602.

Elmore JR et al: Myocardial revascularization before abdominal aortic aneurysmorrhaphy: Effect of coronary angioplasty. Mayo Clin Proc 1993;68:637.

Epstein SE, Quyyumi AA, Bonow RO: Medical intelligence: Current concepts. Myocardial ischemia: Silent or symptomatic. N Engl J Med 1988;318:1038.

Fleisher LA, Barash PG: Preoperative cardiac evaluation for noncardiac surgery: A functional approach. Anesth Analg 1992;74:586.

Franco CD, Veith FJ: Letter to the editor. J Vasc Surg 1991;13:174.

Franco CD et al: Resting gated pool ejection fraction: A poor predictor of perioperative myocardial infarction in patients undergoing vascular surgery for infrainguinal bypass grafting. J Vasc Surg 1989;10:656.

Freeman WK, Gersh BJ, Gloviczki P: Abdominal aortic aneurysm and coronary artery disease: Frequent companions, but an uneasy relationship. J Vasc Surg 1990;12:73.

Gersh BJ, Rihal CS, Rooke TW, Ballard DJ: Evaluation and management of patients with both peripheral vascular and coronary artery disease. J Am Coll Cardiol 1991; 18:203.

Gewertz BL et al: Transesophageal echocardio-graphic monitoring of myocardial ischemia during vascular surgery. J Vasc Surg 1987;5:607.

Goldman L: Cardiac risks and complications of noncardiac surgery. Ann Intern Med 1983;98:504.

Haggmark S et al: Comparison of hemodynamic, electrocardiographic, mechanical, and metabolic indicators of intraoperative myocardial ischemia in vascular surgical patients with coronary artery disease. Anaesthesia 1989; 70:19

Hertzer NR: Basic data concerning associated coronary disease in peripheral vascular patients. Ann Vasc Surg 1987; 1:616.

Hertzer NR et al: Late results of coronary bypass in patients with peripheral vascular disease. I. Five-year survival according to age and clinical cardiac status. Cleve Clin Q 1986;53:133.

Hollier LH, Spittell JA Jr, Puga FJ: Intra-aortic balloon counterpulsation as adjunct to aneurysmectomy in high-risk patients. Mayo Clin Proc 1981;56:565.

Johnston KW: Multicenter prospective study of nonruptured abdominal aortic aneurysm. Part II: Variables predicting morbidity and mortality. J Vasc Surg 1989;9:437.

Kalman PG et al: Cardiac dysfunction during abdominal aortic operation: The limitations of pulmonary wedge pressures. J Vasc Surg 1986;3:773.

Kazmers A, Cerqueira MD, Zierler RE: The role of preoperative radionuclide ejection fraction in direct abdominal aortic aneurysm repair. J Vasc Surg 1988;8:128.

Kazmers A, Cerqueira MD, Zierler RE: The role of preoperative radionuclide left ventricular ejection fraction for risk assessment in carotid surgery. Arch Surg 1988; 123:416.

Krupski WC et al: Comparison of cardiac morbidity between aortic and infrainguinal operations. J Vasc Surg 1992; 15:354.

Lane SE et al: Predictive value of quantitative dipyridamole-thallium scintigraphy in assessing cardiovascular risk after vascular surgery in diabetes mellitus. Am J Cardiol 1989;64:1275.

Leppo JA: Dipyridamole-thallium imaging: The lazy man's stress test. J Nucl Med 1989;30:281.

Lette J et al: Multivariate clinical models and quantitative dipyridamole-thallium imaging to predict cardiac morbidity and death after vascular reconstruction. J Vasc Surg 1991;14:160.

Lette J et al: Postoperative myocardial infarction and cardiac death. Ann Surg 1990;211:84.

Lette J et al: Usefulness of the severity and extent of reversible perfusion defects during thallium-dipyridamole imaging for cardiac risk assessment before noncardiac surgery. Am J Cardiol 1989;64:276.

Levinson JR et al: Usefulness of semiquantitative analysis of dipyridamole-thallium-201 redistribution for improving risk stratification before vascular surgery. Am J Cardiol 1990;66:406.

London MJ et al: The "natural history" of segmental wall motion abnormalities in patients undergoing noncardiac surgery. Anaesthesia 1990;73:644.

Mangano DT et al: Association of perioperative myocardial ischemia with cardiac morbidity and mortality in men undergoing noncardiac surgery. N Engl J Med 1990;323: 1781.

Mangano DT et al: Dipyridamole thallium-201 scintigraphy as a preoperative screening test: A reexamination of its predictive potential. Circulation 1991;84:493.

McCabe CJ et al: The value of electrocardiogram monitoring during treadmill testing for peripheral vascular disease. Surgery 1982;89:183.

McCann RL, Wolfe WG: Resection of abdominal aortic aneurysm in patients with low ejection fractions. J Vasc Surg 1989;10:240.

McEnroe CS et al: Comparison of ejection fraction and Goldman risk factor analysis to dipyridamole-thallium 201 studies in the evaluation of cardiac morbidity after aortic aneurysm surgery. J Vasc Surg 1990;11:497.

McPhail NV et al: A comparison of dipyridamole-thallium imaging and exercise testing in the prediction of postoperative cardiac complications in patients requiring arterial reconstruction. J Vasc Surg 1989;10:51.

McPhail NV et al: Comparison of left ventricular function and myocardial perfusion for evaluating perioperative cardiac risk of abdominal aortic surgery. Can J Surg 1990;33:224.

McPhail NV et al: The use of preoperative exercise testing to predict cardiac complications after arterial reconstruction. J Vasc Surg 1988;7:60-68.

Mosley JG, Clarke JMF, Marston A: Assessment of myocardial function before aortic surgery by radionuclide angiocardiography. Br J Surg 1985;72:886.

Nussmeier NA: Anesthetic management of the patient with ischemic heart disease. Lecture from the University of Southern California Review Course in Anesthesiology. March 1987.

Orecchia PM et al: Coronary artery disease in aortic surgery. Ann Vasc Surg 1988;2:28.

Ouyang P et al: Frequency and significance of early postoperative silent myocardial ischemia in patients having peripheral vascular surgery. Am J Cardiol 1989;64:1113.

Pasternack PF et al: The value of radionuclide angiography as a predictor of perioperative myocardial infarction in patients undergoing abdominal aortic aneurysm resection. J Vasc Surg 1984;1:320.

Pasternack PF et al: The value of the radionuclide angiogram in the prediction of perioperative myocardial infarction in patients undergoing lower extremity revascularization procedures. Circulation 1985;72:II13.

Pasternack PF et al: Am J Surg 1989;158:113.

Poldermans D et al: Dobutamine stress echocardiography for assessment of perioperative cardiac risk in patients undergoing major vascular surgery. Circulation 1993;87:1506.

Raby KE et al: Long-term prognosis of myocardial ischemia detected by Holter monitoring in peripheral vascular disease. Am J Cardiol 1990;66:1309.

Reifsnyder T et al: Use of stress thallium imaging to stratify cardiac risk in patients undergoing vascular surgery. J Surg Res 1992;52:147.

Reul GJ Jr et al: The effect of coronary bypass on the outcome of peripheral vascular operations in 1093 patients. J Vasc Surg 1986;3:788.

Rivers SP, Scher LA, Gupta SK, Veith FJ: Safety of peripheral vascular surgery after recent acute myocardial infarction. J Vasc Surg 1990;11:70.

Rivers SP, Scher LA, Sheehan E, Veith FJ: Epidural versus general anesthesia for infrainguinal arterial reconstruction. J Vasc Surg 1991;14:764.

Ruby ST et al: Coronary artery disease in patients requiring abdominal aortic aneurysm repair: Selective use of a combined operation. Ann Surg 1985;201:758.

Salem DN, Chuttani K, Isner JM: Assessment and management of cardiac disease in the surgical patient. Curr Probl Cardiol 1989;14:165.

Toal KW, Jacocks MA, Elkins RC: Preoperative coronary artery bypass grafting in patients undergoing abdominal aortic reconstruction. Am J Surg 1984;148:825.

Whittemore AD et al: Aortic aneurysm repair: Reduced operative mortality associated with maintenance of optimal cardiac performance. Ann Surg 1980;192:414.

Wong T, Detsky AS: Preoperative cardiac risk assessment for patients having peripheral vascular surgery. Ann Intern Med 1992;116:743.

Yeager RA et al: Application of clinically valid cardiac risk factors to aortic aneurysm surgery. Arch Surg 1986;121:278.

Younis LT et al: Perioperative long-term prognostic value of intravenous dipyridamole thallium scintigraphy in patients with peripheral vascular disease. Am Heart J 1990;119:1287.

Bleeding & Clotting Disorders 6

Arun Chervu, MD, & G. Patrick Clagett, MD

I. PHYSIOLOGIC BASIS OF HEMOSTASIS

Hemostatic mechanisms are designed to prevent hemorrhage from breaks in the vascular system. Regardless of whether the damage to a blood vessel is mechanical, chemical, biologic, or cellular in origin, focal generation of thrombin produces a fibrin-platelet clot at the site of vascular injury. In addition to localizing clot formation to the site of local injury, hemostatic mechanisms maintain the fluidity of blood in the native circulation. Thrombosis may occur when the hemostatic stimulus is unregulated or the natural anticoagulant mechanisms are overwhelmed by the degree of the stimulus. Bleeding may occur in the presence of quantitative and qualitative problems in the coagulation cascade. The components of hemostasis include the endothelium, platelets, coagulation cascade, and fibrin formation and fibrinolysis (Fig 6–1).

VASCULAR ENDOTHELIUM

The vascular endothelium plays an important role in the regulation of coagulation, fibrinolysis, vascular tone, cellular growth, and differentiation as well as immune and inflammatory responses. The endothelium is strikingly nonthrombogenic and in its normal state does not react with either platelets or circulating coagulation factors. Blood-contacting artificial devices such as vascular prostheses, arterial and venous catheters, prosthetic heart valves, and hemodialysis machines all have thromboembolic complications due to the lack of an endothelialized flow surface. Antithrombotic properties of endothelium are outlined in Figure 6–2. Endothelial cells synthesize prostacyclin (prostaglandin I_2 [PGI_2]), which inhibits platelet aggregation and causes both smooth muscle relaxation as well as vasodilation. Prostacyclin increases platelet adenylate cyclase activity, and therefore raises platelet cyclic adenosine monophosphate (cAMP) levels. High levels of cAMP prevent platelet activation. Local increases in blood flow from vasodilatation caused by prostacyclin may help to wash away the

forming platelet aggregates, thus limiting the intravascular hemostatic response. Lipoxygenase products of endothelial prostaglandin metabolism also inhibit platelet adhesion. Endothelial ectonucleotidase enzyme activity also affects platelet function by degrading plasma adenosine diphosphate (ADP), a compound that activates platelets and stimulates their aggregation.

Endothelial cells also produce endothelium-derived relaxing factor (EDRF), which has been identified as nitric oxide (NO). Like prostacyclin, EDRF-NO is a potent inhibitor of smooth muscle cell contractions and causes vasodilatation. EDRF-NO also inhibits platelet aggregation, stimulates disaggregation, inhibits platelet and monocyte adhesion to endothelial surfaces, and inhibits smooth muscle cell proliferation.

In addition to inhibiting platelet adhesion and aggregation, the vascular endothelium also counteracts coagulation enzymatic reactions. Endothelial cells synthesize heparin-like glycosaminoglycans that possess anticoagulant activity. Heparan sulfate activates circulating antithrombin III (ATIII), which then effectively neutralizes activated factors XII, XI, X, IX, and II (thrombin) at the cell surface level, thus limiting thrombin production. Thrombomodulin is an endothelial surface receptor that binds thrombin and inhibits the ability of the enzyme to cleave fibrinogen, while it accelerates the activation of protein C by thrombin by greater than 1000-fold. Activated protein C in turn inactivates factors Va and VIIIa and enhances fibrinolysis, probably by binding an inhibitor of plasminogen activators. Protein C activity is facilitated by protein S, which functions as a cofactor. Circulating ATIII also inactivates thrombin bound to thrombomodulin, and this is accelerated by heparan sulfate. The binding of thrombin to thrombomodulin results in loss of its coagulant effects and enhancement of its ability to activate protein C, which acts as an anticoagulant and inhibits thrombogenesis.

The endothelium synthesizes and secretes plasminogen activators. It is the principal in vivo source of tissue plasminogen activator (tPA), which converts plasminogen to plasmin, which in turn lyses fibrin. The efficiency of local fibrinolysis is also enhanced by endothelial cell surface receptors that bind plasminogen. This local fibrinolysis may aggravate bleeding in some susceptible patients, as in patients without nor-

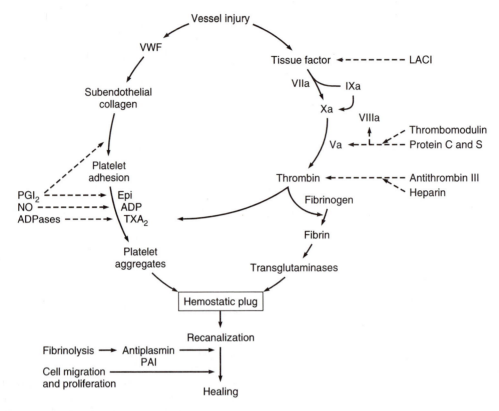

Figure 6–1. Global view of hemostasis with platelet and tissue factor participation in thrombus formation. Following vessel injury, exposure of subendothelial collagen results in immediate platelet adherence to basement membrane in the presence of von Willebrand factor and glycoprotein Ib. Platelet adhesion results in release of dense and α-granule constituents. These cause platelet recruitment and aggregation to form a hemostatic plug. Concurrently, tissue factor is induced on endothelial cells after vessel injury. The extrinsic coagulation system results in production of thrombin with initiation of fibrin formation and consolidation of the thrombus. Dissolution of the clot leads to deposition of collagen, formation of fibrous tissue, and wound healing. (Reproduced, with permission, from Colman RW, Marder VJ, Salzman EW, Hirsh J: Overview of hemostasis. In: *Hemostasis and Thrombosis: Basic Principles and Clinical Practice,* 3rd ed. Colman RW, Hirsh J, Marder VJ, Salzman EW [editors]. JB Lippincott, 1994:4.)

mal production of plasminogen activator inhibitors (PAI-1).

Damage to the vessel wall can lead to endothelial cell injury and dysfunction or loss and subsequent thrombus formation. Direct injury includes vascular trauma, interventional radiologic and endovascular procedures, thermal injury, and surgical procedures. Indirect injury to the endothelial cell can occur from bacteria, viruses, immune complexes, byproducts of smoking, cholesterol, elevated blood homocysteine, localized turbulence around areas of stenosis, and enzymes from activated platelets and leukocytes. Loss of antithrombotic properties of endothelium is compounded by activation of endothelial procoagulant activity. This can be induced by bacterial endotoxins, thrombin, interleukin-1, and tumor necrosis factor. The damaged endothelial cell expresses tissue factor, which then acts as a cofactor with factor VII to activate the extrinsic coagulation cascade. In addition, the

endothelial cell also induces expression of receptors that bind coagulation factors that can generate thrombin and increase local cell surface clotting.

PLATELETS

Following vessel wall injury, subendothelial structures are exposed to the circulation, which leads to platelet adhesion, the initial step in thrombus formation. Platelets contain several glycoprotein (GP) receptor molecules on their surface that bind with collagen and adhesive proteins located in the vessel wall. The main adhesive proteins include von Willebrand factor (vWF), fibronectin, laminin, thrombospondin, and vitronectin. The platelet receptor, glycoprotein Ib (GPIb), of an unactivated platelet binds with vWF that is present in the subendothelium. This binding does not require platelet activation and is thus activation in-

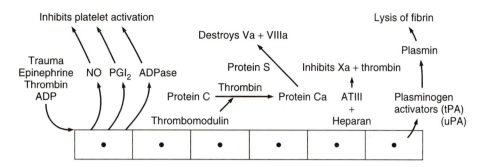

Figure 6–2. Endothelial cells synthesize substances that prevent platelet activation and aggregation (PGI$_2$ or prostacyclin) and nitric oxide (NO or EDRF), disaggregate platelets (tPA and EDRF) and inactivates platelet agonists (TM or thrombomodulin and heparin-like glycosaminoglycans that inactivate thrombin, and the ectonucleotidase that degrades ADP). In addition, prostacyclin and NO relax smooth muscle and bring about vasodilatation.(Reproduced, with permission, from Colman RW, Marder VJ, Salzman EW, Hirsh J: Overview of hemostasis. In: *Hemostasis and Thrombosis: Basic Principles and Clinical Practice,* 3rd ed. Colman RW, Hirsh J, Marder VJ, Salzman EW [editors]. JB Lippincott, 1994:4.)

dependent. The platelet GPIb-vWF interaction depends on shear rate as well as transport of the platelet to the vessel wall. Therefore, shear rates in veins below 650 s^{-1} do not generate the GPIb-vWF-dependent adhesion mechanism, as occurs in the arterial system. Platelet adhesion is also supported by other GPs, with fibrin and subendothelial collagen serving as the substrates. Direct binding of GPIa to collagen ultimately results in platelet activation and secretion. Platelet adhesion to polymerizing fibrin is required for thrombus formation and growth. The GPIIb:IIIa complex is the fibrinogen receptor and is responsible for platelet adhesion to a fibrin network.

Platelet secretion is induced by a number of agents that cause platelet aggregation. Platelet secretion and aggregation probably occur together in vivo and should be collectively referred to as **platelet activation.** Substances released by platelet secretion cause recruitment of other platelets and contribute to the growth of the thrombus. The initial event in platelet activation is binding of an agonist such as thrombin or ADP to the extracellular domain of a specific platelet membrane receptor, which then activates phospholipase C (PLC). PLC then initiates the phosphoinositide pathway through hydrolysis of the membrane phospholipid phosphatidylinositol 4,5-biphosphate (PIP$_2$), which gives rise to 2 platelet second messengers, inositol 1,4,5-triphosphate (IP$_3$) and diacylglycerol (DAG). IP$_3$ induces calcium release from the platelet dense tubular system causing an increase in cytosolic calcium, which is an important component in platelet activation. DAG activates protein kinase C, which in turn promotes protein phosphorylation. This leads to platelet secretion, with expression of the fibrinogen receptor, GPIIb:IIIa, causing platelet aggregation. Other agonists of platelet activation include collagen, epinephrine, thromboxane A$_2$, and platelet activating factor (PAF), which cause platelets to empty contents of dense and α-granules.

Platelet aggregation occurs simultaneously with platelet secretion, with ADP stimulating the expression of the GPIIb:IIIa receptor. Fibrinogen serves as a link between aggregated platelets and the binding of fibrinogen to its receptor is a prerequisite for platelet aggregation. This bridging link is calcium dependent and involves some of the platelet α-granule products including fibronectin, thrombospondin, vitronectin, and vWF. Other agonists of platelet aggregation are thromboxane A$_2$, collagen, thrombin, and PAF. The pathways of both secretion and aggregation probably act through a final common pathway, involving intracellular mobilization of calcium from the platelet-dense tubular system in the cytosol and the binding of calcium to calmodulin. This results in activation of protein kinases leading to aggregation. Re-uptake of calcium into the dense tubules is dependent on cAMP. Drugs that increase cAMP will reduce calcium mobilization from all agonists and thus inhibit platelet activation.

COAGULATION CASCADE

Coagulation is the sequence of events leading to the generation of thrombin and the formation of a fibrin clot. This was initially conceived as 2 distinct pathways, the intrinsic and the extrinsic, based on in vitro analysis (Fig 6–3). In the intrinsic pathway, factor XII is activated by surface contact and binding, followed by the sequential activation of factors XI, IX, X, and prothrombin. The function of the intrinsic pathway is measured by the activated partial thromboplastin time (aPTT). In the extrinsic pathway, there is formation of a complex between tissue factor and factor VII, which is then followed by sequential activation of factors VII, X, and prothrombin. The function of the extrinsic pathway is measured by the prothrombin time (PT). The common pathway occurs from factor X activation.

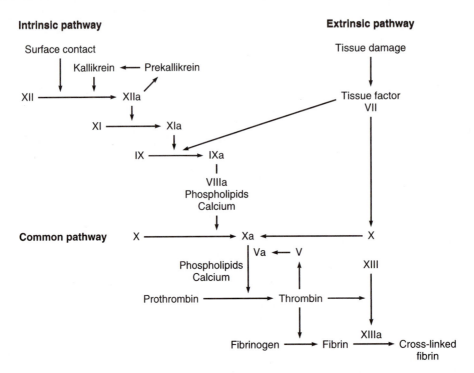

Figure 6–3. Schematic representation of the clotting cascade. Intrinsic and extrinsic pathways lead to production of activated factor X (Xa). The common pathway proceeds to generation of thrombin, which cleaves fibrinogen to monomeric fibrin. See text for further details.

In vivo, the coagulation factors involved in clot formation from tissue factor are the most important in hemostasis and thrombosis. Tissue factor is a normal component on the surface of nonvascular cells and is expressed on the surface of stimulated monocytes and endothelial cells. The extracellular domain of tissue factor is the factor VII receptor, and the exposure of cell surface expressing tissue factor to circulating plasma proteins leads to the binding of factor VII to tissue factor. This generates the activated form of factor VII, factor VIIa, which activates factors IX and X. Factor Xa in complex with factor Va then activates prothrombin, also bound to the cell membrane. This leads to the generation of thrombin, which cleaves fibrinogen to monomeric fibrin. The monomeric fibrin then polymerizes to form the fibrin clot.

FIBRINOLYTIC SYSTEM

Fibrinolysis is a natural process directed at maintaining the patency of the blood vessel by lysing the fibrin deposits. In circulating blood, fibrinolytic activity occurs when the β-globulin plasminogen is converted to the active proteolytic enzyme, **plasmin,** by a number of plasminogen activators synthesized by endothelial cells and other tissues. Plasmin then degrades

the fibrin by hydrolyzing it into soluble polypeptides called **fibrin degradation products.**

The interactions between components of the fibrinolytic system take place within the local environment of the blood clot. Both plasminogen and tPA are derived from the adjacent endothelium and bind specifically to fibrin, with tPA converting the clot-bound plasminogen to plasmin. Native circulating Glu-plasminogen is also cleaved to Lys-plasminogen, and this has a greater affinity for fibrin. After being bound to the clot, Lys-plasminogen is more easily activated to plasmin than is Glu-plasminogen. Plasmin that is bound to fibrin is partially protected from inhibition by α_2-antiplasmin, which is the main circulating inhibitor of plasmin. Plasmin is released after fibrinolysis, where it is rapidly neutralized by α_2-antiplasmin, with excess plasmin inactivated by α_2-macroglobulin. When both of these inhibitors are overwhelmed, which may occur during thrombolytic therapy, degradation of plasma coagulation factors and fibrinogen occurs.

Endothelium plays an important role in modulation of fibrinolysis in vivo. Endothelial cells that are exposed to thrombin are stimulated to synthesize both tPA as well as plaminogen activator inhibitor PAI-1. Of these effects, PAI-1 synthesis is greater leading to down-regulation of fibrinolytic activity.

Colman RW et al: Overview of hemostasis. In: *Hemostasis and Thrombosis: Basic Principles and Clinical Practice,* 3rd ed. Colman RW, Hirsh J, Marder VJ, Salzman EW (editors). JB Lippincott, 1994.

Davies MG, Hagen P: The vascular endothelium: A new horizon. Ann Surg 1993;218:593.

Furie B, Furie BC: Molecular and cellular biology of blood coagulation. N Engl J Med 1992;326:800.

Hantgan RR et al: Glycoprotein Ib, von Willebrand factor, and glycoprotein IIb:IIIa are all involved in platelet adhesion to fibrin in flowing whole blood. Blood 1990;76:345.

Ware JA, Heistad DD: Platelet-endothelium interactions. N Engl J Med 1993;328:628.

II. BLEEDING DISORDERS

Preoperative evaluation of hemostatic competence is mandatory in all patients regardless of the magnitude of their interventional or surgical procedure. Even a minor procedure in a patient with a hemostatic defect can be a major undertaking with disastrous consequences. A detailed history should be taken and a physical examination performed in all patients, with specific questions directed at a history of abnormal bleeding. The history should elicit whether the patient bleeds spontaneously or in response to minor trauma. In addition, the response to dental extractions and minor and major operations is extremely helpful. The manifestations of bleeding may give a clue as to the nature of the defect. Thrombocytopenia or a qualitative platelet disorder may be suggested by easy bruisability, ecchymoses, nosebleeds, or oral mucosal bleeding. On the other hand, joint hemorrhages, deep muscular hematomas, and retroperitoneal bleeds are usually signs of a coagulation defect. A family history of bleeding tendencies is very important and may help to identify the specific defect.

In a patient undergoing elective surgery, the platelet count is the most important laboratory test, since thrombocytopenia is the most common cause of abnormal bleeding in general practice. Other general screening tests should be based on the history and physical examination and include PT, aPTT, bleeding time, and fibrinogen tests (Table 6–1). Guidelines have been proposed by Rappaport (1983) to assign patients to the level of risk of bleeding as follows:

Level 1. Bleeding history is negative and the procedure is minor. No screening tests are recommended.

Level 2. Bleeding history is negative but the procedure is major. Platelet count and aPTT done to detect thrombocytopenia or the presence of an anticoagulant that may have developed without any challenge to hemostasis in the form of recent trauma or surgery.

Level 3. Bleeding history raises the possibility of a bleeding disorder or a major procedure with multiple

Table 6–1. Tests of hemostasis and blood coagulation.

Platelet count
Bleeding time
Platelet aggregation
Prothrombin time (PT)
Activated partial thromboplastin time (aPTT)
Thrombin time (TT)
Fibrinogen
Fibrin degradation products (FDP)

transfusions is anticipated or patients in whom even minor bleeding could be hazardous (ie, intracranial surgery, open prostatectomy). Bleeding time, PT, and a test of clot solubility to screen for factor XIII deficiency are done in addition to a platelet count and an aPTT.

Level 4. Bleeding history is strongly positive for a bleeding disorder. In addition to the screening tests used in Level 3, platelet aggregometry, specific factor VIII and IX assays to detect hemophilia A or B, a bleeding time to detect von Willebrand's disease or other qualitative platelet disorders, and a thrombin time to detect dysfibrinogemia or a circulating anticoagulant.

Clagett GP: Preoperative assessment of hemostasis. In: *Principles of Transfusion Medicine.* Rossi EC, Simon TL, Moss GS (editors). Williams & Wilkins, 1991.

Rappaport SI: Preoperative hemostatic evaluation: Which tests, if any? Blood 1983;61:229.

CONGENITAL BLEEDING DISORDERS

Congenital bleeding disorders include hemophilia A and B, von Willebrand's disease and other factor deficiencies, disorders of prothrombin conversion, abnormalities in fibrinogen, and congenital platelet disorders (Table 6–2). Patients with these disorders generally have either a positive family history or a personal history of bleeding problems.

HEMOPHILIA A

Essentials of Diagnosis

- X-linked recessive inheritance affecting only males.
- Normal levels of factor VIII antigen.
- Decreased levels of factor VIII procoagulant activity.
- Frequent painful joint and intramuscular hemorrhages.

Table 6–2. Congenital bleeding disorders.

Hemophilia A (factor VIII deficiency)
Hemophilia B (factor IX deficiency)
Von Willebrand's disease
Other Factor deficiencies
    Factor XI (Rosenthal's syndrome)
    Factor V (proaccelerin)
    Factor VII (proconvertin)
    Factor X (Stuart-Prower)
    Factor XIII
Inherited hypoprothrombinemia (factor II deficiency)
Abnormalities in fibrinogen
Congenital platelet disorders
    Glanzmann's thrombasthenia
    Bernard-Soulier syndrome
    Storage pool disease

General Considerations

Hemophilia A (factor VIII deficiency—classic hemophilia) is an X-linked hereditary recessive disorder with bleeding due to deficiency or dysfunction of the procoagulant portion of factor VIII (VIII:C). Twenty percent of cases arise from spontaneous mutation. The disease occurs almost exclusively in males, with an incidence of 1 in 10,000 male births. Sons of affected males are free of disease, and daughters are asymptomatic carriers. Females with a hemophiliac father and a carrier mother may become affected.

Those with factor VIII:C levels of less than 1% have severe disease and major bleeding episodes requiring therapy 2–4 times monthly. Those with factor VIII:C levels of 1–5% suffer multiple spontaneous bleeding episodes and are classified as having moderate disease. Hemophiliacs with factor VIII:C levels greater than 5% are usually only mildly affected and have bleeding only from trauma or surgical intervention.

Clinical Findings

A. Signs and Symptoms: Hemophilia A is the most common severe bleeding disorder and is second only to von Willebrand's disease as the most common congenital bleeding disorder. Levels of factor VIII antigen are normal as measured by immunologic methods. However, the severity of bleeding correlates with factor VIII:C levels measured by functional assays (normal, 50–100%).

Clinically, abnormal bleeding in patients with hemophilia A is most often into joints, muscles, and the gastrointestinal tract. Hemarthroses begin to appear when the child begins to walk. The joints most frequently affected are the knees, elbows, ankles, shoulders, hips, and wrists. Joint hemorrhages can lead to chronic synovitis and ultimately to hemophilic arthropathy, which is characterized by chronic pain, limitation of motion, disuse atrophy of associated muscles, bony cysts, and later fibrous or bony ankylosis of the large joints. Aggressive factor replacement with local cold packing at the first sign of hemarthroses is important in preventing these complications. Active physiotherapy is also important in preventing immobility.

Aspiration of blood from the hemophilic joint is not uniformly endorsed. Intramuscular bleeding is common in hemophiliacs and may lead to compression of adjacent nerves and other important structures. Bleeding into the psoas muscle may mimic appendicitis and other intra-abdominal surgical emergencies because of the abdominal pain, fever, and leukocytosis. Bleeding into myofascial structures may lead to a compartment syndrome; in the forearm this could lead to Volkmann's ischemic contracture of the hand. Compartment syndrome in the lower extremity can present as pain and loss of dorsiflexion of the foot secondary to bleeding into the anterior calf compartment. Intracranial bleeding in hemophiliacs may be subdural, epidural, subarachnoid, or intracerebral and accounts for up to 25% of deaths in hemophiliacs.

B. Laboratory Findings: Typical findings are a prolonged aPTT, but normal PT, bleeding time, platelet count, and fibrinogen level. Factor VIII:C levels depend on the severity of the disease. Mixing plasma from a hemophiliac with normal plasma should normalize the aPTT; if not, this indicates the presence of an inhibitor of factor VIII, rather than hemophilia.

Differential Diagnosis

The finding of decreased factor VIII:C levels is the hallmark of hemophilia A. Clinically, it is difficult to distinguish hemophilia A from hemophilia B, and this can be performed only with assay of the specific factors. Differentiation from von Willebrand's disease can be made on the basis of a normal factor VIII antigen level in hemophiliacs.

Treatment

Patients with hemophilia can often lead normal lives until they either have a traumatic episode or undergo surgery. Although patients with as little as 2–3% of factor VIII:C do not bleed spontaneously, they need much higher factor levels after bleeding starts. Most treatment is currently based on the infusion of factor VIII concentrates that have been pretreated to reduce the risk of transmission of AIDS. One unit of factor VIII activity is considered that amount present in 1 mL of normal plasma. The volume of distribution for factor VIII:C is 60 mg/kg, 1.5 times the plasma volume (40 mL/kg). The half-life of factor VIII:C is about 8–12 hours. Recombinant factor VIII is comparable to plasma-derived factor VIII in efficacy, but does not carry the risk of transmission of viruses. However, it is manufactured at greater expense and may cause a higher incidence of antibodies to factor VIII.

The amount of factor VIII administered depends on the severity of the bleeding diathesis. For mild hemorrhages, the minimum hemostatic level of factor VIII is 30%. For moderate bleeding, such as deep muscle hematomas, the minimum level of factor VIII should be 50% initially and should be maintained at levels greater than 30% for at least the next 2–3 days. Pa-

Table 6–3. Circulating hemostatic elements.

| | | | | Minimum Levels Required in Surgical Patients | | |
Factors	In Vivo Half-Life	Stability in Bank Blood	Agents Available for Replacement	Maintenance	Minor Surgery	Major Surgery
I (fibrinogen)	4–5 days	Stable	Cryoprecipitate, FFP, fibrinogen concentrates	(>50 mg/dL)	(>100 mg/dL)	(>200 mg/dL)
II (prothrombin)	3–4 days	Stable	FFP, prothrombin complex concentrates	>20%	>40%	>50%
V (proaccelerin)	1–3 days	Labile (50% activity at 1 wk)	FFP; whole blood <1 wk old	>10%	>25%	>50%
VII (proconvertin)	2–5 hr	Stable	Whole blood, FFP, VII concentrates	>10%	>20%	>20%
VIII (antihemophilic factor AHF)	8–12 hr	Labile (30% activity at 1 week	VIII concentrate, cryoprecipitate, FFP	>50%	>50%	>100%
IX (Christmas factor)	18 hr	Stable	Whole blood, FFP IX concentrates	>50%	>50%	>80%
X (Stuart-Prower)	2–3 days	Stable	Whole blood, FFP X concentrates	>10%	>20%	>50%
XI (plasma thromboplastin antecedent, PTA)	60 hr	Stable	Whole blood, FFP	>10%	>20%	>50%
XII (Hageman factor)	50–70 hr	Stable	Replacement unnecessary			
XIII (fibrin stabilizing factor)	3–5 days	Stable	Whole blood, FFP cryoprecipitate, XIII concentrate	2–3% of normal (?)	?	?
Platelets	8–11 days life span	Labile (no effective platelets at 48 hr)	Platelet concentrate	>10,000/mm³	60,000–100,000/mm³	>100,000/mm³

FFP, fresh frozen plasma.

tients with severe bleeding problems or those requiring surgical intervention should be taken care of by an experienced team including a surgeon, hematologist, and blood bank and coagulation laboratory personnel.

Prior to surgical intervention, factor VIII levels should be raised to 100%, then maintained for 10–14 days at levels greater than 50%. Table 6–3 outlines all the circulating hemostatic factors and the levels required for surgical hemostasis. For a 70-kg man with 0% factor VIII activity, this would equate to about 4000 units (70 kg × 60 units[U]/kg) initially followed by 2000 U every 12 hours. Aspirin should be avoided by hemophiliacs, because it produces a marked increase in the bleeding time. Intramuscular medications should also be avoided, since they may lead to further bleeding problems. Careful intraoperative hemostasis is critical for the prevention of postoperative hemorrhage, and ligation of small vessels is preferable to electrocautery. Wounds should be well healed and all drains removed prior to termination of the factor VIII transfusions.

Desmopressin acetate (DDAVP), 0.3 µg/kg, is useful only in mild hemophiliacs, because it causes release of endogenously produced factor VIII from storage sites and can produce a two- to fourfold increase in factor VIII:C levels. It is not effective in patients with severe hemophilia. If persistent bleeding continues after transfusion of factor VIII:C to appropriate levels, patients may be treated with ε-aminocaproic acid (EACA), 4 g orally every 4 hours for several days.

Factor VIII levels are monitored after initial transfusion and on a daily basis to modify the transfusion requirements. If levels fail to rise, an inhibitor of factor VIII should be suspected. This occurs in 8–15% of patients with severe hemophilia, and these patients may require plasmapheresis and other complex interventions.

Prognosis

The prognosis of patients with hemophilia is limited mainly by recurrent joint bleeding and its sequelae, and the development of viral infections from recurrent transfusions. In addition, the development of inhibitors to factor VIII may severely increase the possibility of death from bleeding.

Brettler DB, Levine PH: Factor concentrates for treatment of hemophilia: Which one to choose? Blood 1989;73:2067.
Hoyer LW: Hemophilia A. N Engl J Med 1994;330:38.
Mannucci PM: Desmopressin: A nontransfusional hemostatic agent. Annu Rev Med 1990;41:55.

HEMOPHILIA B

Essentials of Diagnosis

- X-linked recessive inheritance affecting only males.
- Low or absent factor IX activity.
- Frequent painful joint and muscle hemorrhages.

General Considerations

Hemophilia B (factor IX deficiency, Christmas disease) is clinically indistinguishable from hemophilia A and is also an X-linked recessive bleeding disorder. The disorder is most often due to a quantitative reduction in factor IX, but one-third of patients have an abnormally functioning protein. Hemophilia B accounts for about 20% of all hemophiliacs. It also occurs in mild, moderate, and severe forms of the disease. Fifty percent of the patients have the severe form with less than 1% of the factor IX level.

Clinical Findings

Clinical signs and symptoms of hemophilia B are indistinguishable from those of hemophilia A. Laboratory findings include reduced factor IX activity and a prolonged aPTT, with other tests being normal.

Treatment

Treatment is directed at replacement with factor IX concentrates. For major surgery, factor IX levels of greater than 80% should be achieved (see Table 6–3). The half-life of factor IX is 18 hours, and the volume of distribution is twice that of plasma. For this reason, 80 U per kg or about 5600 U would be the initial dose followed by 2800 U every 18 hours in a 70-kg man with 0% factor IX activity. As with factor VIII levels, factor IX levels need to be carefully followed up, and up to 10% of patients may develop inhibitors. Factor IX concentrates can contain a number of other proteins including activated clotting factors; thromboembolic complications have been reported. This has improved with more recent concentrates. The prognosis for hemophilia B patients is similar to that of those with classic hemophilia.

Brettler DB, Levine PH: Factor concentrates for treatment of hemophilia: Which one to choose? Blood 1989:73:2067.

VON WILLEBRAND'S DISEASE

Essentials of Diagnosis

- Family history with disease transmitted as an autosomal trait with dominant and recessive modes of inheritance.
- Usually reduced levels of factor VIII coagulant activity.
- Reduced levels of factor VIII antigen or ristocetin cofactor.
- Prolonged bleeding time.

General Considerations

Von Willebrand's disease is the most common congenital bleeding disorder. It is most often transmitted as an autosomal dominant trait, but recessive inheritance may occur. The disease is characterized by a dual hemostatic defect. First, there is a deficiency or dysfunction of von Willebrand factor (vWF), which is important in platelet adhesion to the subendothelial surface. This is mediated by the platelet receptor, GPIb, of an unactivated platelet that binds with vWF that is present in the subendothelium. This defect causes prolongation of the bleeding time because of impaired platelet plug formation. Although platelet adhesion is abnormal in von Willebrand's disease patients, platelet secretion and aggregation are not affected. Second, there is a deficiency of factor VIII coagulant activity (primary defect of hemophilia A) that contributes to the hemostatic defect. The reduction in factor VIII:C activity is not as great as that seen in hemophilia A and is usually variable.

The most common subtype of von Willebrand's disease is type I, which is present in 80% of cases. Type I is caused by a quantitative decrease in vWF antigen and in ristocetin cofactor activity. A qualitative abnormality in the protein that prevents multimer formation is present in subtype IIa, whereas type IIb is caused by a qualitative abnormality in the protein that causes rapid clearance of the large multimeric forms. Type IIa has a marked decrease in ristocetin cofactor activity and can thus be differentiated from the other subtypes. In type III von Willebrand's disease, vWF antigen and ristocetin cofactor activity are virtually absent; this is a rare autosomal recessive disorder. Platelet-type or pseudo-von Willebrand's disease is characterized by rapid clearance of the large multimers of vWF from the plasma because of an abnormality in platelet GPIb. Affected patients develop a mild thrombocytopenia.

Clinical Findings

A. Signs and Symptoms: Patients with severe von Willebrand's disease present with abnormal bleeding in childhood. In those with less severe forms, the disease may not be apparent before adulthood. Patients may need to be studied on several occasions to pinpoint von Willebrand's disease as the cause of minor bleeding, since vWF is an acute phase reactant and is increased during stress and pregnancy or after surgery. Mucocutaneous hemorrhages are characteristic of the disorder. Epistaxis, gingival bleeding, menorrhagia, and gastrointestinal bleeding are common. Excessive bleeding after dental procedures, tonsillectomy, other surgery, and normal pregnancy and delivery may be the first manifestation of the disease. Joint and intramuscular hemorrhages are rare in contrast to the hemophilias. Spontaneous bleeding is not seen as commonly as in hemophilia A.

B. Laboratory Findings: Screening laboratory tests include a prolonged aPTT with normal PT, platelet count, and platelet aggregation to ADP and epinephrine. Patients usually demonstrate a prolonged bleeding time. In patients with normal bleeding times, challenge with aspirin greatly increases the bleeding time. This is not entirely specific, because this response is also present in patients with other platelet function abnormalities. In type I von Willebrand's disease, there is a decrease in both factor VIII antigen and ristocetin cofactor activity. In addition, when there is decrease of the factor VIII antigen, there may also be a decrease in the factor VIII coagulant activity. More complex analyses including vWF multimeric assays and ristocetin- and cryoprecipitate-induced platelet aggregation may be necessary to differentiate the various subtypes to direct therapeutic measures.

Differential Diagnosis

When patients present with abnormal bleeding, it is important to differentiate von Willebrand's disease from other qualitative platelet disorders, both congenital and acquired. This can be done based on a thorough history and physical examination, including the family history. Patients with von Willebrand's disease also have an elevated aPTT, and the presence of reduced factor VIII:C levels allows them to be differentiated from those with other bleeding disorders except hemophilia, in which vWF antigen levels and ristocetin cofactor activity are normal.

Treatment

Most patients with von Willebrand's disease have mild symptoms and may require treatment only prior to surgery or after severe trauma. They should refrain from all aspirin use. DDAVP, 0.3 mg/kg intravenously over 30 minutes, is useful for mild type I von Willebrand's disease patients. It is thought to release factor VIII and vWF from storage sites in the endothelial cell, although the mechanism is not fully understood. Most patients respond with a three- to fourfold increase in vWF, with repeat doses given every 12–24 hours. A new highly concentrated intranasal formulation of DDAVP (1.5 mg/mL) has shown efficacy in clinical trials, but the response is variable. DDAVP is not effective in patients with von Willebrand's disease type IIa and may be harmful in those with type IIb .

Transfusion of plasma cryoprecipitate has been the standard therapy for von Willebrand's disease patients. Cryoprecipitate should be given every 12 hours in dosages of 10–15 U/kg, beginning the day before any surgical procedure. Cryoprecipitate corrects the bleeding time and restores adequate levels of factor VIII coagulant activity. The bleeding time best correlates with the risk of bleeding but may be an impractical frequent test. If the factor VIII is very low, it should be monitored to ensure adequate levels of both vWF and factor VIII. If the vWF is abnormal, as is subtype II, ristocetin cofactor activity can be followed up to determine adequacy of transfusion. The frequency of monitoring should be dictated by the severity of the hemostatic insult, the clinical response, and the site of bleeding. Commercial factor VIII concentrates have been either heat treated or detergent treated to reduce the risk of viral transmission seen with cryoprecipitate. Humate-P (Armour) contains normal vWF multimers and is the most widely used product.

Prognosis

Prognosis is usually very good because most cases of von Willebrand's disease are mild. In serious forms of the disease, replacement therapy is very effective and inhibitors develop rarely.

Gill FM: Congenital bleeding disorders: Hemophilia and von Willebrand's disease. Med Clin North Am 1984;68:601.
Lethagen S, Harris AS, Sjorin E, Nilsson IM: Intranasal and intravenous administration of desmopressin: Effect on factor VIII/vWF, pharmacokinetics and reproducibility. Thromb Haemost 1987; 58:1033.

FACTOR XI DEFICIENCY (Rosenthal's Syndrome)

Factor XI deficiency appears most frequently among persons of Jewish extraction and is transmitted as an incompletely recessive autosomal dominant trait. Spontaneous bleeding is rare, and bleeding is seen mainly after surgery or trauma. The aPTT is prolonged; the level of factor XI does not correlate with the bleeding tendency. Treatment is transfusion with fresh frozen plasma, 10 mL/kg, to maintain levels greater than 20% for minor surgery and greater than 50% for major procedures (see Table 6–3).

FACTOR V (Proaccelerin) DEFICIENCY

Essentials of Diagnosis

- Ecchymoses, epistaxis, menorrhagia, gastrointestinal tract bleeding.
- Occasionally no symptoms.

General Considerations

Factor V deficiency is extremely rare and is transmitted as an autosomal recessive trait in both males and females. Factor V is synthesized in the liver, but its synthesis does not depend on vitamin K. Both PT and aPTT are prolonged, but diagnosis is made by specific assay for factor V. Bleeding time is prolonged in one-third of patients. Hemorrhagic manifestations of factor V deficiency include ecchymoses, epistaxis, menorrhagia, and gastrointestinal tract bleeding. Patients even with low levels of factor V (<10%) may be asymptomatic for long periods of time.

Treatment

Excessive bleeding can occur in patients with factor V deficiency at the time of surgery, especially if factor V levels are below 1%. The factor V level should be raised to 25% with 15 mL/kg of fresh frozen plasma for minor surgery and to 50% for major surgical procedures (see Table 6–3). Maintenance infusion at 7–10 mL/kg every 24 hours is done until healing is complete. Only plasma frozen fresh is suitable for transfusion, since factor V is labile and loses activity during storage. Aspirin should be avoided in all patients with factor V deficiency.

FACTOR VII
(Proconvertin) DEFICIENCY

Essentials of Diagnosis
- Mucocutaneous hemorrhages.
- Easy bruising.
- Occasional hemarthroses.

General Considerations

Factor VII deficiency is an uncommon but not rare disorder, which is transmitted in an autosomal recessive fashion. Severe deficiency of factor VII occurs in the homozygote and may be associated with severe bleeding. Heterozygotes may have few clinical manifestations of the disease. In general, patients with factor VII levels of less than 1% have severe hemorrhagic complications, similar to those seen in severe hemophilia. Patients with factor VII levels above 5% generally have mild bleeding episodes. Typical manifestations of factor VII deficiency are mucocutaneous hemorrhages, easy bruising, and occasional hemarthroses. Even severely affected patients appear to do well with surgical procedures, except dental extractions.

Laboratory Findings

PT is elevated in patients with factor VII deficiency and in those who have deficiencies of factors II and X as well. However, since factor VII is important only in the extrinsic pathway of the coagulation cascade, aPTT and thrombin clotting time are normal. The Stypven time (Russell's viper venom time) is normal in factor VII deficiency and can be used to distinguish it from factor X deficiency.

Treatment

Replacement therapy in patients with factor VII deficiency depends on the severity of the hemorrhage. Patients should receive prophylaxis prior to dental extractions and other surgical procedures. The biologic half-life of factor VII is 2–5 hours. It is unclear what level of factor VII is required to prevent bleeding, but patients are treated with banked plasma, 10 mL/kg of body weight, to maintain levels above 20% (see Table 6–3). A pure recombinant factor VIIa is currently being tested. Some investigators recommend using factor VII-containing prothrombin complex concentrates for treatment. Vitamin K has no value in the treatment of hereditary factor VII deficiency.

Kelleher JF, Gomperts E, Davis W et al: Selection of replacement therapy for patients with severe factor VII deficiency. Am J Pediatr Hematol 1986;8:318.

Nemerson Y: Tissue factor and hemostasis. Blood 1988; 71:1.

FACTOR X
(Stuart-Prower) DEFICIENCY

Essentials of Diagnosis
- Possible hemarthroses.
- Exsanguinating postoperative hemorrhage.
- CNS bleeding episodes.

General Considerations

Factor X deficiency is relatively rare and is inherited as a highly penetrant, incompletely recessive, autosomal recessive trait. An association exists between the disease and amyloidosis, as well as familial carotid body tumors. Clinical manifestations are more severe in homozygotes and can include hemarthroses, exsanguinating postoperative hemorrhage, and central nervous system bleeding episodes. Diagnosis of factor X deficiency can be made with prolonged PT and aPTT and an appropriate family history. The bleeding time is generally normal. Acquired deficiencies should be excluded.

Treatment

Treatment for factor X deficiency consists of fresh frozen plasma or prothrombin-complex concentrates, guided by the severity of the bleeding episode. A factor level of 10–50% is considered adequate for hemostasis. Postoperative maintenance should be continued for at least 5 days (see Table 6–3).

Girolami A: Tentative and updated classification of factor X variants. Acta Haematol 1986;75:58.
Kroll AJ, Alexander B, Cochizo F, Pechet L: Hereditary deficiencies of clotting factors VII and X associated with carotid body tumors. N Engl J Med 1964;270:6.

CONGENITAL FACTOR
XIII DEFICIENCY

General Considerations

Factor XIII deficiency is a rare autosomal recessive disorder with the homozygous deficiency state resulting in a moderate-to-severe hemorrhagic diathesis. This disorder is often manifested by bleeding from the umbilical stump and thus may be detected shortly after birth. The most serious form of bleeding is in the central nervous system, and patients have a high incidence of deaths from intracranial bleeds. The screening test for factor XIII deficiency is solubility of the patient's recalcified plasma clot in urea or monochloroacetic acid. This does not differentiate congenital from acquired deficiency. Acquired partial deficiency of factor XIII has been seen in patients with leukemias, severe liver disease, and disseminated intravascular coagulation.

Treatment

Bleeding in factor XIII deficiency can be controlled with fresh frozen plasma, cryoprecipitate, or factor XIII concentrate prepared from placenta (see Table 6–3).

Karges HE, Clemens R: Factor XIII: Enzymatic and clinical aspects. Behring Inst Mitt 1988;82:43.

INHERITED HYPOPROTHROMBINEMIA (Factor II Deficiency)

General Considerations

Inherited hypoprothrombinemia is an extremely rare disorder with an autosomal recessive pattern of inheritance. Functional levels of prothrombin range from 2% to 25% of normal. Clinical manifestations of the disease are based on the level of hypoprothrombinemia, and patients can exhibit easy bruising, epistaxis, menorrhagia, and postoperative hemorrhage. Laboratory findings include variable prolongation of the PT and aPTT, with a normal thrombin time and platelet count. Hypoprothrombinemia should be differentiated from vitamin K deficiency and warfarin intoxication.

Treatment

Mild bleeding does not need to be treated with replacement therapy. Fresh frozen plasma is used for replacement therapy in patients with severe bleeding. The need for replacement therapy is infrequent because the half-life of prothrombin is 3 days. Prothrombin-complex concentrates can also be used for replacement therapy for patients with factor II deficiency (see Table 6–3).

ABNORMALITIES IN FIBRINOGEN

General Considerations

Patients with abnormalities in fibrinogen include those with afibrinogenemia, hypofibrinogenemia, and dysfibrinogenemia. **Afibrinogenemia** is a rare disorder with an autosomal recessive mode of inheritance. There is no measurable fibrinogen in plasma, and the bleeding time may be markedly prolonged because fibrinogen is required for platelet aggregation. Clinically, the disease manifests early in life, and bleeding from the umbilical stump is a common presentation. Patients can also have epistaxis, excessive bleeding after lacerations, and intracranial bleeding after trauma. Patients with **hypofibrinogenemia** can be categorized into 2 groups: those with fibrinogen levels less than 50 mg/dL and those with levels greater than 50 mg/dL. The severity of symptoms depends on the fibrinogen level. Patients with **dysfibrinogenemias** have a defect in the fibrinogen molecule and are often asymptomatic except during an surgical procedure.

These patients also tend to have a higher incidence of thromboembolic complications. The thrombin clotting time is diagnostic for this group of fibrinogen abnormalities, but complex analysis is sometimes required to differentiate among the subtypes.

Treatment

A fibrinogen level of 100 mg/dL is generally believed necessary for hemostasis prior to minor surgery and a level greater than 150 mg/dL for major surgery (see Table 6–3). Replacement therapy is with fresh frozen plasma or cryoprecipitate, with fibrinogen levels monitored to assess correction of the defect. Fibrinogen levels should then be maintained until wound healing is adequate.

McDonagh J, Carrell N, Lee MH: Dysfibrinogenemia and other disorders of fibrinogen structure and function. In: *Hemostasis and Thrombosis: Basic Principles and Clinical Practice,* 3rd ed. Colman RW, Hirsh J, Marder VJ, Salzman EW (editors). JB Lippincott, 1994.

CONGENITAL PLATELET DISORDERS

Glanzmann's Thrombasthenia

Glanzmann's thrombasthenia is a rare autosomal recessive disorder whose hallmark is deficient platelet aggregation. This appears to be secondary to lack of platelet GPIIb:IIIa, which is the fibrinogen receptor. Binding of fibrinogen to its receptor is a prerequisite for platelet aggregation. Clinical manifestations of the disease include purpura, epistaxis, gingival bleeding, and menorrhagia. Laboratory findings include a normal platelet count and platelet morphology with a prolonged bleeding time. Affected patients demonstrate absent platelet aggregation in response to ADP, thrombin, collagen, and epinephrine, but aggregate normally at least initially in response to ristocetin. In addition, many patients have diminished or absent clot retraction. Treatment is with platelet transfusion, but should be judiciously used to minimize the development of antibodies. Prognosis is generally very good.

Bernard-Soulier Syndrome

Bernard-Soulier syndrome is a rare autosomal recessive disorder with clinical manifestations of purpura, gingival bleeding, and menorrhagia. Platelet adhesion to the subendothelium is markedly decreased because Bernard-Soulier platelets lack the GIb receptors for vWF. However, they have normal GPIIb-IIIa, so that fibrinogen binding is normal and platelet aggregation is normal in response to collagen, ADP, and thrombin. Laboratory findings include a moderate-to-severe thrombocytopenia and an abnormal bleeding time. The peripheral blood smear demonstrates very large platelets up to 20 mm in diameter. Treatment consists of platelet transfusion when necessary.

Storage Pool Disease

Storage pool disease comprises a group of diseases characterized by defects in either platelet dense granule or α-granule contents. Most patients are only mildly affected. Laboratory findings include abnormalities in platelet aggregation and, in some cases, prolonged bleeding times. Platelet aggregation may be normal to a concentration of 1 μg/mL of collagen in some patients. Platelet transfusions should be useful in the management of patients with storage pool disease, but should be used carefully. DDAVP appears to shorten the bleeding time in patients with functional platelet defects for unclear reasons, and has been used in some patients.

George JN, Caen JP, Nurden AT: Glanzmann's thrombasthenia: The spectrum of clinical disease. Blood 1990;75: 1383.

Israels SS et al: Platelet storage pool deficiency: Diagnosis in patients with prolonged bleeding times and normal platelet aggregation. Br J Haematol 1990;75:118.

Nurden AT, Jallu V, Hourdille P: GP Ib and Bernard-Soulier platelets. Blood 1989;73:2225.

ACQUIRED BLEEDING DISORDERS

Acquired bleeding disorders include massive transfusion, disseminated intravascular coagulation (DIC), liver disease and vitamin K deficiency states, qualitative and quantitative platelet abnormalities, and hyperfibrinolysis.

In surgical patients, most bleeding disorders are acute and acquired and occur in clinical settings like massive trauma, shock, and sepsis. Early recognition is important, with intraoperative management dictated by the severity of the bleeding. The first sign of intraoperative coagulopathy is usually persistent oozing from raw surfaces that were previously dry. The anesthesiologist may note bleeding from the oropharynx, the endotracheal tube, the nose from nasogastric tube insertion, and intravenous insertion sites. If a coagulopathy is suspected, blood should be immediately drawn for a platelet count, PT, APTT, thrombin time, and fibrinogen level. The results of screening tests in some common acquired bleeding disorders are outlined in Table 6–4.

The initial treatment of a coagulopathy should focus on maintaining blood volume and hemodynamic stability, since hypotension and shock will only worsen the coagulopathy. If blood products are being transfused, they should be stopped immediately in case there has been a major transfusion reaction. Any medications or maintenance solutions being infused into the intravenous lines and into arterial catheters should be inspected and changed.

Further therapy is often empiric and depends on the severity of bleeding. Severe coagulopathy should be treated with whole blood transfusions, because packed red cells (RBCs) do not replenish coagulation factors. Whole blood contains normal amounts of all hemostatic elements except factors V and VIII and platelets. If volume overload is a concern, packed RBCs can be transfused with fresh frozen plasma. Thrombocytopenia and platelet dysfunction are the most common abnormalities seen in unexpected intraoperative bleeding and can be treated with platelet transfusions. Prior to platelet transfusions, coagulation factors should be replaced with fresh frozen plasma. Most acute acquired bleeding should be treatable with component therapy, but some cases may be refractory to treatment. In refractory cases, the operation should be terminated as soon as possible, and the abdominal cavity should be packed and then closed with watertight, running sutures. Abdominal tamponade can be very effective in the control of ongoing hemorrhage. After control of hemostasis in the intensive care unit, the patient can be surgically reexplored in 24–48 hours.

Clagett GP: Preoperative assessment of hemostasis. In: *Principles of Transfusion Medicine*. Rossi EC, Simon TL, Moss GS (editors). Williams & Wilkins, 1991.

MASSIVE TRANSFUSION COAGULOPATHY

Essentials of Diagnosis

- Massive blood loss necessitating massive transfusion.
- Dilutional thrombocytopenia and deficiency of factors V and VIII.
- Control bleeding diathesis.

Table 6–4. Screening tests in common acquired bleeding disorders.

	Platelet Count	PT	aPTT	TT	Bleeding Time	Fibrinogen
Massive transfusion	↓	N/↑	↑	N	↑	N/↓
DIC	↓	↑	↑	↑	↑	↓
Liver disease	N/↓	↑	↑	N/↑	N/↑	N/↓
Vitamin K deficiency & warfarin	N	↑	↑	N		N
Aspirin	N	N	N	N	↑	N
Hyperfibrinolysis	N	↑	↑	↑		↓
Circulating heparin	N	N/↑	↑	↑		↓

PT, prothrombin time; aPTT, activated partial thromboplastin time; TT, thrombin time; N, normal; ↑ increased; ↓ decreased. DIC, disseminated intravascular coagulopathy.

General Considerations

The underlying principle behind **massive transfusion coagulopathy** is dilution. Transfusion with stored blood that is more than 48 hours old is deficient in factors V and VIII as well as platelets. Replacement of shed blood with stored blood thus impairs hemostasis. Rapid transfusion to replace 1 blood volume with stored blood dilutes the autologous blood concentration to 25–30%; replacement of 2 blood volumes reduces the autologous blood concentration to 10%. In most patients, the platelet count falls to 100,000/mm³ after transfusion of 10 U of stored blood. Although thrombocytopenia at this level is generally well tolerated, the combination of this thrombocytopenia and mild clotting factor deficiencies in the face of ongoing blood loss and transfusion will cause rapid decompensation of hemostasis. Up to 30% of patients who receive massive transfusion may have defects of hemostasis. In addition to the dilutional thrombocytopenia, other potential complications of massive transfusion of stored blood include disseminated intravascular coagulation (DIC), immunologic reactions, metabolic and other derangements, and possible transmission of viral agents.

Clinical Findings

A. Signs and Symptoms: Patients with coagulopathy from massive bleeding typically present with diffuse oozing from raw surfaces at the operative site. In addition, patients may have bleeding at intravenous insertion sites—from the nose and the endotracheal tube.

B. Laboratory Findings: Results of screening tests seen in massive transfusion are outlined in Table 6–4. Thrombocytopenia (<100,000/mm³) is the most common abnormality. Because of the body's large reserves of factors V and VIII, deficiencies of these factors after transfusion with stored blood is rarely severe; this explains the minimal increases in PT and APTT in these patients. The bleeding time is also prolonged and may be out of proportion to the thrombocytopenia, suggesting a qualitative platelet abnormality. The fibrinogen level may be normal or slightly decreased.

Differential Diagnosis

The coagulopathy of massive transfusion needs to be differentiated most frequently from DIC. Thrombocytopenia, decreased fibrinogen levels (<125 mg/dL), and the presence of fibrin degradation products (FDP) in the clinical settings of shock, extensive trauma, multiple long-bone fractures, sepsis, or transfusion mismatches suggest DIC. In most other acquired bleeding disorders, the platelet count is normal.

Treatment

Correction of thrombocytopenia is the mainstay of treatment for massive transfusion coagulopathy. In patients with an established massive transfusion coagulopathy, 2–4 U of fresh frozen plasma should be transfused, followed by 8–10 U of a platelet concentrate. A platelet count of at least 100,000/mm³ should be achieved in patients with a coagulopathy and the following formula is useful in guiding transfusion requirements:

**Number of bags of platelet concentrate =
Desired increment × body surface area (m²)/10,000**

Patients with low fibrinogen levels require 4 bags of cryoprecipitate per 10 kg of body weight to raise the fibrinogen level by 100 mg/dL. If bleeding cannot be controlled with the above-mentioned measures, packing the abdominal cavity after repair of all major vessels may be necessary.

Prophylactic use of blood components has been advocated by some when massive bleeding and transfusion are ongoing, prior to the development of a clinically overt coagulopathy. To replenish clotting factor deficiencies, 1 U of fresh frozen plasma should be given for every 3–4 U of transfused blood. In addition, 6–10 U of platelets can be given for every 10 U of blood transfused. However, no benefit of prophylactic platelet transfusions was demonstrated in a prospective trial of patients who received more than 12 U of blood in a short time interval. The coagulopathy could also be potentially prevented by the administration of fresh whole blood in a 1:4 ratio with stored blood, but this is rarely available in emergencies.

Prognosis

Prognosis depends on the severity of the trauma or the cause of intraoperative bleeding, which can be lethal.

Maier RV: The consequences of massive blood transfusion. Surg Rounds 1984;7:58.

Reed RL et al: Prophylactic platelet administration during massive transfusion: A prospective, randomized, double-blind clinical study. Ann Surg 1986;203:40.

DISSEMINATED INTRAVASCULAR COAGULATION

Essentials of Diagnosis

- Decreased fibrinogen level and platelet count, presence of fibrin degradation products, and a prolonged PT.
- Bleeding and/or thrombosis may be present.

General Considerations

Disseminated intravascular coagulation (DIC) is mainly mediated by the activity of thrombin, which is normally localized to the area of local injury by ATIII and heparin cofactor II. Thrombin stimulates proteolytic cleavage of fibrinogen to fibrin monomers, activates factors V and VIII, causes platelet aggregation and secretion and causes release of tPA from endothelial cells leading to generation of plasmin. Plasmin digests fibrin and fibrinogen, generating FDP as well as inactivating factors V and VIII. The balance between thrombin and plasmin determines whether bleeding or thrombosis occurs intravascularly. Bleeding results mainly from consumption of hemostatic factors including fibrinogen, platelets, and factors V and VIII. In addition, stimulation of excessive fibrinolysis and formation of fibrin degradation products is present. The FDPs interfere with polymerization of the fibrin monomers and thus impair platelet function.

DIC is a disease process that has many different underlying causes in surgical patients with a coagulopathy. Severe bacterial infections, mainly from gram-negative but also gram-positive organisms, with associated septicemia and endotoxemia can lead to DIC. Massive tissue trauma, often with associated long-bone fractures can lead to intravascular release of tissue thromboplastin with resulting DIC. Obstetric complications that may result in DIC are abruptio placentae, amniotic fluid embolism, septic abortion, saline-induced abortion, and the retained dead fetus syndrome. Other clinical conditions that may predispose to DIC are liver disease (mainly peritoneovenous shunts or fatty liver of pregnancy), acute hemolysis after transfusion of as little as 25 ml of incompatible blood, the bites of certain vipers and rattlesnakes, and cancer (mucin-secreting adenocarcinomas, acute promyelocytic leukemia).

DIC associated with a hemolytic transfusion reaction may be difficult to detect intraoperatively when the patient is under general anesthesia. This diagnosis needs to be suspected in any operative patient who develops hypotension and sudden bleeding while receiving blood products. DIC associated with malignancy is frequently chronic and partially compensated and may lead to thromboembolic events that require surgical thromboembolectomy. Recurrent migratory superficial and deep venous thromboses (**Trousseau's syndrome**) can also be a sign of subacute DIC in patients with malignancy. Chronic partially compensated DIC also occurs in 4–5% of patients with large aortic aneurysms. Aortic surgery in these patients is associated with severe bleeding, and the use of nonporous vascular grafts that do not require preclotting is mandatory.

Clinical Findings

A. Signs and Symptoms: The clinical presentation of DIC is variable and depends on the nature and intensity of the triggering stimulus (acute/chronic, mild/severe) and the location of the stimulus (intravascular/extravascular, localized/systemic). These factors determine whether there is predominantly bleeding or thrombosis. Bleeding is most common and can occur at any site; it may be mucosal oozing, spontaneous ecchymoses, petechiae, pulmonary hemorrhage, intracranial hemorrhage, and massive gastrointestinal bleeding. Thrombotic occlusions occur first as part of the pathophysiologic process and can cause organ hypoperfusion and even ischemia and infarction. Some of the more devastating complications are ischemic renal cortical necrosis, cerebral infarctions, and hemorrhagic adrenal infarction, which can lead to the Waterhouse-Friderichsen syndrome.

B. Laboratory Findings: Typical findings in DIC patients include a decreased fibrinogen level, thrombocytopenia, elevated fibrin degradation products, and a prolonged PT (see Table 6–4). These laboratory findings need to be considered along with the patient's underlying disease and hepatic function. Fibrinogen levels can be normal in up to 50% of patients, because of increased production during pregnancy and sepsis, even in the presence of DIC. Thrombocytopenia is seen in 98% of patients with DIC, and in 50% the platelet count is less than 50,000/mm^3. Elevated levels of **D-dimer,** a fibrin degradation product, are typically seen in DIC patients but can also be seen in patients with pulmonary embolism or deep venous thrombosis. Fibrin degradation products are cleared by the liver, and elevated levels can also be seen with hepatic dysfunction. The PT is usually prolonged, and this is related to a deficiency mainly in factor V as well as factors II, VII, and X and fibrinogen.

Fibrin deposition in the microvasculature can cause fragmented RBCs on a peripheral smear in some patients and may produce a microangiopathic hemolytic anemia. Other laboratory abnormalities include a prolonged APTT and decreased levels of functional ATIII, heparin cofactor II, and protein C. Plasminogen and α_2-antiplasmin levels may be low if the fibrinolytic system has been activated.

Differential Diagnosis

DIC can be distinguished from the coagulopathy of massive transfusion by the presence of fibrin degradation products with a markedly decreased fibrinogen level. In liver disease, the platelet count and fibrinogen level are usually normal or only slightly decreased, which makes it distinguishable from DIC. Patients with vitamin K deficiency have normal platelet counts and fibrinogen levels, and correction of their coagulopathy is with vitamin K administration. Patients with coagulopathy from aspirin, hyperfibrinolysis, and circulating heparin all have normal platelet counts. In patients with sepsis, the fibrinogen level is usually normal or elevated, since this is an acute-phase reactant.

Treatment

Treatment of patients with DIC should focus on quick and accurate diagnosis of the underlying disorder. Treatment should then consist of aggressive support of normal blood volume and pressure and removal of the stimulus for DIC, if possible. For example, patients who have DIC from a major transfusion reaction should be treated (1) by stopping the transfusion, (2) by restoring normal blood volume and pressure with crystalloid and pharmacologic agents, (3) by alkalinization with sodium bicarbonate, and (4) by administering mannitol to protect against renal tubular necrosis. After the underlying cause of the DIC is identified and supportive therapy has been instituted, it is important to determine whether the patient is continuing to bleed and what hemostatic factors are deficient. Replacement therapy is usually with platelet concentrates, fresh frozen plasma, and cryoprecipitate. Platelet transfusions are given to raise the platelet count higher than 50,000/mm³. The fibrinogen level should be increased to greater than 150 mg/dL with cryoprecipitate, and fresh frozen plasma is given for clotting factor deficiencies. A platelet count and a fibrinogen level should be checked 30–60 minutes after completion of the transfusions and every 6 hours thereafter to assess the need for further therapy.

If the patient has venous thromboembolism or evidence of fibrin deposition such as dermal necrosis seen in purpura fulminans, heparin therapy to control DIC can been used. Purpura fulminans is characterized by a benign infectious process followed in less than 4 weeks by progression of ecchymotic areas of skin to hemorrhagic bullae and then hemorrhagic ischemic necrosis in children. In this disease, heparin administration reduces the mortality rate from 90% to 18%. Other disorders that may benefit from heparin therapy are the retained dead fetus syndrome, giant hemangiomas (Kasabach-Merritt syndrome), aortic aneurysms, and acute promyelocytic leukemia.

Patients with DIC undergoing elective abdominal aortic aneurysm repair should be given heparin to normalize hemostatic factors before surgical repair. If bleeding is present from a leaking aneurysm, the use of heparin is contraindicated. Heparin is used with induction chemotherapy for acute promyelocytic leukemia because of the release of procoagulant material from the abnormal promyelocytes causing DIC. Studies have shown fewer hemorrhagic deaths in patients treated with heparin, with low-dose heparin (5–10 U/kg/hr) being better than high-dose heparin (15–20 U/kg/hr). The dose of heparin (typically 500–750 U/hr) depends on the clinical disorder with the therapeutic efficacy of heparin monitored by serial measurements of the fibrinogen level and the platelet count. Heparin is probably not useful in the treatment of DIC from septicemia, liver disease, and complications of pregnancy. Heparin is contraindicated in patients with bleeding into a closed space, such as intracranial, pericardial, and paratracheal bleeding.

ATIII levels may be low from consumption or decreased synthesis; adequate levels are necessary for the function of heparin. Fresh frozen plasma can be used to raise ATIII levels to greater than 50%. Antifibrinolytic agents are used in patients with DIC complicated by excessive fibrinolysis with resulting bleeding not controlled by replacement therapy and heparin administration. In these patients, ε-aminocaproic acid (EACA) is used to block the accumulation of fibrin degradation products in the blood and to protect hemostatic plugs. The loading dose of EACA is 4–6 g intravenously, then

1 g every 1–2 hours for up to 48 hours to raise the fibrinogen level. The use of EACA without prior administration of heparin is extremely dangerous and risks fatal thrombosis.

Prognosis

The prognosis for DIC patients depends on the underlying disease and its early identification and treatment. DIC can be lethal in severe cases.

Baker WF Jr: Clinical aspects of DIC: A clinician's point of view. Semin Thromb Hemost 1989;15:1.

Fisher DF, Yawn DH, Crawford ES: Preoperative DIC associated with aortic aneurysms: A prospective study of 76 cases. Arch Surg 1983;118:1252.

Hoyle CF et al: Beneficial effect of heparin in the management of patients with acute promyelocytic leukemia. Br J Haematol 1988;68:283.

Thompson RW et al: DIC caused by abdominal aortic aneurysm. J Vasc Surg 1986;4:184.

LIVER DISEASE & VITAMIN K DEFICIENCY STATES

Essentials of Diagnosis

- PT more prolonged than the APTT.
- Rapid correction of the bleeding disorder with vitamin K in vitamin K deficiency states.
- No response to vitamin K in liver disease.

General Considerations

The liver is an important organ in blood coagulation and hemostasis. It is the major site of synthesis for 12 blood coagulation proteins (Table 6–5), components of the fibrinolytic system (plasminogen and α²-antiplasmin), and the serine protease inhibitor, ATIII. The vitamin K-dependent factors (II, VII, IX, and X) and factor V are the first to be affected with hepatic insufficiency. The liver also serves an important filtering function because it clears activated coagulation factors and plasminogen activators from the circulation. The hemostatic derangements that can occur with liver disease can be complex and difficult to manage. Defective synthesis of fibrinogen and other coagulation factors accompanied by hyperfibrinolysis can be further complicated by thrombocytopenia resulting from congestive splenomegaly. Platelet function can also be impaired. DIC may complicate severe liver disease in some cases because of activation of coagulation factors by release of thromboplastin into the circulation during hepatic necrosis, defective clearance of activated coagulation factors, and decreased levels of ATIII.

Liver transplantations are often performed on patients with the coagulopathy of advanced severe liver disease. The operation induces the consumption of hemostatic factors during the anhepatic state, during the reperfusion of the donor liver, and during venovenous bypass. Intraoperative blood transfusion correlates with the preoperative coagulation abnormality.

Table 6–5. Coagulation proteins synthesized in the liver.

Fibrinogen
Prothrombin
Prekallikrein
HMW kininogen
Protein C
Factors V, VII, IX, X, XI, XII, XIII

The vitamin K-dependent coagulation factors include factors II, VII, IX, and X. Vitamin K is supplied in the diet primarily from leafy vegetables and is also synthesized endogenously from the gut flora. Prolonged starvation, malnutrition, biliary obstruction and fistulas, malabsorption syndromes, liver disease, drug therapy with warfarin, and the use of gut-sterilizing and other broad-spectrum antibiotics can deplete vitamin K stores within 1 week. A typical surgical patient who could develop vitamin K deficiency would be one who has taken gut-sterilizing medications preoperatively, is not eating postoperatively, and continues on broad-spectrum antibiotics.

Clinical Findings

Signs and Symptoms: Bleeding may occur at any site and is typically seen as epistaxis, gastrointestinal bleeding, bleeding from biopsy sites, and major bleeding after biliary surgery or portosystemic shunt in patients with liver disease. Patients with vitamin K deficiency have no specific bleeding diathesis.

Laboratory Findings: Patients with liver disease typically have a PT that is more prolonged than the APTT, and early in the course of liver disease may have a normal APTT. Fibrinogen level may be normal or decreased, depending on the severity of the liver disease. The platelet count may be normal or slightly decreased, depending on whether there is congestive splenomegaly. The thrombin time may be normal or prolonged (see Table 6–4).

Patients with vitamin K deficiency typically have a PT that is more prolonged than the APTT. The platelet count, fibrinogen level, and thrombin time are normal (see Table 6–4).

Differential Diagnosis

Vitamin K deficiency can be differentiated from liver disease by means of a normal platelet count, fibrinogen level, and thrombin time. Vitamin K deficiency invariably responds to replacement.

Treatment

Bleeding and coagulopathy that develop from liver disease are usually treated initially with fresh frozen plasma. However, large volumes (1–1.5 L) may be necessary to correct a markedly prolonged PT. In addition, because of the short half-life of factor VII (6 hr), additional fresh frozen plasma may need to be transfused every 6–12 hours. Vitamin K should also be administered to the actively bleeding patient, with assessment of its affect on the PT. If thrombocytopenia

is present, platelet transfusions may be effective. Cryoprecipitate transfusions may be needed if the fibrinogen is low.

While these measures are being instituted, blood should be drawn for determination of the presence of DIC or hyperfibrinolysis (euglobulin lysis time). If no test of fibrinolysis is available, draw 1 mL of whole blood in a glass tube, incubate it at 37°C, and observe it for lysis. A normal clot takes 24 hours to lyse, and spontaneous lysis within 1–2 hours is evidence of severe fibrinolysis. In most cases, component therapy will control the coagulopathy, but EACA may be required if hyperfibrinolysis is present. Be careful with this agent because it may potentiate microcirculatory thrombosis if DIC is present. The use of prothrombin complex concentrates (factors II, VII, IX, and X) is generally contraindicated. These concentrates contain activated coagulation factors that are poorly tolerated in patients with liver disease because of their low levels of ATIII and decreased hepatic clearance of activated factors. DIC can be initiated by the use of these agents, and thromboembolic complications have been reported.

Treatment for vitamin K deficiency is subcutaneous vitamin K (10–15 mg/day for 3–4 days) with daily monitoring of the PT. In urgent situations, 10–25 mg of vitamin K can be administered intravenously. Parenteral vitamin K usually restores effective hemostasis in 6 hours, with normalization of the PT in 24–36 hours. In emergency situations, 2–4 U of fresh frozen plasma can be used to restore immediate hemostasis.

Prognosis

The prognosis in coagulopathy from liver disease depends on the severity of the underlying disease. Vitamin K deficiency is usually corrected with replacement therapy.

Alperin JB: Coagulopathy caused by vitamin K deficiency in critically ill, hospitalized patients. JAMA 1987;258:1916.

Baranski B, Young N: Hematologic consequences of viral infection. Hematol Oncol Clin North Am 1987;1:167.

Furie B, Furie BC: Molecular basis of vitamin-K dependent gamma carboxylation. Blood 1990;75:1753.

Porte RJ, Knot EAR, Bontempo FA: Hemostasis in liver transplantation. Gastroenterology 1989;97:488.

QUANTITATIVE & QUALITATIVE PLATELET ABNORMALITIES

THROMBOCYTOPENIA

General Considerations

A number of acquired platelet disorders lead to changes in platelet count or platelet function. **Throm-**

bocytopenia is the most common abnormality of hemostasis in the surgical patient. Thrombocytopenias can be classified according to disorders of platelet production, destruction, and sequestration. Among surgical patients, defective platelet production is found with aplastic anemia, marrow infiltration (leukemia, carcinoma, myeloproliferative disorders, and tuberculosis), myelosuppressive drugs used in cancer chemotherapy, nutritional deficiencies (vitamin B_{12}, folic acid, and possibly iron), viral infections, and drugs that affect platelet production (estrogens, alcohol, thiazide diuretics). Abnormal destruction of platelets can occur from both immune sources (idiopathic thrombocytopenic purpura, drugs, posttransfusion purpura, and some allergies) and nonimmune sources (infection, DIC, extracorporeal circulation, drugs, thrombotic thrombocytopenic purpura, and hemolytic-uremic syndrome). Platelet sequestration occurs with hypersplenism from multiple causes.

Drug-related thrombocytopenias are particularly noteworthy because platelet transfusion is rarely necessary if the offending agent is removed. Common drugs associated with thrombocytopenia in surgical patients are outlined in Table 6–6.

Treatment

Treatment for surgical patients with thrombocytopenia and bleeding is platelet transfusion. This is determined by the platelet count, the functional capabilities of the platelets (bleeding time), and the magnitude of the operative procedure. In all patients with thrombocytopenia, drugs that impair platelet function should be avoided. Splenectomy is the definitive treatment for patients with idiopathic thrombocytopenic purpura and other splenic sequestration disorders. Large-volume plasmapheresis with fresh frozen plasma replacement is the treatment of choice for thrombotic thrombocytopenic purpura and hemolytic-uremic syndrome.

PLATELET DYSFUNCTION

Acquired platelet dysfunction is common and occurs with several medical illnesses as well as with medications. Clinically significant bleeding from platelet defects has been described in patients with uremia, myeloproliferative disorders (essential thrombocythemia, polycythemia vera, myeloid metaplasia, and chronic myelogenous leukemia), dysproteinemias (multiple myeloma, macroglobulinemia), liver disease, and cardiopulmonary bypass, and after drug ingestion.

Uremia

Surgical procedures on uremic patients are often complicated by abnormal bleeding. The pathogenesis of the defect remains unclear but may be related to the buildup of guanidinosuccinic acid, which is toxic to platelets. Platelet dysfunction and impaired platelet/

Table 6–6. Drugs associated with thrombocytopenia.

Acetaminophen	Meprobamate
Alcohol	Nitrofurantoin
α-methyldopa	Nitroglycerin
Ampicillin	Oxytetracycline
Aspirin	Para-aminosalicylic acid
Cephalothin	Penicillin
Chlorpropamide (Diabenese)	Phenylbutazone
Chlorthalidone (Hygroton)	Phenytoin
Cimetidine	Propylthiouracil
Digoxin	Quinidine
Estrogens	Quinine
Furosemide	Spironolactone
Gold salts	Streptomycin
Heparin	Sulfonamides
Isoniazid	Thiazide diuretics
Lincomycin	Tolbutamide (Orinase)

vessel wall interactions are present in uremic patients. Bleeding is generally mucocutaneous, but can be intracranial or pericardial in rare circumstances. Defective platelet function is corrected by aggressive preoperative and postoperative dialysis (both hemodialysis and peritoneal dialysis) and is mandatory in all patients undergoing surgical procedures. Clinical bleeding roughly correlates with the degree of renal insufficiency. Platelet transfusions are ineffective in uremic patients, even in the presence of thrombocytopenia. Elevation of the hematocrit by the use of erythropoietin or RBC transfusions has been shown to reduce the bleeding time and improve platelet adhesion, probably by displacing the platelets toward the vessel wall. Transfusion of 10 bags of cryoprecipitate immediately corrects the bleeding time in uremic patients and lasts for 24 hours. DDAVP (0.3 µg/kg intravenous) stimulates the release of vWF from endothelial cells and has been seen to reduce the bleeding time in most uremic patients. Conjugated estrogens (0.6 mg/kg intravenous) can shorten the bleeding time in some patients, and the effect lasts up to 72 hours.

Myeloproliferative Disorders

The pathology of the platelet defect in myeloproliferative disorders is not well understood, and clinical bleeding does not always correlate with laboratory abnormalities. Bleeding is typically mucocutaneous, primarily in the gastrointestinal and genitourinary tracts. It is typically controlled with myelosuppressive therapy, which reduces the platelet count. Antiplatelet therapy and phlebotomy have also been successfully used in patients with polycythemia vera.

Cardiopulmonary Bypass

Platelet dysfunction with resultant clinical bleeding is seen in 2–5% of patients after cardiopulmonary bypass. The underlying pathologic process is due to extensive contact between circulating blood and the foreign surfaces of the extracorporeal circuit. This can lead to platelet activation, release of platelet granule products, and decreased platelet aggregation to standard agonists. Platelet dysfunction can also be further impaired by hypothermia, heparin and other drugs, and any preexisting hemostatic defect. The bleeding time may also be prolonged by thrombocytopenia from dilution, consumption, and sequestration of platelets. Other less common causes of bleeding are dilution of clotting factors, activation of fibrinolysis, and incomplete reversal of heparin.

Laboratory abnormalities immediately after cardiac surgery include a moderate thrombocytopenia $(100,000-150,000/mm^3)$ and mild prolongations of PT and aPTT. In most patients, bleeding is not a problem and these mild abnormalities need not be treated. However, if the laboratory values are severely abnormal or the bleeding is severe, further investigation and treatment are necessary. Patients with massive hemorrhage should be immediately taken back to the operating room for a suspected mechanical problem. Marked prolongations of the aPTT and the activated clotting time (ACT) are usually the result of excess heparin and should be treated with protamine sulfate. Platelet transfusions, 8–12 U, should also be administered regardless of whether thrombocytopenia is present. In some cases, fresh frozen plasma and cryoprecipitate need to be given. The key to patient survival is rapid diagnosis and treatment of the coagulopathy.

Drugs

A number of drugs affect platelet function and produce prolongation of bleeding time and a mild hemostatic defect (Table 6–7). Aspirin is the most commonly used drug that impairs platelet function (see Table 6–4). The mode of action of aspirin is through acetylation and inactivation of cyclo-oxygenase. This enzyme is responsible for conversion of membrane arachidonic acid to prostaglandin endoperoxides and thromboxane A_2. Platelet release is inhibited, and platelet aggregation is impaired. All platelets exposed to a single dose of aspirin are affected for their life span, since the acetylation reaction is irreversible and platelets lack a nucleus to replenish the enzyme. Clinically, this means that the potential for bleeding during surgical procedures lasts 3–4 days after the last dose of aspirin.

In most patients, aspirin-induced bleeding is mild. In patients with underlying hemostatic defects such as hemophilia, von Willebrand's disease, and mild platelet dysfunction and in those on oral anticoagulants, serious bleeding may result. Other nonsteroidal anti-inflammatory drugs produce a defect in platelet release similar to that caused by aspirin, but their effects are transient and present only while the drug is circulating. Alcohol may potentiate the effect of aspirin on bleeding time, although it has no effect on platelet function. Bleeding tendencies may increase in an alcoholic who ingests aspirin. The treatment for the deleterious effect of aspirin on hemostasis is transfusion with 6–10 U of platelet concentrates. Patients undergoing elective surgical procedures, such as abdom-

Table 6–7. Drugs that affect platelet function.

Cyclo-oxygenase inhibitors
  Aspirin
  Other nonsteroidal anti-inflammatory agents (NSAIDs)
Phosphodiesterase inhibitors
  Dipyridamole
  Caffeine
  Theophylline
  Papaverine
Antibiotics
  Penicillin G (high dose)
  Piperacillin
  Carbenicillin
  Ticarcillin
  Cephalosporins (Cefoxitin, Moxalactom)
  Nitrofurantoin
  Hydroxychloroquine
Cardiovascular drugs
  Propranolol
  Furosemide
  Quinidine
  Calcium channel blockers
  Nitroprusside, nitroglycerin
Tranquilizers, antipsychotic agents
  Phenothiazines
  Tricyclic antidepressants
Chemotherapeutic agents
  Mithramycin
  Daunorubicin
Miscellaneous agents
  Dextran
  Antihistamines
  Sulfinpyrazone
  Ticlopidine
  Lipid-lowering agents (clofibrate, halofenate)
  General anesthetics (halothane)
  Radiographic contrast agents
  Ethanol

inal aortic aneurysm repair should wait 5–7 days after the last aspirin dose.

Aside from aspirin, antibiotics are the drugs most often associated with bleeding. The penicillins produce a dose-dependent inhibition of platelet receptors for ADP and epinephrine. The platelet dysfunction can take 2–3 days to manifest and can then last 3–10 days after discontinuation of the drug. Urgent treatment is with platelet transfusions. Dextran, used frequently in surgical patients as an antithrombotic agent, can also inhibit platelet function and fibrin polymerization. The effect on platelets is unclear, but may be related to decreases in the level of circulating von Willebrand's factor.

Baker RI, Manoharan A: Platelet function in myeloproliferative disorders and sequential studies show multiple platelet abnormalities and change with time. Eur J Haematol 1988;40:267.

Clagett GP: Preoperative assessment of hemostasis. In: *Principles of Transfusion Medicine.* Rossi EC, Simon TL, Moss GS (editors). Williams & Wilkins, 1991.

Edmunds LH: Blood contact activation during cardiopulmonary bypass. J Vasc Surg 1990;12:213.

Fass RJ et al: Platelet-mediated bleeding caused by broad-spectrum penicillins. J Infect Dis 1987;155:1242.

Ferraris VA et al: Preoperative aspirin ingestion increases operative blood loss after coronary artery bypass grafting. Ann Thorac Surg 1988;45:71.

Remuzzi G: Bleeding in renal failure. Lancet 1988; May:1205.

Salzman EW: Desmopressin and surgical hemostasis. N Engl J Med 1990;322:1085.

Woodman RC, Harker LA: Bleeding complications associated with cardiopulmonary bypass. Blood 1990;76:1680.

HYPERFIBRINOLYSIS

The pathophysiology of systemic hyperfibrinolysis is massive release of endothelial cell plasminogen activator, which converts plasminogen to plasmin, which in turn lyses hemostatic fibrin plugs and degrades fibrinogen. Systemic hyperfibrinolysis has been reported with heatstroke, cardiac arrest, and cardiopulmonary bypass. It is also a frequent manifestation of DIC, particularly in patients with severe hepatic decompensation. In these patients, the patients need systemic heparin therapy before antifibrinolytic therapy with EACA. Abnormal laboratory values in patients with hyperfibrinolysis include prolonged PT, aPTT, and thrombin time with decreased fibrinogen levels (see Table 6–4).

Systemic hyperfibrinolysis is more common with administration of streptokinase and urokinase used to dissolve arterial and venous thrombi. Even with regional use, systemic fibrinolysis can occur with impairment of hemostasis. In patients undergoing this therapy for ischemic syndromes, emergent cardiac and vascular surgery may be required in instances in which the ischemia worsens or bleeding ensues. In these cases, rapid therapy is required to correct the hemostatic defects on the way to the operating room. The goals should be to stop the fibrinolytic process, allow clearance of the FDP by the reticuloendothelial system, and restore normal fibrinogen levels. EACA can be used to halt the free action of plasmin at a loading dose of 5 g intravenously followed by 1 g per hour for 24 hours. Cryoprecipitate is given to restore fibrinogen levels.

III. CLOTTING DISORDERS

Clotting disorders or hypercoagulable states occur under the following circumstances: when deficiencies of serine protease or natural anticoagulants exist, when imbalances occur in the fibrinolytic system, when substances are present that accelerate coagulation or platelet reactions, or when diffuse endothelial dysfunction exists. Hypercoagulable states are classified as either congenital or acquired, with the acquired syndromes being far more common (Table 6–8). In the congenital hypercoagulable states, the biochemical alterations are generally fixed, but the clinical thrombotic events are episodic. Acquired hypercoagulable states often accompany other illnesses. Inherited disorders are frequently characterized by venous thrombosis, especially in unusual sites, and a family history of thrombotic events. On the other hand, patients with acquired disorders may present with venous or arterial thrombosis. An underlying congenital hypercoagulable disorder should be ruled out in the following situations: unexplained venous thrombosis in a person younger than 45 years; recurrent venous thrombosis; thrombosis of the mesenteric, hepatic, portal, renal, or cerebral veins or the inferior vena cava; a positive family history of thrombosis; and diffuse cutaneous microvascular thrombosis. Arterial thrombosis is seen much less commonly as a manifestation of hypercoagulable syndromes.

CONGENITAL HYPERCOAGULABLE STATES

ANTITHROMBIN III DEFICIENCY

Essentials of Diagnosis

- Autosomal dominant trait; equal in males and females.
- Heterozygotes ATIII levels 30–70% of normal.
- Venous thrombosis most common symptom.

General Considerations

Congenital ATIII deficiency is inherited as an autosomal dominant trait, with equal expression in males and females. The estimated incidence in the population is between 1 in 2000 and 1 in 5000 live births. Homozygous ATIII deficiency is lethal in utero.

Table 6–8. Hypercoagulable syndromes.

Congenital
Antithrombin III deficiency
Protein C deficiency
Protein S deficiency
Congenital fibrinolytic disorders
Dysfibrinogenemia
Homocystinuria
Other disorders
Acquired
Heparin-induced thrombocytopenia and thrombosis
Lupus anticoagulant and related antiphospholipid antibodies
Malignancy
Postoperative state
Pregnancy
Oral contraceptives
Other disorders

Heterozygotes have ATIII levels 30–70% of normal. ATIII deficiency can be caused by either decreased synthesis (most common) or by synthesis of a defective molecule. The deficiency causes less inhibition of serine proteinases. ATIII deficiency is found in up to 5% of patients who present with deep vein thrombosis.

The major clinical features of ATIII deficiency are thrombosis at a young age, idiopathic venous thrombosis without an identifying clinical condition, recurrent venous thromboembolism, thrombosis resistant to heparin therapy, thrombosis at an unusual site, and thrombosis during pregnancy. Thrombosis of the superficial or deep veins of the leg occur in over 90% of patients with thromboembolic episodes, with pulmonary emboli in 50% of these cases. The overall incidence of venous thromboembolism is 20% in adult heterozygotes. The risk of thrombosis increases dramatically after 15 years of age. The incidence of venous thrombosis is also increased in carriers, with 85% having episodes of thrombosis by age 55 years.

Decreased levels of ATIII are demonstrated for diagnosis of ATIII deficiency. Short-term therapy includes heparin administration with ATIII replacement. Long-term treatment is with warfarin for patients who have had at least one documented episode of thrombosis.

PROTEIN C DEFICIENCY

Essentials of Diagnosis
- Autosomal dominant trait.
- Variable expression of thrombosis in carriers.
- Venous thrombosis most common.

General Considerations
Protein C deficiency is inherited as an autosomal dominant trait, with heterozygotes suffering venous thromboembolism. Protein C is the zymogen of the serine proteinase Ca, the activated protein that inactivates factors Va and VIIIa. Protein C is activated to protein Ca 20,000 times faster through the interaction of thrombomodulin and thrombin on the endothelial surface than through thrombin alone. Protein C also proteolytically inactivates the inhibitor to tPA, thus increasing the natural antifibrinolytic activity of plasma. Protein S is a cofactor of protein C, with 60% circulating in an inactive form bound to C4b-binding protein (Fig 6–4).

The 2 key differences between deficiency of ATIII and protein C are the variable expression of thrombosis in carriers and the existence of a homozygous state. Homozygous protein C deficiency causes neonatal purpura that is difficult to treat and almost always fatal. As with ATIII deficiency, a moderate reduction to 50% of normal levels of protein C can cause devastating thrombotic complications among heterozygotes.

Clinical manifestations include young age at onset and venous thrombosis at unusual sites. The prevalence of venous thromboembolism is 60–80%. In patients presenting with deep vein thrombosis, protein C deficiency may be more common than ATIII deficiency. In young patients under age 51 requiring arterial revascularization, protein C deficiency has been noted in 15% and protein S deficiency in 20%.

Treatment for thromboembolism in patients with protein C deficiency is with heparin followed by warfarin. Warfarin-induced skin necrosis has been seen in some patients with protein C deficiency. In these patients, warfarin causes marked reduction of protein C levels before anticoagulant levels of factors II, VII, IX, and X are achieved. This can result in necrosis and skin infarction of the trunk, breasts, extremities, or tip of penis. Treatment includes immediate heparin therapy, plasma or protein C infusions, and cessation of warfarin. Because of the possibility of warfarin-induced skin necrosis in those with unrecognized protein C deficiency, heparin should always be administered with warfarin until the PT is in the therapeutic range.

PROTEIN S DEFICIENCY

Protein S is the vitamin K-dependent cofactor of activated protein C (Ca). The clinical manifestations of protein S deficiency are similar to those of protein C deficiency. About 60% of protein S circulates in an inactive form bound to C4b-binding protein, which is an acute-phase reactant (see Fig 6–4). Increased plasma levels of C4b-binding protein, as seen during inflammatory states and the postoperative period, decrease the level of free protein S, thus predisposing to thrombotic complications. Levels of free protein S in heterozygotes range from 15% to 50% of normal. Homozygotes have free protein S levels of less than 5%. Treatment of thromboembolic complications in patients with protein S deficiency is with life-long warfarin.

RESISTANCE TO ACTIVATED PROTEIN C

In young patients with venous thrombosis, resistance to activated Protein C may be the most common (>30%) hypercoagulable disorder. This resistance appears to be caused by an inherited (autosomal dominant) deficiency of an anticoagulant factor that functions as a cofactor to activated protein C. Recent studies show this to be unactivated factor V and suggest that it may be due to a selective defect in the anticoagulant function of factor V, since there are normal levels of factor V procoagulant.

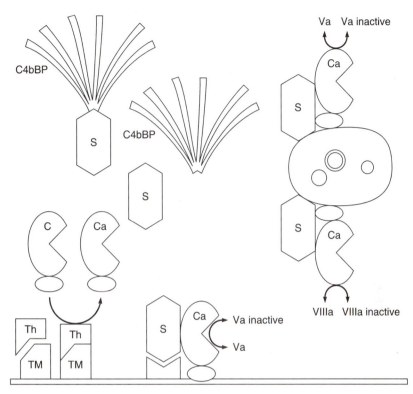

Figure 6–4. Schematic representation of protein C, protein S, and thrombomodulin anticoagulant pathway. Thrombin (Th) generated at the site binds with thrombomodulin (TM) on the endothelial surface. The Th-TM complex then rapidly activates protein C (Ca). At the surface of endothelium or platelets, Ca in combination with its cofactor protein S, functions as an anticoagulant by degrading the activated forms of factors V (Va) and VIII (VIIIa). The complex of Ca and protein S both attach to phospholipid surfaces via their γ-carboxyglutamic acid domains. Only free protein S is able to complex with Ca, with protein S bound to C4b-binding protein (C4bBP) unable to function as a cofactor. (Reproduced, with permission, from Wakefield TW: Hemostasis. In: *Surgery: Scientific Principles and Practice.* Greenfield LJ, Mulholland MW, Oldham KT, Zelenock GB [editors]. JB Lippincott, 1993:108.)

CONGENITAL FIBRINOLYTIC DISORDERS

Impaired fibrin digestion due to abnormalities in the fibrinolytic system can lead to thrombotic complications. Familial deficiencies and functional abnormalities in plasminogen, defective release of plasminogen activator from vessel walls stemming from defective endothelial synthesis of plasminogen activator, and the presence of excess circulating inhibitors to plasminogen activators have been described. These disorders are rare, and their prevalence is unknown. As with the other congenital disorders, fibrinolytic abnormalities are usually manifested clinically as venous thromboembolism, and treatment for recurrent thrombosis involves lifelong anticoagulant therapy.

DYSFIBRINOGENEMIA

Impaired fibrinolysis may be due to the formation of fibrin that is pathologically resistant to plasmin. Some congenital functional abnormalities of fibrinogen cause a hypercoagulable state complicated by thrombosis. The process is transmitted in an autosomal dominant fashion. Patients with dysfibrinogenemia and thrombosis respond to anticoagulant therapy.

HOMOCYSTINURIA (Cystathionine Synthase Deficiency)

The development of premature atherosclerosis, as well as arterial and venous thromboembolism are prominent clinical features of homocystinuria. Homocysteine causes endothelial damage and dysfunction. It down-regulates endothelial thrombomodulin function and may also impair endothelial plasmin generation by inhibiting binding of tPA to its endothelial cell surface receptor. In patients with homozygous cystathionine synthase deficiency, severe vascular disease may appear in childhood; most have thromboembolic events before the age of 40 years. Patients with heterozygous homocystinuria (estimated at 1 in 70 of the normal population) may develop premature atherosclerosis. An estimated 20–40% of patients presenting with premature peripheral vascular disease or stroke have heterozygous homocystinuria. Pyridoxine treatment reduces the incidence of thromboembolic events in homozygous patients. Whether treatment with pyridoxine or other vitamins that influence homocysteine will influence the course of premature atherosclerosis in heterozygotes is not known.

OTHER INHERITED DISORDERS

A variety of other inherited disorders have been reported to be associated with thrombotic manifestations, but the evidence of a true association is lacking. Factor XII deficiency and deficiency of α_2-macroglobulin are among these. Heparin cofactor II is a circulating plasma protein that inhibits thrombin but not factor Xa and whose action is enhanced by heparin. Deficiency of this cofactor was thought to be a cause of thrombophilia, but recent studies suggest that this is not the case. Altered levels of endothelial PAI-1 and tPA have been reported to be associated with thrombosis, but prospective study of levels of these substances concluded that these components of fibrinolysis were not predictive of thrombosis. Histidine-rich glycoprotein binds heparin and complexes with fibrinogen. Increased levels of this material could lead to thrombotic complications. Although increased levels of this substance have been observed in some patients with thrombosis, the association is uncertain. Sickle cell anemia produces obstruction of microvessels by stiff, deformed RBCs, but thrombosis does not appear to play a major role in this process.

Dahlback B, Hildebrand B: Inherited resistance to activated protein C is corrected by anticoagulant factor activity found to be a property of factor V. Proc Natl Acad Sci USA 1994;91:1396.

Clagett GP: Occlusive disease: Thrombosis. In: *Surgery: Scientific Principles and Practice.* Greenfield LJ, Mulholland MW, Oldham KT, Zelenock GB (editors). JB Lippincott, 1993.

Hirsh J, Piovella F, Pini M: Congenital antithrombin III deficiency: Incidence and clinical features. Am J Med 1989;87:34S.

Melissari E, Kakkar VV: Congenital severe protein C deficiency in adults. Br J Haematol 1989;72:222.

Nachman RL, Silverstein R: Hypercoagulable states. Ann Intern Med 1993;119:819.

Rees MM, Rodgers GM: Homocysteinemia: Association of a metabolic disorder with vascular disease and thrombosis. Thromb Res 1993;71: 337.

Rick ME: Protein C and protein S: Vitamin K-dependent inhibitors of blood coagulation. JAMA 1990;263:701.

Svensson PJ, Dahlback B: Resistance to activated protein C as a basis for venous thrombosis. N Engl J Med 1994; 330:517.

ACQUIRED HYPERCOAGULABLE STATES

HEPARIN-INDUCED THROMBOCYTOPENIA AND THROMBOSIS

Essentials of Diagnosis
- Thrombocytopenia after heparin administration.
- Development of arterial and venous thromboses; bleeding uncommon.
- Mortality rate of 20–40% from thrombotic complications.

General Considerations
Heparin-induced thrombocytopenia is uncommon and occurs in about 6% of patients receiving heparin. Unlike thrombocytopenia due to other drugs, bleeding seldom occurs; instead, these patients suffer arterial and venous thromboses. Thrombotic complications occur in less than 1% of patients having a drop in platelet count while on heparin therapy. Neither the dose nor the source (porcine versus bovine) of heparin is related to the severity of the thrombocytopenia or the severity of thrombotic complications. Thrombocytopenia has been reported to occur with all routes of administration of heparin including intravenous, subcutaneous, and even heparin bonded to indwelling venous catheters. The thrombotic complications are diverse and include venous thromboembolism, stroke, myocardial infarction, and peripheral arterial thromboembolism. The mortality rate from thrombotic complications is 20–40%, and the morbidity rate in the form of limb loss is 60–75%. Peripheral thrombosis is frequently manifested in an artery or vein previously damaged by catheterization or instrumentation. The pathogenesis of the disorder appears is related to the development of a heparin-dependent IgG antibody that attaches to platelets via the Fc receptor and triggers platelet secretion and aggregation. In addition, heparin-induced antibody binds to endothelial cells and is associated with the expression of tissue factor on the endothelial cell surface. The combination of a potent stimulus for platelet aggregation and secretion, which also alters the thrombogenicity of endothelium, may be the underlying mechanism for thrombosis in some patients with this disorder.

Treatment
All patients receiving heparin should be monitored with frequent platelet counts. If severe thrombocytopenia or thrombosis develops, heparin should be discontinued. Alternative methods of anticoagulation are necessary in most patients. Substituting a heparin-like compound can be useful. For example, Lomoparin is a

combination of heparan sulfate and dermatan sulfate that cross-reacts very little with most antiheparin antibodies. Iloprost, a prostacyclin analogue, has been used to inhibit platelet activation during short periods of heparin administration such as during cardiopulmonary bypass or vascular reconstructions. Success has also been reported with the use of ancrod, a rapidly acting defibrinogenating agent. In patients presenting with venous thromboembolism as a complication of heparin therapy, placement of a Greenfield filter, systemic thrombolytic therapy, and warfarin therapy are useful.

LUPUS ANTICOAGULANT & RELATED ANTIPHOSPHOLIPID ANTIBODIES

Essentials of Diagnosis

- Venous thromboembolism.
- Stroke, myocardial infarction.
- Postoperative thrombosis of arterial reconstructions.
- Obstetric complications due to thrombosis of placental vessels.

General Considerations

The **lupus anticoagulant** is an antibody that prolongs phospholipid-dependent coagulation tests such as APTT by binding to phospholipid. Although initially described in patients with systemic lupus erythematosus (hence its name), the antibody is more frequently encountered in patients without lupus. The paradoxical nature of the term is further compounded by the fact that patients with lupus anticoagulant appear to have a thrombotic, not hemorrhagic, diathesis. Interest has been directed toward a related antiphospholipid antibody, anticardiolipin antibody. Evidence indicates that lupus anticoagulant and anticardiolipin antibody define 2 distinct but related patient populations, each associated with an increased risk of arterial and venous thrombosis. It has become clear that the lupus anticoagulant and anticardiolipin antibodies are 2 separate entities; many with anticardiolipin antibodies do not have a lupus anticoagulant, and many with the lupus anticoagulant do not have anticardiolipin antibodies. About 1–2% of persons in the general population and higher percentages of patients with autoimmune disorders produce a family of circulating antibodies directed against anionic phospholipids. The true incidence and risk of thrombosis are unknown because of the insufficient number of prospective longitudinal studies on patients with these antibodies to determine how many will develop thrombosis.

Clinical Findings

A. Signs and Symptoms: The clinical manifestations are diverse and include venous thromboembolism, stroke, myocardial infarction, postoperative thrombosis of arterial reconstructions, and obstetric complications due to thrombosis of placental vessels. **Antiphospholipid antibody syndrome** is one of the most common causes of transient cerebral ischemia and stroke in young persons. Various potential mechanisms have been proposed to explain the increased risk of thrombosis, including decreased plasma levels of free protein S, a plasma inhibitor of endothelial activation of protein C, a plasma inhibitor of protein C, a plasma inhibitor of factor Va degradation, increased levels of PAI-1, and inhibition of endothelial cell release or production of prostacyclin. All these biologic activities of the antibodies have been demonstrated in vitro, but it is not clear which mechanisms are responsible for promoting thrombosis in vivo.

B. Laboratory Findings: Diagnostic tests include various coagulation tests (aPTT, the kaolin clotting time, and the dilute phospholipid test), assay for anticardiolipin antibodies, and other assays for antibodies against phospholipids. No single test has been demonstrated to be the best predictor of thrombosis. Because the tests may be transiently positive, a positive test result should be repeated after a period of weeks. In patients with systemic lupus erythematosus, persistently positive assays are predictive of thrombosis.

Treatment

In patients who have experienced arterial or venous thrombosis, long-term oral anticoagulant therapy is usually indicated. Antiplatelet therapy with aspirin or ticlopidine may also be useful.

MALIGNANCY

The overall prevalence of thrombosis in patients with malignancy is about 5–15%, but may be as high as 50% with some tumors, notably pancreatic carcinoma. Thrombosis is not equally common in all types of malignancy. The highest incidence of thrombotic manifestations is found in patients with acute promyelocytic leukemia, myeloproliferative disorders, primary tumors of the brain, and mucin-secreting adenocarcinomas of the pancreas (especially the body and tail of the pancreas), gastrointestinal tract, lung, and ovary. The overall incidence of thromboembolic manifestations in malignancy bears some relation to the frequency of tumors of particular types. Thus, although an especially high proportion of patients with cancer of the pancreas develop clinically evident thromboembolic disease, cancer of the pancreas is relatively uncommon compared with carcinoma of the lung, which, because of its relatively greater rate of occurrence, is the tumor most commonly associated with clinically evident thromboembolic disease. Episodes of thrombosis, particularly migratory superficial thrombophlebitis, may antedate by months the clinical diagnosis of cancer in some patients and may be the first clinical indication of the underlying cancer. In addition to venous thromboembolism, arterial embolism from nonbacterial thrombotic endocarditis may develop.

Many coagulation abnormalities predisposing to thrombosis have been described in patients with malignancy. These include thrombocytosis, shortening of the PT and aPTT, elevation of plasma coagulation factors (increases in fibrinogen and factors V, VIII, IX, and XI) and fibrinogen-fibrin degradation products, shortened platelet and fibrinogen survival, decreased ATIII levels, and increased PAI-1 activity. Many of these changes reflect generalized activation of the clotting system, resulting in chronic, partially compensated DIC. The clinical expression of these abnormalities may include bleeding and large vessel thrombosis in complex cases. In addition to these hemostatic abnormalities, there is evidence of platelet activation by tumor cells, the expression of tissue factor by monocytes and macrophages stimulated by tumor antigens, endothelial cell expression of tissue factor by cytokines produced by tumors, and the production of procoagulants by tumor cells that activate factor X. Other procoagulants may be released, such as thromboplastic substances contained in the granules of leukemic progranulocytes.

Cytotoxic chemotherapy can also cause release of thromboplastic substances from tumor cells and precipitate thrombotic events. An increased risk of thrombosis has been reported in patients undergoing chemotherapy for leukemias, breast cancer, and prostate cancer. In some cases, cytotoxic agents themselves appear to contribute to thrombosis.

POSTOPERATIVE STATE

After major surgery or trauma of any nature, several hemostatic changes occur that predispose patients to thrombosis. These are elevations in coagulation factors (fibrinogen and factor VIII), moderate (20–30%) depression of ATIII levels, decreases in free protein S levels (due to increases in C4b-binding protein levels), thrombocytosis, increased platelet reactivity or stickiness, and release of tissue thromboplastin into the bloodstream. In addition, defective fibrinolysis may occur 48–72 hours postoperatively because of elevations in α_2-macroglobulin and other inhibitory proteins. Recent evidence suggests that postoperative fibrinolytic shutdown is mediated by plasma factors that stimulate endothelial cell PAI-1 biosynthesis. Increases in blood viscosity are also common and are related to fluid shifts and dehydration. When these changes are combined with immobilization and venous pooling in the lower extremities from anesthetics

and narcotics, postoperative venous thromboembolism may result.

PREGNANCY

Although pregnancy is associated with an increased risk of venous thromboembolism, the risk increases many times immediately after delivery. Multiple anatomic, physiologic, and biochemical changes during pregnancy and the postpartum period predispose the patient to venous thromboembolism. Venous compression by the gravid uterus and increased intra-abdominal pressure along with venous smooth muscle relaxation induced by estrogen and other hormonal effects bring about venous pooling of blood in the lower extremities. Fibrinogen levels increase along with concentrations of factors VII, VIII, IX, X, and XII, whereas ATIII levels and protein S levels are mildly decreased. Depression of fibrinolytic activity further enhances hypercoagulability.

ORAL CONTRACEPTIVES

An increased risk of mortality from cardiovascular disease and particularly venous thromboembolism is seen in persons who use oral contraceptives. Use of new, lower-dose estrogen combination pills reduces but does not eliminate this risk. The systemic effect induced by oral contraceptives is similar to that seen in pregnancy and includes increased levels of clotting factors and decreases in ATIII levels.

OTHER ACQUIRED HYPERCOAGULABLE STATES

Several hematologic conditions predispose to thrombotic complications. Polycythemia vera causes marked increases in blood viscosity due to increased RBC mass and abnormalities in platelets, leading to platelet activation. Other myeloproliferative disorders such as essential thrombocythemia, chronic myelogenous leukemia, myelofibrosis, and myeloid metaplasia are also associated with thrombosis. Along with common sites of arterial and venous thrombosis, patients with myeloproliferative disorders may develop thrombosis at unusual sites such as the splenic, portal, hepatic, and mesenteric veins. A high incidence of thrombotic complications has also been described in patients with paroxysmal nocturnal hemoglobinuria, diabetes mellitus, nephrotic syndrome, some hyperlipidemias, and chronic elevations in fibrinogen levels.

Bick RL, Baker WF: Anticardiolipin antibodies and thrombosis. Hematol Oncol Clin N Am 1992;6:1287.

Clagett GP: Thrombosis and antithrombotic therapy. In: *Textbook of Vascular Surgery.* Callow AD, Ernst CB (editors). Appleton & Lange (in press).

Ey FS, Goodnight SH: Bleeding disorders in cancer. Semin Oncol 1990;17:187.

Kassis J, Hrish J, Podor TJ: Evidence that postoperative fibrinolytic shutdown is mediated by plasma factors that stimulate endothelial cell type I plasminogen activator inhibitor biosynthesis. Blood 1992;80:1758.

Schmitt BP, Adelman B: Heparin-associated thrombocytopenia: a critical review and pooled analysis. Am J Med Sci 1993;305:208.

7

Fluid Shifts & Renal Dysfunction in Vascular Surgery

David Robaczewski, MD, & Richard H. Dean, MD

Our knowledge of fluid shifts and renal function is fragmentary, and therapeutic regimens for prevention or correction of renal dysfunction remain imperfect. Examination of the nomenclature used for description of renal dysfunction underscores the relative simplicity with which the medical community views renal injury and its management. For instance, the term "acute tubular necrosis" (ATN) is commonly used by clinicians as the single term to describe the kidney's response to injury. The implication that an insult to renal function must produce tubular cell death to be considered clinically important connotes a level of understanding that is both naive and erroneous. An understanding of normal renal physiology is needed to appreciate the mechanisms responsible for renal dysfunction and failure following aortic surgery.

NORMAL RENAL FUNCTION

The regulation of extracellular fluid and electrolyte balance depends on the delivery of adequate blood volume to the kidney and the efficient filtration, reabsorption, secretion, and excretion by the nephron. Under normal physiologic conditions, the kidneys receive 25% of cardiac output. Although this amount far exceeds the minimal metabolic needs of the individual renal cell, the high flow is necessary for adequate systemic homeostasis. Based on a 5 L/min cardiac output and a hematocrit of 45 mL/dL, about 900 L of plasma flow through the kidneys each day. Normally, the kidneys filter 20% of this plasma, or 180 L, into the tubular system, where appropriate fluid balance is achieved through reabsorption and waste excretion. Considering that the normal 24-hour urine output for a 70-kg man is less than 1.8 L, the impressiveness of the reabsorption and excretion ability of the renal system becomes apparent. The major structures responsible for this process are the glomerulus, Bowman's capsule, the tubular system, and the collecting ducts.

The Nephron

The functional unit of the renal system is the nephron, which consists of the glomerulus and the tubular system. Each human kidney contains an estimated 1 million nephrons. The starting point for each nephron is

the glomerulus. As seen in Figure 7–1, the glomerulus is made up of the glomerular capillary tuft and the Bowman's capsule. The significance of this configuration exists in the interface of these 2 structures. Three layers make up this interface: the fenestrated glomerular capillary endothelium, the basement membrane, and the mesangial cells of Bowman's capsule. Each mesangial cell contains contractile filaments and extends numerous foot processes to partially envelop adjacent glomerular capillary loops. The relation between these interfacing cells is dynamic. An increase in the tone of the mesangial cells diminishes the glomerular filtration surface area, whereas a decrease in tone allows for increased filtration across the glomerular capillaries. In addition to these cellular components, negatively charged glycosaminoglycans of the basement membrane serve to repel passage of similarly charged molecules and proteins of varying sizes. Finally, intrarenal regulatory mechanisms control the amount of blood delivered to the glomerulus and the degree of filtration of plasma into the tubular system.

The tubular system of the nephron has several specialized areas that serve to reabsorb water and electrolytes into the circulation and concentrate the urine (Fig 7–2). The proximal tubule is the first specialized segment of the nephron encountered by the ultrafiltrate. Reabsorption of electrolytes from the tubular fluid occurs both by active transport and passive backdiffusion. The sodium ion is reabsorbed in the early proximal tubule by its cotransportation with organic solutes and bicarbonate through an active transport mechanism. Similarly, sodium is actively transported in the late proximal tubule in linkage with chloride transport. Prior to entering the descending loop of Henle, about two-thirds of the ultrafiltrate is reabsorbed from the tubular system. Furthermore, since water freely follows this movement of solutes and ions, the tubular fluid is isosmotic to plasma as it enters the loop of Henle.

The descending loop of Henle is permeable to water but relatively impermeable to sodium and chloride, whereas the ascending loop of Henle is impermeable to water but relatively permeable to sodium and chloride. The thick ascending loop of Henle is impermeable to water but actively transports Na^+, K^+ and Cl^- via a $Na^+/K^+/2Cl^-$-ATPase pump. The vasa recta ap-

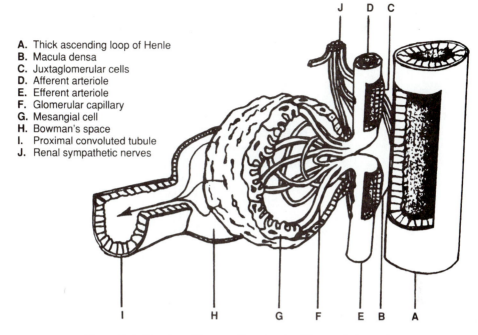

A. Thick ascending loop of Henle
B. Macula densa
C. Juxtaglomerular cells
D. Afferent arteriole
E. Efferent arteriole
F. Glomerular capillary
G. Mesangial cell
H. Bowman's space
I. Proximal convoluted tubule
J. Renal sympathetic nerves

Figure 7–1. Drawing of the constituent parts of the renal glomerulus.

proximate the tubules throughout their descent into the medullary interstitium. This medullary tubule/capillary design results in countercurrent multiplication and exchange mechanisms, which produce a medullary osmotic gradient that can regulate urine osmolarity from 50 to 1200 mOsm. Filtered potassium is almost totally reabsorbed in the proximal tubule and the loop of Henle. However, reabsorption of this ion is influenced by the electronegatively of the tubular fluid, the intracellular concentration of potassium, and the presence of aldosterone.

Dean RH, Tribble RW: Renal failure and fluid shifts following vascular surgery. In: *Complications in Vascular Surgery.* Bernhard VM, Towne JB (editors). Quality Medical Publishing, 1991:42.

Gann DS, Amaral JF: Preoperative electrolyte management. In: *Sabiston's Essentials of Surgery.* Sabiston DC Jr (editor). WB Saunders, 1987:29.

Robaczewski DL, Dean RH: Pathophysiology of renovascular hypertension. In: *Vascular Surgery: Basic Science & Clinical Correlations.* White RA, Hollier LH (editors). JB Lippincott, 1994:263.

Shires TG, Canizaro PC, Shires TC III, Lowry SF: Fluid, electrolyte, and nutritional management of the surgical patient. In: *Principles of Surgery,* 5th ed. Schwartz SI (editor). McGraw-Hill, 1989:68.

FLUID SHIFTS ASSOCIATED WITH SURGERY

Intra-abdominal vascular surgery appropriately can be considered a major insult, trauma, or injury. To ap-

preciate the response to such an insult and the impact on the fluid balance within the respective fluid compartments of the body, examination of the factors influencing transcapillary and transcellular migration of fluid is necessary. Normally, water and its respective solutes move from the plasma into the interstitial space at the precapillary level due to the net hydrostatic pressure at that level. Reentry into the intravascular space at the distal capillary level is predominantly governed by the net intravascular oncotic pressure produced by plasma proteins. Among these proteins, albumin is the most plentiful and the most important. Normally, about 7% of intravascular albumin arriving at the capillary level crosses the capillary membrane into the interstitial space. This is a unidirectional flow of albumin, and it ultimately returns to the intravascular pool by transport through the lymphatic system.

Following trauma to a specific tissue and as a net result of multiple complex hemodynamic mechanisms induced by any major insult, capillary membrane permeability to albumin is dramatically enhanced. This net egress of albumin into the interstitial space is further enhanced by interruption or alteration of poorly understood complex mechanisms governing the lymphatic transport of albumin following systemic or local trauma. Therefore, the increased albumin that is transported across the capillary membranes stays in the interstitial space longer. The effect of the increased migration of albumin into the interstitial fluid space is a decrease in distal capillary oncotic pressure and a resultant decrease in the reabsorption of water into the intravascular compartment. This in turn decreases in-

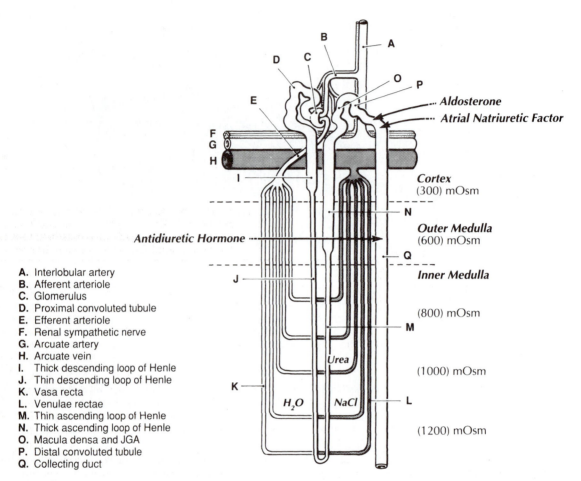

Figure 7–2. Schematic depiction of the nephron unit and its respective parts. Note the progressive increase in concentration of the urine as it passes from the outer cortex through the inner medulla.

A. Interlobular artery
B. Afferent arteriole
C. Glomerulus
D. Proximal convoluted tubule
E. Efferent arteriole
F. Renal sympathetic nerve
G. Arcuate artery
H. Arcuate vein
I. Thick descending loop of Henle
J. Thin descending loop of Henle
K. Vasa recta
L. Venulae rectae
M. Thin ascending loop of Henle
N. Thick ascending loop of Henle
O. Macula densa and JGA
P. Distal convoluted tubule
Q. Collecting duct

travascular volume and enhances the neuroendocrine mechanisms to decrease renal excretion of sodium and free water.

The normal homeostatic mechanism to contend with a decreased circulating intravascular volume is mobilization of the extracellular interstitial (third-space) fluid. Indeed, the extracellular fluid space is expanded as a consequence of the aforementioned response to the stress of major intra-abdominal surgery. Unfortunately, this excess extracellular third-space fluid might be described as "entrapped" by its greater oncotic pressure, and the functional reserve of fluid available for return to the plasma for expansion of the contracted intravascular volume is severely reduced. Considering the additive impact of temporary ischemia to tissue beds during major vascular surgery, the ensuring shift in the acid-base balance within the involved tissue beds, the adverse impact of unreplaced blood loss, the potential reductions in cardiac performance during aortic cross-clamping, and the stimula-

tion of stress response neuroendocrine mechanisms, the vicious cycle of events leading to a shifting of total body water out of the functional circulation blood volume into the third space can easily be visualized.

This obligatory loss of circulating free water and its associated solutes following major surgery only recently has been appreciated. The impact of such knowledge has been dramatically beneficial for the intraoperative and early postoperative fluid management of patients undergoing major vascular surgery. Recognition of increased obligatory losses of intravascular volume associated with major surgery has led to the current use of balanced salt solutions for replenishment. Although formulas for calculation of required intraoperative and postoperative fluid administration are available, of greatest importance is the appreciation that hourly parenteral fluid replacement requirements during surgery are several-fold more than what is required during a resting state and may vary from 100 to 500 mL/hr. Even this range of additional replacement fluids is inadequate during and after acute blood loss. These increased fluid replacement requirements continue in the immediate postoperative period because of continued sequestration of fluid into the areas of the operative site.

Mobilization of the sequestered third-space fluid is delayed for a variable period of days, depending on the magnitude of ongoing postoperative stress, cardiac performance, and intravascular oncotic pressure. Usually, the reabsorption of this third-space fluid begins on the second or third postoperative day. If not managed with appropriate reduction in maintenance parenteral fluid administration or addition of diuretic therapy, this mobilization phase of third-space fluid can lead to intravascular volume overload and acute congestive heart failure.

Granger H, Dhar J, Chen HI: Structure and function of the interstitium. In: *Proceedings of the Workshop on Albumin.* Squoris JT, Rene A (editors). National Institutes of Health, 1976;114.

Lucas CE, Ledgerwood AM: The fluid problem in the critically ill. Surg Clin North Am 1983;63:439.

Taylor AE, Granger DN: A model of protein and fluid exchange between plasma and interstitium. In: *Proceedings of the Workshop of Albumin.* Squoris JT, Rene A (editors). National Institutes of Health, 1976;93.

Valtin H: Renal function: Mechanisms preserving fluid and solute balance in health. In: *Renal Dysfunction: Mechanisms Involved in Fluid and Solute Imbalance.* Valtin H (editor). Little, Brown, 1983.

RENAL DYSFUNCTION AFTER VASCULAR SURGERY

The severity of renal dysfunction following vascular surgery may range from minor inappropriate loss of sodium in the urine to anuric acute renal failure. Similarly, its causes range from prerenal to postrenal to parenchymal (Table 7–1). Fortunately, the incidence of clinically severe acute renal failure after major surgery has dramatically decreased over the last 50 years as knowledge of the factors affecting fluid and electrolyte balance has increased and as early intervention to abort underlying causes has been implemented. Nevertheless, the mortality rate of patients with postoperative acute renal failure remains high and varies from 10% to 80%, depending on the associated presence of multiorgan system failure.

Prerenal Causes

Prerenal causes are the most common source of acute renal dysfunction in the early postoperative period. Usually, renal failure from a prerenal cause is a direct result of a contracted intravascular volume secondary to inadequate fluid replacement following intraoperative and immediate postoperative fluid losses or fluid sequestration into the third space. Less commonly, it is secondary to reduced cardiac performance,

which likewise triggers the neurohormonal reflexes to increase intravascular volume by increasing tubular reabsorption of sodium and water. In their pure forms, these 2 causes of reduced renal function are easily discernible. Whereas hypovolemia is associated with flat neck veins and dry mucous membranes, reduced dysfunction secondary to poor cardiac performance is associated with distended neck veins, apparent fluid overload (evident when the lungs are auscultated), elevated central venous pressure, and elevated pulmonary artery wedge pressure. Obviously, therapy for hypovolemic prerenal azotemia is to increase intravascular volume by administration of a balanced salt solution and red blood cells as needed. Conversely, therapy for renal dysfunction of cardiogenic origin is directed at improving myocardial performance by administering afterload reducing agents and inotropic agents and by instituting diuretic therapy as needed to diminish preloading of the failing myocardium.

Unfortunately, the diffusely atherosclerotic patient who is undergoing major vascular surgery frequently has associated coronary artery disease and impaired myocardial function. Segregation of the 2 causes of renal dysfunction (hypovolemic and cardiogenic) can be problematic. In this circumstance, preexisting heart disease may alter the euvolemic level for a person at higher central filling pressures, and apparently normal or low cardiac filling pressures may in fact reflect hypovolemia. In this clinical setting, a constant infusion of afterload reducing agents (eg, nitroprusside or nitroglycerin) and inotropic agents (eg, dobutamine) should be maintained, and sequential boluses of balanced salt solutions should be cautiously administered while monitoring cardiac output and left atrial filling pressure (pulmonary artery wedge pressure). If no urinary response is noted once filling pressures begin to rise, begin diuretic therapy as an added measure to treat the cardiac origin of the reduced urinary output.

The final variety of prerenal causes of renal failure is occlusive disease of the renal arteries. Because occlusive disease is initially a diagnosis made by exclusion of other causes, first evaluate the patient for other sources of renal failure. When other causes have been excluded, the initial study recommended to determine the presence of occlusive disease of the renal arteries is a technetium-99m-pertechnetate perfusion scan of the kidneys. Since intense interstitial swelling from parenchymal causes of ATN may dramatically increase renal parenchymal resistance, a slow renal perfusion as determined by isotope renography may be misleading. In all instances in which correction of a renovascular occlusion may be contemplated, contrast arteriography should be performed to clarify the presence of the occlusion and to plan its correction.

Postrenal Causes

Although an uncommon cause of postoperative oliguria and apparent renal failure, postrenal obstruc-

Table 7–1. Sites and causes of acute renal failure.

Prerenal	Parenchymal	Postrenal
Low cardiac	Nephrotoxic drugs	Catheter kinking
Output/cardiogenic		
Shock increased vascular	Radiologic contrast	Catheter clot
Space		
Septic shock	Myoglobinuria	Bladder clot
Hypovolemia	Acute tubular necrosis	Ureteral obstruction
Blood loss	Any cause	Renal pelvic obstruction
Dehydration		
Third-space		
Sequestration		

tion of urine flow may be the easiest to overcome and embarrassing when not excluded. Kinking or obstruction of the indwelling urinary catheter may produce sudden cessation to urinary flow. For this reason, irrigate the catheter as the first maneuver for diagnostic evaluation and potential therapy. Obstruction by clotted blood in the bladder can follow a traumatic catheter insertion. Therefore, be especially sensitive to this cause following such a difficult bladder catheterization. Finally, ureteral or renal pelvic obstructions also can cause postrenal oliguria. If other causes of oliguria have been excluded, preliminary screening of their cause can be obtained with isotope renography. Definitive diagnosis is obtained by retrograde urography. When identified, placement of an ureteral stent frequently can relieve such an obstruction.

Renal Parenchymal Causes

Parenchymal causes of acute renal dysfunction represent a wide range of causes and have the greatest potential for permanent compromise of renal function. The pathophysiology of the dysfunction is dependent on the specific cause.

A. Ischemic Injury: Caused by either temporary periods of interruption of perfusion to the kidney or periods of shock during or after major vascular procedures, ischemic injury is 2-fold. First, as a consequence of the magnitude and duration of ischemia, tubular cell swelling occurs following reperfusion. This in turn can cause tubular obstruction and lead to further reduction or cessation of glomerular filtration in the nephron. Second, tubular cells can either lose their basement membrane attachment secondary to the interstitial edema that develops after reperfusion or undergo cell death during ischemia and subsequently be sloughed into the tubule. The finding of tubular cells in the urinary sediment is the genesis of the term **acute tubular necrosis** (ATN). Although it is a poor pathologic description of this form of injury, ATN is commonly used to describe all renal parenchymal causes of acute renal failure. The medullary thick ascending loop of Henle and the pars recta of the proxi-

mal tubule appear to be the segments of the tubular epithelium most sensitive to ischemia. Following loss of the tubular cell, a back-leak of glomerular filtrate into the renal parenchyma then develops.

B. Toxic Injury: Chemical injury to the kidney can have many sources. The most common compounds responsible for such injury in the postoperative period are aminoglycosides, but myoglobin and radiologic contrast media have also been implicated. Aminoglycosides appear primarily to exert their toxicity on the tubular cell in relation to their trough level of plasma concentration. Because of this relation and the frequent history of reduced renal function in postoperative vascular surgery patients requiring the administration of aminoglycosides, it is important to monitor the peak and trough levels of the antibiotic to establish appropriate dosing levels.

Myoglobinuria is an important cause of renal failure in patients submitted to revascularization of limbs with prolonged extreme ischemia. Circulating as a breakdown product of muscle death, myoglobin is freely filtered by the glomerulus. Myoglobin exerts its toxicity through direct tubular cell injury and through precipitation and obstruction of the tubule. Therefore, prevention of injury to the kidney is directed toward maximizing urine flow rate with intravenous crystalloid infusion and diuretics and alkalinizing the urine.

Although a multitude of other parenchymal causes of acute renal failure exist, most are uncommon in surgical patients. Causes that are peculiar to vascular surgery and vascular contrast imaging have special pertinence and are discussed separately.

Brezis M, Rosen S, Silva P, Epstein FH: Renal ischemia: A new perspective. Kidney Int 1984;26:275.

Eneas JF, Schoenfeld PY, Humphreys MH: The effect of infusion of mannitol-sodium bicarbonate on the clinical course of myoglobinuria. Arch Intern Med 1979;139:801.

Jones DB: Ultrastructure of human acute renal failure. Lab Invest 1982;46:254.

Matzke GR, Lucarotti RL, Shapiro HS: Controlled comparison of gentamicin and tobramycin nephrotoxicity. Am J Nephrol 1983;3:11.

RENAL FAILURE ASSOCIATED WITH AORTIC SURGERY

Acute renal failure following aortic surgery continues to be a complication that is associated with an extremely high mortality rate. Although it is reported to have an incidence ranging from 1% to 13% in elective aortic surgery, its occurrence depends on the clinical circumstances of the operation, the intraoperative and postoperative events, and the overall prior health status of the patient.

The incidence of acute renal failure following elective abdominal aortic aneurysm surgery is around 2–5%. In contrast, operations performed for ruptured abdominal aortic aneurysms have an associated 20–50% incidence of acute renal failure among operative survivors. The mortality rate associated with postoperative renal failure has remained formidable over the past 20 years. Nevertheless, recognition of the clinical syndrome of multiorgan system failure has shed some light on factors that increase the mortality rate associated with postoperative renal failure.

In patients with postoperative renal failure as an isolated system failure, the associated mortality rate is low. In contrast, when renal failure is only one of several system failures, the mortality rate is extremely high. It might be surmised that all that is needed is simply to prevent or provide improved treatment of multiorgan system failure to improve the probability of survival in the group with renal failure. To date, the prevention of multiorgan system failure has been an unachieved goal of allied research and clinical care.

Pathophysiology of Postaortic Surgery Renal Failure

The development of acute renal failure after procedures involving the juxtarenal aorta seldom parallels pure pathophysiologic models, but stems from a mixture of underlying causes. However, the respective causes are addressed here (for the sake of understanding) as independent sources of acute renal failure, although all these mechanisms may be active in the production of postoperative renal failure in an individual patient.

A temporary, isolated period of renal ischemia caused by suprarenal aortic cross-clamping, temporary renal artery occlusion, a single episode of hypovolemic shock, declamping hypotension, or cardiogenic shock in the perioperative period are the most common causes of acute renal dysfunction and renal failure associated with aortic surgery. Postischemic acute renal failure probably is initiated through tubular luminal obstruction caused by sloughed tubular cells. The resultant tubular obstruction is postulated first to cause a transtubular back leak of glomerular filtrate. Since obstruction of tubular flow also leads to an increase in the tubular luminal hydrostatic pressure above the obstruction, less hydrostatic pressure differential exists between the glomerular capillary lumen and the tubular space within Bowman's capsule. This reduced hydrostatic pressure differential leads to reduction in glomerular filtration. Then, because of the increased permeability of the tubular lining and the resultant increased interstitial oncotic pressure, further back-diffusion of filtered water occurs. This increased back-diffusion of glomerular filtrate further spurs the progression of oliguria.

The final mechanism that leads to filtration failure and oliguria is the impact of an increased solute load presented to the macula densa as a consequence of the dramatic back-diffusion of fluid. This solute load is believed to stimulate the macula densa to activate the renin-angiotensin-aldosterone system. Through this mechanism, afferent or preglomerular arteriolar vasoconstriction is triggered, which decreases the glomerular capillary hydrostatic pressure and further encourages filtration failure. The magnitude and duration of the ischemic result are the predominant factors that determine the clinical severity and duration of this type of acute renal failure.

An alternate cause of acute renal failure in aortic surgery that might be considered as a permanent form of ischemic insult is microscopic embolization of cholesterol-rich atheromatous debris into the renal vasculature during the act of cross-clamping or declamping of the juxtarenal aorta. Although this receives much less attention in the literature than the pathophysiologic consequences of temporary ischemia, it is suggested as the dominant cause of acute renal failure in patients without prolonged renal ischemia, excessive blood loss, and hypotension or other recognized nephrotoxic insults to renal function. Obviously, the quantity of microembolization produced by clamping or declamping the aorta and by manipulation of the juxtarenal aorta during dissection depends on the embologenic potential of the atheromatous debris and the operative techniques used to prevent such an event. Furthermore, the clinical impact of such renal microembolization depends on the quantity of functioning renal parenchyma embolized and the presence of other causes of acute renal failure.

In the absence of other causes of acute renal failure and a normal mass of functioning nephron units, relatively large amounts of atheromatous microemboli can occur without immediate impact on the adequacy of renal function. In contrast, if there is a minimal renal reserve as in the azotemic patient, the added insult of even minor losses of nephron units by microembolization can lead to decompensation and acute renal failure.

Diagnosis of Renal Dysfunction

The patient with postoperative renal dysfunction or failure usually is identified by oliguria or increases in serum creatinine. Consideration of the many possible causes of postoperative renal dysfunction helps the clinician to develop an organized plan of diagnosis and treatment. In the oliguric patient, the first step involves physical examination of the patient. Observation of the patient and his or her vital signs for evidence of vascular depletion, hemodynamic instability, sepsis, and congestive heart failure allows the clinician to focus the differential diagnosis on possible prerenal, renal, and postrenal causes of renal dysfunction. For the sake of ease and simplicity, the status of the Foley catheter is then evaluated. As mentioned, prerenal causes are the most common source of acute renal dysfunction in the early postoperative period. An evaluation of the patient's intravascular volume status and cardiac performance is then carried out.

In the patient with signs of volume depletion (flat neck veins, dry mucous membranes, reduced filling pressures), replenish intravascular volume with saline. In light of the possibility of renal failure, initially avoid infusing potassium-containing solutions and blood products. On the other hand, if the examination reveals that diminished cardiac performance (distended neck veins, S3 gallop, pulmonary edema, acute electrocardiographic changes, dysrhythmias, decreased cardiac output, and elevated central venous pressure) is responsible for the oliguria, proceed by ruling out a possible myocardial infarction and provide judicious inotropic support, monitoring the patient closely with Swan-Ganz catheter monitoring (if not already in place).

If correction of filling pressures or myocardial performance fails to improve urinary output, obtain samples of urine and blood and begin diuretic therapy. Serum electrolytes, blood counts, and urine studies (urinalysis; urine sodium, urea, and creatinine concentrations; urine osmolality; and the fractional excretion of sodium) allow evaluation of other possible sources of oliguria and renal failure (ATN, myoglobinuria, nephrolithiasis). When these sources of renal dysfunction are ruled out, consider the possibility of renal artery occlusive disease. The approach to evaluating this was mentioned earlier.

In general, screen for renal artery occlusive disease with a technetium-99m-pertechnetate scan of the kidneys. This scan should be carried out only when followed up by angiographic confirmation and surgical intervention.

Protection of Renal Function

Several fundamental concepts for protection of renal function during aortic surgery are widely understood and practiced. These include provision of adequate circulating blood volume prior to operation by preoperative intravenous fluid hydration, adequate blood volume replacement during and immediately after surgery, avoidance of repetitive or prolonged renal ischemia, and maintenance of maximal parameters of cardiac performance. Additional modalities include the use of mannitol and other diuretics, renal hy-

pothermia, renal vasodilator drugs, and other more investigational techniques.

Conceptually, all these modalities are directed toward reduction of the severity or duration of renal tubular ischemia, reduction of renal tubular metabolic needs during periods of ischemia, or prevention of tubular obstruction by sloughed tubular cells. No single modality or combination prevents the insult of aortic surgery on renal function, but by maximizing the impact of each of these preventive measures, the severity and duration of renal dysfunction can be significantly reduced.

The intravenous administration of mannitol, 12.5 to 25 g, before aortic cross-clamping is widely practiced as a routine measure to prevent acute renal failure. Extensive investigation of its actions suggests that mannitol not only acts as an osmotic diuretic to increase urine flow rate, but also may attenuate the reduction in cortical blood flow that occurs during and immediately after aortic cross-clamping and may beneficially function as a free radical scavenger.

Careful attention should be given to limiting the period of warm renal ischemia. For the normally perfused kidney, anything less than 45 minutes of warm ischemia is generally safe. For the chronically ischemic kidney, the duration of safe warm ischemia time is extended for an unknown period, depending on the amount of collateral flow that has been developed. Meticulous preoperative evaluation, planning, and intraoperative setup can help reduce necessary cross-clamp time and diminish the changes for time-consuming intraoperative complications.

Regional renal hypothermia has been used sporadically for many years to protect renal function during periods of ischemia. Its use is based on the valid premise that even modest decreases in core temperature will create major reductions in metabolic needs. These unmet metabolic needs during ischemia lead to the cascade of events producing acute renal failure. The technique usually uses the infusion of 500 mL to 1 L of cold (4–5°C) crystalloid solution with or without other additives into the isolated segment of the aorta containing the renal arteries or directly into the renal artery ostia using a hand-held cannula. The protective effect of minimal changes in core temperature have recently been evaluated in rats. Postoperative serum creatinine levels and renal tubular morphology findings revealed a protective effect with a minimal, sustained decrease in core temperature to 35°C. It would be interesting to see whether a similar well-controlled study in humans would reveal like findings.

Finally, the importance of operative technique in prevention of microembolization of atheromatous debris during juxtarenal aortic manipulation or clamping cannot be overstated. Since the embologenic potential of the debris cannot be judged definitively until after the aorta is opened, assume the worst until proved otherwise. For this reason, it is recommended to temporarily occlude renal artery flow immediately before the application of the aortic clamp whenever the aortogram suggests the presence of succulent atheromatous debris. This applies to both cross-clamping immediately below the renal arteries as well as suprarenal aortic cross-clamping.

For infrarenal cross-clamping, it is recommended to "flash-unclamp" the proximal aortic clamp after opening the aorta to flush out any loose debris. Then, reapply the aortic clamp, remove the renal artery-occluding device, and reestablish renal perfusion. Although only antidotal support can be provided for this maneuver, it has been an important adjunct in minimizing the incidence of postoperative acute renal failure among many patients.

Abbott WM, Abel RM, Beck CH: The reversal of renal cortical ischemia during aortic occlusion by mannitol. J Surg Res 1974;16:482.

Bergqvist D et al: Renal failure as a complication to aortoiliac and iliac reconstructive surgery. Acta Chir Scand 1983;149:37.

D'Alecy LG et al: Minimal physiologic temperature variations during renal ischemia alter functional and morphologic outcome. J Vasc Surg 1992;15:619.

Hanley MJ, Davidson K: Prior mannitol and furosemide infusion in a model of ischemic acute renal failure. Am J Physiol 1981;241:F556.

McCombs PR, Roberts B: Acute renal failure following resection of abdominal aortic aneurysm. Surg Gynecol Obstet 1979;148:175.

Miller DC, Myers BD: Pathophysiology and prevention of acute renal failure associated with thoracoabdominal or abdominal aortic surgery. J Vasc Surg 1987;5:518.

Myers BD, Moran SM: Hemodynamically mediated acute renal failure. N Engl J Med 1986;314:97.

O'Donnell D, Clarke G, Hurst P: Acute renal failure following surgery for abdominal aortic aneurysm. Aust NZ J Surg 1989;59:405.

8   Carotid Artery Occlusive Disease

Robert W. Hobson II, MD

General Considerations

Cerebrovascular disease constitutes the third leading cause of death in this country, resulting in over 150,000 deaths, which were attributed to stroke. Although epidemiologic evidence has confirmed a 50% reduction in mortality rate from stroke over the last 2 decades (Fig 8–1), it is a major source of disability among elderly Americans. In a recent report from the Framingham study of 394 stroke victims, 84 or 21% of elderly stroke patients had second strokes and 27 or 7% had third strokes, which also contributed to increased disability.

Thromboembolic disease accounts for about 75% of new strokes each year (Fig 8–2). Of these, carotid artery occlusive disease is probably the single most important causal factor in the development of cerebrovascular ischemia (Fig 8–3). Although transient monocular blindness (TMB) or amaurosis fugax and transient ischemic attack (TIA) constitute important warning signs of impending stroke, many patients do not report or sustain these warning signs. Nevertheless, stroke prevention includes the recognition of these events during a careful history and interpretation of important physical findings.

Management of identifiable risk factors and careful selection of patients for operative intervention constitute the approach toward reducing morbidity and mortality associated with stroke. Identification of subsets of patients who will benefit from carotid endarterectomy naturally progresses from those with asymptomatic carotid disease, to those with transient neurologic symptoms, to those with more severe neurologic deficits including completed stroke. The role of carotid endarterectomy requires careful review of each of these 3 groups of patients.

Valuable epidemiologic information has been obtained from the Framingham study. The relative incidence of stroke by type confirms that no significant differences in stroke manifestations are related to gender. A variety of risk factors contributes to an increased likelihood of stroke: age, systolic blood pressure, diabetes, smoking, history of cardiovascular disease, and electrocardiographic abnormality (left ventricular hypertrophy or atrial fibrillation).

Of the various independent variables, hypertension (brachial blood pressure of 160/95 mmHg or greater) and its management are of paramount importance in stroke prevention. The age-adjusted relative risk of stroke among hypertensive persons compared with normotensive ($<$140/90 mmHg) persons is 3.0 in men and 2.9 in women; even borderline hypertension carries a 50% increase in risk for stroke. Despite some historical emphasis on the greater importance of diastolic hypertension, the levels of both systolic and diastolic pressures are comparable in their impact on the development of stroke. As documented by the Fram-

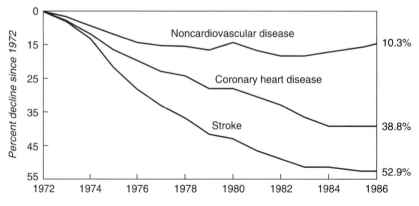

Figure 8–1. Decline in age-adjusted mortality rates for cardiovascular disease, United States, 1972 to 1986. (Reproduced, with permission, from White MF: Reducing cardiovascular risk factors in the United States: An overview of the National Educational Programs. Cardiovasc Risk F 1991;1:277.)

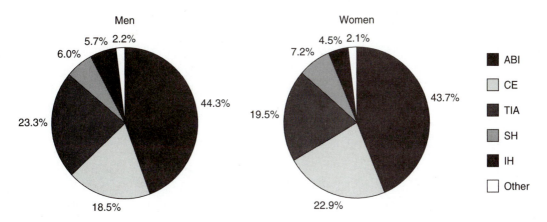

Figure 8–2. Frequency of stroke by type in men and women: 36-year follow-up. ABI, atherothrombotic brain infarction; CE, cerebral embolism; TIA, transient ischemic attack; SH, subarachnoid hemorrhage; IH, intracerebral hemorrhage. (Reproduced, with permission, from Wolf PA Cobb JL, D'Agostino RB: Epidemiology of stroke. In: *Stroke: Pathophysiology, Diagnosis, and Management.* Barnett HJM et al (editors). Churchill Livingstone, 1992.)

ingham study, the incidence of stroke and coronary heart disease has been related to the incidence and severity of hypertension. These data also emphasize the importance of impaired cardiac function on the incidence of stroke (Fig 8–4).

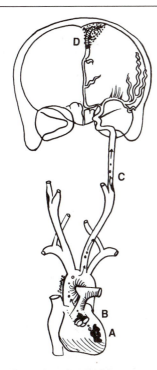

Figure 8–3. Examples of potential sources of embolism: **A:** Cardiac mural thrombus, **B:** Vegetations on heart valve, **C:** Emboli from carotid plaque. Also shown: **D:** Infarcted cortex in area supplied by terminal anterior cerebral artery due to embolism. (Reproduced, with permission, from Caplan LR: *Stroke.* Butterworth-Heinemann, 1993.)

Although blood lipids are correlated with the incidence of coronary heart disease, they are not directly related to the incidence of stroke. Although the relation between lipids and the size of the carotid atheroma have been established, this factor does not translate into a greater overall stroke rate except in patients with increasingly severe degrees of stenosis. Diabetics are known to have a 2–4 times higher incidence of stroke than nondiabetics.

Cigarette smoking is another major risk factor for stroke in addition to being a powerful risk factor for myocardial infarction and sudden death as well as brain infarction. It has been speculated that smoking causes temporary increases in blood pressure, which might then be related to a heightened incidence of atheroembolic stroke as well as subarachnoid, intracranial, or intracerebral hemorrhage. A meta-analysis estimated that smokers have about a 50% increased overall risk for atheroembolic brain infarction compared with nonsmokers. In turn, smoking cessation leads to marked reduction in stroke risk. Furthermore, the risk of coronary disease decreased by about 50% within 1 year of smoking cessation and reached a level comparable to those who had not smoked within 5 years.

ANATOMY & PHYSIOLOGY

The principal vascular supply for the head and neck originates from the right common carotid branch of the innominate artery, the left common carotid artery rising directly from the aortic arch, and the bilateral vertebral arteries (Fig 8–5). The bifurcation of the common carotid artery occurs in the midcervical region within a sheath derived from the deep cervical fascia, which encloses the common carotid, internal jugular

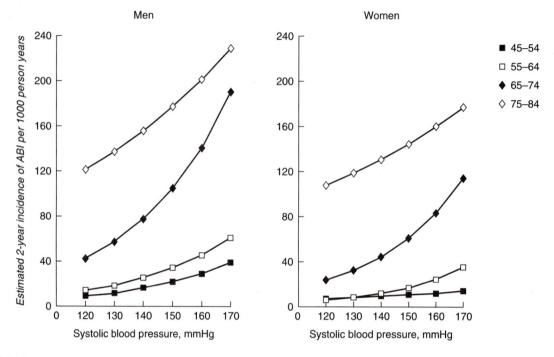

Figure 8–4. Incidence of brain infarction according to systolic blood pressure in men and women, ages 45–84 years, diastolic blood pressure is below 95 mmHg: 36-year follow-up. ABI, atherothrombotic brain infarction. (Data from the Framingham study.)

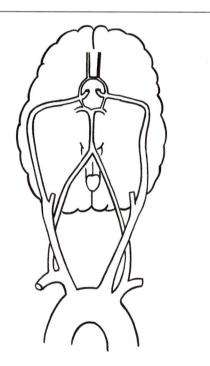

Figure 8–5. Vascular supply for the head and neck originates from major aortic arch branches.

vein, and vagus nerve. The anatomic relation between the external and internal carotid arteries at the carotid bifurcation and the unique hemodynamics of blood flow have been reported as predisposing factors in the development of the carotid atherosclerotic plaque (Figs 8–6 and 8–7).

The vertebral artery is the first branch of the subclavian artery, and the collateralization between the internal carotid and vertebral arteries results in the formation of the **circle of Willis** (Fig 8–8). This structure is composed of the posterior cerebral artery arising from the basilar artery and of the internal carotid and its 2 terminal branches, the middle and anterior cerebral arteries. This classic anatomic description known as a "complete circle of Willis" occurs in about 50% of persons.

When the blood supply from the internal carotid artery is inadequate for its distal territory, several sources of collateralization may develop. One of the most common sources of collateral blood flow is the anastomosis with the internal carotid artery through the orbit. Collateral blood passes through the external carotid and into the intracranial internal carotid by way of periorbital collaterals. These anastomoses also occur between the maxillary branches of the external carotid artery and the ophthalmic artery in the floor orbit. From the intracranial carotid artery, blood flow then extends to the circle of Willis and its intracranial

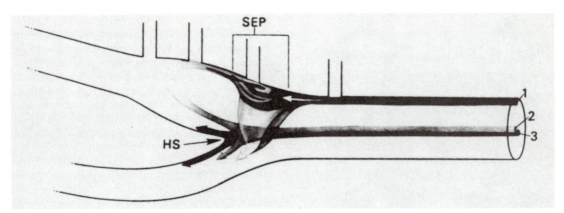

Figure 8–6. Dye flow visualization technique in an acrylic model human carotid bifurcation shows boundary layer separation at the level of the outer wall of the bulb where the atherosclerotic plaque localizes. (Reproduced, with permission, from LoGerfo et al: Structural details of boundary layer separation in a model human carotid bifurcation under steady and pulsatile flow conditions. J Vasc Surg 1989;2:263.)

distribution. The obvious other important collateral in the presence of a unilateral internal carotid occlusion is the contralateral internal carotid artery, which supplies the circle of Willis and then goes across to the opposite intracranial branches of the internal carotid artery.

Obviously, the form of the collateralization depends on an intact anterior half of the circle of Willis. Variations occur, and the adequacy of the collateralization in the presence of unilateral occlusion is a major determinant in the occurrence of stroke with total occlusion of a single internal carotid artery. The vertebrobasilar system may also collateralize to the anterior circulation through the posterior communicating arteries. Rarely, patients tolerate bilateral internal carotid artery occlusions because of redistribution of blood flow from the vertebrobasilar system through the posterior communicating arteries.

The cerebral circulation exhibits autoregulation of its flow to maintain relatively constant blood flow over a range of physiologic variations in blood pressures, cardiac output, and circulating blood volume. Loss of autoregulation, a consequence of stroke, results in areas of the cerebral circulation, which then are regulated only passively through changes in systemic blood pressure. Under these circumstances after stroke, the physiologic alterations influence the conduct of operative intervention mandating use of a shunt and pharmacologic support of systemic blood pressure during carotid endarterectomy.

DETERMINING THE SEVERITY OF STENOSIS

Characterizing the severity of carotid stenosis, particularly in the asymptomatic and symptomatic groups, continues to be a point of some contention. The definition of clinically significant but asymptomatic carotid stenosis is usually related to the magni-

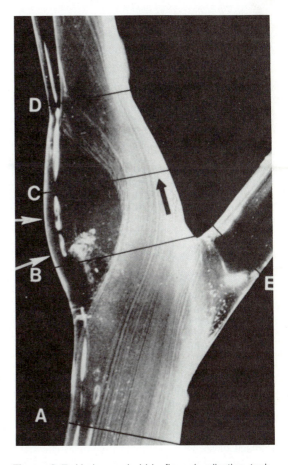

Figure 8–7. Hydrogen bubble flow visualization technique in a glass model human carotid bifurcation shows laminar flow in the inner wall of the bulb and area of flow separation in the outer wall where the atherosclerotic plaque localizes. (Reproduced, with permission, from Zarins et al: Carotid bifurcation atherosclerosis: Quantitative correaltion of plaque localisation with flow velocity profiles and wall shear stress. Circ Res 1983;53:502.)

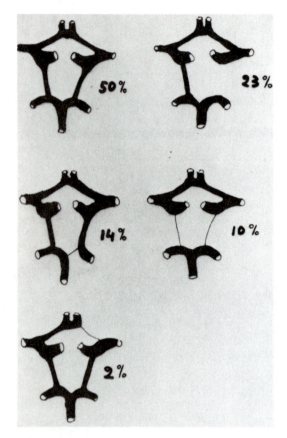

Figure 8–8. Diagram showing the variations in the patterns of the circle of Willis. (From Mohr JP: *Stroke: Pathophysiology, Diagnosis, and Management.* Barnett HJM, Mohr JP, Stein BM, Yatsu FM [editors]. Churchill Livingstone, 1992.)

tude of stenosis present at the carotid bifurcation and the proximal internal carotid artery. By convention, this has been defined as a 50% reduction in the luminal diameter of the artery or a 75% reduction in the cross-sectional area when accompanied by positive noninvasive studies such as ocular pneumoplethysmography (OPG) or duplex scan.

The percentage of stenosis is determined by comparing the least transverse diameter at the stenosis with the diameter of the distal uninvolved internal carotid artery (Fig 8–9). This arteriographic methodology was adopted by the investigators in the VA Asymptomatic trial and subsequently adopted by the investigators in the North American Symptomatic trial (NASCET), the VA Symptomatic trial, and the Asymptomatic Carotid Atherosclerosis Study (ACAS) trial.

The values obtained in duplex scanning and the degree of stenosis as defined by the University of Washington criteria require modification to correlate with arteriographic estimates of stenosis as defined. However, these rigid cut-off points may be unrealistic in

clinical practice and are not recommended because some patients would be eliminated who might benefit from operation and because many patients would be needlessly subjected to the invasive procedure of arteriography. A possible solution is to use as a basis the 50% diameter-reducing stenosis accompanied by positive OPG or duplex scan (area-reducing stenosis of 75%) as the threshold lesion for intervention in asymptomatic as well as symptomatic patients.

Clinical data have confirmed that high-grade stenosis associated with the least transverse diameter (<1.0 mm) at the stenosis predicts stroke risk in symptomatic and asymptomatic patients. However, it has been suggested that other factors need to be considered along with percentage of stenosis, since subsets of patients are identified as benefitting from operative intervention. Additional factors include ultrasonic plaque morphology, incidence of silent computed tomography (CT)-confirmed cerebral infarction, status of the collateral cerebral circulation, and a combination of clinical risk factors such as hypertension, coronary artery, history of smoking, and peripheral vascular disease. The latter factors combined with the threshold degree of stenosis may result in a higher risk of neurologic events.

Although it is incumbent on the clinical vascular surgeon to be aware of all these factors, adoption of a plan to consider operative intervention in selected patients with symptomatic and asymptomatic carotid stenosis (area reduction > 70–75%) can be recommended with confidence.

ASYMPTOMATIC CAROTID ARTERY DISEASE

Asymptomatic Carotid Artery Stenosis

Because of the morbidity and mortality of symptomatic extracranial carotid occlusive disease in terms of transient and permanent neurologic deficits, one of the goals of management is to identify patients before neurologic symptomatology develops. Asymptomatic carotid disease is suggested in the high-risk atherosclerotic population because of the important physical sign of carotid bruit or nonlateralizing symptoms such as lightheadedness and nonspecific visual aberrations. Although carotid bruit alone is not an accurate predictor of stroke risk a significant relation exists between high-grade asymptomatic carotid stenosis (area-reducing stenoses > 75%) and increased neurologic event rates (Fig 8–10, Table 8–1). Confirmation of this association comes from randomized clinical trial data in Table 8–2. Further studies on the natural history of significant carotid disease also include useful retrospective analyses.

Data in Tables 8–3 and 8–4 emphasize the importance of accurate clinical audits concerning the perioperative risk of carotid endarterectomy. The effec-

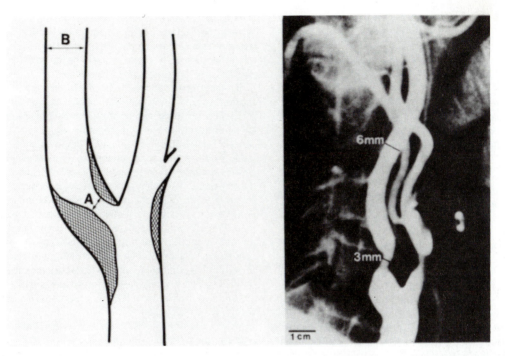

Figure 8–9. The percentage of stenosis is calculated by dividing the least transverse diameter of the internal carotid artery at the stenosis (A), by the diameter of the distal, uninvolved artery (B). The minimum residual lumen diameter is equivalent to the least transverse diameter (A) divided by the magnification factor (MagF) of the arteriogram. The example (*right*) illustrates a 50% stenosis by diameter and a minimum residual lumen diameter of 2.2 mm. (Reproduced, with permission, from Lynch TG, Hobson RW: Noninvasive cerebrovascular diagnostic techniques. In: *Vascular Surgery: Principles and Practice*. Wilson SE, Veith FJ, Hobson RW, Williams RA [editors]. McGraw-Hill, 1987:105.)

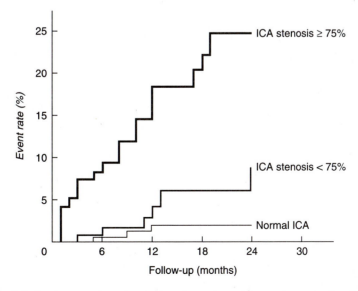

Figure 8–10. Neurologic ischemic events in patients with an internal carotid stenosis greater than 75% occurred at a rate of 15% per year. In patients with stenoses of less than 75%, however, the rate was less than 3% per year. (Reproduced, with permission, from Chamber BR, Norris JW: The case against surgery for asymptomatic carotid stenosis. Stroke 1984;15:964.)

Table 8–1. Annual percentage of vascular events over period of follow-up.

Degree of Stenosis	TIA	Stroke	Cardiac	Vascular Deaths
<50% (mild)	1.0	1.3	2.7	1.8
50–75% (moderate)	3.0	1.3	6.6	3.3
>75% (severe)	7.2	3.3	8.3	6.5

TIA, transient ischemic attack.

(From Norris JW et al: Vascular risk of asymptomatic carotid stenosis. Stroke 1991;22:1485.)

tiveness of this operation ultimately depends on maintaining low complication rates as the surgical group is compared with natural history data from the medical group.

Surgeons encounter patients with asymptomatic carotid stenosis under 3 different clinical circumstances: (1) referral because of cervical bruit in the absence of lateralizing neurologic symptoms; (2) presence of a symptomatic unilateral carotid stenosis treated by carotid endarterectomy with an asymptomatic contralateral stenosis noted arteriographically; and (3) presence of a significant stenosis in a patient scheduled for another major operative surgical procedure.

A. Asymptomatic with Cervical Bruit: The most common clinical situation is that of the patient referred with cervical bruit who is either asymptomatic or has occasional and intermittent episodes of nonspecific global symptomatology such as lightheadedness, dizziness, and possibly nonspecific visual irregularities. These patients are generally referred for cerebrovascular noninvasive testing; with positive results, they become candidates for arteriography and possible operation.

The incidence of asymptomatic carotid stenosis is difficult to define for a population. For example, over 2000 neurologically asymptomatic patients were screened using direct continuous-wave Doppler techniques. Significant extracranial carotid occlusive disease was identified in 32.8% of patients with peripheral vascular disease, in 6.8% of patients with coronary disease, and in 5.9% of patients with significant risk factors. In a survey evaluating the prevalence of carotid arterial stenosis in an nonselected asymptomatic population over 50 years of age, carotid occlu-

sive disease was identified in about 10% of the group. In addition, stenoses of increasing significance were noted with each passing decade of life. The incidence of carotid stenosis has been found to be increased in all subjects who have associated risk factors.

B. Asymptomatic with Contralateral Symptomatic Lesion: The second clinically important group of patients presents with asymptomatic carotid stenosis contralateral to a symptomatic lesion that has caused a lateralizing neurologic complication. Data from 5 clinical series on asymptomatic contralateral carotid stenosis are presented in Table 8–5. However, these studies included only a few patients with stenoses exceeding 75%, and some selected nonrandomly those patients with stenotic lesions of greater than 75% for prophylactic endarterectomy. Furthermore, as emphasized by one recent clinical trial, the occurrence of warning TIA may be unusual or absent. In addition, a clinical recommendation to await development of TIA presupposes that these transient events are innocuous. A clinical TIA may also be associated with a 30–40% incidence of positive CT or magnetic resonance imaging (MRI) scans. Consequently, the concept that a transient neurologic event is of no significance may be erroneous, suggesting that stroke prevention also may be related to prevention of TIAs. Although contralateral asymptomatic stenoses of less than a 75% area-reducing level can be followed clinically, stenoses greater than 75% need to be considered for prophylactic endarterectomy (based on data from randomized clinical trials).

C. Asymptomatic Prior to Cardiovascular Procedure: The third group includes patients identified as having asymptomatic carotid stenoses prior to a major cardiovascular surgical procedure. Intraoperative hypotension combined with carotid stenosis may predispose a patient to carotid arterial occlusion and has been suggested as a mechanism for cerebral hypoperfusion and stroke. Nevertheless, the overall risk of perioperative stroke is about 0.3% in general surgical patients, 1% in patients undergoing peripheral vascular surgery, and 1% to 5% in patients following coronary bypass grafting. No well-documented relation exists between the presence of carotid bruit and subsequent incidence of perioperative stroke, but the perioperative risk of stroke in the asymptomatic patient with a hemodynamically significant stenosis has

Table 8–2. Ipsilateral stroke and 30-day operative stroke/mortality for VA & ACAS trials.

| | VA (n = 444) | | ACAS (n = 1662) | |
	Medical (%)	Surgical (%)	Medical (%)	Surgical (%)
Ipsilateral stroke	9.4	4.7*	10.6	4.8†
Operative complications	—	4.3	—	2.3

* Benefit for carotid endarterectomy; P = 0.056.
† Benefit for carotid endarterectomy; P = 0.006.
(Data taken from Hobson RW et al and the Veterans Affairs Cooperative Study Group: Efficacy of carotid endarterectomy for asymptomatic carotid stenosis. N Engl J Med 1993; 328:221; and The Asymptomatic Carotid Atherosclerosis Study Group: Study design for randomized prospective trial of carotid endarterectomy for asymptomatic atherosclerosis. Stroke 1989;20:844.)

Table 8–3. Recommended upper limits of combined stroke morbidity & mortality for carotid endarterectomy.

Indication	Percentage
Asymptomatic carotid stenosis	<3%
Transient ischemic attack	<5%
Stroke with fixed neurologic deficit	<7%
Restenosis	<10%
Mortality	≤2%

(From Callow AD et al: Carotid endarterectomy: What is its current status? Am J Med 1988;85:835.)

Table 8–5. Follow up of asymptomatic contralateral carotid artery disease.

Study	Follow-up (Yr)	Number of Arteries	TIAs	Cerebro-vascular Accidents
Podore et al	5	22	3 (14%)	2 (9%)
Humphries et al	0–13	182	29 (16%)	1 (0.5%)
Durward et al	4	31	4 (13%)	0
Levin et al	0–20	147	9 (6%)	0
Johnson et al	1–4	22	2 (9%)	0
Total		404	47 (12%)	3 (0.7%)

TIA, transient ischemic attack.

not been definitively evaluated. The incidence of postoperative death from myocardial infarction, however, was significantly increased in this group of patients.

In a noninvasive study of patients prior to coronary bypass, 2.5% were identified as having hemodynamically significant lesions. There was a 15% incidence of perioperative neurologic deficits in patients with significant carotid occlusive disease compared with a 2% incidence in patients with no carotid disease. Nevertheless, the investigators recommended against prophylactic carotid endarterectomy in this population because of a comparably higher incidence of perioperative complications. Other investigators have performed the operation with lesser morbidity and recommend routine carotid endarterectomy under these circumstances. No firm recommendation will be possible until a randomized trial is conducted.

Asymptomatic Ulcerative Disease

Although diagnostic procedures designed to interrogate the cervical carotid artery have had their greatest accuracy in the identification of high-grade stenosis, asymptomatic ulcerative nonstenotic disease has also been implicated as a significant stroke risk. Recent analysis has demonstrated the direct relation of plaque ulceration and increased risk of stroke.

A. Size of Ulcer: Ulcer size has been categorized as an area measurement determined by multiplying the length and width of the ulcer in millimeters. An "A" ulcer measures less than 10.0 mm^2, a "B" ulcer ranges from 10.0 to 44.0 mm^2, and a "C" ulcer exceeds 40.0 mm^2. The presence of a C ulcer, independent of associated carotid stenosis, identified a group of patients with a 7.5% per year stroke risk, whereas the smaller

Table 8–4. Morbidity & mortality of carotid endarterectomy for asymptomatic carotid disease.

Author	Operations	Mortality	Morbidity Transient	Morbidity Permanent
Thompson et al	167	0	2 (1.2%)	2 (1.2%)
Moore et al	78	0	2 (2.6%)	0
Hertzer et al	95	1 (1.1%)	—	4 (4.2%)
Whitney et al	279	3 (1.1%)	5 (1.8%)	6 (2.2%)
Javid et al	65	1 (1.5%)	1 (1.5%)	1 (1.5%)
Anderson et al	120	0	2 (1.7%)	0

A ulcerations were not associated with an increased stroke risk. However, it has been reported that the definition of ulceration is imprecise and that smooth shallow depressions in the atherosclerotic plaque noted at operation can be misinterpreted as significant ulcerations preoperatively.

Controversy also exists concerning the natural history of intermediate-sized ulcers and their effect on stroke risk. Some reports suggest a modest increase in stroke risk to as high as 4.5% per year, whereas other reports show no relation between the presence of a B ulcer and subsequent stroke risk.

B. Pathogenesis of Ulceration: The evolution of the carotid plaque relates in no small measure to risk factors outlined earlier in this chapter including hypertension, cigarette smoking, and cardiac disease. The local hemodynamics of blood flow at the carotid bifurcation predisposes the development of a atherosclerotic plaque. Ultimate fracture and hemorrhage or ulceration within the plaque become an important part of an increasingly complex lesion. For example, the importance of the plaque's fibrous cap and its deterioration with exposure of mixed areas of lipids and intraplaque hemorrhage to the carotid circulation have been emphasized. Emboli associated with such ulceration may give rise to retinal and cerebral ischemia and infarction with or without symptoms. Some of these symptoms may result in "silent" infarction, which becomes part of the presentation of asymptomatic carotid stenosis. Patients with CT-confirmed silent infarctions have a higher incidence of subsequent stroke. Many of these factors are considered important in the conversion of an asymptomatic carotid plaque to one associated with neurologic symptoms. The factors include the severity of stenosis, the effects of plaque morphology, the status of collateral cerebral circulation, and the presence of various systemic risk factors.

C. Other Risk Factors: Rapidly progressing asymptomatic carotid stenoses are also associated with increased risk of neurologic events. The transition of an asymptomatic carotid stenosis to a symptomatic lesion can be caused by embolization from an altered plaque or occlusion of a critical stenosis. Some reports have emphasized that stroke occurs in 20–30% of acute occlusions of the internal carotid.

The impact of plaque morphology depends on its diagnosis by duplex scanning. The heterogenic plaque is more significantly associated with stroke than the homogenous plaque. Presence of echolucent or heterogenic plaques are probably related to deposition of cholesterol and intraplaque hemorrhage, which are associated with instability of the plaque. Although the diagnosis of the ulcerative lesion is less than satisfactory by duplex scan or arteriography when compared with that for explanted carotid atheroma, its presence can be assumed to increase the likelihood of neurologic events. This was confirmed from a recent report from the NASCET investigators among symptomatic patients, in whom the incidence of stroke was progressively increased with each degree of stenosis in the presence of ulceration.

The impact of collateral circulation relates to a knowledge of the anatomy of the circle of Willis and the quality of collateral circulation, as detected by techniques such as transcranial Doppler analysis. In severe asymptomatic stenosis, occlusion of the carotid artery is more likely to result in stroke in the absence of adequate collateral circulation from the opposite carotid artery. However, further study of this question is required.

Asymptomatic brain infarction carries with it a risk of subsequent stroke. Therefore, patients with high-grade asymptomatic carotid stenosis who are being considered for carotid endarterectomy should undergo CT scanning. for patients with a silent cerebral infarct, the recommendation for operative intervention is increased.

Finally, a combination of clinical risk factors has been considered to be most important in these patients. This emphasizes the importance of risk factor management.

SYMPTOMATIC CAROTID ARTERY DISEASE

Transient Cerebral Ischemia

Transient cerebral ischemia includes transient monocular blindness (TMB) or amaurosis fugax and the lateralizing transient ischemic attack (TIA). TMB has been recognized as an important manifestation of carotid artery occlusive disease. Described as a brief impairment in visual acuity as noted in patients' description of a "fog," a "blur," or the more classic "shade" or "curtain over the eye," it clears in several seconds to minutes. The occurrence of TMB should prompt investigation of the carotid bifurcation as well as other sources of atheroemboli. TIA manifests as weakness or the presence of paresthesias over part or all of the contralateral body with or without speech disturbances, depending on whether or not the more dominant hemisphere has been affected. Although by definition, the duration of TIAs is less than 24 hours, most last only several minutes to 1 hour before resolving without neurologic deficits. The accuracy of the history in defining the presence of TIA has stimulated

considerable controversy because these symptoms can be underreported or underestimated by patients and misinterpreted by clinicians. Differentiation of TIA and nondisabling stroke may be unnecessarily rigid. Toole and colleagues have reported on the continuum between these neurologic events.

Data also emphasize the importance of using TMB and TIA as indicators for investigation of the patient's cardiovascular status. Sources of atheroemboli include mural thrombi from recent myocardial infarction, vegetations or atherosclerotic debris from valvular heart disease, and embolization from carotid atheroma (see Fig 8–3). Once the differential diagnosis of cardiac disease has been excluded, the identification of significant carotid occlusive disease becomes of paramount importance, particularly in the presence of a high-grade stenosis. Although the overall risk of stroke in TIA patients is 24–29% over 5 years, these numbers increase significantly to more than 40% in 2 years in TIA patients with carotid stenosis over 70%. Consequently, these patients deserve prompt workup and evaluation including arteriography and carotid endarterectomy as indicated by the severity of their carotid stenosis.

Stroke

The term **completed stroke** is ordinarily used to describe the focal neurologic deficit that is abrupt in onset and persists beyond 24 hours without immediate improvement. Stroke severity scores have been used to characterize deficits (Table 8–6). Although patients

Table 8–6. Stroke severity scale.

Severity Level	Impairment*	Neurologic Symptoms	Neurologic Signs
1	None	Present	Absent
2	None	Absent	Present
3	None	Present	Present
4	Minor (in 1 or more domains)	Present	Present
5	Major (in only 1 domain)	Present	Present
6	Major (in any 2 domains)		
7	Major (in any 3 domains)		
8	Major (in any 4 domains)		
9	Major (in all 5 domains)		
10	Reduced level of consciousness		
11	Death		

* Impairment in the domains of swallowing, self-care ambulation, communication, and comprehension. If independence is maintained despite the impairment, it is classified as *minor*; if independence is lost, it is classified as *major* (Barnett's method).

(From The EC/IC Bypass Study Group: Failure of extracranial-intracranial arterial bypass to reduce the risk of ischemic stroke: Results of an international randomized trial. N Engl J Med 1985;313:1191.)

with nondisabling stroke become candidates for carotid endarterectomy, patients with acute stroke and severe neurologic deficits have an unacceptably high mortality rate from operation. The variability in symptoms and severity of complications as well as recovery of function relate to many factors including adequacy of collateral circulation, state of cardiorespiratory function, and presence of major systemic illness.

Another intermediate neurologic syndrome is **reversible ischemic neurologic deficit (RIND)**. This may simply represent a continuum of TIA, which is somewhat more severe and associated with clearing of neurologic deficit after the traditional and perhaps arbitrary duration of 24 hours as applies to TIA. The so-called **stroke-in-evolution** or the **stuttering stroke** must be included as a clinical variant. Again, the return to a near baseline neurologic examination characterizes these stepwise progressive evolutions and creates an opportunity for operative intervention in selected patients, occasionally described as also having frequent or "crescendo" TIAs. Description of these cases is variable enough that final statements regarding their care must be regarded as largely anecdotal.

Finally, stroke may be associated with acute carotid occlusion, and a few of such patients may be candidates for urgent operative intervention, particularly if hospitalized at the time of the event or if geographically close to a medical center. Each case must be evaluated independently, but this circumstance may represent an exception to the usual recommendation against carotid endarterectomy for acute stroke.

Some medical trials have also considered use of lytic agents in patients with acute stroke or acute carotid occlusions. However, complications of intracerebral bleeding have been reported, and these data are still being analyzed prospectively.

MEDICAL MANAGEMENT

Antiplatelet Therapy

A. Aspirin: Antiplatelet therapy, principally aspirin, has been recommended as a therapeutic intervention for patients with TIAs or nondisabling stroke because of its ability to reduce platelet aggregation. When platelets interact with the atherosclerotic plaque, their aggregation and subsequent embolization account for some neurologic events. Aspirin is a cyclo-oxygenase inhibitor, which prevents platelet aggregation and reduces the incidence of neurologic events. Reduction in the incidence of TIAs was confirmed in the American aspirin study, whereas reduction in stroke and cardiovascular death was reported in the Canadian aspirin trial. Dipyridamole, another platelet suppressant, had no added benefit over aspirin. Both prior trials used the higher dose aspirins protocol (1300 mg/day), however, a dosage of 325 mg/day to reduce platelet activity by 90% without as significant an inhibition of prostacyclin production by the vascu-

lar endothelium is the current recommendation. Gastrointestinal complaints are minimized at this dose. However, a recent meta-analysis demonstrated an only modest difference in the antiplatelet drug treatment group, the incidence of new nonfatal strokes was 8.2%, whereas in the control group the incidence was 10.2%. The impact of aspirin appeared to be more profound with regard to cardiovascular death than to stroke alone.

B. Ticlopidine: Ticlopidine hydrochloride is a newer platelet antiaggregator, which functions primarily as an inhibitor of the adenosine diphosphate pathway of platelet aggregation. Although it does not inhibit the cyclo-oxygenase pathway and does not block the production of thromboxane by platelets or the production of prostacyclin by endothelial cells, ticlopidine does alter platelet function for the normal life span of the platelets. In a recently published trial, ticlopidine showed modest superiority over aspirin. However, an associated risk of gastrointestinal upset as well as bone marrow suppression was reported, which ultimately limits its clinical applicability.

CAROTID ENDARTERECTOMY: RESULTS OF RANDOMIZED CLINICAL TRIALS

Carotid endarterectomy is one of the most commonly performed vascular procedures in this country. Historically, the case reported by Eastcott, Pickering, and Rob in 1954 resulted in the greatest impetus for operative intervention for carotid occlusive disease.

For Asymptomatic Carotid Stenosis

Results of a published clinical trial conducted within the Veterans Administration demonstrated the efficacy of carotid endarterectomy in reducing the combined neurologic events of TIA and stroke. Although stroke alone was reduced by a factor of 2:1 in the surgical group, addition of perioperative mortality resulted in the loss of statistical significance for this endpoint. It now appears that the ongoing and largest clinical trial on asymptomatic carotid stenosis has reached a preliminary conclusion regarding reduction in stroke alone in favor of carotid endarterectomy over medical management.

The asymptomatic carotid atherosclerosis study (ACAS) found that by using Kaplan-Meier projections at 5 years, the primary outcome of ipsilateral stroke, including perioperative mortality, was 4.8% for the surgical group and 10.6% for the medical group (see Table 8–2). These trials have defined the indications for carotid endarterectomy in patients with asymptomatic stenosis. Patients with diameter-reducing stenoses of >60% should be considered for operative intervention, provided the risk of coronary artery disease is identified and the operations are performed by surgeons who have confirmed a low risk for perioperative complications.

For Symptomatic Carotid Stenosis

In patients with recent TIA or nondisabling stroke and high-grade ($\geq$70% diameter reducing stenosis) ipsilateral stenosis, carotid endarterectomy, and optimal medical management significantly reduce stroke and death when compared with optimal medical care only. In the North American (NASCET) trial, after a mean follow-up of 2 years, 26% of the medical care group and 9% of the surgical group experienced a fatal or nonfatal ipsilateral stroke. The European (ECST) trialists have published confirmatory data. These studies have established the significant benefit offered symptomatic patients by carotid endarterectomy. Further study of patients with 30–69% stenoses is required before definitive recommendations can be made on this group with lesser degrees of stenosis.

SURGICAL PROCEDURE

Performance of carotid endarterectomy permits some variations depending on the surgeon's preferences and experience. Although several technical considerations are acceptable, this section reviews the author's preferred technique.

Patient Preparation

General anesthesia is recommended for carotid endarterectomy, although some surgeons have recommended local or cervical block anesthesia. Since the complication rates from operation are difficult to relate to the anesthetic management, informed surgical judgment combined with recommendations from an anesthesiologist should be followed.

The patient is placed in the supine position on the operating table with the shoulders elevated on a rolled sheet and the neck extended and rotated toward the side opposite the proposed endarterectomy. A radial artery cannula is placed routinely for monitoring preanesthetic, operative, and 24-hour postoperative arterial blood pressures. Significant hypotension is managed with intravenous fluids and occasionally with vasopressors. However, significant hypertension is more common, observed in about 20% of cases, and can be managed with intravenous nitroprusside or nitroglycerin.

Operative Technique

With the patient stabilized under endotracheal anesthesia, a longitudinal incision anterior to the sternocleidomastoid muscle is preferred (Fig 8–11, 1). The incision is deepened through the platysma muscle layer anterior to the sternocleidomastoid muscle.

The internal jugular vein is encountered and is a key anatomic feature that directs further dissection toward the underlying carotid artery. Identification and divi-

sion of the major common facial vein between suture ligatures or ligation of multiple venous tributaries from the facial area provide easy lateral retraction of the jugular vein and open the neck to further dissection of the common, internal, and external carotid arteries (Fig 8–11, 2). The dissection is developed around the common carotid artery initially and the vagus nerve identified posteriorly. Gentle dissection in this area is emphasized, and avoidance of electrocautery, which can result in neural injury, is recommended. Dissection is then carried superiorly, and the superior thyroid artery is identified at the junction of the common and external carotid arteries. Its blood flow is controlled by passage of a silk Potts tie (Fig 8–11, 4), and the dissection is then carried superiorly for identification and mobilization of the external carotid artery; dissection is maintained in close proximity to the artery, behind which is located the superior laryngeal nerve. Injury to this nerve can cause troublesome voice fatigue and an unpleasant posterior pharyngeal sensation. The internal carotid artery is then dissected well above the area of the bifurcation and atheroma. Care is taken to avoid dissection of the bifurcation posterolaterally, and the internal carotid is dissected free and surrounded with the vascular tape, taking additional care to avoid trauma to the vagus nerve. Some additional superior dissection is recommended to have complete mobilization of the internal carotid well above the most distal extent of the atherosclerotic plaque. In this dissection, the hypoglossal nerve and its descendens branch are identified. The nerve may be mobilized medially after division of 1 or 2 arterial and venous branches to the sternocleidomastoid muscle. Traction on the divided descendens hypoglossal nerve can also facilitate this medial retraction. Occasionally, division of the tendon of the digastric muscle also facilitates exposure of the more distal internal carotid artery. However, take care to avoid injury to the glossopharyngeal nerve, which is located posterior and somewhat superior to this dissection.

After the appropriate segment of internal carotid artery has been surrounded with a vascular tape, vascular clamps (see Fig 8–11, 5) or Rummel tourniquets (Fig 8–12, 10) can be used for arterial control. Routine use of an intra-arterial shunt is recommended. An appropriate-sized plastic tubing may be used (Fig 8–12, 11); however, recent preference is an armored Silastic shunt (Sundt external endarterectomy shunt, V. Mueller, Chicago, IL). Other options include shunts (Pruitt-Inahara) with balloon control of the internal and common carotid arteries, thus eliminating the need for tourniquets or vascular clamps. Selective shunting guided by measurement of internal carotid back pressure (Fig 8–11, 4) or electroencephalography in patients under general anesthesia as well as evaluation of sensorium in patients under local or regional anesthesia may also be used successfully.

The patient is given heparin and flow through the carotid bifurcation is interrupted by application of the

Rummel tourniquets. An arteriotomy is placed anterolaterally in the common carotid artery and extended superiorly beyond the most distal extent of the lesion so that normal intima is observed before insertion of the shunt. The upper end of the shunt is first inserted into the internal carotid artery. After appropriate backbleeding, the lower end is inserted into the common carotid. Reestablishment of blood flow can usually be accomplished within 60 seconds.

The endarterectomy plane is developed circumferentially, and the plaque is divided in the common carotid artery (see Fig 8–11, 6 and 7). After this, the endarterectomy is extended into the external carotid artery, which is completed by eversion endarterectomy. Completion of the endarterectomy at an endpoint in the internal carotid artery becomes a very important step in the procedure. Great care is exercised in developing the endpoint in the internal carotid artery. Use of alternating flushing and suction of heparinized saline against this area is important to identify even small intimal flaps. Use of tacking sutures to prevent elevation of an intimal flap (see Fig 8–11, 8) is occasionally necessary. Small debris are also carefully removed circumferentially.

With completion of the endarterectomy, the arteriotomy may be closed primarily (see Fig 8–11, 9); or in cases of anatomically smaller arteries, particularly in women, prosthetic or saphenous vein patch angioplasty is currently recommended. When closure at the patch is nearly completed, the shunt is removed and the last few sutures are placed. After appropriate backbleeding to remove any retained thrombus and air, arterial blood flow is restored first to the external carotid artery and then to the internal carotid artery.

Following closure of the arteriotomy, qualitative hemodynamic assessment of the endarterectomy site is performed by insonation of the operative site with a gas-sterilized transducer of a continuous-wave Doppler device. The unusual findings of high-resistance signals in the internal carotid artery, absence of signals over the external carotid artery, or external evidence of any technical deficiencies are indications for operative arteriography. Heparin is then reversed with intravenous protamine sulfate if persistent local soft tissue oozing is apparent. A closed-system drain is placed in the subplatysmal space, and the platysma muscle layer is approximated with absorbable sutures. The skin is closed with a subcuticular absorbable suture and steristrips.

The drain is removed on the first postoperative day. Arterial blood pressure is monitored postoperatively from the radial arterial line and pharmacologic control is used as needed; however, this is generally not required beyond the first 4–6 hours postoperatively.

Complications

The complications following carotid endarterectomy that are of greatest concern are perioperative stroke and death. Mortalities are frequently associated with postoperative myocardial infarction. The upper limits of combined stroke and death after carotid endarterectomy have generally been defined as 3% for asymptomatic carotid stenosis, 5% for TIA, 7% for stroke with permanent deficit, and 10% for restenosis (see Table 8–3). Overall morbidity should be less than 5% with operative mortality less than 2%.

A. Neurologic Complications:

1. Major neurologic deficit–Most neurologic deficits are noted immediately on recovery from anesthesia. Minor deficits can be observed for their evolution. However, for the patient with a immediate postoperative neurologic deficit, return to the operating room for exploration of the carotid bifurcation is advisable rather than delay for noninvasive or invasive testing. At reoperation, thrombosis of the repair site should result in operative reexploration, thrombectomy, and patch angioplasty. If the artery is patent, intraoperative arteriography should be performed to identify any adherent thrombus or technical abnormality, which, if present, should be repaired. For patients with more subtle neurologic deficits, duplex scanning in the intensive care unit may be useful, and arteriography may be considered. Identification of technical errors at the endarterectomy site would result in the recommendation for reoperation.

2. Cranial nerve injury–Transient neurologic deficits occur after endarterectomy owing to injuries to the recurrent laryngeal, hypoglossal nerves, and marginal mandibular branch of the 7th nerve. Injuries to the vagus or glossopharyngeal nerves may result in more significant deficits such as vocal cord paralysis and hoarseness, change in vocal tone, and difficulty with swallowing or coughing. Injury to the superior laryngeal nerve results in troublesome symptoms such as voice fatigue and posterior pharyngeal irritation. Knowledge of the anatomy of the nerves and their relation to carotid bifurcation is essential for the surgeon performing the operation. Although these transient neurologic injuries result in perioperative deficits, most patients recover during a period of 3–6 months postoperatively.

B. Myocardial Infarction: One of the more significant complications of carotid endarterectomy is myocardial infarction. Mortality rate in most clinical series of carotid endarterectomy is less than 2%; however, as emphasized in the recent cooperative trial on asymptomatic carotid stenosis, all mortalities were related to myocardial infarction, whereas occurrence of stroke was not associated with any deaths.

Assessing the presence and severity of coronary artery disease preoperatively constitutes an important aspect of patient management. Chimowitz and the VA group confirmed that men with carotid stenosis and no history of coronary artery disease had a lower rate of cardiac events than men with carotid stenosis and a history of coronary artery disease. However, a subgroup of patients with carotid stenosis and no history of coronary artery disease who had coexistent in-

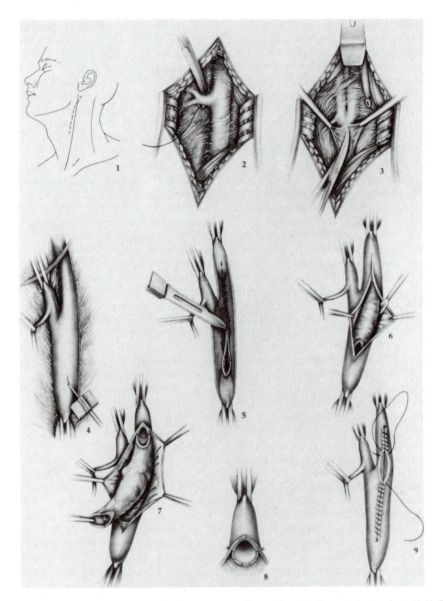

Figures 8–11 and 8–12. Technique of carotid endarterectomy. (Reproduced, with permission, from Veith FJ: Vascular surgical techniques. In: *Vascular Surgery: Principles and Practice,* 2nd ed. Veith FJ, Hobson RW, Williams RA, Wilson SE [editors]. McGraw-Hill, 1994.)

tracranial occlusive disease, diabetes, or peripheral vascular disease were found to have a risk of cardiac events similar to that of patients with a history of coronary disease. These factors have an implication for patients undergoing carotid endarterectomy. In current practice, selective thallium scanning based on clinical criteria is recommended. However, some clinical data emphasize that absence of a history of coronary artery disease is not enough to eliminate this important risk factor in patients selected for carotid endarterectomy.

Although it is acknowledged that screening tests for coronary artery disease will not reduce the currently reported low operative complication rates associated with carotid endarterectomy, these data can be used effectively in identifying patients with significant coronary disease. Data may also indicate further workup for possible coronary angiography, angioplasty, or bypass. In addition, these data may be used to select higher-risk patients for medical management alone, awaiting development of neurologic symptoms before operative intervention. However, this practice should not be adopted as a routine justification for delay.

Further analyses have demonstrated that among adult male patients with high-grade asymptomatic carotid stenosis, an overall mortality rate of 37% was reported at a mean follow-up of 4 years. Multivariate

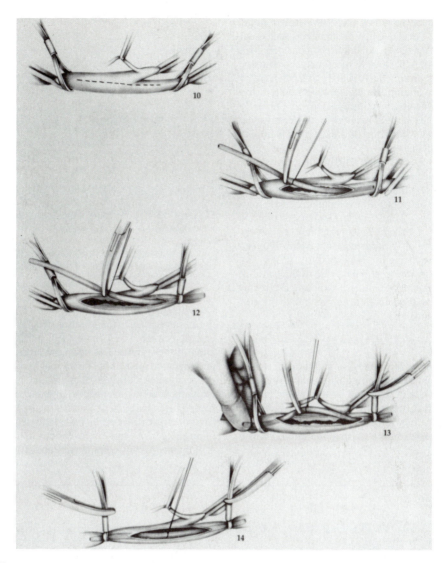

Figure 8–12.

analysis resulted in a demonstrably greater risk for increased mortality rates in the presence of abnormal electrocardiograms, diabetes, and claudication. Patients with 2 or 3 of these risk factors are at high risk of death (see Table 8–2) and may require aggressive treatment of their concurrent medical disease before considering carotid endarterectomy. In this way, risk management assessment becomes a factor in selecting patients for operative intervention. Furthermore, assessment of the risk of stroke in patients with stenoses of more than 75% suggests that this is an appropriate threshold for considering intervention.

Patients with stenoses of less than 50% or between 50% and 75% had a stroke risk of 1.3% annually, whereas those with stenosis of more than 75% had a combined TIA and stroke risk of 10.5% per year (see Table 8–1). Cardiac event rates and vascular deaths correlated with increasing severity of asymptomatic carotid stenosis.

C. Wound Complications: Wound complications including perioperative hematomas develop in about 2–5% of patients undergoing carotid endarterectomy. A large hematoma requires operative evacuation and control of bleeding points. The routine use of suction drains reduces the collection of blood and serum in the wound, but this has not been found to influence the incidence of postoperative hematoma. Wound infections are rare, probably because of the relatively short operative time and the excellent blood supply in the neck.

D. Hypertension/Hypotension: Other complications of moderate concern are hypertension and hypotension, which invariably can be controlled pharmacologically. Note that severe hypertension is associated with an increased incidence of neurologic complications. Consequently, use of agents such as nitroprusside or nitroglycerin should be considered for all patients with hypertensive reactions. Hypotension is less common postoperatively and can be avoided by careful fluid hydration. Rarely, bradycardia and hypotension may be observed intraoperatively caused by stimulation of the carotid body nerve; this can usually be controlled by infiltration of a local anesthetic into the carotid body nerve.

E. Carotid Restenosis: The incidence of symptomatic carotid restenosis following carotid endarterectomy is less than 5%. No consistent association has been found between the development of symptoms and the occurrence of restenosis. Our data established the durability of carotid endarterectomy and documented the cumulative occurrence of restenosis over a 8-year follow-up using life-table analyses (Fig 8–13). Although physicians need to be aware of the possibility of postoperative restenosis, symptomatic recurrences are low and do not directly relate to the degree of recurrent stenosis.

Prognosis

The long-term effectiveness of carotid endarterectomy when combined with optimal medical management has now been confirmed by the results of randomized clinical trials. Stroke risk after carotid endarterectomy has ranged from 0.5% to 1% per year, and the durability of the operation is well established.

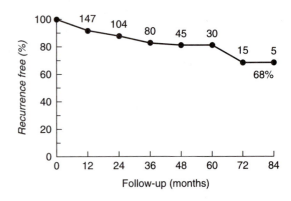

Figure 8–13. The cumulative incidence of hemodynamically significant carotid restenosis after carotid endarterectomy. (Reproduced, with permission, from DeGroote RD et al: Carotid restenosis: Long-term follow-up after carotid endarterectomy. Stroke 1987;18:1031.)

Conclusions

Continued care in the selection of patients for carotid endarterectomy is recommended, particularly as related to the influence of coronary artery disease and perioperative myocardial infarction. Surgical audits on the performance of surgical groups and institutions are recommended to evaluate compliance with recommended standards. In institutions with low postoperative complications, carotid endarterectomy can be recommended for stroke prevention in patients with asymptomatic and symptomatic carotid stenosis.

REFERENCES

Ackerman RH, Candia MR: Identifying clinically relevant carotid disease. Stroke 1994;25:1.

American Heart Association: 1991 Heart and Stroke Facts, 1991.

Anderson RJ, Hobson RW II, Padberg FT Jr et al: Carotid endarterectomy for asymptomatic carotid stenosis: A ten-year experience with 120 procedures in a fellowship training program. Ann Vasc Surg 1991;5:111.

Antiplatelet Trialists Collaboration: Collaborative overview of randomized trials of antiplatelet therapy. I. Prevention of death, myocardial infarction, and stroke by prolonged antiplatelet therapy in various categories of patients. Br Med J 1994;308:81.

Barnes RW et al: The natural history of asymptomatic carotid disease in patients undergoing cardiovascular surgery. Surgery 1981;90:1075.

Barnett HJ, Plum F, Walton JN: Carotid endarterectomy: An expression of concern. Stroke 1984;15:941.

Blackshear WM Jr et al: Detection of carotid occlusive disease by ultrasonic imaging and pulsed Doppler spectrum analysis. Surgery 1979;86:698.

Bove EL et al: Hypotension and hypertension as consequences of baroreceptor dysfunction following carotid endarterectomy. Surg 1971;86:633.

Brener BJ et al: A four-year experience with preoperative noninvasive carotid evaluation of two thousand twenty-six patients undergoing cardiac surgery. J Vasc Surg 1984;1:326.

Brock RW, Lusby RJ: Carotid plaque morphology and interpretation of the echolucent lesion. In: *Diagnostic Vascular Ultrasound.* Labs KH (editor). Edward Arnold, 1992.

Canadian Cooperative Study Group: A randomized trial of aspirin and sulfinpyrazone in threatened stroke. N Engl J Med 1978;299:53.

Chambers BR, Norris JW: Outcome in patients with asymptomatic neck bruits. N Engl J Med 1986;315:860.

Chambers BR, Norris JW: The case against surgery for asymptomatic carotid stenosis. Stroke 1984;15:964.

Chimowitz MI et al: Cardiac prognosis of patients with carotid stenosis and no history of coronary artery disease. Stroke 1994;25:759.

Cohen SN et al: Death associated with asymptomatic carotid artery stenosis: Long-term clinical evaluation. J Vasc Surg 1993;18:100.

Colgan MP, Kingston V, Shanik G: Stenosis following carotid endarterectomy. Arch Surg 1984;119:1033.

Crouse JR et al: Risk factors for extracranial carotid artery atherosclerosis. Stroke 1987;16:990.

DeGroote RD, Lynch TG, Jamil Z, Hobson RW: Carotid restenosis: Long term invasive follow-up after carotid endarterectomy. Stroke 1987;18:1031.

Dennis M, Bamford J, Sandercock P, Warlow C: Prognosis of transient ischemic attacks in the Oxfordshire Community Stroke Project. Stroke 1990;21:848.

Dixson S et al: Natural history of nonstenotic asymptomatic ulcerative lesions of the carotid artery. Arch Surg 1982; 117:1493.

Durward QJ, Ferguson GG, Barr HWK: The natural history of asymptomatic carotid bifurcation plaques. Stroke 1982; 13:459.

Dyken ML, Pokras R: The performance of endarterectomy for disease of the extracranial arteries of the head. Stroke 1984;15:948.

Eastcott HHG, Pickering GW, Rob C: Reconstruction of internal carotid artery in a patient with intermittent attacks of hemiplegia. Lancet 1954;994.

Eliasziw M et al: The North American Symptomatic Carotid Endarterectomy Trial: Significance of plaque ulceration in symptomatic patients with high-grade carotid stenosis. Stroke 1994;25:304.

Feinberg WM et al: Guidelines for the Management of Transient Ischemic Attacks (from the Ad Hoc Committee on Guidelines for the Management of Transient Ischemic Attacks of the Stroke Council of the American Heart Association). Stroke 1994;25:1320.

Fields WS: Symptomatic extracranial vascular disease: Natural history and medical management. In: *Vascular Surgery: Principles and Practice,* 2nd ed. Veith FJ, Hobson RW, Williams RA, Wilson SE (editors). McGraw-Hill, 1994:611.

Fields WS et al: Controlled trial of aspirin in cerebral ischemia. Stroke 1977;8:301.

Gee W, Mehigan JT, Wylie EJ: Measurement of collateral cerebral hemispheric blood pressure by ocular pneumoplethysmography. Am J Surg 1975;130:121.

Goldstone J, Moore WS: Emergency carotid artery surgery in neurologically unstable patients. Arch Surg 1976;111: 1284.

Gross CR et al: Interobserver agreement in the diagnosis of stroke type. Arch Neurol 1986;43:893.

Harward TRS, Kroener JM, Wickbom IG, Bernstein EF: Natural history of asymptomatic ulcerative plaques of the carotid bifurcation. Am J Surg 1983;146:208.

Hass WK et al: A randomized trial comparing ticlopidine hydrochloride with aspirin for the prevention of stroke in high risk patients. N Engl J Med 1989;321:501.

Hennerici M et al: Incidence of asymptomatic extracranial disease. Stroke 1981;12:750.

Hertzer NR, Arison R: Cumulative stroke and survival ten years after carotid endarterectomy. J Vasc Surg 1985;2:661.

Hertzer NR et al: A prospective study of incidence of injury to the cranial nerves during carotid endarterectomy. Surg Gynecol Obstet 1980;151:781.

Heyman A et al: Risk of ischemic heart disease in patients with TIA. Neurology 1984;34:626.

Heyman W et al: Risk of stroke in asymptomatic persons with cervical arterial bruits: A population study in Evans County, Georgia. N Engl J Med 1980;302:838.

Hobson RW, Strandness DE Jr.: Carotid artery stenosis: What's in the measurement? J Vasc Surg 1993;18:1069.

Hobson RW et al and the Veterans Affairs Cooperative Study Group: Efficacy of carotid endarterectomy for asymptomatic carotid stenosis. N Engl J Med 1993;328:221.

Hobson RW et al: Influence of aspirin in the management of asymptomatic carotid artery stenosis. J Vasc Surg 1993; 17:257.

Humphries AW et al: Unoperated asymptomatic significant internal carotid artery stenosis: A review of 182 instances. Surgery 1976;80:695.

Johnson N et al: Carotid endarterectomy: A follow-up study of the contralateral nonoperated carotid artery. Ann Surg 1978;188:748.

Koslow AR et al: Reexploration for thrombosis in carotid endarterectomy. Circulation 1989;80:73.

Langsfeld M, Gray-Weale AC, Lusby RJ: The role of plaque morphology and diameter reduction in the development of new symptoms in asymptomatic carotid arteries. J Vasc Surg 1989;9:548.

Levin SM, Sondheimer FK, Levin JM: The contralateral disease but asymptomatic carotid artery: To operate or not? An update. Am J Surg 1980;140:203.

Levy DE: How transient are transient ischemic attacks? Neurology 1988;38:674.

Lusby RJ et al: Carotid plaque hemorrhage: Its role in production of cerebral ischemia. Arch Surg 1982;117: 1479.

Masotti G et al: Differential inhibition of prostacyclin production and platelet aggregation by aspirin. Lancet 1979; 1:1213.

Mayberg MR et al: Carotid endarterectomy and prevention of cerebral ischemia in symptomatic carotid stenosis. JAMA 1991;266:3289.

Mohr JP, Gautier JC, Pessin MS: Internal carotid artery disease. In: *Stroke: Pathophysiology, Diagnosis, and Management.* Barnett HJM, Mohr JP, Stein BM, Yatsu FM (editors). Churchill Livingstone, 1992:285.

Moneta GL et al: Correlation of North American Carotid Endarterectomy Trial (NASCET) angiographic definition of 70% to 90% internal carotid artery stenosis with Duplex scanning. J Vasc Surg 1993;17:152.

Moore DJ et al: Are strokes predictable with noninvasive methods: A five-year follow-up of 303 unoperated patients. J Vasc Surg 1985;2:654.

Moore WS et al: Natural history of nonstenotic asymptomatic ulcerative lesions of the carotid artery. Arch Surg 1978;113:1352.

Moore WS et al: Indications for carotid endarterectomy: A multidisciplinary consensus statement. Stroke (in press).

Moore WS, Boren C, Malone JM, Goldstone J: Asymptomatic carotid stenosis: Immediate and long-term results after prophylactic endarterectomy. Am J Surg 1979;138: 228.

Nicolaides A: Consensus statement on the management of patients with asymptomatic carotid lesions. Int Angiol (in press).

Norris JW et al: Vascular risks of asymptomatic carotid stenosis. Stroke 1991;22:1485.

O'Leary DH et al: Cholesterol and carotid atherosclerosis in older persons: The Framingham Study. Ann Epidemiol 1992;2:147.

Podore PC et al: Asymptomatic contralateral carotid endarterectomy. Surgery 1980;88:748.

Rich NM, Hobson RW: Carotid endarterectomy under regional anesthesia. Am Surg 1975;41:253.

Roederer GP et al: The natural history of carotid arterial disease in asymptomatic patients with cervical bruits. Stroke 1984;15:605.

Role of carotid endarterectomy in asymptomatic carotid stenosis: A Veterans Administration Cooperative Study. Stroke 1986;17:534.

Rutan GH, McDonald RH, Kuller LH: A historical perspective of elevated systolic vs diastolic blood trial viewpoint. J Clin Epidemiol 1989;42:663.

Salenius JP et al: Rate of carotid restenosis: Etiologic factors for recurrent carotid artery stenosis during long term follow up. Eur J Vasc Surg 1989;3:271.

Salonen R, Seppanen K, Rauramaa R, Salonen JT: Prevalence of carotid atherosclerosis and serum cholesterol levels in eastern Finland. Atherosclerosis 1988;8:788.

Shinton R, Beevers G: Meta-analysis of relation between cigarette smoking and stroke. Br Med J 1989;298:789.

Strandness DE Jr: Extracranial arterial disease. In: *Duplex Scanning in Vascular Disorders.* Strandness DE Jr (editor). Raven Press, 1990:90.

Sze PC et al: Antiplatelet agents in the secondary prevention of stroke: Meta-analysis of the randomized control trials. Stroke 1988;19:436.

The Asymptomatic Carotid Atherosclerosis Study Group: Study design for randomized prospective trial of carotid endarterectomy for asymptomatic atherosclerosis. Stroke 1989;20:844.

The CASANOVA Study Group: Carotid surgery versus medical therapy in asymptomatic carotid stenosis. Stroke 1991;22:1229.

Thompson JE: Carotid surgery: Historial review. In: *Surgery for Stroke,* Greenhalgh RM, Hollier LH (editors). WB Saunders, 1993:3.

Thompson JF, Patman RD, Talking CM: Asymptomatic carotid bruit: Long-term outcome in patients having endarterectomy compared with unoperated controls. Ann Surg 1978;188:308.

Toole JF: NIH Clinical Advisory, National Institute of Neurological Disorders and Stroke. September 1994. NIH, Bethesda, Maryland.

Toole JF: The Willis lecture: Transient ischemic attacks, scientific method, and new realities. Stroke 1991;22:99.

Towne JB, Weiss DG, Hobson RW: First phase report of cooperative VA asymptomatic carotid stenosis study: Operative morbidity and mortality. J Vasc Surg 1990;11:252.

Warlow C: Carotid endarterectomy: Does it work? Stroke 1984;15:1086.

Wechsler LR: Ulceration and carotid artery disease. Stroke 1988;19:650.

White MF: Reducing cardiovascular risk factors in the United States: An overview of the National Educational Programs. Cardiovasc Risk Factors 1991;1:277.

Whitney DG, Kahn EM, Estes JW, Jones CE: Carotid artery surgery without a temporary indwelling shunt. Arch Surg 1980;115:1393.

Wolf PA, Cobb JL, D'Agostino RB: Epidemiology of stroke. In: *Stroke: Pathophysiology, Diagnosis, and Management.* Barnett HJM, Mohr JP, Stein BM, Yatsu FM (editors). Churchill Livingstone, 1992:3.

Wolf PA, D'Agostino RB, Belanger AJ, Kannel WB: Probability of stroke: A risk profile from the Framingham Study. Stroke 1991;22:312.

Wolf PA et al: Asymptomatic carotid bruit and the risk of stroke. JAMA 1981;245:1442.

Zierler BE, Bandyt DF, Thiele BL, Standness DE: Carotid artery stenosis following endarterectomy. Arch Surg 1982;117:1408.

Zukowski AJ et al: Incidence of CT scan cerebral infarction in relation to carotid plaque ulceration. J Vasc Surg 1984;1:782.

Vertebrobasilar Ischemia

9

Ramon Berguer, MD, PhD

Essentials of Diagnosis

- Dizziness, vertigo, diplopia, blurring of vision, alternating paresthesias, tinnitus, and drop attacks.
- Exclusion of systemic causes of symptoms (eg, drug-induced hypotension, cardiac arrhythmias, orthostatism).
- Arteriogram of appropriate anatomic lesion in the vertebral or basilar artery.

General Considerations

The concept of **vertebrobasilar ischemia** (VBI) has changed over the last decade. The term "vertebrobasilar insufficiency" is beginning to disappear, just as the term "carotid insufficiency" did a decade ago. VBI denotes global ischemia of the territory supplied by the basilar artery because of inadequate blood flow. This may result from central hypotension or from a drop in blood pressure within the vertebrobasilar (VB) system because of an occlusion or an obstructing lesion in the proximal subclavian artery, the vertebral artery (VA), or the basilar artery. Vertebrobasilar ischemia is a broader but more appropriate description because it includes global ischemia as well as focal ischemia secondary to embolization from the heart, the proximal left subclavian, the VA, or the basilar artery. This descriptor is more acceptable because it embraces both hemodynamic and embolic mechanisms responsible for the symptoms.

Arterial embolization is a well-recognized mechanism responsible for about 70% of carotid ischemia symptoms. It is the underlying mechanism of VBI in about 30% of cases. Pathologic studies show that in most patients who have a thrombus lodged in a branch of the basilar artery, no plaque is found subjacent to it when the embolus is removed. This suggests that the obstructing thrombus was formed elsewhere and underwent embolization into its resting site.

In some patients, the symptoms of VBI appear only with rotation, extension, or flexion of the neck. In these cases, the VA traveling in an osteomuscular conduit in the neck is compressed when the vertebrae are rotated. The compressing agent is usually an osteophyte in the cervical spine, but occasionally other structures such as the arch of the atlas or the tendon of the longus colli may be responsible (Fig 9–1).

The relevance of embolization in the pathogenesis of transient ischemic attacks (TIAs) and strokes in the posterior cirulation has been underestimated due to a limited understanding of the pathologic mechanisms of VBI.

Surgical correction of VA lesions responsible for VBI developed a decade later than carotid artery surgery because of the limited understanding of the mechanisms involved, the difficulty in visualizing these lesions with standard arteriographic techniques, and the technical problems attending the exposure and repair of a small artery that courses deep in the neck and is covered by bone and muscles. Surgical experience with repair of the VA and longitudinal follow-up of these patients have been substantive for more than a decade. The outcome of operations on the VA, when the indications are strict, is actually better than the outcome of operations done on the carotid artery.

Types of Lesions

Atherosclerosis is the most common underlying problem in VBI. **Plaque formation** results in stenosing lesions that may affect the VA at any level but are most common at its origin from the subclavian. Plaques in the VA show the same degenerative features as plaques that appear elsewhere, such as ulceration, intraplaque hemorrhage, and surface thrombus. The growth of a plaque may ultimately result in thrombosis of the VA.

The VA can also be compressed by bone, mostly by osteophytes, throughout its cervical trajectory. It is subjected to motion and stretching in the segment between C2 and its entrance at the skull. At this level where most of the neck rotation occurs, and traumatic injuries secondary to brisk deceleration or rotation of the head are often seen. Dissections and arteriovenous aneurysms, which are often related to trauma, are particularly common in this segment as well (Fig 9–2).

Clinical Findings

A. Signs and Symptoms: The spectrum of symptoms of VBI patients includes dizziness, diplopia, vertigo, tinnitus, perioral numbness, drop attacks, and alternating paresthesias. Although dizziness is the most common symptom, it is generally associated with other symptoms.

Two patterns of clinical presentation of VBI are recognized, depending on whether the patient has **hemodynamic** or **embolic** ischemia. Hemodynamic symp-

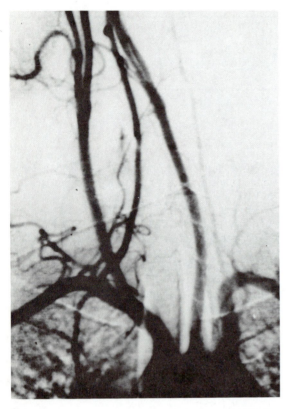

A

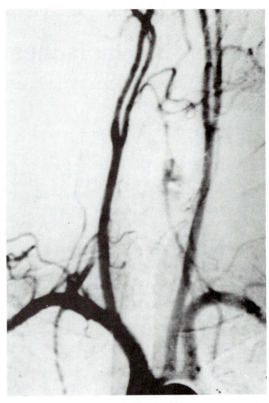

B

Figure 9–1. Arteriogram showing occlusion of a dominant vertebral artery when patient's head is rotated. **A:** With head turning to right, a single right vertebral artery supplies the posterior circulation. **B:** With head turning to left, the dominant right vertebral artery is occluded by the longus colli tendon.

toms tend to be brief in duration and stereotyped. They appear frequently and can generally be triggered by changes in the position of the patient's body or neck and can be relieved by lying down. Thromboembolic symptoms tend to last longer and to be varied in presentation. They are independent of body and neck position and are generally accompanied by findings of small infarctions in magnetic resonance imaging (MRI) of the brain stem (Fig 9–3).

Prognoses associated with the 2 types of ischemia are also different: strokes are uncommon in **hemodynamic** VBI patients, who experience complications derived from loss of balance (mainly falls), automobile accidents, and other mishaps. **Thromboembolic** disease of the VB system has a grim prognosis, carries a high risk of permanent neurologic deficits, and may be life threatening.

B. History: History taking includes ascertaining how often and under what conditions symptoms occur. Patients with hemodynamic VBI can often identify a body position or a particular neck motion that triggers the symptom. The most common trigger is an orthostatic mechanism in which the patient experiences symptoms when changing from a lying or sitting position to a standing position. In VBI patients, symptoms

are often triggered by a fall in central blood pressure as a result of vasomotor paralysis, such as occurs in diabetics and in persons taking ganglion blockers. The postulated mechanism in these patients is that a stenosis or thrombosis of the VA or basilar artery has already caused a blood pressure drop in the VB system under basal conditions. This pressure drop is further accentuated (thus becomes critical and asymptomatic) when the central blood pressure drops as the patient stands up.

In patients who experience symptoms on rotation of the head, the hypotension of the VB system is caused by the temporary occlusion of the VA, usually by extrinsic compression. Although arrhythmias infrequently are seen in patients with VBI, the patient should be questioned regarding a history of irregular heartbeat or palpitations occurring before or in conjunction with bouts of VBI.

C. Physical Examination: Examination should begin with the recording of blood pressure and pulses in both upper extremities. An absent or markedly decreased radial pulse should raise the suspicion of a subclavian stenosis with a subclavian-vertebral steal. This condition should be ruled out as a likely mechanism whenever the pressure difference between both

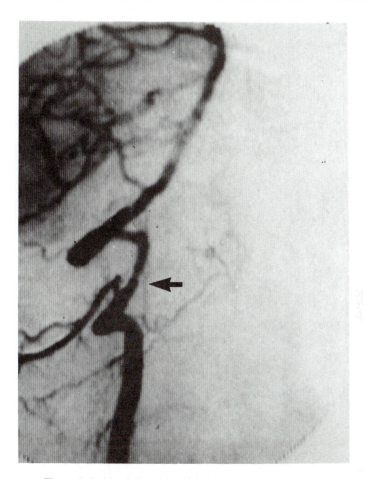

Figure 9–2. Mural dissection of the distal vertebral artery.

brachial arteries is greater than 20 mmHg. Likewise, in a patient who has symptoms on standing, the brachial pressure should be measured when the patient is lying down and immediately after standing up. A systolic pressure difference greater than 20 mmHg suggests orthostatic hypotension. If the symptoms are caused by rotation, flexion, or extension of the neck, they should be reproduced with the patient sitting up. The patient's head should be moved slowly to the trigger position with the physician being ready to assist the patient if loss of consciousness or imbalance occurs.

D. Imaging Studies: Duplex sonography has limited use for evaluation of VA disease, although it can show reversal of flow in cases of subclavian-vertebral steal. This diagnosis can also be made by demonstrating a delay greater than 5 msec during simultaneous recording of both radial artery waveforms with a continuous wave Doppler instrument.

In patients with thromboembolic VBI, the MRI scans of the brain may show small infarctions in the brain stem or cerebellum, which were previously missed by computed tomography (CT). On rare occasions, MRI of the brain may disclose an unexpected tumor as being responsible for the patient's symptoms.

To show the arterial lesion that may be the cause of the problem, obtain a 4-vessel arteriogram with selective injections into both carotids and both subclavian arteries to outline the anterior and posterior circulations. Arteriography of the VA requires special oblique projections to show its origin, usually superimposed partially by the subclavian artery. Patients with VBI triggered by specific head positions need to have the arteriogram performed with the head and neck positioned to provoke symptoms during the injection. Unless this is done, the VA compression and its mechanism will probably not be demonstrated by arteriography (Fig 9–4).

Differential Diagnosis

If VBI symptoms appear only on standing, the presence and degree of orthostatism should be investigated. This can be accomplished by the maneuvers previously discussed in the section on History. Transient hypoglycemia should be ruled out, although pallor and sweating are not part of the VBI syndrome.

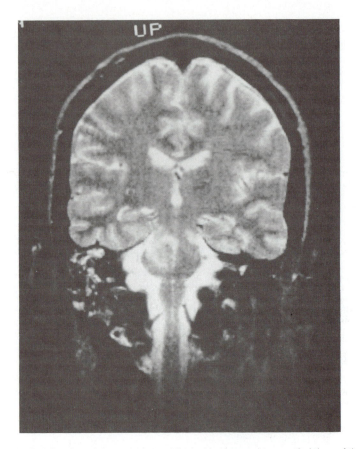

Figure 9–3. Thromboembolic infarction of the pons in a patient with repeated traumatic injury of the vertebral artery by an osteophyte.

Symptomatic subclavian steal syndrome presents as VBI of hemodynamic type. An absent or decreased radial pulse or a systolic difference in pressure in both brachial arteries indicates hemodynamic VBI. Anemia and brain tumors are rare causes of VBI symptoms and can be detected by a complete blood count (CBC) and CT scanning of the brain. Transient arrhythmias are diagnosed by Holter monitoring. In a minority of patients, echocardiography may reveal a potential source of embolization in the heart.

The internal carotid artery system should be thoroughly evaluated. Severe bilateral disease of the internal carotid arteries may result in VB hypotension, particularly in patients with hypoplastic or occluded vertebral arteries. Duplex examination of the carotids should be done in all patients presenting with VBI.

Treatment

Patients with orthostatic VBI symptoms may become asymptomatic when the orthostatic trigger mechanism is abolished. Treatment of affected patients may consist of a readjustment or change in blood pressure medication, the use of elastic stockings, and advice on how to avoid sudden changes in position by learning to use small steps when going from a lying or sitting position to a standing position. Alpha-blockers are used for treatment of this condition by European neurologists.

If symptoms persist despite these simple measures and if the arteriogram shows a critical lesion of the dominant VA or both VAs, consideration should be given to correction of the anatomic blockage. Although the ostial lesions are theoretically amenable to Permtaneous transluminal augioplasty, experience with this procedure is very limited. The plaque in the ostium of the vertebral artery is always a continuation of the plaque in the subclavian artery, and this may cause complications. The limited experience reported with PTA of plaques at the origin of the VA involves only short-term follow-up, and early results are not as good as those obtained by surgical repair.

Stenosing lesions at the origin of the VA are the most common lesions found in patients presenting with VBI. It is empirically accepted that hemodynamic VBI should not be incriminated to a VA stenosis/

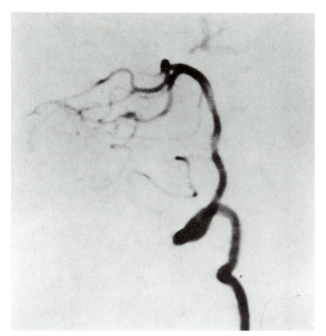
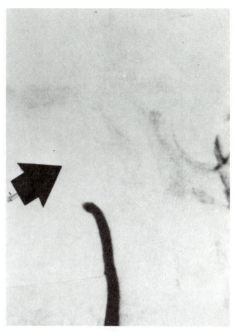

A   **B**

Figure 9–4. Uncommon site of extrinsic compression of the vertebral artery between the atlas and the occipital bone. **A:** Normal arteriogram with the head in neutral position. **B:** Severe compression of VA and poor filling of the basilar artery and its branches when head is rotated to the right. (Reproduced, by permission, from Berguer R, Kieffer E [editors]: *Surgery of the Arteries to the Head.* Springer-Verlag, 1992.)

occlusion if the opposite VA is normal and ends in the basilar artery. The current indications for correction of an ostial lesion require that both VAs (if present) be severely involved (≥75% cross-sectional area). A stenosis greater than 75% in a patient with a single VA is also considered a hemodynamically critical lesion. In thromboembolic VBI, these considerations do not apply. If the source of thromboembolism can be demonstrated, it is excluded by an operation, regardless of the condition of the other VA.

Stenotic lesions at the origin of the VA are most commonly dealt with by dividing the artery above the stenosis and transposing it to the neighboring carotid artery—a **vertebral-to-carotid transposition** (Fig 9–5). Other techniques infrequently used in specific instances are subclavian-VA bypasses with autogenous vein and transposition of an elongated VA to another subclavian site with the stenotic origin left behind.

Compression of the VA in the cervical spine, usually by osteophytes, can be repaired by a bypass or transposition to the level of C2, at which the artery is most accessible. Even when the proximal VA is thrombosed below, it is usually patent at the C2–C1 level. Above this level, the VA is seldom involved by atherosclerosis or compressed extrinsically.

Of the 3 common methods of reconstruction of the VA at the C2–C1 interval, the most frequently used is

a common carotid-to-distal VA bypass using saphenous vein. Other times, the external carotid artery can be dissected with its branches ligated and divided and the artery transposed to the VA (Fig 9–6). Finally, the distal VA itself can be moved forward and anastomosed to the distal cervical internal carotid artery. The rare lesions above the C1 segment are usually aneurysms or external compression. They are difficult to access, since generally part of the atlas has to be removed for exposure.

Prognosis

The operative risk in proximal VA reconstruction is substantially lower than that for distal operations. For patients undergoing only proximal VA reconstruction, the mortality and morbidity rates are less than 1%. The primary patency of these operations after 10 years is 86%. Distal vertebral reconstructions hold a higher risk; the death/stroke rate is 3.5%.

Some persons have combined carotid and VA disease. At first, it made sense to perform both operations at the same time, provided that the lesions were on the same side of the neck to allow a surgical approach through the same incision. Results have shown, however, that the morbidity/mortality rates of combined carotid-VA reconstruction are greater than the sum of the specific death/stroke rates for carotid and proximal

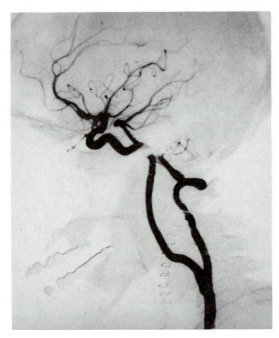

Figure 9–6. Postoperative arteriogram showing an external carotid artery, with all its branches ligated, anastomosed to the distal vertebral artery below C1.

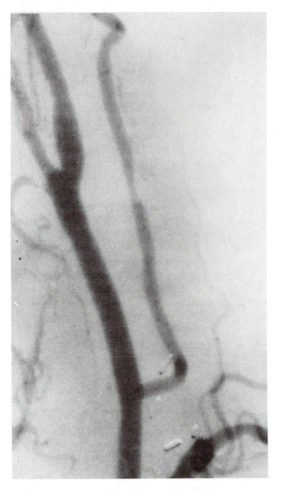

Figure 9–5. Postoperative arteriogram after a vertebral-to-carotid transposition. The vertebral artery was divided above its stenotic origin and anastomosed to the common carotid artery.

VA operations performed separately. The combined operations carry a death/stroke rate of 3.5%. This is probably because patients in this combined group tend to have extensive extracranial disease and are higher surgical risks. In patients with combined symptomatic carotid and VA disease, it is important to determine which of the 2 vessels is the source of symptoms and focus on surgically correcting it.

REFERENCES

Amarenco P et al: Les infarctus du territoire de l'artère cérébelleuse posteroinférieure: Étude clinico-pathologique des 28 cas. Rev Neurol 1989;145:277.

Berguer R: Long-term results of reconstructions of the vertebral artery. In: *Long-term Results in Vascular Surgery*. Yao J, Pierce W (editors). Appleton & Lange, 1993.

Berguer R, Higgins R, Nelson R: Noninvasive diagnosis of reversal of vertebral flow. N Engl J Med 1980;302:1349.

Berguer R, Kieffer E: *Surgery of the Arteries of the Head*. Springer-Verlag, 1992.

Caplan LR, Tettenborn B: Embolism in the posterior circulation. In: *Vertebrobasilar Arterial Disease*. Berguer R, Caplan LR (editors). Quality Medical Publishing, 1992.

Castaigne P et al: Arterial occlusions in the vertebral-basilar system. Brain 1973;96:133.

Davis SM et al: Magnetic resonance imaging in posterior circulation infarction: Impact on diagnosis and management. Aust NZ J Med 1989;19:219.

Rancurel G et al: Hemodynamic vertebrobasilar ischemia: Differentiation of hemodynamic and thromboembolic mechanisms. In: *Vertebrobasilar Arterial Disease*. Berguer R, Caplan LR (editors). Quality Medical Publishing, 1992.

Sypert GW, Alvord EC: Cerebellar infarction: A clinico-pathologic study. Arch Neurol 1975;32:357.

Nonatherosclerotic Disease of the Cerebral Vasculature

10

David H. Deaton, MD, & Wesley S. Moore, MD

Atherosclerotic disease of the extracranial vasculature, particularly the carotid bifurcation, is the primary cause of symptomatic cerebral vascular disease, but a variety of other conditions can lead to symptomatic cerebral ischemia and infarction. Patients with the following conditions often present in a manner similar to or identical with atherosclerotic lesions with symptoms of transient ischemic attack (TIA) or stroke:

- Radiation injury
- Fibromuscular dysplasia
- Temporal arteritis
- Carotid artery dissection
- Carotid coils and kinks
- Takayasu's arteritis
- Carotid body tumors
- Aneurysms of the extracranial cerebral vasculature

Elements of the initial history and physical examination are the keys to identifying these patients, since subsequent evaluation and therapy differ from what is prescribed for a patient with an atherosclerotic lesion. Duplex Doppler examination, contrast-enhanced computed tomography (CT), magnetic resonance imaging (MRI), and arteriography imaging each have their own advantages in the evaluation of these lesions but cannot be efficiently used unless the clinical suspicion for these less common lesions has been aroused.

A careful history and physical examination are imperative for identifying the patient whose symptoms might originate from a disease process other than atherosclerosis. Fibromuscular disease and Takayasu's arteritis typically occur in younger females. Accelerated atherosclerotic changes are seen in patients with a history of radiation therapy. Elderly females with ocular symptoms and headaches may well have temporal or giant cell arteritis. Patients with aneurysms, carotid body tumor, or carotid kinks or coils are identified by careful examination and the finding of a pulsatile neck mass. Intimal dissection of the extracranial cerebral vasculature can occur in patients with a history of blunt trauma or heavy physical exertion. These elements of the initial encounter can narrow the differential diagnosis and indicate the appropriate imaging study necessary to arrive at a final diagnosis.

As with atherosclerotic diseases of the carotid bifurcation, initial medical therapy is directed at the inhibition of platelet aggregation. Aspirin is the first line of therapy and should be prescribed in any patient who has had TIA symptoms prior to surgical intervention. If symptoms are recurrent or if surgical correction is not possible, ticlopidine is the next agent of choice and offers a more complete inhibition of platelet aggregation. For patients unresponsive to platelet inhibition or thought to be at risk for thrombosis, anticoagulation with coumadin can be used to elevate the patient's prothrombin time to a ratio of 1.5–1.7 over normal. Medical therapy offers only partial protection from the potential morbidity of an embolic source. Ablation of the lesion that is the source of the emboli is the most effective and durable therapy.

RADIATION INJURY

Essentials of Diagnosis
- Stenosis years after irradiation.
- Plaques with fibrosis, fatty infiltration, intimal destruction.
- Carotid artery aneurysmal degeneration or rupture.

General Considerations
Therapeutic radiation that affects the extracranial cerebral vasculature is usually performed to eradicate a tumor with or without adjunctive surgery. In general, radiation leads to an acceleration of the affected atherosclerotic lesions. In patients with no risk factors and little evidence of atherosclerotic disease, a lesion of the carotid bifurcation might manifest many years after radiation therapy and without concomitant lesions in the arterial tree.

Clinical Findings
A. Signs and Symptoms: For patients with significant preexisting atherosclerosis, a shorter time period to critical stenosis is seen in the affected area. The average interval between irradiation and cerebrovascular symptoms is nearly 20 years, although a wide variability (5–37 years) is seen. The development of lesions nearly identical with those of atherosclerosis has been confirmed experimentally in dogs that devel-

oped aortic lesions after either x-ray or electron-beam irradiation. Irradiated arteries have an increased permeability to circulating lipids and an impaired ability to repair elastic tissue. The plaques in these lesions are characterized by fibrosis, fatty infiltration, and intimal destruction.

Carotid artery aneurysmal degeneration or rupture ("blow-out") is another manifestation of radiation treatment. This occurs most often in the setting of a large extirpative procedure in the region of the carotid with dissection of the artery followed by radiation therapy. Rupture can occur without surgical intervention as well. Several investigators have noted a late incidence of both extracranial and intracranial cerebrovascular lesions in patients receiving radiation therapy for pituitary tumors. This finding is of particular importance in the treatment of children, whose radiation dosage should be minimized to prevent future cerebrovascular complications. Francfort and associates (1989) reported an increased incidence of airway problems in patients undergoing surgery for vascular lesions after radiation therapy. The cause of these airway problems included (1) endotracheal tube trauma to the fixed irradiated vocal cords, (2) laryngeal edema caused by surgical dissection in an irradiated field, and (3) hypercarbia as a result of bilateral carotid body ablation.

Treatment

The technical aspects of any operation in an irradiated field can be complicated by induration of the soft tissues and concerns about wound healing. These factors have persuaded some investigators to recommend alternative methods for cerebral revascularization. Others note that, once isolated, the vessels can be repaired in a standard fashion. In general, radiation therapy can exacerbate and accelerate the progression of atherosclerosis and complicate the technical aspects of surgical intervention through its effects on soft tissue fibrosis and vascularity.

FIBROMUSCULAR DYSPLASIA

Essentials of Diagnosis

- Lesion in medium-sized vessel.
- Most frequently seen in women.
- Often bilateral lesions.
- "String of beads" stenoses.

Fibromuscular dysplasia (FMD) is a nonatherosclerotic lesion affecting medium-sized vessels first reported in the carotid artery in 1964. The 4 types of FMD are intimal fibroplasia, medial hyperplasia, medial fibroplasia, and perimedial dysplasia. Most patients (~90%) with FMD are women. Although most present with either TIAs or amaurosis fugax, about 22% will present with stroke. As much as 30% of these patients will also have evidence of intracranial disease,

and up to 65% will have bilateral manifestations of FMD. The lesion is most often a series of noncritical stenoses in either one or both carotid arteries, characterized as a "string of beads" angiographically, which are presumably responsible for the embolic phenomena. Other lesions have been described in conjunction with FMD including aneurysms, carotid-cavernous fistula, arterial webs, and intimal dissection.

The standard surgical approach to FMD is open internal carotid arterial dilatation with destruction of the constricting bands of hyperplastic tissue that are responsible for the irregular surface of the artery and that lead to embolization. Percutaneous transluminal angioplasty has also been used to treat this lesion but suffers theoretically in its inability to allow retrograde bleeding after the dilatation to clear any debris. Those who have identified intimal webs in the carotid circulation point out that neurologic symptoms are repetitive in these patients and feel that this lesion represents a greater risk. Fistulas have been treated successfully with detachable balloons, and aneurysms are treated most often by resection and interposition grafting. FMD of the extracranial cerebral vasculature is a lesion with the potential for catastrophic morbidity in a young patient population but is easily treated when diagnosed.

TEMPORAL ARTERITIS

Essentials of Diagnosis

- Aortic inflammatory changes.
- Most common in white women over 55 years.
- Headaches.
- Pain in pelvic and shoulder girdles.
- Visual disturbances.
- Erythema and nodularity over temporal artery.

Temporal arteritis, or systemic giant cell arteritis, is a systemic process with chronic inflammatory changes of the aorta and its major branches. It is most often seen in older (>55 years) white females in conjunction with headaches and pain in both the pelvic and shoulder girdles, often referred to as **polymyalgia rheumatica.** Visual disturbance as a result of either ischemic optic or retrobulbar neuritis or central retinal artery occlusion is a particularly devastating complication of this condition. A recent Danish series recorded that about 3–4% of referred patients had some visual loss and that one patient in their series of 51 patients had bilateral blindness. Visual symptoms can be confusing in this population, which would otherwise be considered at risk for carotid atherosclerotic disease. The condition is often diagnosed by the discovery of erythema and nodularity with tenderness over the course of the temporal artery. An elevated erythrocyte sedimentation rate and a positive temporal artery biopsy confirm the diagnosis. Angiography reveals long smooth stenotic segments interspersed with normal-appearing artery.

Treatment

Steroid administration is the first line of therapy in temporal arteritis and is often effective in preventing significant visual loss and slowing or reversing serious aortic lesions. Surgical therapy is reserved for lesions that are residual after steroid therapy without evidence of active vasculitis. Although peripheral arterial involvement is much less common than aortic involvement, it does occur. Subclavian involvement is more common than carotid or vertebral disease, which is rare. Vein bypass graft from the subclavian to the carotid has been described in the unusual case of significant carotid disease with residual symptoms after steroid therapy. Temporal arteritis should always be considered in elderly white females with visual symptoms regardless of concomitant carotid atherosclerotic disease.

CAROTID ARTERY DISSECTION

Essentials of Diagnosis

- Trauma or heavy exertion 2 weeks to 6 months before symptoms.
- Unilateral headaches.
- Ipsilateral Horner's syndrome.
- Cranial Nerve Palsies.

General Considerations

Intimal dissection of the carotid or vertebral arteries is most often the sequela of blunt trauma but can occur spontaneously with heavy physical exertion as well. Cervical arterial dissection must be suspected in young patients with neurologic symptoms or in any patient with symptoms consistent with embolic phenomena and atypical noninvasive studies. Spontaneous cases often have unrecognized arterial disorders including FMD, cystic medial degeneration, and familial arteriopathies. Although most dissections are diagnosed after the development of neurologic deficits, many patients have an asymptomatic period (2 weeks– 6 months), followed by symptoms that precede neurologic deficits. The delay between injury and symptoms is particularly important because it allows for successful intervention when clinical suspicion and investigation identify this potentially devastating lesion.

Clinical Findings

A. Signs and Symptoms: Common presenting symptoms of carotid artery dissection are (1) unilateral headaches after a period of delay by focal cerebral ischemic symptoms, (2) unilateral headaches and ipsilateral incomplete Horner's syndrome, and more rarely (3) lower cranial nerve palsies with dysphonia, dysarthria, dysphagia, and numbness of the throat. This course of presentation is particularly important to recognize in the trauma victim, who has a lucid interval followed by neurologic symptoms in which CT of the brain is negative.

B. Imaging Studies: Diagnosis of carotid or vertebral dissection has traditionally been made with arteriography. A variety of findings are indicative of arterial dissection and include aneurysm, stenosis of the lumen, occlusion, intimal flap, distal branch occlusion (embolization), and slow ICA-to-middle cerebral artery flow. Technical advances in extracranial and transcranial Doppler sonography and in MRI and arteriography have led some authors to recommend their primary use in the diagnosis and follow-up of this disorder. Mural hematomas and false lumens are particularly well seen on MRI studies.

Treatment

The therapy for cervical arterial dissection is directed at the prevention of further thromboembolic phenomena primarily and at flow-related cerebral ischemia if the remaining collateral supply to the brain is insufficient. Early diagnosis and prompt anticoagulation are the critical factors in achieving a satisfactory outcome. Although surgical management has not been used very often in this condition, recent reports recommend replacement of the injured arterial segment when the dissection is limited to surgically accessible areas of the artery and the patient is symptomatic. Chronic sequelae of carotid intimal dissections include aneurysmal degeneration, which increases the risk for embolic phenomena, may cause pressure symptoms on other vital structures in the neck, and may rupture. Procedures using detachable balloons deposited proximally and distally in the affected artery under angiographic guidance have been reported. Anticoagulation remains the mainstay of treatment for carotid dissection with surgical intervention reserved for complications.

CAROTID COILS & KINKS

General Considerations

Coils and kinks in the course of the extracranial carotid artery are pathologic only when symptomatic, since some degree of tortuosity in the course of the carotid artery is usual. The presence of these anomalies in children is probably the result of embryologic events, whereas symptomatic lesions in adults occur late in life and are probably acquired lesions. An arterial segment is considered kinked if an angle less than 90 degrees exists between adjacent segments. Disturbances in laminar flow and low wall shear stress have been implicated in the development and progression of atherosclerotic plaques. These flow disturbances can be accentuated in coils and kinks, and the coexistence of plaques in these arterial segments is common. Plaques are most likely responsible for symptoms. Pathologic studies reveal destruction of the smooth muscles and elastic fibrils and fragmentation of the internal elastic membrane. Fibrous tissue is seen in all layers of the arterial wall, and microaneurysms with parietal thrombosis have been identified as well.

Clinical Findings

A. Signs and Symptoms: Physical examination may reveal a prominent carotid pulsation or even the impression of a pulsatile mass in the region of the carotid. Carotid coils and kinks most often are seen in patients with a history consistent with carotid occlusive disease with the exception that some patients may note a positional exacerbation of symptoms when turning the head toward the side of the lesion.

B. Imaging Studies: Duplex sonography can identify kinks and coils with a high degree of accuracy and can differentiate carotid body tumors from true aneurysms. Color flow duplex sonography allows more rapid and easier identification of these anomalies. Arteriography allows definitive visualization of the lesion but does not necessarily alter surgical management.

Treatment

The correction of kinks and coils is nearly always performed in conjunction with carotid endarterectomy (CEA). A recent series of 579 patients with CEAs included the concomitant correction of kink or coil in 19 patients (3.3%). In this series, correction of excessive internal carotid length was achieved by resecting a segment with reanastomosis of the back wall and closing the anterior arteriotomy with a patch angioplasty. Other investigators favor reimplantation of the internal carotid to a lower origin off the common carotid artery. Carotid kinks and coils are usually discovered in patients with symptomatic carotid occlusive disease and represent a technical challenge at the time of endarterectomy to reconstruct the internal carotid artery to restore laminar flow.

TAKAYASU'S ARTERITIS

Essentials of Diagnosis

- Rash, fever, myalgia, generalized weakness (first phase).
- Symptoms of arterial occlusive disease (second phase).

Takayasu's arteritis was first described in a 21-year-old female with nonspecific arteritis in 1908. It is characterized by a nonspecific inflammatory process affecting the aorta and its main branches. There are 4 recognized varieties:

- Type 1—involvement of the aortic arch and its branches
- Type 2—involvement of the descending and abdominal aorta only

- Type 3—features of types 1 and 2
- Type 4—any elements of the previous types with pulmonary artery involvement

Takayasu's arteritis most often occurs in females in the second and third decade. It occurs in 2 separate phases. The first is nonspecific in nature with skin rashes, fever, myalgia, arthralgias, pleuritis, generalized weakness, and other nonspecific complaints. The second stage is characterized by symptoms of arterial occlusive disease. Angiography provides a global assessment of the involvement of the aorta and its branches, but other imaging techniques have been used with good success as well. Cerebral blood flow single photon emission computed tomography and transcranial Doppler sonography are used to evaluate intracranial hemodynamics and hypoperfusion which is the predominant cause of neurologic symptoms rather than thromboembolic phenomena. Duplex sonography has been suggested as a useful modality in monitoring carotid occlusive lesions and their response to steroid therapy.

Treatment

Steroids are often used when arterial symptoms are recognized, and they are the first line of therapy in Takayasu's arteritis. Although abdominal aortic involvement with resultant renovascular hypertension is the most common indication for surgical intervention, a significant proportion of affected patients have neurologic symptoms on the basis of cerebral hypoperfusion and are at risk for stroke. Surgical correction of occlusive lesions is not routinely recommended but is necessary in patients unresponsive to steroids with progressive neurologic symptoms. Endarterectomy is not feasible in these lesions, making bypass procedures necessary. A variety of reports have documented successful cerebral revascularization with bypass grafts originating off either the subclavian artery or the ascending aorta. Bypass grafts originating from the subclavian artery are noted to have a higher incidence of anastomotic stenosis. A less common but more serious complication of bypass grafting is anastomotic aneurysmal dilatation. Percutaneous transluminal angioplasty has been reported to have limited success in the treatment of patients with Takayasu's arteritis and would not be expected to work well when occlusion is caused by a fibrotic process rather than a plaque amenable to fracture.

Prognosis

Takayasu's arteritis can threaten the cerebral circulation with multiple extracranial cerebral vessel involvement. The role of bypass surgery is one of salvage after the failure of steroids and other medical therapy to halt the progression of the disease. It is fraught with technical difficulties and complications but can be successful when done for the right indications at the right time in the course of the disease.

CAROTID BODY TUMORS

Essentials of Diagnosis
- Mass below angle of mandible.
- Hoarseness, dysphagia, tinnitus.

General Considerations
Carotid body tumors are neoplasms of the carotid body located at the bifurcation of the carotid artery. These indolent neoplasms have also been described as chemodectomas and glomus tumors but are most accurately termed **paragangliomas** because they represent the neoplastic growth of tissue derived from neural crest cells. Their intimate association with the carotid artery in most cases brings them into the domain of the vascular surgeon, since their primary morbidity is related to vascular complications when they are resected. Although most carotid body tumors occur in the posteromedial aspect of the carotid bifurcation, they can occur along the course of the vagus nerve up to the level of the skull base. Bilaterality is found in about 8% of cases, and a familial origin in 9%. Of patients with a family history of carotid body tumors, about one-third will have bilateral tumors. Carotid body tumors rarely may be active secretors of catecholamines and thus belong to the amine precursor uptake decarboxylase group of tumors.

Clinical Findings
A. Signs and Symptoms: The most common presentation is simply that of a mass just below the angle of the mandible. Other symptoms of carotid body tumors are largely referable to cranial nerve palsies as a result of compression by the tumor (eg, hoarseness, dysphagia, tinnitus). Screening for pheochromocytoma is warranted in the hypertensive patient with a carotid body tumor.

B. Imaging Studies: A variety of techniques (CT, MRI, duplex sonography) can document the presence of a carotid body tumor by the appropriate location and rich vascularity. Separation of the external and internal arteries into the typical "saddle deformity," where the normally acute angle between these 2 arteries is broadened and smoothed, is also indicative of a carotid body tumor. Contrast-enhanced CT is particularly helpful in identifying the tumor with bright enhancement due to the tumor's vascularity and in providing details of its proximity to the skull base and other vital structures. Angiography continues to be an important diagnostic study in the hands of most clinicians because it confirms the diagnosis and defines the details of the pertinent arterial anatomy.

Treatment
The best therapy for carotid body tumors is surgical resection. Resection is necessary because about 7% exhibit malignant behavior with direct extension and metastatic spread. Their growth rate is slow but incessant, and even without malignant degeneration they can cause a variety of serious symptoms as a result of compression of vital structures in the neck. Resection is best and most easily accomplished when the tumor is small. Larger tumors in proximity to the skull base considerably increase the vascular and cranial nerve complications of resection. Angiographic embolization has been reported both as definitive therapy and adjunct therapy to surgical resection. Embolization is currently used by some as a preoperative adjunct to surgical resection only. Radiation therapy has been used with moderate success and is best suited to patients at high risk for a surgical procedure because of a tumor in a relatively inaccessible location. Surgical resection is possible without dividing the carotid vasculature when the tumor is in a relatively early stage and is not encasing the vessels.

In more advanced cases, the carotid bifurcation often needs to be resected and a venous interposition graft used to reconstruct the vessels. The use of an indwelling shunt is preferred in these cases to protect the cerebral area and to exclude the blood supply to the tumor during dissection, thus minimizing hemorrhage. Although they are relatively uncommon, carotid body tumors should be dealt with promptly to avoid the morbidity of resection seen with large tumors. When a family history is obtained, a careful evaluation for bilaterality and multiple tumors is warranted.

ANEURYSMS OF THE EXTRACRANIAL CEREBRAL VASCULATURE

Essentials of Diagnosis
- Mass in neck.
- Pain or cranial nerve palsies.

General Considerations
Aneurysms of the extracranial cerebral vasculature are rare but serious problems. One major clinical center reported 8 cases out of a total of 1500 carotid procedures. Carotid aneurysms are of concern because they pose a thromboembolic risk to the cerebral circulation similar to that of a symptomatic carotid plaque. The causes of carotid aneurysm include the following:

- Atherosclerosis
- Intimal dissection
- Congenital, mycotic
- Secondary (false aneurysms) after previous carotid surgery
- Cystic medial necrosis
- Fibromuscular dysplasia
- Marfan's syndrome
- Posttraumatic complication

Several familial, bilateral, and multiple aneurysms in a single patient have also been reported.

A. Signs and Symptoms: Persons with aneurysms of the extracranial cerebral vasculature usually present with a mass in the neck or less frequently with pain or cranial nerve palsies as a result of pressure from the enlarging mass.

B. Imaging Studies: These aneurysms can be imaged with all of the usual vascular imaging modalities with accuracy. Angiography is desirable prior to operation to determine the extent of the aneurysm and relevant arterial anatomy.

Treatment

The standard therapeutic approach to aneurysms that are surgically accessible is resection with either reanastomosis or interposition grafting with vein. Recent experimental evidence with stent placement in artificial aneurysms in dogs raises the hopes that either stents or stent graft combinations will be available in the future. Attempts to exclude saccular aneurysms with filaments of varying composition have been only modestly successful. Several interesting presentations of carotid aneurysm are worth special mention. One presentation is that of the carotid aneurysm ipsilateral to a previous CEA. In acute cases, this usually results from suture line disruption, infection, or both. Chronically, the combination of recurrent carotid stenosis and aneurysmal degeneration of the endarterectomy site has been reported to generate neurologic symptoms in up to 50% of patients cases. Carotid aneurysms demand prompt intervention when recognized, and a flexible operative plan if interposition grafting is necessary.

REFERENCES

Adiseshiah M, Hobsley M: A technique for safe resection of extensive tumours associated with the extracranial internal carotid artery. J Cardiovasc Surg 1992;33(6):735.

Barry R et al: Duplex Doppler investigation of suspected vascular lesions at the carotid bifurcation. Ann Vasc Surg 1993;7(2):140.

Bellot J et al: Fibromuscular dysplasia of cervico-cephalic arteries with multiple dissections and a carotid-cavernous fistula: A pathological study. Stroke 1985;16(2):255.

Bergamini TM et al: Symptomatic recurrent carotid stenosis and aneurysmal degeneration after endarterectomy. Surgery 1993;113(5):580.

Bergqvist D et al: Treatment of arterial lesions after radiation therapy. Surg Gynecol Obstet 1987;165(2):116.

Bour P et al: Aneurysms of the extracranial internal carotid artery due to fibromuscular dysplasia: Results of surgical management. Ann Vasc Surg 1992;6(3):205.

Bowen J, Paulsen CA: Stroke after pituitary irradiation. Stroke 1992;23(6):908.

Collins PS, Orecchia P, Gomez E: A technique for correction of carotid kinks and coils following endarterectomy. Ann Vasc Surg 1991;5(2):116.

de Jong KP, Zondervan PE, van Urk H: Extracranial carotid artery aneurysms. Eur J Vasc Surg 1989;3(6):557.

Dolmatov EA, Diuzhikov AA: Reconstructive vascular surgery in stenosis and kinking of the internal carotid artery. Grudn Serdechnososudistaia Khir 1990;10:15.

Early TF et al: Spontaneous carotid dissection: Duplex scanning in diagnosis and management. J Vasc Surg 1991; 14(3):391.

Effeney DJ et al: Fibromuscular dysplasia of the carotid artery. Aust N Z J Surg 1983;53(6):527.

Fernandez JM et al: Spontaneous intrapetrous dissection of the internal carotid in muscular fibrodysplasia. (Letter). Neurologia 1993;8(1):30.

Fledelius HC, Nissen KR: Giant cell arteritis and visual loss: A 3-year retrospective hospital investigation in a Danish county. Acta Ophthalmol 1992;70(6):801.

Fortner GS, Thiele BL: Giant cell arteritis involving the carotid artery. Surg 1984;95(6):759.

Francfort JW et al: Airway compromise after carotid surgery in patients with cervical irradiation. J Cardiovasc Surg 1989;30(6):877.

Fukazawa S et al: Fibromuscular dysplasia of the cervical arteries associated with a distal vertebral trunk aneurysm: Case report. Neurol Med Chir 1990;30(11 Spec No):899.

Gersdorff M et al: Clinical aspects and surgical treatment of carotid body tumors. Acta Otorhinolaryngol Belg 1985; 39(6):907.

Giordano JM et al: Experience with surgical treatment of Takayasu's disease. Surgery 1991;109(3 Pt 1):252.

Graves VB, Strother CM, Rappe AH: Treatment of experimental canine carotid aneurysms with platinum coils. AJNR 1993;14(4):787.

Grosset DG, Patterson J, Bone I: Intracranial haemodynamics in Takayasu's arteritis. Acta Neurochir 1992;119 (1-4):161.

Guedea F et al: Radiotherapy for chemodectoma of the carotid body and ganglion nodosum. Head Neck 1991; 13(6):509.

Hanakita J et al: Bilateral aneurysms of extracranial internal carotid arteries: Case report. Neurol Med Chir 1991;31 (13):972.

Hieshima GB et al: Spontaneous arteriovenous fistulas of cerebral vessels in association with fibromuscular dysplasia. Neurosurgery 1986;18(4):454.

Hirata Y et al: Occlusion of the internal carotid artery after radiation therapy for the chiasmal lesion. Acta Neurochir 1985;74(3–4):141.

Hodgins GW, Dutton JW: Transluminal dilatation for Takayasu's arteritis. Can J Surg 1984;27(4):355.

Humphrey PW et al: Spontaneous common carotid artery dissection. J Vasc Surg 1993;18(1):95.

Hupp T, Kretzschmar U, Allenberg JR: Surgical therapy of radiation-induced arterial vascular damage. Chirurg 1987; 58(5):328.

Iaccarino V et al: Embolization of glomus tumors of the carotid: Temporary or definitive? Cardiovasc Intervent Radiol 1985;8(4):206.

Iannuzzi R, Metson R, Lofgren R: Carotid artery rupture after twice-a-day radiation therapy. Otolaryngol Head Neck Surg 1989;100(6):621.

Jones TR, Frusha JD: Carotid revascularization after cervical irradiation. South Med J 1986;79(12):1517.

Kubo S, Nakagawa H, Imaoka S: Systemic multiple aneurysms of the extracranial internal carotid artery, intracranial vertebral artery, and visceral arteries: Case report. Neurosurgery 1992;30(4):600.

Kuroda S et al: Magnetic resonance findings in spontaneous dissection of the cervical internal carotid artery: Case report. Neurol Med Chir 1992;32(10):773.

Kwan ES, Heilman CB, Roth PA: Endovascular packing of carotid bifurcation aneurysm with polyester fiber-coated platinum coils in a rabbit model. AJNR 1993;14(2):323.

Lagneau P, Michel JB, Vuong PN: Surgical treatment of Takayasu's disease. Ann Surg 1987;205(2):157.

Landre E, Roux FX, Cioloca C: Spontaneous dissection of the exocranial internal carotid artery: Therapeutic aspects. Presse Med 1987;16(26):1273.

Latter DA et al: Internal carotid artery aneurysm and Marfan's syndrome. Can J Surg 1989;32(6):463.

Leipzig TJ, Dohrmann GJ: The tortuous or kinked carotid artery: Pathogenesis and clinical considerations: A historical review. Surg Neurol 1986;25(5):478.

Lin FY et al: Pseudoaneurysm of common carotid artery after irradiation: Report of a case. Taiwan I Hsueh Hui Tsa Chih 1988;87(8):828.

Linder F et al: Tumors of the glomus caroticum. Chirurg 1984;55(1):19.

Lindsay S: Aortic arteriosclerosis in the dog after localized aortic irradiation with electrons. Circ Res 1962;10(61).

Lupi-Herrera E et al: Takayasu's arteritis: Clinical study of 107 cases. Am Heart J 1977;93:94.

Mas JL et al: Extracranial vertebral artery dissections: A review of 13 cases. Stroke 1987;18(6):1037.

Matskevichus ZK, Pauliukas PA: The morphological changes in the wall of the carotid and vertebral arteries in pathological kinks and loops. Arkh Patol 1990;52(10):53.

Maurizi M et al: Carotid body tumors: The clinical, diagnostic and surgical aspects. Acta Otorhinolaryngol Ital 1992;12(6):527.

McCready RA et al: Radiation-induced arterial injuries. Surgery 1983;93(2):306.

Mokri B, Piepgras DG, Houser OW: Traumatic dissections of the extracranial internal carotid artery. J Neurosurg 1988;68(2):189.

Mokri B et al: Familial occurrence of spontaneous dissection of the internal carotid artery. Stroke 1987;18(1):246.

Mokri B et al: Spontaneous dissection of the cervical internal carotid artery: Presentation with lower cranial nerve palsies. Arch Otolaryngol Head Neck Surg 1992;118(4):431.

Moore W: Extracranial cerebrovascular disease: The carotid artery. In: *Vascular Surgery: A Comprehensive Review.* Moore W (editor). WB Saunders, 1993:532.

Morgenlander JC, Goldstein LB: Recurrent transient ischemic attacks and stroke in association with an internal carotid artery web see comments. Stroke 1991;22(1):94.

Mullges W, Ringelstein EB, Leibold M: Non-invasive diagnosis of internal carotid artery dissections. J Neurol Neurosurg Psychiatr 1992;55(2):98.

Nishiyama K et al: A case of fibromuscular dysplasia presenting with Wallenberg syndrome, and developing a giant aneurysm of the internal carotid artery in the cavernous sinus. Rinsho Shinkeigaku 1992;32(10):1117.

Nordestgaard AG et al: Blunt traumatic dissection of the internal carotid artery treated by balloon occlusion. Ann Vasc Surg 1987;1(5):610.

Osborn A, Anderson R: Angiographic spectrum of cervical and intracranial fibromuscular dysplasia. Stroke 1977;8:617.

Painter TA et al: Extracranial carotid aneurysms: Report of six cases and review of the literature. J Vasc Surg 1985;2(2):312.

Palubinskas A, Ripley H: Fibromuscular hyperplasia in extrarenal arteries. Radiology 1964;82:451.

Pauliukas PA, Matskevichus ZK, Barkauskas EM: Changes in the internal carotid artery in its loop-shaped kinking and their clinical significance. Khirurgiia 1989;9:47.

Petrovic P et al: Surgical management of extracranial carotid artery aneurysms. Ann Vasc Surg 1991;5(6):506.

Porter J, Taylor L Jr, Harris E Jr: Nonatherosclerotic vascular disease. In: *Vascular Surgery: A Comprehensive Review.* Moore W (editor). WB Saunders 1993:117.

Powell S, Peters N, Harmer C: Chemodectoma of the head and neck: Results of treatment in 84 patients. Int J Radiat Oncol Biol Phys 1992;22(5):919.

Pozzati E et al: Blunt traumatic carotid dissection with delayed symptoms. Stroke 1989;20(3):412.

Redaelli C, Carrel T, Turina M: Surgery of extracranial aneurysms of the carotid artery: Analysis of 8 cases. Chirurg 1991;62(8):620.

Ridge BA et al: Familial carotid body tumors: Incidence and implications. Ann Vasc Surg 1993;7(2):190.

Robbs JV, Human RR, Rajaruthnam P: Operative treatment of nonspecific aortoarteritis (Takayasu's arteritis). J Vasc Surg 1986;3(4):605.

Schwaber MK et al: Diagnosis and management of catecholamine secreting glomus tumors. Laryngoscope 1984;94(8):1008.

Smith L, Ajalat G: Tumors of the carotid body: Diagnosis, prognosis, and surgical management. In: *Surgery for Cerebrovascular Disease.* Moore W (editor). Churchill Livingstone, 1987:579.

Stanley J: Arterial fibrodysplasia: Histopathologic character and current etiologic concepts. Arch Surg 1975;110:56.

Steiger HJ: Treatment of traumatic carotid dissection. Neurochirurgia 1988;31(4):128.

Sumner DS: Use of color-flow imaging technique in carotid artery disease. Surg Clin North Am 1990;70(1):201.

Tada Y et al: Surgical treatment of Takayasu arteritis. Heart Vessels 1992;7(Suppl 1):159.

Taguchi J et al: Bypass surgery for aortitis syndrome: Aortocarotid bypass with saphenous vein graft. Surg Neurol 1992;37(4):300.

Takayasu M: Case with unusual changes of the central vessels of the retina. Acta Soc Ophthalmol Jpn 1908;12:554.

Turjman F et al: Treatment of experimental carotid aneurysms by endoprosthesis implantation: Preliminary report. Neurol Res 1993;15(3):181.

van der Mey AG et al: Does intervention improve the natural course of glomus tumors? A series of 108 patients seen in a 32-year period. Ann Otol Rhinol Laryngol 1992;101(8):635.

Verlato F et al: Takayasu's arteritis: Anatomic change before and after steroid therapy evaluated by angiography and echo-Doppler color-flow. Int Angiol 1992;11(3):233.

Watanabe S et al: Fibromuscular dysplasia at the internal carotid origin: A case of carotid web. No Shinkei Geka 1993;21(5):449.

Weaver FA et al: Surgical procedures in the management of Takayasu's arteritis. J Vasc Surg 1990;12(4):429.

Zarins C: Hemodynamic factors in atherosclerosis. In: *Vascular Surgery: A Comprehensive Review.* Moore W (editor). WB Saunders, 1993:96.

11

Diseases of the Thoracic Aorta

Joseph S. Coselli, MD, & Scott A. LeMaire, MD

The large volume of blood that flows through the thoracic aorta at high pressure is unparalleled by any other vascular structure. For this reason, any condition that disrupts the integrity of the thoracic aorta, such as aortic dissection, rupture, and traumatic injury, will have catastrophic consequences.

Aortic aneurysm is defined as a permanent, localized dilatation resulting in at least a 50% increase in diameter compared with the normal expected aortic diameter at the same anatomic level. Thoracic aortic aneurysms, which account for less than 10% of all aortic aneurysms, have several causes: degenerative disease of the aortic wall, aortic dissection, aortitis, infection, and trauma. Poststenotic dilatation with aneurysm formation may occur in patients with coarctation or aortic valvular stenosis. The clinical manifestations, methods of treatment, and treatment results in patients with aortic aneurysms vary according to the cause and aortic segment involved.

The ascending aorta is the segment between the aortic valve and the origin of the innominate artery. This portion of the thoracic aorta can be further subdivided into three segments: (1) the annular region, which includes the valve leaflets; (2) the sinus segment, including the sinuses of Valsalva and coronary arterial ostia; and (3) the supracoronary tubular portion. Aneurysmal dilatation of the annular segment is referred to as **annuloaortic ectasia.**

Immediately distal to the ascending aorta is the transverse aortic arch, which is the segment from which the brachiocephalic vessels arise. Forty-three percent of transverse aortic arch aneurysms involve only the distal arch. In general, these aneurysms are saccular in nature and arise from the lesser curvature of the arch, opposite the origins of the left subclavian artery and the left common carotid artery. The remaining 57% involve the ascending aorta and all or most of the transverse arch. They are most often fusiform, involving the entire aortic circumference.

The descending thoracic aorta is the segment between the left subclavian artery and the diaphragm. Aneurysms at this site are fusiform in 95% of cases and saccular in 5%.

Thoracoabdominal aortic aneurysms always involve the segment of abdominal aorta from which the visceral vessels arise. The Crawford classification of thoracoabdominal aortic aneurysms is based on the extent of aortic involvement (Fig 11–1). Type I thoracoabdominal aortic aneurysms usually involve all of the descending thoracic aorta and extend down through the visceral vessels in the abdomen. A type II thoracoabdominal aortic aneurysm extends from the left subclavian artery to the aortic bifurcation; a subtype also involves the ascending aorta and transverse arch. Type III thoracoabdominal aortic aneurysms involve the distal half of descending thoracic aorta and most or all of the abdominal aorta. Type IV thoracoabdominal aortic aneurysms begin near the diaphragm and usually extend to the aortic bifurcation.

Aneurysmal dilatation of multiple segments of the aorta is not uncommon among patients with thoracic aortic aneurysms. Any combination of aortic aneurysms occurring in various aortic segments is possible. In the most extreme case, the entire aorta is aneurysmal (mega-aorta).

THORACIC AORTIC ANEURYSMS CAUSED BY DEGENERATIVE DISEASE

Essentials of Diagnosis

- Thoracic aortic aneurysms are often asymptomatic.
- Physical examination is imprecise; therefore, imaging studies are required.
- Associated aortic valvular insufficiency when the ascending aorta is involved.
- Associated symptoms and signs of concomitant occlusive disease of the cerebral, coronary, or peripheral vascular systems.

General Considerations

Degenerative disease of the aortic wall is the cause of most thoracic aortic aneurysms, including 66% of descending thoracic aneurysms and 83% of thoracoabdominal aortic aneurysms. Two types of degenerative disease lead to thoracic aortic aneurysms: medial degenerative disease and arteriosclerosis.

Medial degenerative disease (also known as mucoid degeneration, myxomatous degeneration, and cystic medial necrosis) is responsible for at least 95% of ascending thoracic aortic aneurysms and most fusiform aneurysms involving the descending or transverse aortic arch segments. In medial degenerative disease, the smooth muscle cells and elastic laminae in the aortic media are replaced by cystic spaces filled

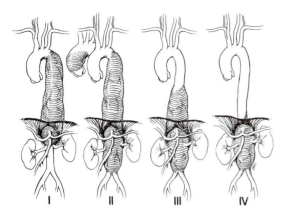

Figure 11–1. The Crawford classification of thoracoabdominal aortic aneuyrsms.

with mucoid material. The disease, frequently involving multiple segments of the aorta, produces progressive weakening and dilatation of the aortic wall, with eventual aneurysm formation and subsequent complications including aortic valvular insufficiency, intimal laceration with dissection, and rupture.

Medial degenerative disease is also responsible for thoracic aortic aneurysms in patients with **Marfan syndrome,** an autosomal dominant connective tissue disorder with associated cardiovascular, skeletal, and ocular abnormalities. Marfan syndrome is caused by a mutation involving a gene located on the 15th chromosome that codes for the microfibrillar protein, fibrillin. The resulting connective tissue defect weakens the aortic wall. The ascending aorta is most commonly affected with the development of generalized aortic root dilatation (annuloaortic ectasia) and aortic valvular insufficiency. Cardiovascular complications, especially thoracic aortic aneurysms, are primarily responsible for the reduced life expectancy in patients with Marfan syndrome: without surgical treatment patients die at an average age of 32 years.

Arteriosclerosis, in contrast to medial degenerative disease, is a process that primarily involves the aortic intima. It is characterized by raised atheromatous intimal plaques consisting of a lipid core and fibrous cap, which eventually compromise blood flow and weaken the vessel wall. Arteriosclerosis is the most common cause of aneurysms of the infrarenal abdominal aorta. In the thoracic aorta, however, it is more commonly a process superimposed on aneurysmal disease rather than the primary cause. Those thoracic aneurysms that are caused by atherosclerosis are frequently saccular.

Although small thoracic aortic aneurysms may change very little over time, most thoracic aortic aneurysms are life threatening. Up to 78% of untreated patients with thoracic aortic aneurysms die within five years after diagnosis, most often from rupture of the aneurysm. The prognosis is worse for patients with untreated thoracoabdominal aortic aneurysms, at least

75% of whom die within two years of diagnosis—one-half due to rupture.

Clinical Findings

A. Signs and Symptoms: Physical examination rarely provides direct evidence of a thoracic aortic aneurysm. A pulsatile abdominal mass may be present in a patient with a thoracoabdominal aortic aneurysm, and tenderness of such a mass signifies impending rupture. Most physical findings are nonspecific and are usually related to complications and cardiovascular disease. A diastolic cardiac murmur is present in patients with aortic insufficiency. An ascending aortic aneurysm may compress the superior vena cava, producing jugular venous distention and upper extremity edema. Findings secondary to associated cerebrovascular or peripheral arterial occlusive disease are common.

Patients with thoracic aortic aneurysms are usually asymptomatic at the time of diagnosis. The aneurysm is frequently discovered serendipitously during either routine examination or evaluation for an unrelated problem. A patient presenting with pain related to a thoracic aortic aneurysm should be considered to have actual or impending rupture, an indication for emergency surgery. Anterior chest pain suggests an ascending aortic aneurysm, whereas back pain is suggestive of a descending thoracic aortic aneurysm, and abdominal pain may signify a be caused by a rupturing thoracoabdominal aortic aneurysm. Compression of the trachea may cause cough, dyspnea, or stridor, whereas rupture into the tracheobronchial tree produces massive hemoptysis. Involvement of the gastrointestinal tract can include compression of the esophagus resulting in dysphagia, or erosion into the viscera leading to either hematemesis or hematochezia. Neurologic symptoms include a hoarse voice due to pressure on the left recurrent laryngeal nerve. Symptoms characteristic of associated conditions, such as aortic valvular insufficiency and congestive heart failure, are commonly present in patients with thoracic aneurysms.

B. Imaging Studies: Because history and physical examination are imprecise in the diagnosis of thoracic aortic aneurysms, various imaging studies play a critical role in detection and follow-up.

1. Radiography–In many cases, the initial suspicion of a thoracic aortic aneurysm is raised by findings on a chest radiograph. The presence of a mediastinal mass or generalized mediastinal widening is suggestive of an aneurysm. Ascending aortic aneurysms tend to produce convexity of the right heart border. A prominent aortic knob is consistent with an aneurysm involving the transverse aortic arch. The trachea or left mainstream bronchus may be displaced or compressed. Descending thoracic aortic aneurysms often manifest as posterior or left lateral thoracic masses. Although a chest radiograph is helpful, (1) it cannot precisely define the extent of aortic involvement; (2) it cannot always differentiate between an aneurysm and simple aortic tortuosity; and (3) it cannot identify an aneurysm of the sinus segment that is hidden within the cardiac silhouette.

Other radiographic studies can occasionally show signs of aortic aneurysmal disease. In the presence of a radiopaque, calcified aortic wall, radiographs of the abdomen may demonstrate a thoracoabdominal aortic aneurysm. Barium studies of the upper gastrointestinal tract may reveal displacement or obstruction of the esophagus.

2. Transthoracic echocardiography–Transthoracic echocardiography is useful in diagnosing ascending aortic aneurysms and in evaluating cardiac valve function. Unfortunately, transthoracic echocardiography cannot be used to evaluate the entire thoracic aorta.

3. Transesophageal echocardiography (TEE)–Preoperative ultrasound evaluation of the thoracic aorta is far better with TEE, which produces high-resolution images of the cardiac structures, entire thoracic aorta, and other great vessels. Transesophageal echocardiography is highly accurate in the detection of intraluminal thrombus, fistulization, aortic valvular insufficiency, and pericardial effusion or tamponade. This method also is useful for intraoperative cardiac monitoring. It can evaluate left ventricular volume and compliance to help refine anesthetic management and can confirm the surgical correction of aortic valvular insufficiency. Like transthoracic echocardiography, TEE provides no information concerning coronary artery patency and its usefulness depends on the skill of the operator. These two methods share the advantage of being able to be performed at the bedside or in the operating room.

4. Computed tomography (CT)–CT is highly accurate for determining the aortic diameter, the extent of aneurysmal disease, and the presence of intraluminal thrombus. CT images can identify aortic rupture contained by periaortic tissues, a pulmonary lesion, a nonfunctioning atretic kidney, and a horseshoe kidney—conditions that affect operative strategy. Additional advantages of CT are standardization of scale and resolution, near-ubiquitous availability, nonoperator dependence, speed of performance, and relative cost-effectiveness. CT scans are not helpful in evaluating cardiac function, or major branch vessel patency. With CT, a risk of renal dysfunction exists secondary to the administration of intravenous contrast.

5. Magnetic resonance imaging (MRI)–MRI is also effective in evaluating the entire aorta and allows visualization in the transverse, sagittal, and coronal planes. Specialized magnetic resonance angiography (MRA) techniques greatly enhance the imaging of the aorta. Gated scans offer semiquantification of aortic valvular insufficiency and left ventricular function. MRI shares with CT the disadvantage of being performed in a nonintensive care area of the hospital. Monitoring equipment and ventilators required for critically ill patients are generally not compatible with the magnetic environment. The high cost, limited availability, and greater time requirements are further disadvantages of MRI.

6. Aortography–Although not absolutely essential for the planning of an operation, aortography is the single most informative method of evaluating the thoracic aorta. It precisely defines aortic anatomy and is the superior method of evaluating all the major branch vessels for patency and anatomic anomalies. This capability cannot be underemphasized in light of the common occurrence of concomitant branch vessel occlusive disease and its impact on the operative plan. For example, 20% of patients with thoracoabdominal aortic aneurysms have visceral arterial occlusive disease that requires surgical treatment. Evaluation of the brachiocephalic vessels is critical in patients with transverse aortic arch aneurysms to detect arterial aneurysms, anomalies, or occlusive disease that require special intraoperative attention. Aortography may underestimate the diameter of an aneurysm because of the nonopacification of luminal thrombus. Thoracic aortography can be performed as part of cardiac catheterization in patients with known or suspected coronary artery occlusive disease.

Differential Diagnosis

The differential diagnosis of a mediastinal mass discovered on a chest radiograph includes thoracic aortic aneurysm, pericardial cyst, substernal goiter, hiatal hernia, esophageal carcinoma, esophageal dilatation due to achalasia or scleroderma, lymphadenopathy, and metastatic disease. Other mediastinal neoplasms include bronchogenic carcinoma, thymoma, teratoma, lymphoma, and multiple neurologic tumors.

Treatment

Aneurysms of the thoracic aorta consistently increase in size and progress to serious complications including rupture, which is usually a fatal event. Therefore, aggressive treatment is indicated in all but the poorest surgical candidates.

A. Medical Treatment: Small asymptomatic thoracic aortic aneurysms can be followed, especially in poor risk patients, and later treated surgically if the patient develops symptoms or complications, or if progressive enlargement occurs. Meticulous control of hypertension is the primary medical treatment.

B. Surgical Treatment: Elective resection with graft replacement is indicated in asymptomatic patients with an aortic diameter of at least twice the normal diameter for the involved segment (5–6 cm in most thoracic segments). Contraindications to elective repair are extreme operative risk because of severe coexisting cardiac or pulmonary disease, or a limited life expectancy due to other conditions, such as malignancy. An emergency operation is required for any patient in whom a ruptured aneurysm is suspected.

Patients with a thoracic aortic aneurysm often have coexisting aneurysms of other aortic segments. A common cause of death following repair of a thoracic aortic aneurysm is rupture of a different aortic aneurysm. Therefore, staged repair of multiple aortic segments is often necessary.

1. Preoperative evaluation–As with any major operative procedure, careful preoperative evaluation regarding coexisting disease and subsequent medical optimization are essential for successful surgical treatment.

The decision to proceed with cardiac catheterization is based on symptomatology and the results of the noninvasive testing. The presence of an ascending aortic aneurysm mandates careful preoperative evaluation of the coronary arteries and the aortic valve so that concomitant coronary artery bypass or aortic valve replacement can be planned, as needed.

Pulmonary function is evaluated based on clinical examination, chest radiography, arterial blood gas testing, and routine screening spirometry. Patients exhibiting an FEV1 of less than 1.40 L per second are at greatest risk for postoperative respiratory failure. Spirometry predicts a patient's response to perioperative bronchodilators. Ideally, patients who smoke should stop smoking before surgery to aid in pulmonary optimization.

The most significant predictors of postoperative renal failure are preexisting renal dysfunction and diffuse atherosclerosis. Patients with documented preoperative renal dysfunction receive intravenous hydration prior to arteriography. If the blood urea nitrogen or creatinine levels are elevated following aortography, surgery should be delayed in asymptomatic patients until these values return to baseline.

2. General techniques–Several general technical details apply to any operation on the thoracic aorta. (1) A cell-saving device is used to collect shed blood for reinfusion. (2) Intraoperative monitoring should include an arterial line, a pulmonary artery catheter, rectal and esophageal temperature probes, and an indwelling bladder catheter. (3) The maintenance of normal cardiovascular hemodynamics during aortic cross-clamping is achieved by using a sodium nitroprusside or nitroglycerine infusion to prevent cardiac strain and promote collateral circulation. Clamp release hypotension is avoided by administering adequate volumes of colloid and crystalloid fluids prior to unclamping. Removal of the cross-clamp should be gradual.

3. Ascending aortic replacement–The repair of aneurysms of the ascending aorta requires cardiopulmonary bypass. The technique of aortic replacement varies according to the extent of the aneurysm and the condition of the aortic valve. Simple Dacron graft replacement of the tubular portion is indicated when the sinus segment is normal and the aortic valve is competent (Fig 11–2, A–D). When aortic valvular disease is present and the sinus segment is normal, separate re-

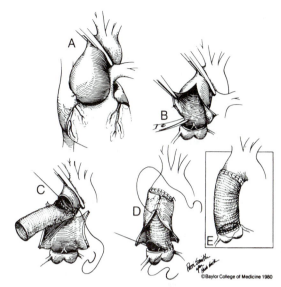

©Baylor College of Medicine 1980

Figure 11–2. Technique for replacement of ascending aortic aneurysm, showing sequential steps A through E.

placement of the aortic valve and tubular ascending aorta is carried out. In patients with Marfan syndrome, separate replacement of the aortic valve and ascending aorta without replacement of the sinus segment, consistently leads to progressive dilatation of the sinus segment and subsequent complications. Therefore, a composite valve graft is always used in patients with Marfan syndrome. Composite valve grafts are also used to replace the entire aortic root in patients with aortic valvular dysfunction and an aneurysmal sinus segment (annuloaortic ectasia) (Fig 11–2E).

4. Transverse aortic arch replacement–The approach to transverse aortic arch aneurysms depends on the extent of involvement and the need for cardiac or cerebral protection during replacement. Aneurysms involving the distal arch can be controlled by clamping distal to the innominate artery; consequently, they do not require cardiopulmonary bypass. Dacron patch aortoplasty is performed for saccular aneurysms when they involve less than 50% of aortic circumference.

The repair of fusiform or extensive saccular aneurysms involving the proximal transverse arch requires cerebral protection, which is achieved by profound hypothermic circulatory arrest and reversed cerebral perfusion through the superior vena cava. These aneurysms are replaced with Dacron tube grafts with the brachiocephalic vessels reattached to an opening in the graft. The operative mortality rate for resection and graft replacement of nondissecting transverse aortic arch aneurysms is 5%.

5. Descending thoracic aortic replacement–In the descending thoracic aorta, saccular aneurysms are repaired with Dacron patch aortoplasty, whereas fusiform aneurysms are treated with tube graft replacement (Fig 11–3) with reattachment of the vital intercostal arteries in the region of T8–T12. The operative mortality rate for this procedure ranges from 5% to 15% with a 5–10% risk of paraplegia, depending on the extent of the aneurysm.

6. Thoracoabdominal aortic replacement– The repair of thoracoabdominal aortic aneurysms is performed through a thoracoabdominal incision— a left thoracotomy that extends into the abdominal midline. Resection and graft replacement involves reattaching the critical intercostal and lumbar arteries supplying the spinal cord (T8–L2) to openings in the graft. Likewise, the celiac, superior mesenteric, and renal arteries are also reattached. Up to 20% of patients undergoing repair of a thoracoabdominal aortic aneurysm have celiac, superior mesenteric, or renal arterial occlusive disease requiring concomitant endarterectomy or bypass.

Postoperative Management

A. Immediate Care: The careful hemodynamic monitoring initiated in the operating room is continued in the surgical intensive care unit. Serum electrolytes, hematocrit, coagulation parameters, and arterial blood gases are monitored regularly. Stress gastritis and ulceration are prevented by administering histamine antagonists. Perioperative antibiotics are necessary to avert graft infection. Following extubation, early mobilization and aggressive pulmonary therapy should be initiated to prevent pulmonary complications.

B. Complications:

1. Paraplegia and paraparesis–The blood supply to the spinal cord can become compromised during the repair of descending thoracic or thoracoabdominal aortic aneurysms. The incidence of resulting paraplegia or paraparesis at centers with experienced surgical teams is about 4% for descending thoracic aortic replacement and 16% for thoracoabdominal aortic replacement. Significant risk factors include a long total aortic clamp time, periods of perioperative hypotension, aortic rupture, advanced age, and—perhaps most important—the extent of aortic repair. Repair of type I and II thoracoabdominal aortic aneurysms carry the highest risk.

The best technique for preventing paraplegia and paraparesis is a topic of considerable debate. Distal aortic perfusion with cardiofemoral bypass is used in some centers. A combination of careful control of intraoperative hemodynamics, preservation of intercostal collateral circulation, and techniques to limit aortic occlusion time provides favorable results. Intraoperative cerebral spinal fluid drainage has not been proven to be beneficial.

2. Acute renal failure–Acute renal failure occurs in 5.7% of patients undergoing replacement of the descending thoracic aorta and up to 18% of patients following surgery for thoracoabdominal aortic aneurysms. Up to one-third of these patients with acute renal failure require hemodialysis. Acute renal failure after thoracic aortic aneurysm surgery is associated with a mortality rate of up to 75%. Significant risk factors are preoperative renal dysfunction, perioperative hypotension, the extent of aneurysm repair, renal ischemic time, and advanced age. Expeditious surgery and the maintenance of perioperative normovolemia are therefore imperative. Cold lactated Ringer's infusion into the renal arteries is used for hypothermic renal protection in patients with preoperative renal dysfunction or anticipated extended clamp times. Concomitant renal endarterectomy or bypass is performed if occlusive renal arterial disease is present.

3. Vocal cord paralysis–Injury to the left recurrent laryngeal nerve causes paralysis of the left vocal cord, which manifests as persistent postoperative hoarseness. Excellent results have been obtained with corrective thyroplasty.

4. Other complications–Pulmonary and cardiac complications are common causes of morbidity and mortality following thoracic aortic surgery. Less common complications are hemorrhage, embolic events, stroke, infection, and graft occlusion.

C. Follow-up Care: Many patients, especially those with Marfan syndrome, develop new aneurysms at other sites and therefore require regular evaluation of the aorta. Evaluation with a yearly echocardiogram and CT or MRI may be reasonable for those at highest risk. Strict prophylaxis against graft infection using parenteral antibiotics is mandatory during invasive procedures and dental work. Patients with mechanical valves require lifelong anticoagulation.

Prognosis

The 30-day survival rate following surgical correction of thoracic or thoracoabdominal aortic aneurysms exceeds 90%. Important predictors of early mortality are advanced age, renal dysfunction, concurrent aneurysms, coronary artery occlusive disease, chronic

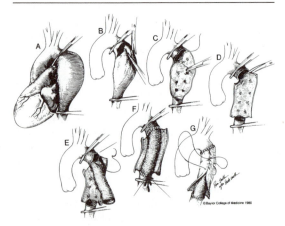

Figure 11–3. Technique for replacement of descending thoracic aortic aneurysm.

obstructive pulmonary disease, and prolonged aortic cross-clamp time. In contrast to the 25% 5-year survival rate for patients with untreated thoracic aortic aneurysms, the 5-year survival rate following operative repair ranges from 60–66%.

Cabrol C et al: Long-term results with total replacement of the ascending aorta and reimplantation of the coronary arteries. J Thorac Cardiovasc Surg 1986;91:17.

Crawford ES, Coselli JS: Replacement of the aortic arch. Semin Thorac Cardiovasc Surg 1991;3:194.

Crawford ES, Crawford JL: *Diseases of the Aorta: Including an Atlas of Angiographic Pathology and Surgical Technique*. Williams & Wilkins, 1984.

Crawford ES, DeNatale RW: Thoracoabdominal aortic aneurysm: Observations regarding the natural course of the disease. J Vasc Surg 1986;3:578.

Crawford ES, Svensson LG, Coselli JS, Hess KR: Surgical treatment of aneurysm and/or dissection of the ascending aorta, transverse aortic arch, and ascending aorta with transverse aortic arch: Factors influencing survival in 717 patients. J Thorac Cardiovasc Surg 1989;98:659.

Crawford ES et al: Aortic arch aneurysm: A sentinel of extensive aortic disease requiring subtotal and total aortic replacement. Ann Surg 1984;199:742.

Crawford ES et al: Diffuse aneurysmal disease (chronic aortic dissection, Marfan, and mega aorta syndromes) and multiple aneurysm: Treatment by subtotal and total aortic replacement emphasizing the elephant trunk operation. Ann Surg 1990;211:521.

Gerry JL Jr, Morris L, Pyeritz RE: Clinical management of the cardiovascular complications of the Marfan syndrome. J LA State Med Soc 1991;143:43.

Golden MA, Donaldson MC, Whittemore AD, Mannick JA: Evolving experience with thoracoabdominal aortic aneurysm repairs at a single institution. J Vasc Surg 1991; 13:792.

Miller DC, Myers BD: Pathophysiology and prevention of acute renal failure associated with thoracoabdominal or abdominal surgery. J Vasc Surg 1987;5:518.

Svensson LG et al: Experience with 1509 patients undergoing thoracoabdominal aortic operations. J Vasc Surg 1993;17(2):357.

AORTIC DISSECTION

Essentials of Diagnosis

- A history of hypertension, existing aortic aneurysm, or Marfan syndrome.
- Sudden severe chest pain, often radiating to the back, neck, or abdomen.
- Coexisting findings of branch vessel occlusion, aortic insufficiency, and an abnormal chest radiograph.
- A normal electrocardiogram and normal cardiac enzymes, differentiating aortic dissection from acute myocardial infarction. (A confirmed diagnosis of acute myocardial infarction does not rule out the concomitant presence of dissection.)
- Imaging studies—including echocardiography, CT, and MRI—revealing an aortic intimal flap.

General Considerations

Acute aortic dissection, the most common catastrophic process affecting the aorta, is a serious condition requiring emergency medical and surgical management. Forces generated by pulsatile aortic pressure and flow cause an intimal tear, which extends into the aortic media. The initial intimal tear usually begins just above the aortic valve (2–4 cm beyond the coronary artery ostia) or distal to the left subclavian artery. Pulsatile extravasation of blood into the aortic wall leads to progressive separation of the intimal flap, most often in a distal direction. The resulting false channel generally occupies at least one-half of the aortic circumference and compresses the true lumen. Reentry sites, in which the blood flow in the false lumen ruptures through the intimal flap and back into the true lumen, are often multiple. The outer layers of the false channel being composed of only adventitia and a portion of the tunica media, are attenuated; therefore, progressive dilatation occurs. The portion of aortic wall that is adjacent to the initial intimal tear is the weakest point and the most common site of rupture.

The chronicity of dissection is an important factor in determining appropriate management. Acute aortic dissections are arbitrarily defined as those presenting with 14 days of the initial dissection. After 14 days, dissections are considered chronic. Two classifications focus on the extent of aortic involvement, which determines prognosis and treatment; they disregard the site of intimal tear, which is less important.

The **DeBakey classification of aortic dissections** describes three distinct types (Fig 11–4). In a DeBakey type I aortic dissection the ascending, transverse arch, and descending thoracic segments are involved; the dissection frequently extends into the abdominal aorta. DeBakey type II dissections also arise in the ascending aorta, but terminate just proximal to the origin of the innominate artery. Finally, DeBakey type III dissections are subdivided into two subtypes: type IIIA, which begins just distal to the left subclavian artery and terminates above the diaphragm, and type IIIB, which begins at the same point but extends into the abdominal aorta. A DeBakey type III dissection will rarely later extend proximally to reach the aortic valve, converting it to a type I dissection.

The **Stanford classification** divides aortic dissection into only two groups: type A and type B. Stanford type A dissections involve the ascending aorta and account for about 74% of all cases, whereas type B dissections do not involve the ascending aorta, usually arising just distal to the left subclavian artery.

Aortic dissection is more common in men. The usual cause is medial degenerative disease; dissection is rarely caused by atherosclerosis. Distal dissection (DeBakey III, Stanford B) tends to develop in the older patients, whereas proximal or total aortic dissection (DeBakey I or II, Stanford A) tend to develop in younger patients such as those with Marfan syndrome.

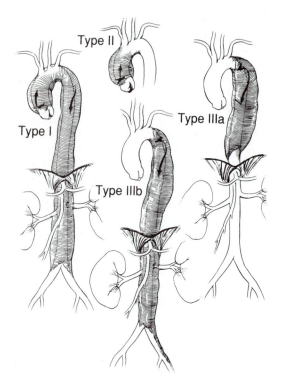

Figure 11–4. The DeBakey classification of aortic dissection.

Dissections can also result from direct injury, such as blunt thoracic trauma or iatrogenic injuries. Aortic dissection has been reported as a complication of cardiac and aortic surgery, pregnancy, and aortitis.

Most untreated patients with acute proximal aortic dissection die from complications within two weeks of onset. The mortality rates in these patients are 20% within the first 24 hours, 50% within 48 hours, and 70% within one week. Untreated distal aortic dissection is associated with a 40% mortality rate at one month, followed by a 20% yearly mortality rate in the chronic state. As with thoracic aneurysms of degenerative cause, death is usually secondary to rupture. Although large dissecting aortic aneurysms are especially prone to rupture, nearly 25% of ruptured dissecting thoracic aortic aneurysms are smaller than 6 cm in diameter.

Acute dissecting thoracic aortic aneurysms can rupture into the pericardial sac, pleural cavity, mediastinum, abdomen, or adjacent cardiac chamber or great vessel; depending on the location, rupture can result in cardiac tamponade, exsanguinating hemorrhage, or acute congestive heart failure. The ascending aorta is the most common site of rupture. Rupture of a distal segment usually produces hemorrhage into the left chest. A left pleural effusion, however, is ubiquitously present in patients with acute DeBakey type I and III dissections within 72 hours after onset and, de-

spite being blood-tinged, should not be confused with rupture. The progression of the false channel hematoma can extend proximally to the aortic valve and cause dehiscence of the valvular commissures, resulting in acute aortic valvular insufficiency. Likewise, extension into the coronary artery ostia can cause sudden coronary artery occlusion and an acute myocardial infarction. The expanding intramural hematoma can compress the superior vena cava or pulmonary artery, causing superior vena cava syndrome or severe congestive heart failure. Aortic branch vessels can also become occluded, manifesting as stroke, renal failure, visceral ischemia, upper or lower extremity ischemia, or spinal ischemia.

In the chronic stage, the primary complication remains rupture resulting from progressive false lumen dilatation.

Clinical Findings

Because the early mortality rates are so high for untreated aortic dissection, improvement in survival rates can only be achieved with earlier diagnosis and treatment.

A. Signs and Symptoms: Physical examination reveals only indirect evidence of aortic dissection. Blood pressure can be elevated, normal, or low. Hypotension is related to either rupture or loss of circulating blood volume into the false lumen. Blood pressures and pulses in the extremities may be asymmetric. A diastolic murmur suggestive of aortic valvular insufficiency and findings consistent with a pleural effusion are both common. Diminished cardiac tones, jugular venous distention, and pulsus paradoxus are suggestive of cardiac tamponade caused by rupture.

Severe sudden, persistent chest or back pain is the most common presenting symptom in the acute stage, occurring in at least 90% of patients. It is commonly temporally and topographically related to the initial intimal tear and subsequent formation of the false channel. Therefore, dissections involving the ascending aorta typically produce chest pain, whereas those occurring in the descending thoracic aorta usually cause back pain. The pain is classically described as having a "tearing" quality and may radiate to the neck, arms, abdomen, or hips. Abdominal pain may be present because of either the dissection itself or secondary visceral ischemia.

Acute congestive heart failure occurs in the setting of aortic valvular insufficiency. Obstruction of the brachiocephalic vessels can cause syncope or focal neurologic deficits. Other potential neurologic complaints include hoarseness caused by recurrent laryngeal nerve compression and lower extremity paralysis (in 1% of cases) due to spinal cord ischemia from occlusion of intercostal or lumbar arteries. Tracheobronchial compression manifests as stridor, dyspnea, or symptoms from a resulting pneumonia. Hemoptysis, hematemesis, or hematochezia raises concern about rupture into a pulmonary or gastrointestinal structure.

B. Imaging Studies: A combination of imaging studies is often required for precise diagnosis, delineation of the full extent of aortic involvement, and planning of surgical treatment.

1. Radiography–Although a chest radiograph cannot diagnose dissection or precisely localize the lesion, abnormal findings are usually present. A widened superior mediastinum and an enlarged or abnormal aortic contour are the most suggestive signs of dissection. Associated findings include cardiomegaly, a pericardial effusion, pulmonary edema, pleural effusions, and postobstructive pneumonia resulting from tracheobronchial occlusion.

2. Echocardiography–Transthoracic echocardiography may demonstrate a dilated ascending aorta with interruption of wall continuity and an adjacent echo-free space (the false lumen), which is diagnostic of dissection. Transesophageal echocardiography, unlike the transthoracic method, can evaluate the entire thoracic aorta and identifies aortic dissection with a significantly higher sensitivity. Both types of echocardiography reveal information concerning ventricular and valvular function. Therefore, in many instances, combined transthoracic and transesophageal echocardiography can provide all the needed information for diagnosis and operative planning. Because both methods can be performed at the bedside or in the operating room, they are ideal for patients who are too unstable to be transported to a nonintensive care area of the hospital.

3. Computed tomography (CT)–Contrast-enhanced CT is more than 90% sensitive for aortic dissection, which appears as two or more columns of contrast in the aorta, separated by an intimal flap. The diameter of the aneurysm can be precisely determined, and the true and false lumina can be differentiated based on their different opacification rates.

4. Magnetic resonance imaging (MRI)–MRI is also at least 90% sensitive for aortic dissection and can distinguish between the true and false lumina, identify the site of intimal tear, and display blood flow characteristics within the aorta without the use of contrast.

5. Aortography–Aortography remains the gold standard for aortic imaging, primarily because of its ability to evaluate branch vessel involvement. Although false-negative aortograms can occur in a setting of a totally thrombosed false lumen, aortography can often accurately reveal the extent of dissection and identify the site of intimal laceration.

C. Laboratory Findings: Electrocardiograms are often normal but may exhibit various associated abnormalities, such as left ventricular hypertrophy due to chronic hypertension, myocardial infarction due to dissection into the coronary arteries, or dysrhythmias caused by either chamber enlargement or direct disruption of the intracardiac conduction system by a spreading septal hematoma. An electrocardiogram that is not consistent with an acute myocardial infarction is strongly suggestive of aortic dissection in a patient presenting with severe chest pain.

Differential Diagnosis

Acute chest, back, or abdominal pain, evidence of branch vessel occlusion, and aortic valvular insufficiency are indicative of aortic dissection. Chest pain, especially with coexisting hemodynamic instability, is often initially attributed to an acute myocardial infarction or pulmonary embolism. Patients with aortic dissection usually have an electrocardiogram without ischemic changes and normal cardiac enzyme levels. A confirmed diagnosis of myocardial infarction, however, does not rule out concomitant aortic dissection. It is essential to evaluate all the signs, symptoms, and test results in order to make an accurate diagnosis.

Treatment

A. Medical Treatment: Patients with acute aortic dissections are at an extremely high risk for developing life-threatening complications. Prevention of these complications is primarily achieved by means of aggressive control of hypertension. The patient must be admitted to an intensive care unit where arterial blood pressure, hemodynamic parameters, urine output, peripheral pulses, and neurologic status are meticulously monitored. Systolic blood pressure is monitored continuously by an intra-arterial catheter and ideally maintained at 100–120 mmHg. In hypertensive patients, sodium nitroprusside (50 mg in 500 mL of 5% dextrose in water) is started at a rate of 0.5 µg/kg/min and titrated to maintain the systolic blood pressure within desired limits. If sodium nitroprusside treatment is continued for 48 hours, thiocyanate levels should be evaluated; the drug is discontinued if the level reaches or exceeds 10 mg/dL. Sodium nitroprusside should only be used in conjunction with β-blockers in patients with dissection; the former drug can cause progression of dissection when used alone.

β-Blockers reduce the heart rate, blood pressure, and pulsatile aortic load, thereby limiting the progression of dissection and reducing the risk of rupture. Effective β-blocking agents include propranolol (1 mg IV, repeated in 5-minute intervals until a heart rate of 60–70 beats/min is achieved; then repeated every 4–6 hours), atenolol and esmolol. Intravenous labetalol has both α- and β-blocking actions and can be administered instead of a sodium nitroprusside and β-blocker combination. In patients with contraindications to β-blockers, such as heart failure or a high degree of atrioventricular block, reserpine may be used. Pain is controlled with adequate narcotics.

Uncomplicated chronic DeBakey type III dissections without significant aortic dilatation are treated medically with β-blockers and antihypertensives. Without treatment, chronic distal aortic dissection carries a yearly mortality rate of 20%. Progressive aortic dilatation reaching 6 cm and the development of complications related to the dissecting aortic aneurysm are indications for operative repair. At least one-third of patients with chronic distal aortic dissection require surgical treatment within 5 years of diagnosis.

B. Surgical Treatment: Urgent surgery is indicated for patients with acute or chronic DeBakey type I or II aortic dissections. The indications for surgical repair of DeBakey type III dissections include (1) evidence of leak or rupture; (2) neurologic deficits or any other signs of aortic branch vessel compromise; (3) failed blood pressure control, especially in the presence of continued pain despite medical treatment; and (4) progressive enlargement of the false lumen. In patients with chronic dissections who are reasonable operative candidates, staged replacement of all segments measuring more than 6 cm in diameter is recommended. In patients with Marfan syndrome, this threshold is lowered to 5.5 cm.

Following stabilization in the intensive care unit, patients with an acute DeBakey type I or II aortic dissection must undergo urgent graft replacement of the ascending aorta. The dissection usually progresses distally to involve at least the proximal transverse arch; therefore, placement of a cross-clamp across the distal ascending aorta can cause laceration of the friable intimal flap, creating a new entry into the false lumen distal to the proposed graft. Use of profound hypothermic circulatory arrest obviates the need for such a cross-clamp. In acute dissection, the distal anastomotic suture line between the graft and the aorta is placed so that the false lumen is obliterated and all blood flow is directed into the true lumen, potentially minimizing the distal progression of dissection.

If the sinus segment and aortic valve are not involved, and the proximal aorta was previously normal, simple graft replacement of the tubular segment is performed. In most patients, this aortic resection includes the site of the original intimal tear. If there is calcific aortic valve disease with significant stenosis and a normal sinus segment, concomitant separate aortic valve replacement is performed. Aortic valve resuspension, rather than replacement, is attempted when aortic valvular insufficiency is secondary to dehiscence of one or more commissures from the aortic wall. In patients with annuloaortic ectasia and in all patients with Marfan syndrome, a composite valve graft is inserted. Concomitant coronary artery bypass is performed if the dissection extends into a coronary artery.

In DeBakey type I dissections, the entire transverse arch is involved. The mortality rate of transverse aortic arch replacement in acute dissections is 15.8%, contrasted to a 3.5% mortality for the same repair in chronic dissections. Therefore, in the acute setting, the transverse arch is addressed through "hemi-arch" replacement, which is fashioned by beveling the distal anastomosis under the brachiocephalic vessels; the entire arch is replaced only if the transverse aortic arch is ruptured, contains the initiating intimal tear, or is severely dilated.

Surgery is indicated for patients with acute DeBakey type III dissections only when complications develop or medical management is unsatisfactory. Distal aortic repair in the presence of dissection is more complicated than in cases of fusiform degenerative aneurysms, and thus requires longer aortic clamp times and carries a higher risk of paraplegia and paraparesis. Therefore, cardiofemoral bypass is often used; this provides visceral and renal protection and may reduce spinal cord ischemia. The segment of dissecting aorta is isolated between clamps (Fig 11–5). Graft replacement of the dissecting aneurysm includes resection of the weakest aortic segment (ie, the site of the initial intimal tear) and the obliteration of the false lumen at the distal suture line. The resulting decompression of the false lumen frequently relieves arterial branch obstruction and prevents progression of the dissection. A thoracoabdominal aortic replacement, with reattachment of intercostal, lumbar, visceral, and renal vessels may be necessary, particularly if dissection is superimposed on a previously existing fusiform thoracoabdominal aortic aneurysm.

Graft replacement of chronic DeBakey type III dissections is performed when complications develop or when the false lumen expands to a diameter of 6 cm (5.5 cm in patients with Marfan syndrome). Because major arteries may branch off of the false lumen, the distal anastomosis must direct blood flow into both lumina—otherwise, ischemic complications may result.

Postoperative Management

A. Immediate Care: Most patients with dissections involving the ascending aorta have extension into the descending aorta (ie, Debakey type I aortic dissection). Following surgical treatment of their ascending segment, at least 75% of these patients maintain some patency of the distal false lumen, despite reestablish-

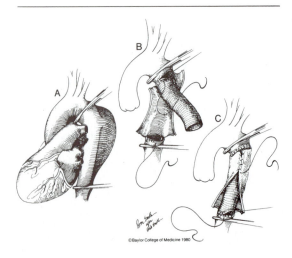

Figure 11–5. Repair of DeBakey type III aortic dissection, showing sequential steps A through C.

ment of flow into the proximal true lumen. Proximal aortic repair, therefore, essentially converts a De-Bakey type I dissection into an acute type III dissection, which requires continued meticulous blood pressure control to prevent further progression. Otherwise, the care of patients after operative repair of aortic dissection is essentially identical to that described above for patients following nondissecting thoracic aortic aneurysms.

B. Follow-up Care: Patients who have aortic dissection often develop aneurysms at unreplaced segments and therefore require evaluation of the aorta by CT or MRI scans at three and six months following the acute event, and yearly thereafter for life. Even with satisfactory blood pressure control, about 30% of patients with chronic distal aortic dissections will require an operation for aneurysmal dilatation of the false lumen. Prophylaxis against graft infection is important.

Prognosis

In the context of the extraordinarily poor prognosis of patients with untreated aortic dissections, survival following surgical repair is excellent. The overall 30-day, 5-year, and 10-year survival rates following operative repair of aortic dissection are 94%, 57%, and 41%, respectively. Aortic reoperation has been necessary in 13% of patients with dissection (all types) within 5 years, and in 23% within 10 years. Survival rates for the medical treatment of uncomplicated De-Bakey Type III dissections are 73%, 58%, and 25% at 1, 5, and 10 years, respectively. The surgical repair of DeBakey type III dissections has a 30-day survival rate of 67% when repair is performed during the acute phase and 91% when performed during the chronic stage. This forms the basis for the selection of careful medical management of acute DeBakey type III dissections in patients without complications such as branch vessel occlusion or suspected rupture.

Crawford ES: The diagnosis and management of aortic dissection. JAMA 1990;264;2537.

Crawford ES et al: Diffuse aneurysmal disease (chronic aortic dissection, Marfan, and mega-aorta syndromes) and multiple aneurysm: Treatment by subtotal and total aortic replacement emphasizing the elephant trunk technique. Ann Surg 1990;211:521.

Crawford ES et al: Surgery for acute ascending aortic dissection: Should the arch be included? J Thorac Cardiovasc Surg 1992;104:46.

Crawford ES, Svensson LG, Coselli JS, Safi HJ: Aortic dissection and dissecting aortic aneurysms. Ann Surg 1988;208:254.

Crawford ES, Svensson LG, Coselli JS, Safi HJ: Surgical treatment of aneurysm and/or dissection of the ascending aorta, transverse aortic arch, and ascending aorta and transverse aortic arch: Factors influencing survival in 717 patients. J Thorac Cardiovasc Surg 1989;98:659.

DeBakey ME, Lawrie GM, Crawford ES, Morris GC Jr: Surgical treatment of dissecting aortic aneurysms: 28 years experience with 527 cases. Contemp Surg 1984;25:13.

Fuster V, Ip JH: Medical aspects of acute aortic dissection. Semin Thorac Cardiovasc Surg 1991;3:219.

Khandheria BK: Aortic dissection, the last frontier. Circulation 1993;87(5):1765.

Svensson LG, Crawford ES, Hess KR, Coselli JS, Safi HJ: Dissection of the aorta and dissecting aortic aneurysms: Improving early and long-term surgical results. Circulation 1990;82 [Suppll IV]:IV-24–IV-38.

AORTITIS

Essentials of Diagnosis

- Autoimmune disorders, namely Takayasu's arteritis, giant cell arteritis, rheumatoid arthritis, and ankylosing spondylitis.
- Extensive thickening of the wall of an aortic aneurysm.

General Considerations

Aortitis can occur as either a localized or systemic process.

A. Inflammatory Aneurysms: Inflammatory aneurysms, which are characterized by localized swelling at sites of preexisting arteriosclerotic or aneurysmal disease can involve the thoracic aorta, but are more common in the infrarenal abdominal aorta. The specific cause is unknown. The inciting event leading to the inflammatory reaction may be mural hemorrhage, sclerosis of the vasa vasorum, or the mural changes secondary to arteriosclerosis. The ultimate result is dense infiltration of the full thickness of aortic wall by lymphocytes, plasma cells, and giant cells with subsequent fibrosis. The medial smooth muscle and elastic tissues are obliterated.

B. Takayasu's Arteritis: Takayasu's arteritis is a systemic autoimmune disorder that primarily affects the aorta, its branches, and the pulmonary artery. It is characterized by an acute inflammatory reaction with degeneration of the elastic tissue and proliferation of the connective tissue. This results in thickening of the intima, and necrosis with fibrosis involving both the medial and adventitial layers. When the intimal thickening is the predominant manifestation, occlusion of the aorta and its branches results. Less frequently, the medial necrosis predominates, causing attenuation of the vessel wall and aneurysm formation. Aortic dissection may occur as a superimposed process. Takayasu's arteritis typically involves young female patients with a mean age at onset of 24 years. Within ten years after diagnosis, nearly 40% of patients suffer cardiovascular complications such as stroke, aortic valvular insufficiency, myocardial infarction, cardiac failure, and ruptured aneurysm.

C. Giant Cell Arteritis: Also known as temporal arteritis, giant cell arteritis is another systemic autoimmune disorder of unknown cause that affects the aorta and its branches. It typically occurs in patients over 50 years of age, with a female to male ratio of about 3:1. Granulomatous inflammation of the entire thickness of the vessel wall leads to intimal thickening and medial destruction. Vessel occlusion and aneurysm formation are the respective sequelae, and dissection may be superimposed. Despite the name, giant cells are absent histologically in over 50% of cases.

D. Rheumatoid Aortitis: Rheumatoid aortitis is an uncommon systemic condition associated with rheumatoid arthritis and ankylosing spondylitis. The inflammatory process primarily involves the medial layer, which is ultimately replaced by fibrotic scar tissue, resulting in aortic annular dilatation and subsequent aortic valvular insufficiency. Ascending aortic aneurysms resulting from rheumatoid aortitis are extraordinarily rare.

Clinical Findings

A. Inflammatory Aneurysms: Patients with localized inflammatory thoracic aneurysms usually present with back or abdominal pain. Involvement of the abdominal aorta may result in a pulsatile, abdominal mass, which is tender (even in the absence of rupture), ureteral obstruction, and various gastrointestinal symptoms including nausea and early satiety.

On CT scan, an aortic aneurysm with an extensive "halo" of thickening beyond the ring of calcification is diagnostic of an inflammatory aneurysm.

B. Takayasu's Arteritis: During the acute phase of Takayasu's arteritis, patients experience fever, malaise, arthralgias, nausea, vomiting, chest pain, and tachycardia. The white blood cell count, erythrocyte sedimentation rate, and C-reactive protein levels are elevated. In addition to the aorta, involvement can include the coronary, pulmonary, brachiocephalic, visceral, renal, and peripheral arteries. Therefore, signs and symptoms secondary to either occlusion or aneurysmal dilatation of these vessels are often present and include loss of peripheral pulses, neurologic deficits, and heart failure. Specific findings on ophthalmologic examination are a fundal cap flush, a circular arteriovenous anastomosis around the papillae, and associated cataracts.

C. Giant Cell Arteritis: The onset of giant cell arteritis is associated with sudden fever, malaise, myalgias, anorexia, severe headaches, jaw pain, visual disturbances, tenderness of the temporal arteries, and an elevated erythrocyte sedimentation rate. Blindness occurs in 50% of untreated patients with involvement of the cranial vessels. Clinical evidence of aortic and major branch vessel involvement typically occurs later, after the acute manifestations have abated. During the acute phase, giant cell arteritis can be diagnosed by biopsy of the temporal artery, which will reveal granulomatous changes. Such a biopsy during the chronic phase, however, shows only nonspecific inflammatory changes and fibrosis.

Differential Diagnosis

The above mentioned clinical findings distinguish aortic disease due to aortitis from that caused by degenerative disease or infection. Like Takayasu's arteritis, Marfan syndrome and Ehlers-Danlos syndrome (Type IV) cause severe cardiovascular complications in young patients; these connective tissue disorders can be ruled-out based on established diagnostic criteria. The diagnosis of aortitis is confirmed by histologic examination of aortic tissue acquired during operative treatment.

Treatment

Like all other thoracic aortic aneurysms, those secondary to aortitis carry a high risk of rupture and other life-threatening complications. They therefore warrant surgical resection and graft replacement whenever they cause symptoms or are of significant diameter.

A. Inflammatory Aneurysms: The indications and methods for treatment of localized inflammatory thoracic aneurysms are identical with those described for thoracic aneurysms caused by degenerative disease.

B. Takayasu's Arteritis: The initial management of patients with acute Takayasu's arteritis involves control of hypertension and the use of steroids to provide symptomatic relief. Corticosteroids are of very limited use during the chronic phase. Patients presenting with cardiovascular symptoms require an operation. Although Takayasu's arteritis may affect a single aortic segment or arterial branch, it most frequently involves a combination of multiple segments and vessels and often requires multiple staged operations. Therefore, preoperative evaluation of the entire aorta and all its branches, including the coronary arteries, is critical. If a patient presents with signs of right heart failure, a right heart catheterization is indicated to rule out pulmonary arterial involvement.

In addition to graft replacement of aneurysmal aorta and branch vessels, significant obstructive lesions are bypassed with vein or prosthetic grafts. For example, proximal occlusion of the left subclavian artery is treated by a carotid to subclavian artery bypass. A large graft from the ascending aorta to the abdominal aorta may be used to treat obstructive lesions of the descending thoracic or upper abdominal aorta. Occlusive pulmonary arterial lesions may be repaired by replacement, bypass, or patch graft angioplasty.

C. Giant Cell Arteritis: For patients with giant cell arteritis, early diagnosis is essential because prompt corticosteroid therapy may restore pulses and prevent blindness. The aortic manifestations are not affected by corticosteroid therapy and require surgical intervention to avoid serious complications.

Prognosis

The surgical treatment of aortitis has an early survival rate exceeding 90% in centers experienced in aortic surgery. Long-term survival rates are also excellent. Because of their propensity for the development of further cardiovascular complications, these patients require lifelong follow-up.

Austen WG, Blennerhassett JB: Giant-cell aortitis causing aneurysm of the ascending aorta and aortic regurgitation. N Engl J Med 1965;272:80.

Huston KA et al: Temporal arteritis: A 25-year epidemiologic, clinical, and pathologic study. Ann Intern Med 1978;88:162.

Ishikawa K: Natural history and classification of occlusive thromboaortopathy, Takayasu's disease. Circulation 1978; 57:27.

Lande A, Berkmen YM: Aortitis: Pathologic, clinical and arteriographic review. Radiol Clin North Am 1976;14:219.

Lupi-Herrera E et al: Takayasu's arteritis: Clinical study of 107 cases. Am Heart J 1977;93:94.

Nasu T: Pathology of pulseless disease: A systematic study and critical review of twenty-one autopsy cases reported in Japan. Angiology 1962;14:225.

Robbs JV, Human RR, Rajaruthnam P: Operative treatment of nonspecific aortitis (Takayasu's arteritis). J Vasc Surg 1986;3:605.

THORACIC AORTIC INFECTION

Essentials of Diagnosis

- Aneurysmal disease associated with a current or previous febrile illness.
- The combination of clinical systemic infection, histologic findings consistent with aortic infection, and positive blood or aortic tissue cultures.
- A history of sepsis, syphilis, endocarditis, thoracic trauma, or previous cardiac or aortic surgery.

General Considerations

Primary infections of aortic tissue result from bacteremia or embolic seeding and can occur in a normal, atherosclerotic, or aneurysmal aorta. Sources of bacteremia include bacterial endocarditis, osteomyelitis, cellulitis, pneumonia, and dental, gastrointestinal, or genitourinary procedures. Direct mediastinal contamination due to trauma or surgery causes secondary aortic infection. Previously placed prosthetic aortic grafts can also become infected; this serious complication occurs in less than 2% of all aortic graft replacement operations. Infected grafts result from intraoperative contamination, wound and venous catheter infections, postoperative bacteremia, and erosion of the graft into the gastrointestinal tract.

Infection of the aortic wall produces destruction of the tunica media, resulting in weakening and aneurysm formation. Infected aneurysms are called **mycotic aneurysms,** which, despite the name, are usually caused by bacteria and very rarely by fungi. Less than 1% of all aortic aneurysms are mycotic. Syphilitic aneurysms are rare today because of the early effective antibiotic treatment of syphilis. Syphilitic infection of the aortic tunica media causes chronic inflammation with subsequent fibrosis, mural attenuation, and aneurysmal dilatation. These aneurysms most frequently involve the ascending and transverse arch segments, are usually saccular, and are known to erode the sternum or chest wall. Mycotic aneurysms caused by pyogenic bacteria—usually *Staphylococcus, Streptococcus, Salmonella,* or *Escherichia coli*—are much more common. Pyogenic bacteria produce mural abscesses, which result in aortic wall destruction and aneurysm formation.

Prevention of graft infection requires the use of broad-spectrum parenteral antibiotics in all patients with vascular grafts undergoing procedures that can cause significant bacteremia.

Clinical Findings

Patients with thoracic aortic infection usually present with pain, fever and other manifestations of systemic infection. They may have a history of syphilis or previous febrile illness, although the original inciting infection is often not identified. Because multiple aortic segments can be simultaneously involved, evaluation of the entire aorta is very important. The presence of accumulating fluid or air in perigraft tissues, which is diagnostic for graft infection may be noted on radiographs, ultrasound, CT, or MRI. Blood cultures may reveal the identity of the pathogen.

Treatment

Because graft infection does not occur secondary to *Treponema pallidum,* the operative repair of syphilitic thoracic aortic aneurysms is identical to the repair of aneurysms of degenerative cause. Pyogenic thoracic aortic aneurysms and infected grafts, however, are treated by wide debridement followed by restoration of aortic continuity. Preoperative treatment with intravenous antibiotics is guided by the results of blood cultures. When the infection is limited to the abdominal aorta or peripheral arteries, an extra-anatomic bypass may be performed to avoid infection of the new graft. This approach is exceedingly more difficult for infections involving the thoracic aorta, therefore, Dacron patch angioplasty or in situ tube graft replacement is used after wide excision and debridement of the infected tissues. The inclusion technique (suturing the aneurysmal wall around the graft) is not used. The resulting periaortic dead space is filled with viable, well-vascularized tissue, such as the omentum or a muscle flap, wrapped around the graft. Flaps of the pectoralis major, rectus abdominus, latissimus dorsi, and serratus all have been used. To reduce the risk of prosthetic graft reinfection, the use of a tissue homograft to replace the involved segment has also been advocated. Otherwise, the details of the specific operation generally parallel those for degenerative thoracic aortic aneurysms.

Postoperative Care

Postoperatively, patients with thoracic aortic infection are treated with high-dose intravenous antibiotics for 4–6 weeks, based on the results of blood or aortic wall cultures. Resected aortic or graft tissue cultures are often negative because of intensive antibiotic treatment. Lifelong oral suppressive antibiotic therapy is mandatory to prevent recurrence.

Prognosis

Debridement and graft replacement of mycotic thoracic aortic aneurysms are associated with short- and long-term survival rates of 83% and 70%, respectively.

Brow SL et al: Bacteriologic and surgical determinants of survival in patients with mycotic aneurysms. J Vasc Surg 1984;1:541.

Chan FY et al: In-situ prosthetic graft replacement for mycotic aneurysm of the aorta. Ann Thorac Surg 1989;47:193.

Coselli JS et al: Treatment of postoperative infection of ascending aorta and transverse aortic arch. Ann Thorac Surg 1990;50:868.

James EC, Gillespie JT: Aortic mycotic abdominal aneurysm involving all visceral branches: Excision and Dacron graft replacement. J Cardiovasc Surg 1977;18:353.

Johansen K, Devin J: Mycotic aortic aneurysms. Arch Surg 1983;118:583.

TRAUMATIC AORTIC INJURY

Essentials of Diagnosis

- Penetrating chest injury or blunt trauma with rapid deceleration.
- No specific symptoms or physical signs.
- External chest wounds are suggestive.
- Widening of superior mediastinum or obliteration of aortic knob on upright chest x-ray.
- High index of suspicion and liberal aortography required.

General Considerations

Traumatic aortic injuries occur frequently. Unfortunately, survival in patients with an aortic injury is extremely rare. In patients who die following an automobile accident, aortic injury is present in 16% of cases and is the primary cause of death in 5%. Ninety percent of traumatic aortic injuries are fatal at the accident scene. At least 40% of patients with a thoracic aortic injury die within 24 hours if not operated upon. Patients with unrecognized aortic injuries rarely survive the acute event. Those few who do survive will develop traumatic thoracic aortic aneurysms, which eventually rupture. When a chronic traumatic thoracic aortic aneurysm is diagnosed, it should be treated in the same aggressive manner as other aneurysms in order to prevent life-threatening complications.

Aortic injury can occur in the setting of penetrating trauma, blunt trauma, and iatrogenic injury. Penetrating thoracic trauma is the most common cause of great vessel injury and usually involves simple laceration of the aorta. Blast effect from a missile can also result in an aortic disruption. Following blunt trauma such as a fall from a great height or a motor vehicle accident, the most common cause of instantaneous death is traumatic aortic rupture. Several mechanisms are felt to contribute to blunt traumatic aortic rupture. Sudden deceleration results in shear forces between mobile and fixed segments of the aorta. The descending thoracic aorta is relatively fixed at two sites—the ligamentum arteriosum and the level of the diaphragm—making this segment extremely susceptible to rupture. Indeed, 58–71% of traumatic aortic ruptures involve the descending thoracic segment. Blunt trauma can also cause direct compression of the aorta against the vertebral column. The marked intravascular hypertension that occurs during a severe traumatic event contributes to the disruption of aortic integrity. Iatrogenic injuries to the aorta usually result in aortic dissection and occur at sites of aortotomy, anastomosis, cross-clamping, or contact by an intra-aortic catheter.

Following aortic injury, the continuity of the aortic wall may be maintained by an intact adventitial layer, which prevents sudden death. Injuries to the ascending aorta or proximal transverse arch often bleed into the pericardial sac, causing tamponade, whereas injuries to the descending segment usually bleed into the mediastinum or left chest. If hemorrhage into the mediastinum occurs, the hematoma must remain contained to allow survival. Free rupture of the aorta into the left thorax produces rapidly fatal exsanguination. When a penetrating aortic injury also involves an adjacent venous structure, such as the superior vena cava or innominate vein, an aortovenous fistula may result.

When evaluating a patient following trauma, the degree of suspicion for an aortic injury should be based initially on the mechanism of injury. Aortic disruption must be considered following any event that produces rapid deceleration, such as a high-speed automobile collision. Because of the extremely high mortality of unrecognized aortic injuries, a high index of suspicion and a meticulous clinical evaluation are mandatory in all trauma patients.

Clinical Findings

A. Signs and Symptoms: No specific symptoms result from aortic injury. Patients may complain of difficulty breathing, lower extremity weakness or paralysis, or symptoms related to hypovolemic shock.

At least 50% of patients with an aortic disruption present without physical signs of the injury. Although hemodynamic instability or respiratory distress may be the only signs, several other findings are suggestive of aortic injury. Inspection and palpation of the chest may reveal external chest wounds, such as a steering wheel imprint or other contusions and abrasions; subcutaneous emphysema; an expanding thoracic outlet hematoma; or palpable fractures involving the sternum, thoracic spine, or left ribs with flail chest. Crush injuries of the chest can cause superior vena caval compression resulting in edema and petechia of the upper torso, face, and arms. Peripheral pulses may be unequal, diminished, or absent. In light of the high risk of developing paraplegia after surgical repair of aortic injuries, the importance of documenting the patient's neurologic status during the initial physical examination cannot be overstated.

B. Imaging Studies:

1. Radiography—In patients with penetrating chest wounds, radiopaque wound clips mark entry and exit sites to help suggest the trajectory. The radiographic findings that are suggestive of an aortic injury in patients with penetrating thoracic trauma are hemothorax, pneumothorax, and proximity of a foreign body or missile trajectory to the aorta. If the foreign body appears within the cardiac silhouette and is out of focus with respect to the rest of the radiograph, it may be located within the heart. A confusing bullet trajectory may indicate embolization of the missile.

In patients sustaining blunt thoracic trauma, several findings on chest radiography raise the suspicion of an aortic disruption. Widening of the superior mediastinum to greater than 8 cm is the most consistent finding. The most reliable marker of aortic transection is obliteration of the aortic knob. Other suggestive findings are hemothorax; a left apical hematoma or "pleural cap"; an aortic double contour; calcium layering in the region of the aortic knob; obliteration of the aortopulmonary window or anterior displacement of the trachea on a lateral chest film; rightward deviation of the trachea, an endotracheal tube, or a nasogastric tube; depression of the left main stem bronchus; elevation or rightward shift of the right main stem bronchus; fractures involving the first rib, second rib, multiple ribs, thoracic spine, scapula, or sternum; and dislocation of the thoracic spine. In 7.3% of patients with traumatic rupture of the thoracic aorta or brachiocephalic arteries, the chest radiograph reveals no signs of mediastinal abnormality.

2. Aortography—Because no single radiographic sign reliably predicts or excludes an aortic injury, liberal aortography is mandatory. Aortography is the gold standard for detecting aortic disruption and is indicated in all hemodynamically stable patients with a significant mechanism and either physical signs of chest trauma or any radiographic signs suggestive of aortic injury. When all trauma patients with a widened mediastinum on a chest radiograph undergo aortography, about 10% of aortograms are positive for aortic injury. False-positive aortograms can occur owing to either a ductus diverticulum or vascular ring remnant.

3. Other imaging studies—Aortography remains superior to both CT and MRI for the diagnosis of aortic injury; therefore, CT and MRI have no practical role in the evaluation of the thoracic aortic in the trauma setting. The usefulness of TEE in the diagnosis of thoracic aortic injury is currently under evaluation.

C. Laboratory Findings: The initial evaluation of any patient with significant thoracic trauma should include hematocrit level, urinalysis, electrocardiogram, and arterial blood gas values.

Differential Diagnosis

Besides aortic injury, several other life-threatening thoracic injuries are associated with respiratory distress, hemodynamic instability, and an abnormal chest radiograph. In fact, thoracic trauma often results in multiple injuries within the chest. Therefore, an aortic disruption may occur along with any of the following injuries:

- Airway obstruction.
- Tracheobronchial disruption.
- Tension pneumothorax.
- Massive hemothorax.
- Flail chest.
- Cardiac injury and tamponade.
- Traumatic diaphragmatic hernia.
- Esophageal disruption.
- Vascular injuries involving the subclavian vessels, innominate vessels, left common carotid artery, pulmonary vessels, thoracic vena cava, azygos vein, internal mammary arteries, or intercostal arteries.

Other associated thoracic injuries are pulmonary contusions, myocardial contusion, thoracic duct injuries, and air embolism secondary to pulmonary injuries.

Treatment

A. Medical Treatment: The initial evaluation and resuscitation of persons with aortic injury follows Advanced Trauma Life Support protocol. All patients with thoracic trauma should receive 100% oxygen through a face mask or, if indicated, an endotracheal tube. Large-caliber intravenous lines need to be placed to facilitate volume replacement. Immediate tube thoracostomy is performed for patients in respiratory distress if pneumothorax or hemothorax is suspected. Use of a cell-saving repository should be considered in the setting of large hemothorax. If bleeding persists after a chest tube is inserted and output is greater than 1 L, the patient must be transported directly to the operating room for an emergency thoracotomy.

Packed red blood cell transfusion for severe shock is initiated (using type-specific, non-cross-matched blood, if necessary). Central venous pressure and urine output are monitored with a subclavian venous catheter and an indwelling bladder catheter, respectively. In patients with aortic injuries who have survived transport to the hospital, the periaortic hemorrhage is contained by the adventitial layer, adjacent mediastinal structures, and clotting mechanisms. Hypotension protects these patients from free rupture by keeping the hematoma contained. Intravenous fluid administration should therefore be limited, maintaining an acceptable degree of hypotension until the hemorrhage can be directly controlled during surgery.

A patient with significant mechanism of injury who is hemodynamically stable and has no physical or radiographic signs of aortic injury may be followed with serial chest radiographs, obtained at 4 hours and 24 hours after presentation.

B. Surgical Treatment: Ideally, thoracotomy is delayed until it can be performed in the operating room. Immediate left anteriolateral thoracotomy performed in the emergency center, however, is indicated for patients presenting with penetrating thoracic trauma and hypovolemic cardiac arrest. This procedure allows descending aortic cross clamping which stops distal hemorrhage and improves cerebral and myocardial perfusion. In addition to the control of active bleeding, emergency center thoracotomy facilitates pericardiotomy for treatment of cardiac tamponade, repair of cardiac or vascular injuries, and open cardiac massage. It is rarely indicted in patients sustaining blunt trauma.

In cases in which the patient requires surgery before arteriograms are obtained, such as hemodynamic instability, suspected thoracic aortic injuries of unknown location are approached via a left anterolateral thoracotomy with the patient in a supine position. Ascending aortic injuries are approached through a median sternotomy. Unless there is a posterior ascending aortic injury, the repair of penetrating injuries to the ascending aorta is usually possible without adjuncts, whereas the repair of ascending aortic rupture due to blunt trauma requires cardiopulmonary bypass.

A posterolateral thoracotomy through the 4th intercostal space is used to approach descending thoracic aortic injuries. The most common site of injury occurs along the medial aspect of the proximal descending aorta at level of the ligamentum arteriosum. The proximal aorta is cross clamped between the left common carotid artery and left subclavian artery. Great care must be taken to avoid entering the site of injury until this proximal control has been obtained. The aortic disruption is repaired with either direct primarily suturing, end-to-end anastomosis, or graft interposition. The use of adjuncts for spinal cord protection during descending thoracic aortic repair is controversial.

Postoperative Management

A. Immediate Care: The postoperative management of these patients is essentially identical to that described above for surgical treatment of degenerative aneurysms and dissection. In addition, all other concomitant injuries must also be addressed appropriately.

B. Complications:

1. Paraplegia and paraparesis—Careful preoperative documentation of neurologic status and communication of the potential for paraplegia to the patient and family are extremely important. The incidence of neurologic deficits involving the lower extremities following repair of a descending aortic injury resulting from blunt trauma approximates 7%. The extent of the aortic injury is the most important predisposing factor.

2. Pulmonary complications—Pulmonary complications including atelectasis, respiratory insufficiency, pneumonia, and adult respiratory distress syndrome are the most common complications following the repair of aortic injuries. Aggressive pulmonary therapy and early patient mobilization following extubation are important protective measures.

3. Other complications—Postoperative hemorrhage is generally a result of either technical problems or a coagulopathy caused by massive transfusion of blood products. Acute renal failure, left vocal cord paralysis, vascular stenosis or thrombosis, and formation of an arteriovenous fistula are additional complications. Complications from concomitant head, abdominal, or other injuries are also common.

C. Follow-up Care: Patients with aortic grafts need antibiotic prophylaxis during all invasive or dental procedures.

Prognosis

With appropriate surgical treatment, the in-hospital mortality rate of an acute traumatic aortic disruption ranges from 11% to 19%. A significant portion of in-hospital mortality results from either associated injuries or complications of multisystem trauma, including head injury, infection, and respiratory or renal insufficiency.

American College of Surgeons Committee on Trauma: Thoracic trauma. In: *Advanced trauma life support course.* American College of Surgeons, 1989:89.

Duhaylongsod FG et al: Acute traumatic aortic aneurysm: The Duke experience from 1970 to 1990. J Vasc Surg 1992;15:331.

Hilgenberg AD et al: Blunt injuries of the thoracic aorta. Ann Thorac Surg 1992;53:233.

Mattox KL: Thoracic great vessel injury. Surg Clin North Am 1988;68:693.

Mattox KL, O'Gorman RB: Injury to the thoracic great vessels. In: *Trauma.* Mattox KL, Moore EE, Feliciano DV (editors). Appleton & Lange, 1988;384.

Meyer DM: Thoracic and great vessel injury. In: *The Parkland Trauma Handbook.* Lopez-Viego MA (editor). Mosby-Yearbook, 1994:217.

Woodring JH: The normal mediastinum in blunt traumatic rupture of the thoracic aorta and brachiocephalic arteries. J Emerg Med 1990;8:467.

Thoracic Outlet Syndrome

12

Richard J. Sanders, MD, & Michael A. Cooper, MD

What today is called thoracic outlet syndrome (TOS) was known historically as scalenus anticus syndrome. In the early 1900s, this was thought to be a vascular problem due to congenital cervical ribs. TOS is now regarded primarily as a neurogenic disease most commonly a result of neck trauma.

TOS os defined as symptoms in the upper extrimity caused by neurovascular compression in the thoracic outlet area. Because the neurovascular bundle includes nerve, artery, and vein, there are three types of TOS: neurogenic, arterial, and venous. From the clinical viewpoint, neurogenic TOS is the most common, accounting for over 95% of all TOS cases. Together, arterial and venous TOS account for less than 5%. It is not unusual for neurogenic TOS to accompany either arterial or venous TOS, but arterial and venous TOS rarely coexist. The three types of TOS are summarized in Table 12–1.

NEUROGENIC TYPE

Essentials of Diagnosis
- History of neck injury.
- Neck pain, headache, shoulder and arm pain.
- Numbness and tingling in the fingers.
- Arm weakness resulting from brachial pressure compression.

General Considerations

The major spaces in the thoracic outlet area are the scalene triangle and the costoclavicular space. The pectoralis minor space is lateral to these 2 areas and is seldom involved in TOS (Fig 12–1). The scalene triangle is the most important structure. While standard anatomy texts describe the brachial plexus nerve roots as emerging in the space between anterior and middle scalene muscles, observations in the operating room demonstrate the roots pushing their way between groups of muscle fibers rather than lying in a open space. The close relationship between nerve and muscle is probably the underlying factor for the development of neurogenic TOS in many patients. Anatomic variations in the scalene triangle are illustrated in Figure 12–2.

A. Cause: The cause of neurogenic TOS is probably a combination of congenital narrowing of the scalene triangle and neck trauma. Several investigators have noted variations in muscle anatomy of the scalene muscles as well as a large variety of congenital ligaments and bands that attach to the first rib. It is surprising to discover how high the incidence of neck trauma is in patients presenting with TOS symptoms. It is in these same patients, a large number of muscle anomalies or anatomic variations have been seen, such as scalene minimus muscles and splits of the anterior scalene muscle around the C5 and C6 nerve roots. These anatomic variations have been present since birth, yet patients did not develop symptoms until some type of neck injury occurred. Table 12–2 summarizes the different causes.

Cervical ribs are only one of several anatomic variations that can narrow the scalene triangle. Less than 5% of neurogenic TOS patients were noted to have cervical ribs. This is several times higher than the 0.7% incidence of cervical ribs in the normal population, suggesting that cervical ribs contribute to neurogenic TOS. However, most patients with cervical ribs do not develop symptoms until neck trauma occurs. The incidence of symptoms in patients with cervical ribs is 11%.

Many patients acquire neurogenic TOS symptoms through their work. The common denominator is repetitive hand motions such as on assembly lines. Their hands may be tied to the job, so the worker cannot turn his or her body around to talk. Instead, they twist and hyperextend their necks to talk to people, hold a telephone against their shoulders, or look at a computer monitor that is positioned above or to the side of their keyboard. These motions cause minor neck trauma, which can be repeated many times per hour or even per minute. The cumulative small traumata to the scalene muscles eventually leads to muscle fibrosis.

B. Pathophysiology: Microscopic examination of the scalene muscles of TOS patients has demonstrated 2 types of abnormalities. In the first type of abnormality, type II muscle fibers are reduced in number and become pleomorphic, and type I fibers are dominant, and in the second type, the amount of connective tissue around each muscle fiber increases. The increase was significant, from 14% in control patients to 36% in neurogenic TOS patients. The type I fiber predominance is a nonspecific change seen in a variety of muscle diseases and dysfunctions. However, the increase in connective tissue has not been seen in other

Table 12–1. Types of TOS.

Type	Incidence	Cause	Symptoms	Physical Examination	Treatment
Neurogenic	95+%	Congenital anatomic narrowing plus neck trauma	Paresthesia in fingers; neck pain; occipital headaches; arm pain	Supraclavic; tenderness; Duplication symptoms with arms in 90 degree AER position	Scalenectomy, 1st rib resection or combined scalectomy & 1st rib resection
Arterial	1+%	Cervical rib or anomalous 1st rib	Digital ischemia; coldness; digital numbness claudication; hand pain	Decreased BP; decreased pulses; pallor; digital gangrene	Replace or bypass aneurysm; resect cervical or abnormal 1st rib thrombectomy; dorsal sympathectomy
Venous	2+%	Venous compression at costoclavic angle	Swelling; arm pain	Swelling; cyanosis; distended veins over chest	Remove thrombus; resect 1st rib; endo-venectomy or venous bypass plus temporary AVF

AVF, arteriovenous fistula.

muscle abnormalities; it has only been observed in neurogenic TOS patients. This connective tissue represents intramuscular scarring and supports the theory that trauma and scalene muscle fibrosis are the cause of many neurogenic TOS cases (Fig 12–3).

Clinical Findings

A. Signs and Symptoms: The most common progression of symptoms begins with a history of neck injury, followed by neck pain, headache, and shoulder and arm pain with numbness and tingling in the fingers developing within a few days to weeks. However, there are many variations on this pattern.

Occasionally, symptoms do not follow the typical progression. The previously mentioned symptoms can indicate brachial pressure compression. Patients often complain of numbness in their hands at night, especially when they sleep with their arms over their head. Even angina needs to be ruled out when the patient experiences anterior chest pain. Some patients give no history of trauma.

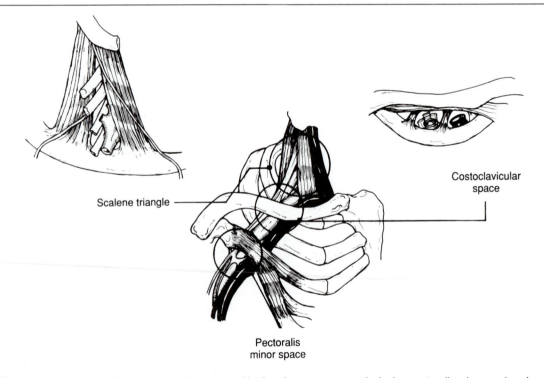

Scalene triangle

Costoclavicular space

Pectoralis minor space

Figure 12–1. Anatomy of the thoracic outlet area and its 3 main spaces: costoclavicular, pectoralis minor, and scalene triangle. (Reproduced, with permission, from Sanders RJ, Haug CE: *Thoracic Outlet Syndrome: A Common Sequela of Neck Injuries.* JB Lippincott, 1991:34.)

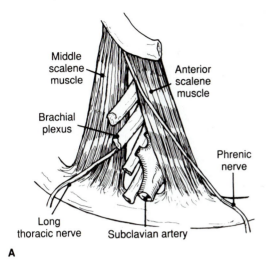

Middle scalene muscle

Anterior scalene muscle

Brachial plexus

Phrenic nerve

Long thoracic nerve

Subclavian artery

A

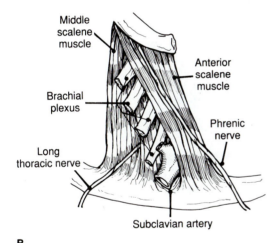

Middle scalene muscle

Anterior scalene muscle

Brachial plexus

Phrenic nerve

Long thoracic nerve

Subclavian artery

B

Figure 12–2. Variations in the relations within the scalene triangle. **A:** The relations found in most cadavers. The triangle is wider and the nerves emerge a little lower in the triangle than in most TOS patients. **B:** The nerves emerge high in the triangle, touching the scalene muscles as they emerge. (Reproduced, with permission, from Sanders RJ, Roos DB: The surgical anatomy of the scalene triangle. Contemp Surg 1989;35:11.)

Paresthesia is often described as being in the ulnar nerve distribution, involving the 4th and 5th fingers. However, involvement of all 5 fingers seems to be a more common distribution; ulnar nerve distribution is the next most common finding. Usually, paresthesia involves just the fingers, but in some patients the entire upper extremity is affected. Weakness of the arm and hand often manifests by the person's dropping things such as glasses and coffee cups. Symptoms typically appear when combing, setting, or blow drying hair; driving a car; or working with the arms overhead.

There are very few positive findings on physical ex-

Table 12–2. Causes of 668 operated cases of TOS.

Trauma		86%
Auto accident	32%	
Work injury	22%	
Other trauma	8%	
Cervical or rudimentary first rib (without trauma)		2%
Axillary vein occlusion		1%
Arterial occlusion		1%
Soft tissue/unknown (no history of trauma)		10%
		100%

(Reprinted, with permission, from Sanders RJ, Haug CE: *Thoracic Outlet Syndrome: A Common Sequela of Neck Injuries.* JB Lippincott 1991:26.)

amination. The most consistent are supraclavicular tenderness over the anterior scalene muscles and duplication of the patient's symptoms with the arms abducted to 90 degrees in external rotation ("stick-em-up" position). Other findings include eliciting paresthesia in the hand or arm by pressing over the scalene muscles in the neck; a positive Tinel's sign elicited by tapping over the brachial plexus in the supraclavicular area; tilting the head to one side and noting pain or paresthesia in the contralateral neck or shoulder; and a positive upper limb tension test. None of these findings is pathognomonic for neurogenic TOS, but the combination of most of these findings on physical examination with a typical history is strong clinical evidence supporting a diagnosis.

The **Adson test** is historically known, but is not a good test. Adson's sign is a positional cut-off of the radial pulse by turning the head toward the ipsilateral side and inhaling deeply. This sign, as well as demonstrating radial pulse deficits with other positional maneuvers, are unreliable because many normal people lose their radial pulses during these maneuvers and most TOS patients do not exhibit pulse loss. Therefore, positional pulse deficits cannot be used to confirm or eliminate a diagnosis of neurogenic TOS.

In an occasional, a patient atrophy of the thenar muscles of the hand. This can be associated with weakness of other intrinsic hand muscles and wasting of muscles of the inner aspect of the forearm.

B. Laboratory Findings: In patients with clinical neurogenic TOS, several tests of neurophysiologic function have been tried in a effort to find a reliable objective diagnostic test. The tests include electromyography, nerve conduction velocities, late F-wave responses, sensory-evoked potentials, and cervical root stimulation. Unfortunately, the results have been normal or reveal nonspecific changes. Only an occasional patient, with muscle wasting in the hand, has demonstrated a typical abnormality for neurogenic TOS: A reduction in amplitude of ulnar sensory action potentials without a comparable change in velocity.

The **scalene muscle block** (injection of the anterior scalene muscle with local anesthetic) is a helpful diagnostic test. The test is performed by extending the neck and injecting 4 mL of 1% lidocaine into the belly of the anterior scalene muscle. Loss of tenderness over

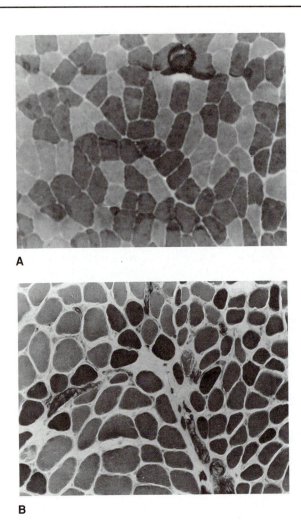

A

B

Figure 12–3. Connective tissue stain in control patient (**A**) and TOS patient. (**B**) Note the increase in connective tissue around individual muscle fibers in TOS patient. (Reproduced, with permission, from Sanders RJ, Jackson CGR, Banchero N, Pearce WH: Scalene muscle abnormalities in traumatic thoracic outlet syndrome. Am J Surg. 1990;159:231.)

the scalene muscle indicates a good block. If the brachial plexus is anesthetized, the block is regarded as inconclusive. In neurogenic TOS patients, there is improvement in the following physical findings a few minutes after the block: the neck is more mobile; less pain on head tilting; 180-degree abduction is easier; there is less tenderness around the shoulder tendons; and abducting the arms to 90 degrees in external rotation results in fewer or less intense symptoms. A good result is defined as improvement in some of these findings, not necessarily all of them. Failure to improve after the block suggests that neurogenic TOS is not the diagnosis. The test is fairly reliable but not infallible.

C. Imaging Studies: Cervical spine x-ray films may show a cervical rib or anomalous first rib; on occasion, a healed fracture of the clavicle or first rib may be seen. Such findings provide an objective anatomic explanation for a narrow neurovascular space (Fig 12–4).

The primary use of magnetic resonance imaging (MRI) in patients with upper extremity symptoms is to identify cervical spine disease such as a herniated disk or arthritis. MRI is also helpful in diagnosing shoulder pathology. Although some investigation of the use of MRI to detect scalene muscle abnormalities is currently in process, no definitive patterns have been established.

Differential Diagnosis

In addition to neurogenic TOS, patients with several other conditions can present with pain and paresthesia in the upper extremity. In patients with a history of trauma, it is usual for more than one condition to exist; and multiple diagnoses are common. It is important to be aware of these conditions and to know how to distinguish them from TOS.

A. Cumulative Trauma Syndrome: This interesting name has been applied to a combination of nerve compressions in the upper extremity that devel-

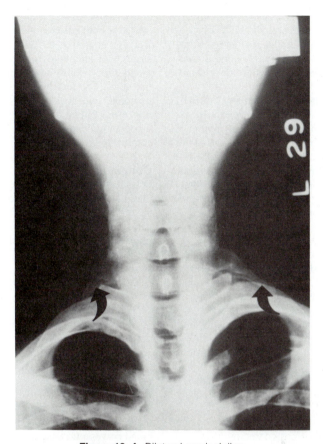

Figure 12–4. Bilateral cervical ribs.

ops in patients who work long hours of each day with their hands. Symptoms of pain and paresthesia develop in the hands, forearms, elbows, and arms, often bilaterally. The pathology is nerve compression at more than one point—wrist, forearm, elbow, or thoracic outlet area. Each of these areas must be evaluated by history, physical examination, and neuroelectric studies where applicable. Treatment is directed toward each individual compression point.

B. Carpal Tunnel Syndrome: Pain and paresthesia in the hand, usually the first 3 fingers (median nerve distribution), is characteristic of carpal tunnel compression. It can also involve all 5 fingers and may be associated with neurogenic TOS or mistaken for it. Carpal tunnel compression is a frequent finding among people who work on keyboards or assembly lines all day, as is neurogenic TOS. Median nerve, and sometimes ulnar nerve, conduction velocities are prolonged across the wrist. When symptoms are limited to the hands and forearms, carpal tunnel syndrome is a more likely diagnosis than neurogenic TOS.

C. Other Nerve Compression Syndromes: Peripheral nerve compression can occur in several places in the upper extremity including the wrist, pronator tunnel, radial nerve tunnel beneath the supinator, and ulnar nerve tunnel at the elbow. Diagnoses are made by precise location of symptoms, points of local tenderness, positive Tinel's sign, and positive neurophysiologic studies.

D. Shoulder Tendinitis: Injury and inflammation of the biceps and rotator cuff tendons around the shoulder, as well as acromioclavicular joint impingement, are frequently associated with TOS, especially if a shoulder injury was the cause of the symptoms. Tenderness on physical examination over the shoulder tendons and reduced range of motion of the shoulder joint should arouse suspicion of shoulder joint pathology. Abnormalities on MRI or arthrogram support the diagnosis.

E. Fibromyositis: Pain over the trapezius, rhomboid, infraspinatus, supraspinatus, and muscles over the back of the neck is a common complaint in neurogenic TOS patients. The cause is inflammation of these muscles caused by trauma. The only diagnostic sign is tenderness over the muscles. This finding frequently coexists with TOS and is treated with physical therapy.

F. Cervical Spine or Disk Disease: Nerve root irritation by abnormalities within the cervical spine can produce cervical radiculopathy with symptoms similar to neurogenic TOS. It most often involves the

C6 or C7 nerve roots, whereas TOS more commonly involves the lower plexus, C8 and T1. MRI is probably the best diagnostic tool although myelograms may still be needed. Cervical spine disease is not as common a differential as carpal tunnel syndrome or shoulder tendinitis.

G. Reflex Sympathetic Dystrophy (RSD): Burning pain in the arm, out of proportion to the extent of an arm injury, is the characteristic symptom of RSD of the upper extremity. It may be associated with paresthesia and may accompany neurogenic TOS. The diagnosis is made by noting relief of pain after stellate ganglion block. When RSD coexists with TOS, dorsal sympathectomy can be performed at the time of thoracic outlet decompression.

Treatment

Initial treatment of neurogenic TOS is a physical therapy program of neck stretching, abdominal breathing, and posture exercises. These should be performed on a home program at least once a day for several months. A physical therapist should supervise the exercise program, particularly early in the course of therapy.

Diagnosis and treatment of associated conditions should be done at the beginning of therapy. Fibromyositis, tendinitis, and peripheral nerve entrapment syndromes can all be treated simultaneously with TOS.

Surgery is the last resort for treating neurogenic TOS patients and should be considered only after all other conservative methods have been exhausted. The patient should understand that the results of surgery cannot be guaranteed and that a good result is improvement, but seldom total relief, of symptoms.

First rib resection, anterior and middle scalenectomy, or combined first rib resection and scalenectomy are all accepted surgical procedures for relief of neurogenic TOS symptoms. They each enlarge the space through which the neurovascular bundle travels. First rib resection can be performed through any 1 of 4 approaches: transaxillary, infraclavicular, supraclavicular, and posterior. The posterior route is rarely used today because it requires cutting too many muscles and postoperative recovery is more painful. The supraclavicular approach has the advantage of permitting scalenectomy and first rib resection through the same incision.

Transaxillary and infraclavicular approaches permit resection of the first rib, but require dissecting deep through narrow tunnels, where good exposure may be difficult to obtain. The techniques are hard to teach and not easy to learn. However, once learned, the skills are readily applied. In patients with arm swelling along with neurologic symptoms, the anterior end of the first rib should be resected and the subclavian vein dissected free, something that can be achieved through each of these 2 approaches but cannot be done via the supraclavicular route.

The supraclavicular approach permits complete removal of both anterior and middle scalene muscles as well as recognition and release of many anatomic variations and anomalies of scalene muscles and ligaments. Good results have been obtained after both partial as well as total removal of these muscles. How complete scalenectomy must be has not been determined. In general, scalenectomy is technically an easier operation to perform than first rib resection because surgical exposure is better.

Complications

Injury to the brachial plexus, subclavian vessels, phrenic and long thoracic nerves are the major complications of TOS surgery. The transaxillary approach has accounted for most of the serious nerve and vessel injuries. The incidence of these is 1–2%, and most nerve injuries are temporary. However, they can cause serious disability.

Supraclavicular scalenectomy has fewer major vessel and plexus injuries than transaxillary first rib resection. The most common complication is phrenic nerve injury, with an incidence of 6%, but it is rarely permanent. Thoracic duct injury can occur with left supraclavicular dissections. It is managed by ligation of the duct, and it causes no serious sequelae.

Prognosis

Initially, 90% of patients note significant improvement after first rib resection, scalenectomy, or combined rib resection and scalenectomy. During the first 18 months after surgery, 20% develop recurrent symptoms. All 3 operations have the same long-term success rate of 70% (Fig 12–5). Significant in these results, as well as the results of others, is that first rib resection did not improve the success rate beyond that of anterior and middle scalenectomy. After 2 years, few recurrences are seen, and most of those are the result of another neck injury.

Recurrent Neurogenic TOS

The symptoms of recurrent neurogenic TOS are the same as for primary TOS. The cause contributing to the relapse is postoperative scarring, which occurs after operations around peripheral nerves. Initial treatment of recurrence is neck stretching and other conservative measures. The indications for surgery for recurrent neurogenic TOS are the same as for primary neurogenic TOS. The choice of operations depends on which operation was initially performed. The second operation should be whichever procedure was not performed the first time. If both procedures have been performed already, neurolysis of the brachial plexus through a supraclavicular approach is the next choice.

Operations for recurrence have a 40–50% long-term success rate. By expressing this in terms of secondary success, in the same way repeat operations for bypass grafts are expressed as secondary patency, operations for recurrent neurogenic TOS increase the pri-

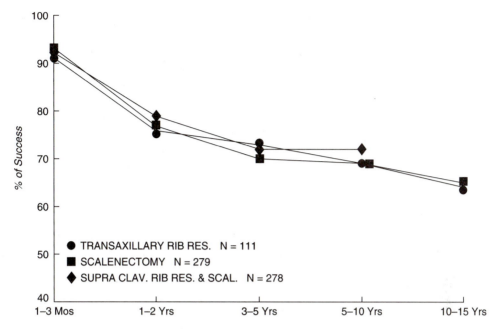

Figure 12–5. Results of 3 primary operations for TOS using life table method. (Reproduced, with permission, from Sanders RJ, Haug CE: *Thoracic Outlet Syndrome: A Common Sequelae of Neck Injuries.* JB Lippincott, 1991:182.)

mary success rate to an 85% secondary success rate (Fig 12–6).

Controversy Over Neurogenic TOS

There are 2 schools of thought regarding the diagnosis of neurogenic TOS. One claims that the condition does not exist because it lacks objective diagnostic criteria. The other states that neurogenic TOS is a mild form of compartment compression, which usually does not cause severe enough nerve disturbances to alter neurophysiologic testing. Support for the clinical diagnosis of neurogenic TOS is that thousands of patients have now been operated upon for this condition, in the absence of positive objective findings, with fairly good success.

The argument against the diagnosis of neurogenic TOS is that the surgical successes are a placebo effect and that in some patients the operation fails. Further, that the complications of surgery can be worse than the disease and therefore no one should be operated on for this condition. Unfortunately, this argument against any type of surgery for neurogenic TOS has resulted in years of suffering for many patients who could have been helped by earlier operation. While there is a risk to any operation, the techniques for thoracic outlet decompression have been developed to a point where in experienced hands, serious complications are under 1%. Over time, more practitioners have learned to diagnose neurogenic TOS on the basis of a characteristic clinical picture.

Cheng SWK, Stoney RJ: Supraclavicular reoperation for neurogenic thoracic outlet syndrome. J Vasc Surg 1994; 19;565–72.

Cheng SWK et al: Neurogenic thoracic outlet decompression: Rationale for sparing the first rib. (Abstract). J Vasc Surg 1993;17;225–6.

Elvey RL: The investigation of arm pain. In: *Modern manual therapy of the vertebral column.* Grieve GP (editor). Churchill Livingstone, 1986:530.

Gage M: Scalenus anticus syndrome: A diagnostic and confirmatory test. Surgery 1939;5:599.

Gilliatt RW, Willison RG, Dietz V, Williams IR: Peripheral nerve conduction in patients with a cervical rib and band. Ann Neurol 1978;4:124.

Gol A, Patrick DW, McNeel DP: Relief of costoclavicular syndrome by infraclavicular removal of first rib. J Neurosurg 1968;28:81.

Love JG: The scalenus anticus syndrome with and without cervical rib. Proc Mayo Clin 1945;20:65.

Makhoul RG, Machleder HI: Developmental anomalies at the thoracic outlet: An analysis of 200 consecutive cases. J Vasc Surg 1992;16:534.

Martinez M: Thoracic outlet syndrome. In: *Current Surgical Therapy.* Cameron JL (editor). BC Decker, 1992:753.

Peet RM, Hendriksen JD, Anderson TP, Martin GM: Thoracic outlet syndrome: Evaluation of a therapeutic exercise program. Proc Mayo Clin 1956;31:281.

Pollak EW: Surgical anatomy of the TOS. Surg Gynecol Obstet 1980;150:97.

Rob CG, Standeven A: Arterial occlusion complicating thoracic outlet compression syndrome. Br Med J 1958;2:709.

Roos DB: New concepts of thoracic outlet syndrome that explain etiology, symptoms, diagnosis, and treatment. Vasc Surg 1979;13:313.

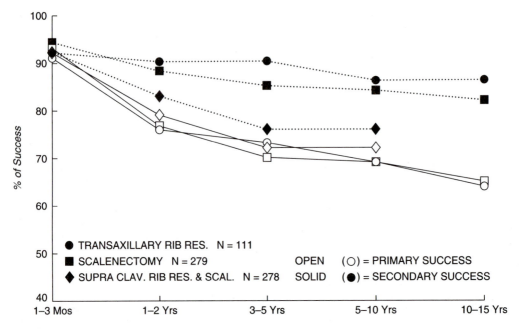

Figure 12–6. Results of reoperation for recurrent or persistent TOS. Curves show success rates of primary and secondary (repeat) operations. (Reproduced, with permission, from Sanders RJ, Haug C, Pearce WH: Recurrent thoracic outlet syndrome. J Vasc Surg 1990;12:396.)

Roos DB: Transaxillary thoracic outlet decompression and sympathectomy. In: *Techniques in arterial surgery.* Bergan JJ, Yao JST (editors). WB Saunders, 1990;305.

Sanders RJ, Haug C, Pearce WH: Recurrent thoracic outlet syndrome. J Vasc Surg 1990;12:390.

Sanders RJ, Jackson CGR, Banchero N, Pearce WH: Scalene muscle abnormalities in traumatic thoracic outlet syndrome. Am J Surg 1990;159:231.

Sanders RJ, Monsour JW, Gerber WJ: Recurrent thoracic outlet syndrome following first rib resection. Vasc Surg 1979;13:325.

Sanders RJ, Pearce WH: The treatment of thoracic outlet syndrome: A comparison of different operations. J Vasc Surg 1989;10:626.

Sanders RJ, Raymer S: The supraclavicular approach to scalenectomy and first rib resection: Description of technique. J Vasc Surg 1985;2:751.

Sanders RJ, Roos DB: The surgical anatomy of the scalene triangle. Contemp Surg 1989;35:11.

ARTERIAL TYPE

Arterial TOS was the first type of TOS to be recognized and treated. In 1821, Sir Astley Cooper described the first patient with arterial TOS, a woman with an ischemic hand and gangrenous spots. He stated correctly that the condition was due to an extra rib pressing against the subclavian artery. It was another 40 years before one of these ribs was removed surgically. This began the development of the field of cervical rib syndrome, which 100 years later expanded into TOS. What started as an arterial compression problem due to cervical ribs has expanded to include brachial plexus and subclavian vein compression, which seldom involve cervical ribs.

Essentials of Diagnosis

- Osseous abnormalities (cervical ribs, anomalous first ribs, compression of subclavian artery).
- Callus formation on clavicle or first rib.
- Tight anterior scalene muscle.
- Fibroligamentous band.
- Occlusion of digital and palmar arterioles.

General Considerations

A. Cause: Arterial TOS is compression of the subclavian artery in the thoracic outlet area. In most arterial TOS patients, either cervical ribs or anomalous first ribs are the structures responsible for the compression. Less common bony abnormalities include callus formation during the healing process of a fracture of the clavicle or first rib. Only 12% have no osseous abnormalities, with a tight anterior scalene muscle or fibroligamentous band probably being the cause.

Although abnormal ribs are the typical causative agent of arterial injury in cases of arterial TOS, most patients with cervical and rudimentary first ribs are asymptomatic. Less than 15% ever develop symptoms, and most of these are neurogenic, not arterial.

B. Pathophysiology: Cervical ribs and rudimentary first ribs damage the subclavian artery by lying immediately under it. Constant pulsation of the artery against the unyielding rib eventually produces intimal damage in the arterial wall above the rib and subsequent arterial stenosis. This is followed by 1 of 2 events: Poststenotic aneurysm formation or poststenotic thrombosis. About 50% of patients have aneurysms. Aneurysms in this location remain asymptomatic until they develop mural thrombus and either release distal emboli or totally thrombose. Even a patient with total occlusion of the subclavian artery may remain asymptomatic until thrombus extends or releases emboli. It is the emboli—usually to the hand and forearm, but sometimes retrograde to the cerebral circulation—that causes the severe morbidity and even mortality from arterial TOS (Fig 12–7).

In 1916, Halsted first observed that arterial stenosis could produce poststenotic aneurysms, although the precise mechanism by which this occurs is still uncertain. The most current explanation is that stenosis produces turbulence in the poststenotic arterial segment and in turn causes vibrations in the arterial wall. If the frequency of the vibrations is within a specific range that produces an audible bruit or thrill, poststenotic dilatation develops. Vibrations in this range apparently alter the composition of the arterial wall. Experimentally, poststenotic dilatation has occurred in less than 2 weeks after banding of the aorta in dogs. Removing the band has resulted in regression of the dilatation if it is less than twice the diameter of the aorta. Very tight or very mild stenoses that do not meet these characteristics are not associated with poststenotic aneurysms.

Clinical Findings

Men and women appear to develop arterial TOS in equal numbers. In one series of 47 patients, 23 were women and 24 were men with an average age of 37 years. Most patients are between 20 and 50 years of age.

A. Signs and Symptoms: Most symptoms of arterial TOS take months or years to develop. The patient may present in an early phase, but more often is seen in an ischemic phase.

Early symptoms are confined to the hand and fingers. They often resemble Raynaud's phenomenon with attacks of coldness, pain, cyanosis, pallor, and numbness. These symptoms are often identical to those of true Raynaud's phenomenon, which occurs in neurogenic TOS. In neurogenic TOS, symptoms are due to compression of the lower nerves of the brachial plexus, which carry sympathetic nerve fibers.

The initial manifestations of arterial TOS are attributed to occlusion of digital and palmar arterioles by emboli from subclavian artery thrombosis, with or without aneurysm formation. In this phase, distal pulses are still present. The natural course of the process includes progression in frequency and intensity of symptoms due to repeated emboli, often to the same areas of the hand.

In the ischemic phase, color changes occur frequently and digital, radial, and ulnar pulses disappear. Pain in the arm becomes pronounced, especially during exercise, and eventually rest pain ensues. Digital gangrene finally develops, which brings the patient to seek medical attention.

Light touch sensation is often diminished. A cervical rib may be palpable in the supraclavicular area, and a thrill or bruit may be present just above or below the clavicle if the artery is still patent. Blood pressure is usually decreased. In chronic cases, muscle atrophy may be present not only in the intrinsic hand muscles, but also in the thenar and hypothenar regions. In advanced cases, the arm and forearm muscles may show

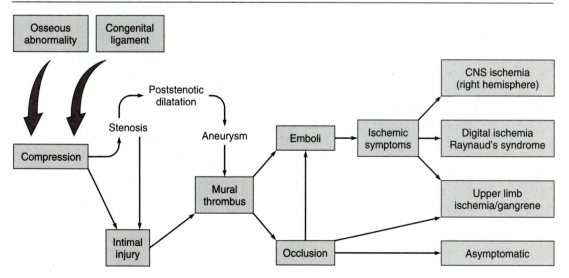

Figure 12–7. Pathophysiology of arterial TOS. (Reproduced, with permission, from Sanders RJ, Haug C: Review of arterial thoracic outlet syndrome with a report of 5 new instances. Surg Gynecol Obstet 1991;173:415.)

similar changes, and fingertips may have ulcers and gangrene. In one series of 29 patients, 37% sustained loss of a phalanx or digit, and 7% experienced major upper extremity amputations. In recent years, gangrene is less common, probably because patients seek medical attention at an earlier stage.

B. Imaging Studies: Cervical spine and neck x-rays disclose cervical ribs, abnormal first ribs, and callus from old fractures (Fig 12–8).

Arteriography and magnetic resonance angiography (MRA) remain the most important diagnostic tools. These demonstrate the point of vessel occlusion and localize occluding emboli in brachial, radial, ulnar, palmar, and digital arteries. Different techniques of arteriography can be used: (1) direct injection via a catheter inserted through the femoral artery and obtaining films either by conventional or digital subtraction arteriographic techniques or (2) intravenous injection with filming after dye has circulated through the heart (Fig 12–9). Magnification of the hand vessels can sometimes aid in visualizing points of occlusion of palmar and digital arteries. This technique may help to differentiate embolic occlusion from arteritis (Fig 12–10).

C. Laboratory Findings: Pulse-volume recordings detect reduction in blood pressure and pulse amplitude; duplex ultrasound scans can localize the point of occlusion and can often visualize vessel walls to detect aneurysms even when they contain mural thrombus. Duplex scans can also measure reduced flow rates.

Differential Diagnosis

Because of the close relationship of cervical ribs to arterial TOS, the question often arises as to how to manage cervical ribs discovered incidently on x-ray film. Cervical ribs can be classified into 4 stages on the basis of symptoms and status of the subclavian artery. Management ranges from doing nothing to doing rib resection and major vascular reconstruction, as described below and in Table 12–3.

Stage 0 Cervical rib, no symptoms; no aneurysm; no palpable mass or thrill; and no bruit. Patients in stage 0 are usually those in whom a cervical rib was noted incidently on chest x-ray. Neither arteriography nor treatment is indicated. However, examination of the area with noninvasive duplex scanning may detect minor poststenotic dilatation or confirm a normal artery. If the artery is normal, no treatment is indicated. If there is mild poststenotic dilatation, the patient falls into stage 1.

Stage 1 Cervical rib, no symptoms; minimal arterial stenosis; and mild poststenotic dilatation. Stage 1 patients are those whose cervical rib shows mild poststenotic dilatation, an early sign of subclavian arterial compression. Although no data support prophylactic cervical rib resection in such patients, knowing that poststenotic dilatation is the first step toward aneurysm formation seems adequate justification to recommend cervical rib resection.

If done before dilatation reaches twice the diameter of the subclavian artery, rib resection alone is adequate treatment because the poststenotic dilatation usually regresses. However, if the aneurysm is twice the diameter of the subclavian artery, resection and repair of the aneurysm is indicated.

Arterial exploration for even minor dilatation (less than twice the arterial diameter) has been recom-

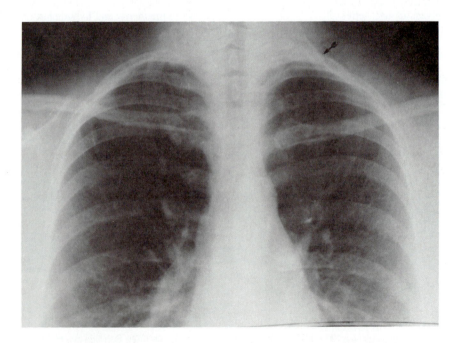

Figure 12–8. Abnormal left first rib (*arrow*). Compare with normal first rib on right side.

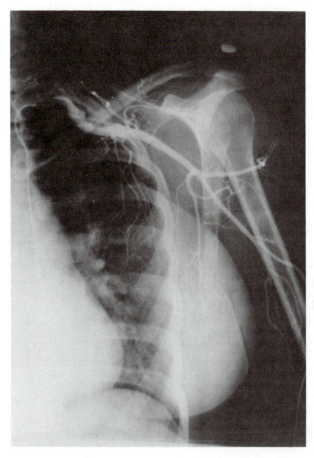

Figure 12–9. Same patient as in Figure 12–8. Arteriogram of subclavian artery aneurysm with mural thrombus and distal emboli. The aneurysm is not evident, although it is suggested by the downward curve in the subclavian artery. At operation, this was found to be a 4-cm aneurysm.

mended by Cormier to detect intimal damage and small mural thrombus. When present, that section of artery is resected. If the intima is normal, the arteriotomy is closed with large bites to restore the artery to normal caliber.

Stage 2 Cervical rib; aneurysm; intimal damage; mural thrombus; thrombotic occlusion; distal emboli. Any arterial complication of a cervical rib beyond poststenotic dilatation advances the patient to Stage 2, which is an indication to remove the rib and repair or replace the artery.

Stage 3 Cervical rib, moderate-to-severe ischemic symptoms, thrombus in artery, or aneurysm with distal emboli. Once emboli have caused ischemia in the hand and arm, gangrene and limb loss are close at hand. Treatment should be instituted immediately. Not only should the osseous abnormality be removed and the artery resected or replaced, but consideration should be given to embolectomy of the brachial artery and dorsal sympathectomy if the digital circulation is occluded.

Treatment

Treatment for arterial TOS begins with the recognition of a cervical rib or an abnormal first rib. Management depends on whether the patient presents with symptoms or an aneurysm. In the absence of symptoms, no treatment is indicated unless the subclavian artery is dilated (Fig 12–11). If an aneurysm or symptoms are present, treatment is aimed at 3 areas: (1) Removing underlying cause of arterial compression (rib resection); (2) repairing or replacing subclavian artery; (3) managing distal emboli.

A. Removing Underlying Cause—Cervical and first rib resection: If rib resection only is planned, cervical ribs or abnormal first ribs can be removed through either transaxillary or supraclavicular routes. The supraclavicular approach is preferred because after both the anterior and middle scalene muscles have been excised, the cervical rib is in the center of the field and can be excised easily.

Extrinsic decompression by resecting the osseous abnormality is the first treatment for patients with ar-

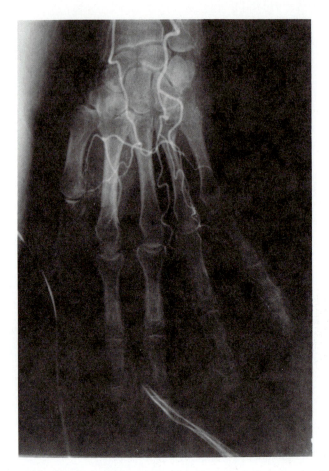

Figure 12–10. Arteriogram of hand with magnification to provide digital arteries in better detail. The radial artery branch to the deep palmar arch is occluded. There is poor filling of the digital arteries of the first 2½ fingers.

terial TOS. Whether or not removal of a normal first rib along with a cervical rib is indicated has not been clearly established. Unless the cervical rib is fused to the first rib and the first rib is deformed after cervical rib removal, removal of a normal first rib is not routinely done. Advocates of routine first rib removal do so to treat patients with associated neurogenic TOS and to prevent recurrent symptoms. However, no data are currently available that compares the two approaches and show that first rib resection is necessary.

B. Repairing or Replacing Artery: As in rib resection, the first choice for arterial repair is the supraclavicular approach. If more exposure is needed, adding an infraclavicular incision will be enough. This

Table 12–3. Stages and management of cervical ribs.

Stage	Signs & Symptoms	Arterial Pathology	Treatment
0	None. No palpable aneurysm	Normal	None
1	None. Possible palpable aneurysm	Mild stenosis & minor poststenotic dilatation	Resect cervical rib or abnormal 1st rib; resect aneurysm if over 2× arterial diameter
2	Possible ischemia, pain, color changes	Intimal damage, thrombus or aneurysm with mural clot and possible emboli	Resect cervical rib or abnormal 1st rib; repair or replace artery
3	Ischemic fingers, severe pain, numbness, threatened limb loss	Thrombus or aneurysm with thrombus and emboli	Resect cervical rib or abnormal 1st rib; repair or replace artery; possible embolectomy; possible dorsal sympathectomy

(From Scher LA et al: Staging of arterial complications of cervical rib: Guidelines for surgical management. Surgery 1984;95:644.)

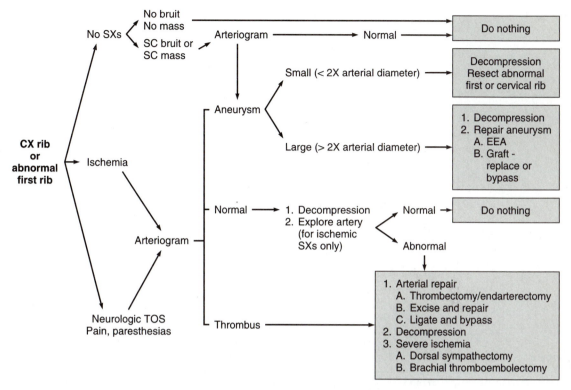

Figure 12–11. Algorithm of treatment options for arterial TOS. (Reprinted, with permission, from Sanders RJ, Haug C: Review of arterial thoracic outlet syndrome with a report of five new instances. Surg Gynecol Obstet 1991;173:415.)

combination of exposures is adequate for managing almost all repairs (Fig 12–12). In addition, cervical ribs and abnormal first ribs can be removed through the same incisions. Dorsal sympathectomy can also be performed through the supraclavicular incision when this procedure is indicated.

1. Claviculectomy–The subclavian artery lies behind the clavicle, which renders complete exposure of the artery difficult without removing the clavicle. Claviculectomy of the medial two-thirds or even the whole clavicle provides the best exposure for arterial repair and bypass. Although some claims that claviculectomy is innocuous, others disagree. In a follow-up of five patients who had claviculectomy to repair subclavian arteries, two patients reported unstable shoulders. Therefore, claviculectomy is performed only in large patients, in whom the artery lies below the level of the clavicle, or in emergency situations.

2. Thrombectomy or endarterectomy– Thrombectomy or endarterectomy of the subclavian artery is indicated when the artery contains thrombus but no aneurysm. Once the thrombus is removed, damaged intima should also be removed. If a smooth arterial intima or media can be left, the artery need not be resected or replaced. However, if there is doubt about the status of the intima, it is advisable to resect and replace the section of subclavian artery with damaged

intima, which is usually the portion of artery immediately distal to the cervical rib. If damaged intima, a patient may continue to form emboli. Thrombectomy should always be accompanied by resection of a cervical rib or abnormal first rib to prevent recurrence.

3. Resection and end-to-end anastomosis– Small aneurysms and injured segments of subclavian artery can be resected and repaired by anastomosing the two ends for defects as long as 2–3 cm. Because the subclavian artery usually lies well above the level of the clavicle in patients with cervical ribs, supraclavicular exposure of the artery is often adequate to perform rib resection, subclavian artery resection, and end-to-end anastomosis. To avoid suture line stenosis, particularly in small diameter subclavian arteries, the vessels should be spatulated and the anastomosis performed with fine interrupted vascular sutures.

4. Bypass graft–For occlusion or aneurysms longer than 2 cm and for shorter resections in which there appears to be any suture line tension, an interposition or bypass graft is indicated. Saphenous vein is the first choice for graft material. However, if it is not available, a prosthesis can be used. Either end-to-end or end-to-side techniques are effective, but with small subclavian arteries or a mismatch in size between graft and artery, end-to-side anastomoses are preferred. When a bypass is used, the artery does not need to be

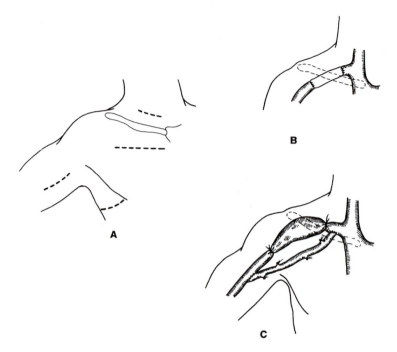

Figure 12–12. Surgical options for subclavian artery repair. **A:** Location of 4 incisions: supraclavicular, infraclavicular, brachial, transaxillary. **B:** Interposition graft with end-to-end anastomoses requiring both supra- and infraclavicular incisions. **C:** Bypass graft with end-to-side anastomoses and ligation of aneurysm at each end requiring supraclavicular and either brachial or transaxillary incisions. (Reproduced, with permission, from Sanders RJ, Haug CE: *Thoracic outlet syndrome: A Common Sequellae of Neck Injuries.* JB Lippincott, 1991:222.)

resected; it is ligated near each anastomotic heel to avoid a cul-de-sac.

C. Managing of Distal Emboli:

1. Chronic ischemia–Removal of old emboli from brachial, ulnar, and radial arteries is often followed by rethrombosis. After extensive experience with attempted embolectomies in these patients, Cormier (1989) has abandoned distal embolectomy. By proximal reconstruction of the subclavian artery and resection of the abnormal rib, patients have experienced symptomatic improvement without attempting to remove distal emboli.

2. Acute ischemia–If a radial or ulnar pulse is still present, proximal reconstruction is the treatment of choice. Collateral circulation should improve blood flow to the hand. However, when the arterial tree below the elbow is occluded, treatment is difficult. Fibrinolytic therapy may work, but positioning the catheter in the Thrombus may cause more complications. Heparin therapy for several hours has been chosen by Cormier because of complications of lytic therapy. Only when this fails is thromboembolectomy of the distal vessels attempted.

3. Embolectomy–Embolectomy of the brachial artery can sometimes be performed through the subclavian artery at the time of subclavian artery repair. If unsuccessful, brachial embolectomy is performed through an antecubital skin incision. The arteriotomy is closed with a patch graft to avoid late stenosis. When available, a segment of excised arterial wall can be used for the patch. Embolectomy below the elbow is often unsuccessful and followed by rethrombosis. In patients with emboli distal to the elbow, proximal disobliteration alone often relieves symptoms without removing the distal emboli.

4. Dorsal sympathectomy–When the distal arterial bed is occluded and symptoms of pain, coldness, and ischemia are present, adding a dorsal sympathectomy to proximal reconstruction has been very effective in improving hand symptoms. Dorsal sympathectomy, removing the 2nd and 3rd dorsal ganglia and sparing the stellate completely, can be performed through the same supraclavicular incision as the arterial repair. Alternately, it can be done thoracoscopically during the same anesthetic as the vascular repair or at a later time.

Results of Treatment

Currently, the results of surgical treatment of arterial TOS are excellent.

During the past 50 years, earlier recognition and treatment of complications of cervical and abnormal first ribs have resulted in progressively better long-term results. Three extensive reviews of the management of arterial TOS, published in 1956, 1972, and 1991, show the progress that has been made in the treatment of this condition. These reviews are virtually a mirror of the history of vascular surgery.

In the earliest review, which included 30 patients treated through 1955, there was only 56% improvement with 7% amputations, 7% strokes, and 3% deaths. Only one patient (3%) had an arterial graft. These results occurred in the infancy of arterial surgery. Between 1957 and 1968, the improvement rate was increased to 71%, amputations fell to 4%, and direct arterial repairs were used in 26% of patients. Between 1969 and 1990, the improvement rate reached 84%, amputation rate 3%, with 1% stroke and 2% deaths. Direct arterial repairs were used in 66% of the patients. In most of the others, decompression by rib resection alone was adequate (Table 12–4).

Thus, over a 30-year period a dramatic change has occurred in the management of arterial TOS and a significant improvement in the results of its treatment.

Cooper A: On exostosis. In: *Surgical Essays,* 3rd ed. Cooper, Cooper, and Travers (editors). 1821;128.

Coote H: Exostosis of the left transverse process of the seventh cervical vertebra, surrounded by blood vessels and nerves: successful removal. Lancet 1861;1:360.

Cormier JM et al: Arterial complications of the thoracic outlet syndrome: Fifty-five operative cases. J Vasc Surg 1989;9:778.

Dobrin PB: Poststenotic dilatation. Surg Gynecol Obstet 1991;172:503.

Halsted WH: An experimental study of circumscribed dilation of an artery immediately distal to a partially occluded band, and its bearing on the dilation of the subclavian artery observed in certain cases of cervical rib. J Exp Med 1916;24:271.

Holman E: The obscure physiology of poststenotic dilatation: Its relationship to the development of aneurysms. J Thorac Surg 1954;28:109.

Judy KL, Heymann RL: Vascular complications of thoracic outlet syndrome. Am J Surg 1972;123:521.

Lord JW Jr, Urschel HC Jr: Total claviculectomy. Surg Rounds 1988;11:17.

Pairolero PC et al: Subclavian-axillary artery aneurysms. Surgery 1981;90:757.

Roach MR: Changes in arterial distensibility as a cause of poststenotic dilatation. Am J Cardiol 1963;12:802.

Sanders RJ, Haug C: Review of arterial thoracic outlet syndrome with a report of five new instances. Surg Gynecol Obstet 1991;173:415.

Sanders RJ, Haug CE: *Thoracic Outlet Syndrome: A Common Sequela of Neck Injuries.* JB Lippincott, 1991:211.

Schein CJ, Haimovici H, Young H: Recent advances in surgery: Arterial thrombosis associated with cervical ribs: Surgical considerations: Report of a case and review of the literature. Surgery 1956;40:428.

Scher LA et al: Staging of arterial complications of cervical rib: Guidelines for surgical management. Surgery 1984;95:644.

VENOUS TYPE

Essentials of Diagnosis

- Subclavian vein obstruction.
- Swelling.
- Pain.
- Cyanosis.

Table 12–4. Comparison of 3 reviews of arterial TOS.

	Schein 1885–1955		Judy 1957–1968		Sanders 1969–90	
	No.	%	No.	%	No.	%
Etiology						
Cervical Rib	30	100	41	80	91	66
Rudimentary first rib	0	0	3	6	26	19
Fracture clavicle/rib	0	0	4	8	4	3
No bony abnormality	0	0	3	6	16	12
Total	30		51		137	
Treatment						
Extrinsic decompression (Rib Resection scalenotomy, clavicular resection)*	15	50	20	39	42	31
Resection or ligation of artery (no repair)*	7	24	3	6	1	1
End to end anastomosis	0	0	3	6	36	26
Graft (vein or prosthesis)	1	3	5	10	30	22
Repair (often endartectomy) with or without patch	0	0	5	10	24	18
Thrombectomy/embolectomy	1	3	12	23	3	2
Dorsal sympathectomy as only Rx	1	3	1	2	0	0
No treatment	5	17	2	4	0	0
Dorsal sympathectomy as adjuvant Rx	0	0	20	39	22	16
Claviculectomy as part of RX					30	22
Results						
Improved	17	56	36	71	108	84
No improvement	9	30	13	25	13	10
Amputation	2	7	2	4	4	3
Stroke (CVA)	2	7	0	0	1	1
Death	1 (CVA)	3	0	0	2 (CVA)	2

*, as primary treatment.

(Reprinted, with permission, from Sanders RJ, Haug C: Review of arterial thoracic outlet syndrome with a report of five new instances. Surg Gynecol Obstet 1991;173:415.)

General Considerations

Venous TOS is caused by partial or complete occulsion of the subclavian vein. It includes all cases of primary venous obstruction plus those instances of secondary venous obstruction that result from extrinsic causes. Primary TOS indicates that the cause is unknown. (The following terms are used interchangeably with "primary venous obstruction:" idiopathic subclavian vein thrombosis, axillary-subclavian vein thrombosis, effort thrombosis, and Paget-Schroetter syndrome.) The secondary group is diversified and includes intimal disturbances (intrinsic causes) as well as extravenous pressures on the vein (extrinsic causes). Treatment depends on whether the obstruction is intrinsic or extrinsic. Table 12–5 shows a more practical classification that divides causes into intrinsic and extrinsic. Extrinsic pressure on the subclavian vein at the costoclavicular angle is the most common cause of idiopathic venous TOS. As observed during surgery, the costoclavicular ligament and subclavius muscles are responsible for compressing the subclavian vein, thereby causing arm swelling.

In contrast, patients operated on for neurogenic TOS with no swelling usually display no indentations and the vein lies a few millimeters lateral to this corner. On the basis of observations in the operating room, almost all patients with arm swelling from extrinsic pressure demonstrate indentation of the subclavian vein by muscle and ligament in the costoclavicular corner.

Clinical Findings

A. Signs and Symptoms: Symptoms of venous compression include swelling, pain, and cyanosis. Patients experience a feeling of heaviness or distention in the arm. In some patients, the symptoms develop suddenly and without warning. However, after careful questioning, many of these patients with acute onset of symptoms can recall minor aching and swelling in the arm for several months prior to acute onset. This suggests that the underlying extrinsic compression existed for some time prior to the final event of acute thrombosis. In patients with mild chronic symptoms, often no abnormal physical findings are found. In the acute phase of venous TOS, the arm is swollen, tender, and blue. Distended veins may be visible on the chest wall and upper arm. In the chronic stage, symptoms and physical findings are often intermittent and present only with use of the arm.

The right side is involved in about two-thirds of all reported series. In most studies, men have involvement more frequently than women, although the gender difference is small.

B. Imaging Studies:

1. Venography–Dye is injected into a medial arm vein to enter the basilic system. Injections into the cephalic system may bypass the brachial and axillary veins and miss demonstrating obstruction of the main venous channel. The initial injection is performed with the arm at rest. If this reveals total obstruction, no more films are necessary. If the films are normal or show mild compression, dynamic venography is indicated. Injections are repeated with the arm at 90 and 180 degrees with the shoulders hyperabducted (military position, thrown backward). The films may demonstrate occlusion or tight stenosis of the vein. These maneuvers are of primarily importance in nonthrombotic cases. If these routine maneuvers do not demonstrate stenosis, venography should be repeated using other dynamic positions, such as anterior placement of the arm.

2. Duplex ultrasonography–Duplex scanning, particularly with color, can noninvasively demonstrate occlusion of the subclavian vein. However, it can miss stenosis and is difficult to use because so much of the vein lies behind the clavicle. It has been particularly helpful in evaluating patients for long-term follow-up after therapy.

3. Magnetic resonance angiography (MRA)–MRA is in its infancy but has already demonstrated an ability to reveal obstruction in the subclavian vein (Fig 12–13). It has the advantage of being noninvasive.

Treatment

Subclavian vein obstruction is best managed by treating separately each of 3 separate problems: acute thrombosis, extrinsic compression, and intrinsic deformity. In nonthrombotic venous obstruction, only the extrinsic and intrinsic problems need to be considered. In thrombosis secondary to intrinsic abnormalities, only the acute clot needs to be considered (Fig 12–14).

A. Acute Thrombosis:

1. Local treatment–Heat and arm elevation give some symptomatic relief for acute thrombosis. In evaluating the effect of local treatment alone for idiopathic thrombosis, 64% of 36 patients remained symp-

Table 12–5. Classification of causes of venous TOS.

Extrinsic compression
Thrombotic
    Idiopathic venous thrombosis
    Callus from healed fractures of first rib or clavicle
    Anterior lying phrenic nerve
    Tumors (Pancoast)
    Irradiation
Nonthrombotic (same as above; these causes
    present with or without thrombosis)
Intrinsic deformity*
Thrombotic
    Indwelling catheters or wires
    Coagulopathies
    Injections of irritating drugs
    Thrombosis secondary to extrinsic causes
Nonthrombotic

* Intrinsic deformities, in the absence of extrinsic compression, seldom cause symptoms unless there is thrombosis or an arteriovenous fistula in the ipsilateral arm.

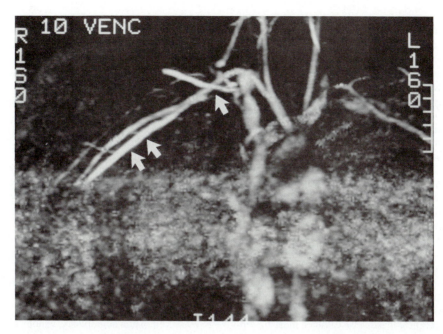

Figure 12–13. Magnetic resonance angiogram in 16-year-old girl with right subclavian vein obstruction. A 2-inch obstruction (*single arrow*) is seen in the right subclavian vein. Double arrow is axillary vein. (Reproduced, with permission, from Sanders RJ, Cooper MA. Venous thoracic outlet syndrome or subclavian vein obstruction. In: *Haimovici's Vascular Surgery,* 4th ed. Haimovici H [editor]. Appleton & Lange, in press.)

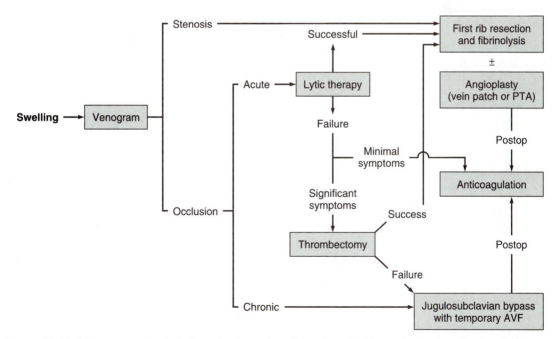

Figure 12–14. Management of subclavian vein obstruction. (Reproduced, with permission, from Sanders RJ, Cooper MA: Surgical management of subclavian vein obstruction: Including 6 cases of subclavian vein bypass. In press.)

tomatic. In comparison, of 126 patients treated with anticoagulants, only 36% remained symptomatic. In the acute state, therapy with anticoagulants or fibrinolytic agents is indicated.

2. Anticoagulants–Continuous-drip intravenous heparin to achieve a partial thromboplastin time (PTT) of twice the control level has been the generally accepted initial treatment for acute thrombosis. However, another approach is to aim for 3½ times the control levels for partial clot lysis. Warfarin is begun a day after heparin is started, and a prothrombin level of 1.5–2 times that of control is sought. Recently, INR levels of 2.0–3.0 times that of control levels have replaced prothrombin times. When the warfarin level is reached, heparin is stopped.

3. Fibrinolysis–When available, the treatment of choice for acute thrombosis has become lysis with agents such as urokinase, because these agents are more likely to dissolve clot than heparin is. Streptokinase is used less often because of antigenicity and systemic reactions; tissue plasminogen activator is an effective fibrinolytic agent but is considerably more expensive than urokinase. The catheter must be embedded in the clot for lytic therapy to be successful. If the catheter cannot be embedded in the clot, lysis should be abandoned because the results of systemic lytic therapy have been disappointing. Heparin is given along with the lytic agent to prevent pericatheter thrombosis.

Fibrinolysis failure. If thrombolysis is unsuccessful and the patient is minimally symptomatic, oral anticoagulants are continued. In these patients, presumably venous collaterals are adequate to make additional therapy unnecessary. In time, recanalization may also improve venous flow and further reduce symptoms.

Surgical thrombectomy is indicated for significant symptoms after failure of lytic therapy. If venous patency is established, vein patch angioplasty is performed if the vein is narrowed; first rib resection and venolysis are added. If thrombectomy does not achieve good outflow, but inflow is adequate, jugular vein transposition bypass is performed. In this scenario, rib resection is unnecessary because there is little value in decompression of a totally occluded vein.

Fibrinolysis success. After successful lytic therapy, there are several options: Anticoagulation, angioplasty, or surgical decompression of the thoracic outlet area. If the underlying problem is intrinsic, anticoagulants are usually administered and continued for a few months. If the underlying problem is extrinsic, surgical decompression is indicated. The role of angioplasty is discussed below.

B. Extrinsic Compression:

First rib resection–The underlying pathology in primary axillosubclavian vein obstruction—both thrombotic and nonthrombotic—is venous compression by rigid structures all of which attach to the first rib. Therefore, removal of the first rib relieves extrin-

sic pressure from several causes. In removing the first rib, it is essential that the anterior portion of the rib be removed at least to the costochondral junction. The subclavian vein is then dissected free of all attachments at this tight corner (**venolysis**). If the vein is not free, removal of additional cartilage may be required.

Both transaxillary and infraclavicular routes provide good exposure for first rib resection with venolysis. The infraclavicular approach is better for subclavian vein exploration, thrombectomy, endovenectomy, and patch closure.

C. Intrinsic Obstruction:

1. Vein patch angioplasty–For either acute or chronic obstruction, vein patch angioplasty offers good relief if the outflow tract of the subclavian vein is open. The procedure can be performed at the time of surgical thrombectomy. It can also be done electively for chronic obstruction. The reported results from 2 series have been excellent.

2. Venous bypass–When the subclavian vein is obstructed at its outflow into the innominate vein and when the obstruction cannot be relieved by thrombectomy or vein patch angioplasty, venous bypass is indicated. An essential ingredient to perform a bypass is adequate inflow into the axillary vein. When inflow is inadequate, thrombectomy can be effective in opening the brachial and axillary veins to permit a bypass. When only the subclavian vein is occluded, **jugular vein transposition** (turning down the jugular vein and anastomosing it to the subclavian vein) has been very successful, more so than with autogenous saphenous vein (Fig 12–15).

Longer obstructions, involving axillary or brachial veins, require a longer bypass. The contralateral cephalic vein is one choice; saphenous vein or 8-mm ePTFE prostheses are other choices. Only antidotal experiences are available for evaluating these bypasses.

3. Bypass in dialysis patients–Patients who have had subclavian catheters for hemodialysis often develop stenosis in that subclavian vein but seldom develop symptoms unless a distal arteriovenous fistula (AVF) is placed in the ipsilateral arm. In this situation, the venous flow rate is greatly augmented by the AVF, and in a few instances, the subclavian vein stenosis is too tight to permit adequate venous outflow. Patients in this situation can develop venous hypertension and severe arm swelling and pain. Relief is possible by switching the AVF to another extremity or by performing a jugular vein transposition or axillo jugular bypass. Since the arm already has a functioning AVF, the bypass should maintain a high flow rate and a high patency rate. A prosthesis can also be used as the bypass conduit.

4. Percutaneous transluminal angioplasty–Percutaneous angioplasty for subclavian vein stenosis has been performed since 1983. The indication for angioplasty is persistent stenosis after fibrinolysis or for nonthrombotic obstruction, but only after extrinsic compression has been treated by first rib resection. In

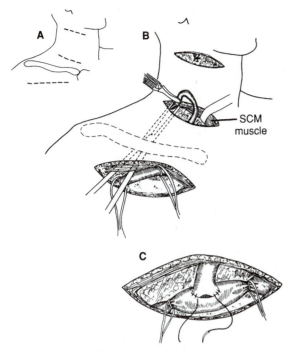

Figure 12–15. Technique of jugulosubclavian vein bypass. **A:** Location of 3 incisions. **B:** Internal jugular vein is mobilized through two 4-6 cm transverse incisions over the SCM muscle and liguted as close to the base of the skull as possible. The vein is passed behind the clorzele, the funnel being opened by elevating the shoulder to left the cloricle. **C:** End to side anostomosis. (Reproduced, with permission, from Sanders RJ: Subclavian vein obstruction. In: *Venous Disorders.* Bergan JJ, Yao ST [editors]. WB Saunders, 1991:269.)

a review of angioplasties, it was noted that 12 of 12 angioplasties failed when performed after successful fibrinolysis. In comparison, 7 of 9 angioplasties remained open when performed after successful lysis and first rib resection. The 2 failures could not be dilated at all. In the presence of extrinsic compression, balloon angioplasty seems destined to failure because the underlying cause has not been treated.

5. Arteriovenous fistula–Whenever a vein is opened for thrombectomy, vein patch angioplasty, or bypass, a temporary AVF should be added. Venous repairs generally are in low-pressure vessels, and postoperative thrombosis is common. To avoid this, a high-pressure, high-flow AVF is added peripheral to all venous repairs and grafts. The AVF is taken down 3 months later.

Prognosis

The natural history of subclavian vein obstruction due to intrinsic deformities is good. Most patients are asymptomatic, some have minimal symptoms, and only a few have significant discomfort or disability. On the other hand, extrinsic compression more often results in significant disability if left untreated.

The success rate after various forms of treatment is summarized in Table 12–6. There is wide variation among the various treatment modalities, because most results are based on subjective improvement, not on venograms. Since most patients develop collaterals and some undergo recanalization, many good results may be unrelated to treatment. Therefore, even though all forms of treatment seem highly effective, most reports are not based on objective standards that evaluate therapy alone.

Contralateral Side: Venograms of the contralateral arm in patients with subclavian vein thrombosis reveal a greater than 50% incidence of stenosis on the contralateral side. Some of these patients have experienced thrombosis of the opposite side during

Table 12–6. Treatment results for subclavian vein occlusion*

Problem	Treatment	No. of Patients	Success (%)[†]	Range
Acute thrombus	Heparin	185	91 (49%)	4–100%
	fibrinolysis	82	65 (79%)	50–100%
	thrombectomy	33	31 (94%)	75–100%
Extrinsic pressure	1st rib resection	114	92 (81%)	50–100%
	soft tissue release[‡]	23	19 (83%)	0–100%
	claviculectomy	6	5 (83%)	NA
Intrinsic stenosis	Endovenectomy with patch	25[§]	24 (96%)	50–100%
	Jugulosubclavian v. bypass with AVF	8	7 (88%)	75–100%
	Jugulosubclavian v. bypass without AVF	7	3 (43%)	0–100%

* Collected results from literature.

[†] Most results are subjective; few patients had venograms to confirm patency. Some venograms revealed rethromboses and recanalization.

[‡] Soft tissue release; division of costoclavicular ligament, subclavius muscle, and anterior scalene muscle.

[§] Includes 15 cases of Molina.

(Reprinted, with permission, from Sanders, RJ; Thoracic Outlet Syndrome. Lippincott, 1991: 247.)

(Reprinted, with permission, from Sanders RJ, Cooper MA. Venous thoracic outlet syndrome or subclavian vein obstruction. In: *Haimovici's Vascular Surgery*, 4th ed. Haimovici H, [editor]. Appleton & Lange, in press.)

the follow up period of the operated side. Other patients were found to already have an occlusion on the contralateral side prior to presentation. As a result, it is recommended that venograms be performed on the contra lateral side. When these show stenosis, the patient is offered prophylactic first rib resection after being informed that there is a greater chance than the normal population of thrombosis of the contralateral side. More data is needed to establish exactly what is the incidence of contralateral symptoms and thrombosis.

Aziz S, Straehley CJ, Whelan TJ Jr: Effort-related axillosubclavian vein thrombosis: A new theory of pathogenesis and a plea for direct surgical intervention. Am J Surg 1986;152:57.

Becker DM, Philbrick JT, Walker FB IV: Axillary and subclavian venous thrombosis: Prognosis and treatment. Arch Intern Med 1991;151:1934.

Conti S, Daschbach BS, Blaisdell FW: A comparison of high dose versus conventional heparin therapy for deep venous thrombosis. Surgery 1982;92:972.

Eklof B et al: The temporary arteriovenous fistula in venous reconstructive surgery. Int Angiol 1985;4:455.

Hashmonai M, Schramek A, Farbstein J: Cephalic vein cross-over bypass for subclavian vein thrombosis: A case report. Surgery 1976;80:563.

Machleder HI: Evaluation of a new treatment strategy for Paget-Schroetter syndrome: Spontaneous thrombosis of the axillary-subclavian vein. J Vasc Surg 1993;17:305.

Molina EJ: Surgery for effort thrombosis of the subclavian vein. J Thorac Cardiovasc Surg 1992;103:341.

Sanders RJ, Haug CE: Subclavian vein obstruction and thoracic outlet syndrome: A review of etiology and management. Ann Vasc Surg 1990;4:397.

Sanders RJ, Rosales C, Pearce WH: Creation and closure of temporary arteriovenous fistulas for venous reconstruction or thrombectomy: Description of technique. J Vasc Surg 1987;6:504.

Thompson RW et al: Circumferential venolysis and paraclavicular thoracic outlet decompression for "effort thrombosis" of the subclavian. J Vasc Surg 1992;16:723.

Witte CL, Smith CA: Single anastomosis vein bypass for subclavian vein obstruction. Arch Surg 1966;93:664.

Upper Extremity Ischemia

13

James S.T. Yao, MD, PhD

Because a wide spectrum of diseases may cause hand ischemia, accurate diagnosis requires a thorough history, careful physical examination, and appropriate diagnostic tests. After the diagnosis is established, treatment varies according to the disease.

General Considerations

Causes of hand ischemia can be divided into proximal arterial and distal arterial lesions. Proximal arterial lesions involve the innominate, subclavian, axillary, and brachial arteries; they are more amenable to reconstructive surgery than distal artery lesions. Distal lesions such as those occurring below the wrist are often difficult or impossible to correct surgically. In patients with distal lesions, the digital arteries are often involved, and many patients so affected are subsequently found to have connective tissue disorders. This chapter reviews the current diagnostic and therapeutic approaches for patients with upper extremity ischemia.

Clinical Findings

A. History: In patients presenting with upper extremity ischemia, history taking is the most important step in guiding the subsequent workup. The history must include occupational, pharmacologic, athletic, and medical information. Unlike patients with lower extremity occlusive disease, patients with upper extremity ischemia are much younger, and atherosclerotic disease is less common. For example, workers using vibratory tools are known to develop the so-called *vibratory white finger.* Similarly, carpenters or mechanics, who often use the hand to strike on hard objects, may develop ulnar occlusion to the hand, a condition known as *hypothenar hammer syndrome.* In young adults presenting with hand ischemia, thoracic-outlet compression of the subclavian artery due to congenital bony anomaly such as cervical rib or anomalous first rib must be suspected. Hand ischemia from athletic injury is not uncommon. The violent and repetitive throwing motion of the shoulder in baseball pitchers can injure the subclavian and axillary arteries.

Questions regarding pharmacologic history are important because many pharmaceutical agents can cause ischemia of the hands. These agents include some of the chemotherapeutic agents, dopamine, and ergot derivatives.

Many causes including medical conditions may be responsible for hand ischemia (Table 13–1). For an explanation of specific conditions giving rise to upper extremity ischemia, see the section on Diagnosis.

B. Signs and Symptoms: Acute ischemia of the hand is often due to cardiac embolization to the brachial artery. The onset is often sudden, with pain and coldness as the dominating symptoms. If the symptoms are unrecognized, the patient may progress to changes of first sensory and then motor function of the hand. Diagnosis is not difficult. It should be suspected in patients with a history of recent myocardial infarction or atrial fibrillation.

In chronic ischemia, presenting symptoms of upper extremity occlusive disease depend on the site of occlusion. For small vessel occlusion, patients often present with Raynaud's phenomenon. Raynaud's phenomenon, first described in 1862, is episodic digital ischemia provoked by stimuli such as cold or emotion. The tricolor changes, first pallor (white) followed by cyanosis (blue) and then redness, have been the hallmark of this phenomenon. Raynaud's phenomenon must be distinguished from acrocyanosis, which is characterized by persistent, diffuse cyanosis of the fingers and hands. In addition, Raynaud's *phenomenon* must not be confused with Raynaud's *disease.* The latter, a primary disease without underlying cause, is diagnosed only after exclusion of all etiologic factors (see Table 13–1) and with symptoms for at least 2 years in the absence of disease that might be causal. In general, in patients with unilateral Raynaud's phenomenon, organic arterial occlusive disease should be suspected. By contrast, bilateral symptoms in patients are often due to systemic disease. The precise classification of primary and secondary Raynaud's phenomenon is often difficult, and many authors prefer to use the term "Raynaud's syndrome" to characterize patients with episodic vasospastic disease of the hands.

In chronic occlusion of major arteries, presenting symptoms often include forearm fatigue after exercise, cold hand and loss of functional use of the hand, pain, and clinical manifestation of arterial emboli. Diagnosis of microemboli may be difficult because presenting symptoms are often subtle. Physical signs such as livedo reticularis, petechiae of the skin, splinter hemorrhage of the nail bed, or gangrene of the tips of the fingers may be confused with other disorders. Mi-

Table 13–1. Upper extremity ischemia related to medical history.

Antiphospholipid syndrome
Aneurysms of the upper extremity
Atherosclerosis
Arteritis
  Collagen disease
    Dermatomyositis
    Rheumatoid arteritis
    Scleroderma
    Systemic lupud erythematosus
  Allergic necrotizing arteritis
  Giant cell arteritis
  Takayasu's disease
Behçet's syndrome
Blood dyscrasias
  Cold agglutinins
  Cryoglobulins
  Polycythemia vera
Thoracic outlet syndrome
Congenital arterial wall defects
  Ehlers-Danlos syndrome
  Pseudoxanthoma elasticum
Fibromuscular dysplasia
Frostbite
Iatrogenic injury
  Arterial blood gas and pressure monitoring
  Arteriography
  Cardiac catheterization
Radiation
  Breast carcinoma
  Hodgkin's disease
Renal transplantation and related problems
  Azotemic arteriopathy
  Hemodialysis shunts

croembolization is a common manifestation in patients with aneurysm of the subclavian or axillary artery and its branches. In a previous review, the incidence of microembolization was found to be about 70% in patients with aneurysm of the subclavian or axillary artery.

C. Physical Examination: Physical examination must include the thoracic outlet and the entire upper extremity. Palpation of the supraclavicular region may help to detect the presence of a subclavian aneurysm or a cervical rib. Place the stethoscope just below the midclavicular region for auscultation of the subclavian artery and listen for the presence of a bruit with the arm placed in neutral or abduction and external rotation or hyperabduction. These procedures help to establish the diagnosis of thoracic outlet compression to the artery. Pulse palpation must begin with the axillary artery under the armpit, brachial artery at the upper arm and elbow, and radial and ulnar arteries at the wrist level. A decrease or absence of a pulse is diagnostic of major artery occlusion.

Examination of hand ischemia is not complete unless Allen's test is performed. The test is done as follows: The examiner stands beside or facing the patient. The radial and ulnar arteries of one wrist are compressed by the examiner's fingers. The patient is asked to open and close the hand rapidly for 1 minute to empty blood from the hand, then to extend the fingers quickly. The radial or the ulnar artery is released, and

the hand is observed for capillary refilling and return of color. The test is judged normal if refilling of the hand is complete within a short period (less than 6 seconds). Any portion of the hand that does not blush is an indication of incomplete continuity of the arch. Hyperextension of the fingers must be avoided because this will give a false-positive result.

In addition to Allen's test, examination of the hand must include palpation of the palm for pulsatile mass or excess scar tissue. Assessment of patency of digital arteries by palpation is often difficult and unreliable.

In patients with severe ischemia, sensory and motor function of the hand must be determined and recorded. The compartment of the forearm must be palpated to determine consistency of the compartment. This is an important examination, especially in patients with penetrating trauma or with fracture and dislocation of the elbow joint.

D. Imaging Studies: Of the noninvasive tests available, the transcutaneous Doppler waveform analysis is the simplest technique. The Doppler examination consists of audible signal interpretation, waveform recording and analysis, and systolic pressure measurements. Bilateral examination should be carried out because many of the diseases affecting the hand are symmetric, and often the asymptomatic hand has significant disease. This is especially true in patients whose hand ischemia is caused by systemic disease.

Because both axillary and brachial arteries are superficially located, they lend themselves to Doppler examination. Any change from normal signals (triphasic) to abnormal signals (monophasic) indicates the presence of an occlusive lesion. Distal to the elbow, however, arterial signals are more difficult to obtain, and both the radial and ulnar arteries become superficial again only at the wrist. Palpation of the ulnar artery can be difficult, and Doppler examination is helpful to determine the patency of this artery. In the hand, the palmar arches are best heard at the midthenar and hypothenar regions. The common digital vessels are heard at the base of the fingers at their division into the proper digital arteries along the shaft of each finger. Waveform recording can be done for analysis and record keeping.

For segmental upper extremity pressures, a pneumatic cuff is placed at the upper arm, as routinely used for blood pressure recording. The arm pressure represents the brachial pressure, which should be within 10–20 mmHg of the opposite extremity. A greater difference signifies innominate, subclavian, axillary, or brachial stenosis. If brachial artery occlusion is suspected, a pressure cuff is then applied to the forearm and the pressure recorded in a similar manner, using the radial artery for signal detection. A pressure drop of 20–30 mmHg signifies an obstruction distal to the brachial artery. For finger pressure measurement, a 2.5-cm cuff is placed at the base of the finger, and the return of Doppler signals following cuff deflation is monitored at the fingertip. An arterial occlusion distal to the palmar arch is defined by a pressure gradient between the fingers of more than 15 mmHg or a wrist-to-digit difference of 30 mmHg.

The Doppler technique is particularly valuable in determining palmar arch patency in a patient who is unconscious or uncooperative in performing an Allen's test. Before arterial line placement, this simple test may help to avoid hand ischemia. The Doppler probe is placed over the radial artery while the ulnar artery is compressed. If the signal disappears, it shows that the arch depends on the ulnar artery for supply. If the signal remains present, it shows that the arch is complete. A similar maneuver is repeated over the ulnar artery while the radial artery is compressed.

Duplex ultrasonography, especially the color-coded mode, offers both velocity and image of an artery under examination. The technique is helpful in detecting aneurysm or arteriovenous fistula after catheterization injury. Occlusion of the axillary or brachial artery can also be detected accurately.

E. Radiographic Findings: Radiologic examination includes soft tissue x-ray of the hand, chest x-ray, and arteriography. The soft tissue x-ray of the hand may reveal calcinosis, which is diagnostic of the CRST syndrome (calcinosis cutis, Raynaud's phenomenon, sclerodactyly, telangiectasia) or diffuse calcified arteries in diabetic or azotemic arteriopathy (Fig 13–1). The chest x-ray is essential for detecting bony anomaly of the thoracic outlet such as cervical rib (Fig 13–2) or anomalous first rib and healed fracture of first rib or clavicle. Pulmonary fibrosis as seen in chest x-ray lends further support to the diagnosis of scleroderma.

Arteriography is often done by the transfemoral catheter technique. Examination must include the innominate artery on the right, the subclavian artery on the left, and the entire upper extremity including detailed exposure of the hand. If thoracic outlet compression is suspected, positional exposure is done by placing the upper extremity in hyperabduction and external rotation or in the position that precipitates compression of the artery. Anatomic variation of palmar arches (superficial and deep) is well known and has been well described by anatomic dissection by several authors.

In general, the deep palmar arch is formed primarily by the terminal part of the radial artery and the superficial arch by the ulnar artery. Variations of the arches, based on the way in which the contributing arteries join, are divided into 2 groups: complete arches and incomplete arches. According to Janevski, who analyzed 500 hand arteriograms, there are many subtypes of variation of superficial and deep palmar arches (Fig 13–3). Since the ulnar artery is the dominant artery in blood supply of the hand, the superficial palmar arch and its completeness are the determining factors in hand ischemia. Janevski found that the deep palmar arch appeared in its complete form in

95.2% of the cases. The finding is close to that reported by Coleman and Anson. There are more variations of the superficial palmar arch, with 6 types of complete arch observed. In contrast to the deep arch, the complete superficial palmar arch occurred in only 42.4% of the cases. This is in contrast to Coleman and Anson, who noted that 78.5% had complete superficial palmar arches.

F. Laboratory Findings: In severe bilateral hand ischemia, a systemic cause of the arterial lesions should be sought. Helpful laboratory evaluations are serologic, immunologic, and hematologic tests.

Diagnosis of connective tissue disorders can be established by (1) an elevation of erythrocyte sedimentation rate (ESR), (2) a positive antinuclear antibody (ANA), (3) an abnormal C3/C4 complement test, and (4) a positive rheumatoid factor. Antibodies to native or double-stranded DNA and to Sm, a ribonuclear pro-

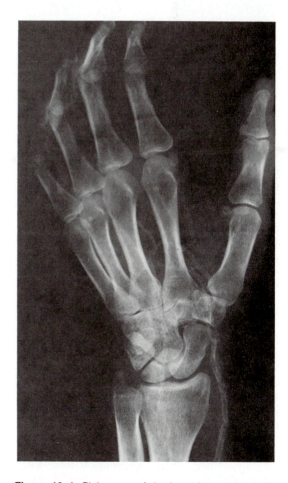

Figure 13–1. Plain x-ray of the hand in a patient with azotemic arteriopathy. Note the calcified pipestem appearance of the radial artery. (Reprinted, with permission, from Yao JST: Arterial surgery of the upper extremity. In: *Haimovici's Vascular Surgery,* 4th ed. Haimovici H et al (editors). Blackwell Scientific, 1994.)

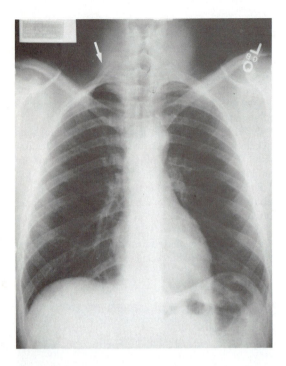

Figure 13–2. Chest x-ray of a patient with right subclavian artery aneurysm. A right cervical rib is present (*arrow*).

tein antigen, are more specific than other ANA for the diagnosis of systemic lupus erythematosus. Antiphospholipid syndrome, a newly recognized clinical entity known to cause thrombosis of small arteries, can be detected by the presence of cardiolipin antibody. Also, not infrequently, the serologic test is negative in patients with recent onset of Raynaud's symptoms, and subsequent follow-up after a longer period of time often turns up a positive serologic test.

Diagnosis

The diagnosis of large artery occlusion is not difficult, and careful pulse examination will establish the diagnosis. In distal arterial lesions causing hand or finger ischemia, the use of noninvasive testing to detect digital artery occlusion helps to distinguish Raynaud's phenomenon from Raynaud's disease. The diagnosis of Raynaud's disease should not be made until all diagnostic tests are exhausted and proven negative. The onset of Raynaud's phenomenon may precede other manifestations of underlying systemic disease by many years. Therefore, the diagnosis of Raynaud's disease must not be made until 2 years have elapsed with no systemic disease appearing. If these strict criteria are followed, most patients will be found to have Raynaud's phenomenon rather than Raynaud's disease.

The following sections on diagnostic evaluation are divided into proximal artery lesions and distal artery lesions.

A. Proximal Arterial Lesions:

1. Atherosclerosis–The common site for atherosclerotic lesions is the first part of the subclavian artery, followed by the innominate artery. Lesions include total occlusion with or without vertebral artery steal and ulcerating plaques causing distal embolization.

2. Arteritis–This includes Takayasu's arteritis, giant cell arteritis, temporal arteritis, and polymyalgia rheumatica. Takayasu's arteritis is a nonspecific inflammatory process of unknown cause, which affects segmentally the aorta and its main branches. The disease process may affect carotid, subclavian, axillary, and pulmonary arteries and is common in young women 10–30 years of age.

The most frequently recognized clinical features of giant cell arteritis (cranial, temporal, and granulomatous arteritis) result from involvement of cranial arteries and occasionally the subclavian axillary artery. Criteria for the classification of giant cell arteritis are being over age 50 years at disease onset, having/displaying headache, temporal artery tenderness, and ESR higher than 50 mm/sec. For temporal arteritis and polymyalgia rheumatica, the subclavian or axillary artery is also a common site of involvement.

Arteriographic examination is often diagnostic of arteritis. Multiple artery involvement and rich collaterals are characteristic of patients with Takayasu's disease. The pulmonary artery is affected in 45% of patients. Typical arteriographic findings in patients with giant cell arteritis include long segments of smooth arterial stenosis alternating with areas of normal or increased caliber; smooth, tapered occlusions; and absence of irregular plaques and ulcerations.

3. Thoracic outlet syndrome–By far the most common vascular complication seen in young adults, thoracic outlet syndrome is manifested by the following compression sites: (1) the costoclavicular space formed by the first thoracic rib and clavicle, (2) the anterior scalene muscle, (3) the angle between the insertion of the pectoralis minor tendon and the coracoid process in the axilla, and (4) the humerus head in extreme external rotation. In addition, thoracic outlet compression may be due to bony anomaly such as cervical rib, first rib, or hypertrophy of the anterior scalene muscle. Recently, compression of the axillary artery, especially in professional athletes such as baseball pitchers, has been reported. In addition to the axillary artery, the circumflex humeral artery may also be injured, causing aneurysm formation.

Arterial complication of thoracic outlet compression includes aneurysm formation, poststenotic dilation, thrombosis, and, most important, distal embolization. The latter can cause digital gangrene or severe hand ischemia. Raynaud's phenomenon, often unilateral, is not uncommon as an initial complaint.

4. Radiation injury–Radiation injury often occurs to arteries supplying the upper limb following radiation treatment for breast carcinoma or Hodgkin's

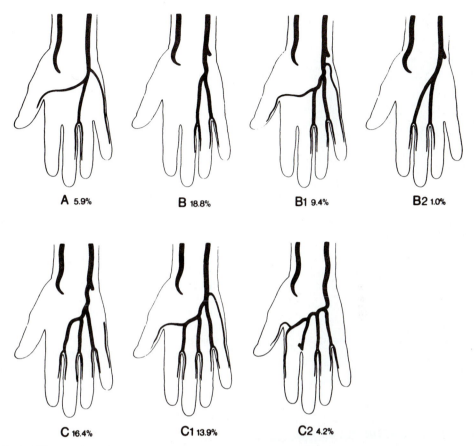

Figure 13–3. Different types of incomplete superficial arch. (Reproduced, with permission, from Janevski BK: *Angiography of the Upper Extremity.* The Hague: Martinus Nijhoff, 1982.)

disease. The most commonly affected artery is the subclavian artery, followed by the axillary artery. The pathogenesis consists of 3 processes:

- Endothelial injury and disruption of the internal elastic lamina followed by intimal fibrosis and plaque formation.
- Occlusion of the vasa vasorum by proliferation and hyaline thickening of the intima, which in turn causes fibrosis of the media.
- Periarterial fibrosis, which brings about extrinsic constriction of the artery.

Clinically, the disease manifests in 1 of 4 patterns. First, fatal hemorrhage can occur from acute rupture due to necrosis of the arterial wall. Second, mural thrombosis in the arterial segment at the site of irradiation usually presents thromboembolic phenomenon within 5 years of exposure. Third, fibrotic occlusion may lead to delayed ischemia symptoms within 10 years of radiation exposure. The 4th group manifests more than 20 years after radiation therapy, with symptoms initiated by periarterial fibrosis and "accelerated atherosclerosis." The diagnosis is established by a history of radi-

ation exposure and the characteristic arteriographic finding of diffuse, long narrowing of the artery.

5. Fibromuscular dysplasia–Fibromuscular dysplasia is probably the rarest form of arterial occlusive disease of the upper extremity. The commonly affected artery in the upper extremity is the brachial artery. Only a few of cases have been reported, and females appear more likely to be affected. Fibromuscular dysplasia is a nonatherosclerotic and noninflammatory vascular disease of unknown cause, which affects primary medium-sized and small arteries. Three predominant types of fibromuscular dysplasia have been identified. Of reported cases of brachial artery involvement, intimal fibroplasia appears to be the most common.

B. Distal Arterial Lesions:

1. Connective tissue disorder–This disorder includes scleroderma, rheumatoid arthritis, systemic lupus erythematosus, polyarteritis nodosa, and dermatomyositis. All these diseases have systemic symptoms. Presenting symptoms include Raynaud's phenomenon to gangrene of the digits. Extensive involvement of palmar arches or digital arteries is common (Fig 13–4).

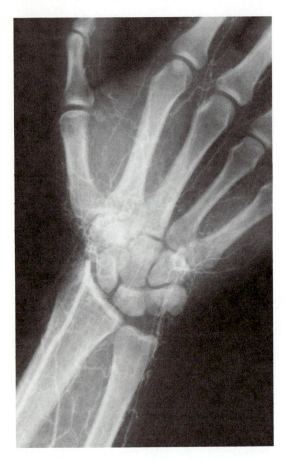

Figure 13–4. Artery of the hand in a patient with advanced scleroderma and gangrene of the fingers. The ulnar and radial arteries are occluded with extensive occlusion of all digital arteries.

2. Buerger's disease (thromboangiitis obliterans)–Buerger's disease was first described by von Winiwarter in 1879. In 1908, Buerger described the disease in Jewish patients who presented with digital gangrene without occlusion of larger arteries. The disease is strongly associated with heavy smoking. Diagnosis of Buerger's disease depends on histologic examination, with involvement not only of arteries but also of veins. The latter may be manifested clinically as migrating phlebitis. Characteristic arteriographic findings are occlusion of small arteries of the digits, with abundant collaterals. Not only does the symptomatic hand demonstrate digital artery occlusion, but the asymptomatic hand may show it as well.

3. Blood dyscrasias–Cold agglutinins, cryoglobulin, and polycythemia vera are the most common forms of blood dyscrasias that may be associated with occlusion of the arteries of the hand. The cause of small artery occlusion is generally thought to be local thrombosis or embolism. Specific blood tests help to establish the diagnosis.

4. Catheter injury–With increasing use of diagnostic and therapeutic procedures involving catheterization, damage of the radial and brachial artery has become more common, especially when an incomplete palmar arch is not recognized before placement of a catheter in the radial artery. Gangrene or severe ischemia can occur as a result of the injury.

5. Vibration syndrome–Blanching and numbness of the hands after using pneumatic drills is now a recognized clinical entity of hand ischemia. Vibratory white finger is a form of occupational trauma. Repetitive trauma to the digital arteries is the primary causal factor.

6. Hypothenar hammer syndrome–This is another form of occupational trauma commonly seen in mechanics or carpenters. The mechanism of injury is the repetitive use of the palm of the hand in activities that involve pushing, pounding, or twisting. The anatomic location of the ulnar artery at the area of hypothenar eminence places it in a vulnerable position. When this area is repeatedly traumatized, ulnar artery occlusion or aneurysm formation can result. Digital artery occlusion as a result of embolization is common in this form of injury.

7. Calciphylactic arteriopathy–Diabetic patients or patients with chronic renal failure may develop heavily calcified arteries leading to gangrene or severe ischemia of the hand. The so-called azotemic arteriography is characterized by calcification of the media of the digital arteries, resulting in a pipestem pattern on plain x-ray film.

Treatment

Treatment of patients with upper extremity ischemia is directed at the underlying disease process for ischemia. In acute ischemia due to embolic occlusion, immediate heparinization must be instantly instituted if there is no contraindication for anticoagulant therapy. Recently, intra-arterial infusion of urokinase has been shown to be effective to lyse the emboli. Even in subacute ischemia, urokinase infusion may help to dissolve clots within the digital arteries. Corticosteroid therapy may be needed for patients with systemic symptoms of arteritis. Drug-induced ischemia must be treated by cessation of the drug. Dramatic improvement has been noted in patients with ergot poisoning. Tobacco is known to aggravate ischemia; therefore, smoking cessation is an important step in treatment.

In general, patients with severe ischemia due to proximal lesions need surgical correction. By contrast, distal lesions with occlusion at or distal to the palmar arch are most unlikely to be amenable to surgical treatment. In these patients, conservative treatment with the use of a calcium blocker (nifedipine) may reduce the severity and frequency of attacks. Many medications have been recommended. Unfortunately, medical treatment is not always successful.

The type of surgical reconstructive procedure depends on the nature and location of the lesion. Arterial complication due to thoracic outlet frequently requires bypass procedure following resection of the subclavian aneurysm and removal of the cervical rib. Bypass graft using autogenous vein (saphenous or cephalic), first proposed by Garrett and colleagues, often yields gratifying results for occlusion of the brachial artery and its major branches. A short segmental occlusion of either the radial or the ulnar artery is best treated by thrombectomy or endarterectomy with vein patch. Aneurysm in the hand can be resected, with continuity restored by end-to-end anastomosis or interposed vein graft.

Prognosis

Results of bypass graft for upper extremity are similar to those for lower extremity revascularization; that is, proximal grafts fared better than distal grafts. In a series of 43 patients who underwent upper extremity bypasses, the operative mortality rate was 0%. Overall patency rate at 5 years was 52.2%. The patency for anastomosis proximal to brachial artery bifurcation was better than more distal placement (61.9% versus 34.8%). Unlike lower extremity surgery, major amputation was not required in any of the cases, even after graft occlusion.

REFERENCES

Benjamin ME, Yao JST: Aneurysms of secondary and tertiary branches of major arteries. In: *Aneurysms: New Findings and Treatments.* Yao JST, Pearce WH (editors). Appleton & Lange, 1994:509.

Butler MS, Lane RHS, Webster JHH: Irradiation injury to large arteries. Br J Surg 1980;67:341.

Coleman SS, Anson BJ: Arterial patterns in the hand based upon a study of 650 specimens. Surg Gynecol Obstet 1961;113:409.

Edwards JM, Porter JM: Long-term outcome of Raynaud's syndrome. In: *Long-Term Results in Vascular Surgery.* Yao JST, Pearce WH (editors). Appleton & Lange, 1993: 345.

Garrett HE et al: Revascularization of upper extremity with autogenous vein bypass graft. Arch Surg 1965;91:751.

Janevski BK: *Angiography of the Upper Extremity.* Martinus Nijhoff Publishers, 1982.

Lie JT: Illustrated histopathologic classification criteria for selected vasculitis syndromes. Arthritis Rheum 1990;33: 1074.

Lin WW, McGee GS, Patterson BK, Yao JST, Pearce WH: Fibromuscular dysplasia of the brachial artery: Case report and review of the literature. J Vasc Surg 1992;16:66.

McCarthy WJ et al: Upper extremity arterial injury in athletes. J Vasc Surg 1989;9:317.

Mesh CL, Yao JST: Upper extremity bypass: Five-year follow-up. In: *Long-Term Results in Vascular Surgery.* Yao JST, Pearce WH (editors). Appleton & Lange, 1993:353.

Mills JA: Systemic lupus erythematosus. N Engl J Med 1994;330:1871.

Palmar RA, Collin J: Vibratory white finger. Br J Surg 1993;80:705.

Raynaud M: *De l'Asphyxie et de la Gangrene Symétrique des Extrémités.* Rignoux, 1862.

Rohrer MJ et al: Axillary artery compression and thrombosis in throwing athletes. J Vasc Surg 1990;11:761.

14

Vasospastic Disorders

R. Donald Patman, MD, & William P. Shutze, MD

The pathophysiology of vasospastic disorders is for the most part unknown. Most of these disorders display alterations in the normal function of the sympathetic nervous system. Many vasospastic conditions are no less incapacitating than limb-threatening atherosclerotic arterial occlusions, but they are frequently overlooked and neglected and almost always misunderstood. These circumstances usually beget a delay in diagnosis and optimal management. Many patients with Raynaud's syndrome do not have an underlying associated disease, whereas the presence of this syndrome may be one of the first symptoms of a wide variety of disease states. An attempt to outline a simple classification of Raynaud's syndrome will be presented to alert the reader to suspect associated disease processes.

The posttraumatic pain syndromes remain poorly understood and therefore create an alarming delay in diagnosis and proper treatment. Hyperhidrosis is an infrequently encountered, incapacitating condition. The neurovascular compression syndromes (thoracic outlet syndrome) are associated with vasospasm and are covered in Chapter 12.

RAYNAUD'S SYNDROME

Essentials of Diagnosis

- Periodic digital vasospasm associated with numbness, tingling, and skin color changes, which vary from pallor to cyanosis to rubor.
- Attacks reproduced after exposure to cold and can be elicited by the ice water immersion test.
- More common in women than men; pulses present or absent.
- Sometimes associated with certain systemic illnesses.

General Considerations

Raynaud's syndrome is defined as the presence of periodic digital vasospasm associated with numbness, tingling, and skin color changes varying from pallor to cyanosis to rubor. The initial pallor is believed to be caused by profound vasospasm, and as the vasospasm gradually resolves the small amount of blood entering the capillaries rapidly desaturates and causes cyanosis. With resolution of the vasospasm, arteriolar relaxation

occurs with resultant hyperemia and rubor. The degree of severity of this tricolor phenomenon varies from person to person. Hyperhidrosis may or may not be apparent, and a small number of patients may have no visible color changes at all. The usual episodic changes are most often precipitated by emotional stress, exposure to cold, and smoking. Raynaud's syndrome is usually seen in the upper extremities but may also affect the feet and toes.

Maurice Raynaud first described this condition in 1862 and suggested that the changes were caused by vasospasm. Allen and Brown (1932) were the first to recognize that the syndrome may occur with a variety of underlying conditions, many of which produce digital artery occlusion. They suggested that the term "Raynaud's disease" be used to categorize those patients with benign disease and without any recognized associated disease process. The term "Raynaud's phenomenon" would be used for the more virulent cases, exhibiting the syndrome but also demonstrating identifiable underlying disease processes such as arteriosclerosis and the collagen-vascular disorders.

The distinction between the "disease" and the "phenomenon" of patients exhibiting Raynaud's syndrome is artificial and unfounded for many reasons. Long periods of clinical observation are often required before associated diseases may manifest and therefore be diagnosed (Table 14–1). Undoubtedly, a benign form of Raynaud's syndrome exists, and it may subside spontaneously or with proper treatment. Most patients should be diagnosed with Raynaud's syndrome without being categorized into the older terminology. Manifestations of associated disorders may appear long after the onset of typical symptoms. The surgeon must be familiar with the existence of these vasospastic disorders because they commonly coexist with many surgical conditions described later in this chapter.

The mechanism of this overactive arterial vasoconstriction is unknown but may be precipitated by cold exposure, anxiety, certain drugs, and smoking. Such patients may have normal digital arterial pressure but diminished blood flow at room temperature. Exposure to even modest decreases in temperature may cause a profound drop in digital pressure and flow. Typical attacks are readily reproducible by exposing the patient to cold. External warming of the extremity gradually increases the flow to normal and usually demonstrates the classic triphasic digital color changes.

Table 14–1. Diseases associated with Raynaud's syndrome.

Connective Tissue Disorders	**Obstructive**
Scleroderma	**Arterial Disease**
SLE	Arteriosclerosis
Rheumatoid arthritis	Peripheral emboli
CREST syndrome	Thromboangiitis obliterans
Mixed connective tissue disease	**Drugs**
Polymyositis	Ergots
Sjögren's syndrome	β-blockers
Reiter's syndrome	Oral contraceptives
Polyarteritis	Bleomycin
Exposure/Trauma	Vinblastine
Vibratory tools	Imipramine
Vinyl chloride	Bromocriptine
Thoracic outlet syndrome	Clonidine
Carpal tunnel syndrome	Cyclosporine
Endocrine	**Hematologic**
Hypothyroidism	Leukemia
Graves' disease	Myeloid metaplasia
Addison's disease	Myeloma
Cushing's disease	Polycythemia
Hypofunctioning pituitary tumors	DIC
Neurologic	Cryoglobulinemia
Polyneuropathy	**Other**
Neurofibromatosis	Chronic renal failure
	Neoplasms
	Hemolytic uremic
	syndrome

Patients with Raynaud's syndrome associated with digital artery obstruction (atherosclerotic) may have attacks limited to one or several fingers, but the florid manifestations may be less dramatic. Certain patients may develop Raynaud's syndrome attacks after the frequent use of high-frequency vibrating equipment such as pneumatic drills, electric hand drills, and chain saws. The development of Raynaud's syndrome in persons using such tools is not clearly understood, and this type of Raynaud's syndrome is referred to as "vibration-induced white finger." In this particular condition, there is widespread palmar and digital artery obstruction.

The body's normal response to cold exposure is mediated through the sympathetic nervous system, which has received the greatest amount of attention in searching for the exact cause of this disorder. It is easy to see how a normally functioning sympathetic nervous system could precipitate cold-induced attacks in patients with small vessel obstruction. However, research also makes it clear that the exact mechanisms responsible for Raynaud's attacks are much more complex than can be explained by simple hypersympathetic function or sympathetic activity superimposed upon circulatory insufficiency. Investigators have identified abnormalities in disparate but interrelated areas such as vasoactive peptides, adrenoreceptors, serotonin activity, platelet aggregation, and viscosity. The biochemical basis for the abnormal or exaggerated response of the sympathetic activity remains for the most part enigmatic.

Clinical Findings

A. Signs and Symptoms: The Raynaud's attacks may vary greatly in severity and distribution. The hands and fingers are most commonly involved. The feet, toes, ears, cheeks, and nose can be affected. The attacks may affect only a single digit in a unilateral fashion, but they may affect all extremity digits in a symmetric fashion (Fig 14–1). The patient may complain of numbness, tingling, burning sensations, and severe blanching of the digits with exposure to cold. The cyanosis and recovery period from rubor may go unnoticed by the patient. Attacks may last from several minutes to several hours. Extensive historical data should be obtained from the patient including occupational and social history and a list of all medications being taken. The patient's emotional status is vital. Specific questions regarding symptoms frequently seen with the enumerated common associated diseases should be detailed for future reference (see Table 14–1).

Between the classic attacks, the physical examination may be completely normal in patients with Raynaud's syndrome. It is important to evaluate the peripheral pulses for their presence and quality. Prominent subclavian artery pulsations should not be overlooked because these may signify aneurysms at this location and be the source of emboli. The digits are inspected for trophic changes, signs of emboli, and the presence of tissue ischemia or necrosis. The entire patient should be assessed for signs of systemic comorbid conditions. Pay particular attention to the skin and joints, especially for telangiectasias, taut skin, or joint abnormalities (Fig 14–2).

Nearly 4 times as many females as males are affected with Raynaud's syndrome. The reason for this gender difference remains unclear.

B. Laboratory Findings: Laboratory testing varies considerably based on the severity, frequency, and duration of symptoms together with any suggestions of underlying conditions detected from the history and physical examination. In most patients displaying significant symptoms, baseline laboratory testing should be obtained. These tests include sedimentation rate (sed rate), complete blood count, chemistry profile, urinalysis, and x-ray films of the hands. Based on clinical suspicions, selected patients require a symptom-directed assay evaluation and perhaps even nerve conduction velocity testing or skin and muscle biopsies (Table 14–2). Certain patients exhibiting symptoms related to intense emotional stimuli are best served by proper counseling rather than laboratory tests.

Digital circulation can be evaluated by Doppler and photoplethysmography. In patients with suspected proximal arterial lesions or in refractory patients, arteriography is often helpful because duplex scanning techniques are of questionable value in the most distal portions of the extremities.

Differential Diagnosis

The diagnosis of Raynaud's syndrome is usually not difficult except in a small group of patients who have subtle or no color changes at all. Most often, the diag-

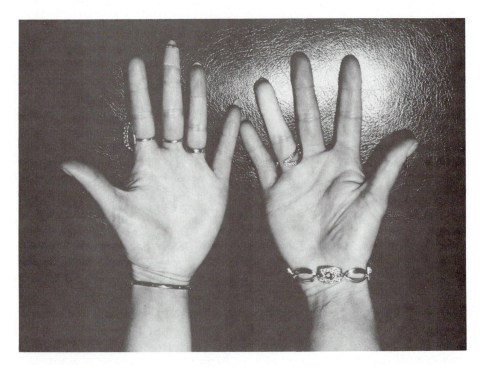

Figure 14–1. Raynaud's syndrome in a young female with localized symptoms. She has a band-aid covering the left middle finger. Note extreme blanching of the right 4th finger.

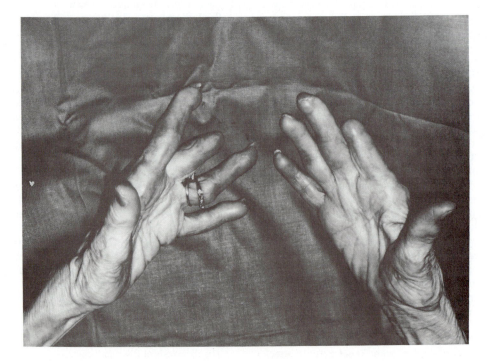

Figure 14–2. Patient with severe Raynaud's syndrome associated with rheumatoid arthritis. The distal phalanx of the right index and left 3rd finger have required amputation.

Table 14–2. Laboratory evaluation
in Raynaud's disease patients.

Rheumatoid factor assay	LE preparation
Antinuclear antibody assay	Immunoglobulin
Anti-DNA antibody assay	Complement C3 and C4
Hepatitis B serologies	Cryoglobulin assay
Serum protein electropheresis	

nosis is made simply by the history of digital color changes, which occur repeatedly to exposure to cold or emotional stimuli. An ice water immersion test usually confirms the diagnosis.

At this point, it may be difficult or impossible to determine whether Raynaud's syndrome is a benign, self-limiting process or an early manifestation of one of the varied underlying diseases associated with this syndrome (see Table 14–1). Discussion of these diseases and their diagnosis are beyond the scope of this chapter. It may take years of observation before associated diseases can be definitively diagnosed. The most common entities to differentiate from Raynaud's syndrome are advanced fixed arterial ischemia, hyperhidrosis, cold hypersensitivity, livedo reticularis, acrocyanosis, and certain types of arteritis.

It is usually easy to differentiate persons with Raynaud's syndrome from those with fixed arterial ischemia because the latter condition is usually present for a shorter length of time, remains continuously symptomatic, and manifests signs of ischemia. Hyperhidrosis lacks the color changes of Raynaud's syndrome. In persons with cold hypersensitivity, the predominant symptom is intense pain, and the duration of the attack is much longer than in Raynaud's syndrome. Livedo reticularis and acrocyanosis are characterized by fixed discoloration without any of the other symptoms present in Raynaud's syndrome.

Treatment

The initial and perhaps most important management plan in the treatment of patients with Raynaud's syndrome is education and reassurance of the patient. Many patients have the misconception that this disorder is invariably associated with cancer, strokes, paralysis, loss of digits or extremities, and other incurable illnesses. The treatments vary as much as the cause of the syndrome.

Avoiding cold, abstaining from tobacco, and instituting an exercise program are helpful to most patients and may inhibit the recurrence of symptoms. Occupational changes should be considered if prolonged exposure to cold, direct occupational arterial trauma, or the use of vibratory tools are thought to play a role in the onset of symptoms. Certain drugs that are known to aggravate Raynaud's symptoms, such as ergotamine preparations, birth control pills, and β-adrenergic blocking agents, are to be avoided. If the attacks are primarily precipitated by emotional stimuli, professional counseling may be successful. Adjunctive

use of relaxants and selected tranquilizers are often indicated. The optimal treatment for any documented associated disease often has a salutary effect on Raynaud's syndrome patients. The presence of neurovascular compression syndromes, carpal tunnel syndrome, and other associated neurovascular disorders must be treated to eliminate this trigger mechanism. All proximal arterial occlusive disease should be dealt with surgically when appropriate.

Drug therapy for Raynaud's syndrome may require multiple trials or combination therapy to obtain the desired result. The sympatholytic agents, calcium channel blocking agents, and direct vasodilators are used singularly or in combination with positive symptomatic results. Following are the drugs most commonly used today:

- Nifedipene
- Guanethidine
- Reserpine
- Prazocin
- Tolazoline
- Phenoxybenzamine

Ketanserin, a serotonin antagonist, and thymoxamime are currently under investigation.

In difficult cases that display intractable pain, digital ulcers, or the not infrequent pharmacologic failures, attempts to alter the abnormal sympathetic activity by surgical intervention is still advised. Surgery is not curative in a definitive sense but may afford significant palliation, relieve pain, and enhance healing of skin ulcerations if local measures do not suffice. Cervicothoracic sympathectomy is used particularly in patients who have a significant amount of arterial obstruction and who respond to diagnostic preoperative sympathetic blocks.

Other modalities of management of patients with intractable and advanced Raynaud's syndrome include intra-arterial reserpine injections, intravenous reserpine by Bier block, plasmapheresis, and prostaglandin infusion with varying results.

Prognosis

Raynaud's syndrome is notable for symptom-free intervals interrupted by episodic attacks. Tissue loss infrequently occurs, and if ulcerations do develop they usually heal well with conservative therapy. Digital loss usually happens only with advanced ischemia associated with severe underlying arterial obstruction (see Fig 14–2).

Abboud FM, Eckstein JW, Lawrence MS: Preliminary observations on the use of the intra-arterial reserpine in Raynaud's phenomenon. Circulation 1967;35;11.

Allen EV, Brown GE: Raynaud's disease: A critical review of minimal requisites for diagnosis. Am J Med Sci 1932; 183:187.

Belch JJ: The phenomenon, syndrome and disease of Maurice Raynaud. Br J Rheumatol 1990;29:162.

Cardelli MB, Kleinsmith DM: Raynaud's phenomenon and disease. Med Clin North Am 1989;73:1127.

Clophas TJM, Niemeyer MG: Raynaud's syndrome, an enigma after 130 years. Angiology 1993;44:196.

Coffman JD: Pathogenesis and treatment of Raynaud's phenomenon. Cardiovasc Drugs Ther 1990;4:45.

Kallenberg CG: Early detection of connective tissue disease in patients with Raynaud's phenomenon. Rheum Dis Clin North Am 1990;16:11.

Raynaud M: On local asphyxia and symmetrical gangrene of the extremities. In: *Selected Monographs,* New Sydenham Society, 1888:99.

Taylor LM Jr et al: Digital ischemia as a manifestation of malignancy. Ann Surg 1987;206:62.

Taylor W, Pelmear PL (editors): *Vibration White Fingers in Industry.* Academic Press, 1975.

Taylor W, Pelmear PL: The hand-arm vibrating syndrome: An update. Br J Ind Med 1990;47:577.

Warmsley D, Goodfield MJ: Evidence for an abnormal peripherally mediated vascular response to temperature in Raynaud's phenomenon. Br J Rheumatol 1990:29:181.

HYPERHIDROSIS

Essentials of Diagnosis

- Inappropriate excessive diaphoresis limited to the hands or soles.

General Considerations

Hyperhidrosis is a condition of unknown cause characterized by increased sweating. It is often confused with Raynaud's syndrome but lacks the intense vascular changes previously described. Hyperhidrosis is an important entity to identify and distinguish from Raynaud's syndrome because surgical sympathetic interruption has been the only method that produces long-lasting relief from this otherwise benign condition.

Clinical Findings

In hyperhidrosis, the palms, axillae, and plantar surfaces are most commonly involved. Areas of involvement are usually symmetric and display profuse sweating far beyond that required to cool the body. Classic symptoms of Raynaud's syndrome are absent. Socially and economically disabling symptoms occur particularly in palmar hyperhidrosis. The incidence of this condition is slightly higher in women than in men, and most patients seek medical attention in their early 20s. This condition may develop in 25–50% of the siblings of affected persons.

Treatment

Nonoperative treatment of hyperhidrosis includes anticholinergics, antiperspirants, absorbing powders, hypnosis, sedation, biofeedback, iontophoresis, and acupuncture. Anticholinergics are occasionally effective, but their side effects have precluded long-term use. Many patients are neglected for years because treating physicians are unfamiliar with the condition and its treatment.

The surgical treatment is directed toward denervation of the sympathetic nerves of the upper extremity (T2 and T3 ganglia) for palmar hyperhidrosis (Fig 14–3). In the lower extremity, the removal of L2 and L3 sympathetic ganglia is usually sufficient. The distribution of sympathetic nerves to each organ or region is only approximate; however, most patients can expect complete and durable improvement after adequate sympathectomy.

Edmondson RA, Banerjee AK, Rennie JA: Endoscopic transthoracic sympathectomy in the treatment of hyperhidrosis. Ann Surg 1992;215:289.

Moran KT, Brady MP: Surgical management of primary hyperhidrosis. Br J Surg 1991;78:279.

White JW: Treatment of primary hyperhidrosis. Mayo Clin Proc 1986;61:951.

COLD HYPERSENSITIVITY

Patients exhibit sensitivity of a digit or entire extremity that is exposed to cold repeatedly. This is particularly true of patients who have a history of documented frostbite. However, many patients exhibit this phenomena with no history of frostbite. However, minor frostbite most likely occurred during childhood.

The affected areas are predictable, repetitive, and seldom symmetric. Patients with cold hypersensitivity display a bluish discoloration of the skin in the exposed area and often complain of severe burning, which may last for hours or days. The pain is similar to that seen in causalgia or mimo-causalgia. If attacks are frequent and uncontrolled, surgical sympathectomy is indicated, and results are comparable to those achieved with posttraumatic pain syndromes.

Jacob JR et al: Chronic pernio: A historical perspective of cold-induced vascular disease. Arch Intern Med 1986; 146:1589.

Spittell Jr JA, Spittell PC: Chronic pernio: Another cause of blue toes. Int Angiol 1992;11:46.

LIVEDO RETICULARIS

Livedo reticularis is often confused with Raynaud's syndrome. It is characterized by persistent reticulated reddish-blue mottling of the skin. Livedo reticularis is accentuated by exposure to cold, but it is often present continuously, regardless of the existing environmental temperature. Livedo reticularis is seen primarily in the lower legs and feet and has a symmetric distribution. Occasionally, involvement is seen in the hands and arms, but this is rare unless the lower extremities are involved.

Livedo reticularis has been described in association with such conditions as periarteritis nodosa, lupus erythematosus, dermatomyositis, and cholesterol emboli. It is thought to be caused by random spasm of cuta-

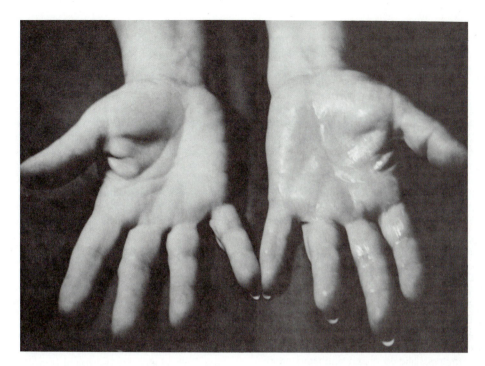

Figure 14–3. Palmar hyperhidrosis. Patient has undergone dorsal sympathectomy on the right with complete relief of symptoms. Note continued excessive sweating of the left hand and palm. (Patient subsequently underwent left dorsal sympathectomy with relief of symptoms on this side.)

neous arterioles with secondary dilatation of associated capillaries and the creation of arteriovenous fistulas at the capillary level. The condition is benign, and no treatment is indicated other than avoidance of cold. Patients with livedo reticularis rarely complain of discomfort or pain but remain concerned about the appearance. After patients are reassured that it is a benign condition and not a grave illness, it is often accepted and the vague presenting complaints disappear. The rare patients with livedo reticularis associated with pain or skin ulceration should be screened for the presence of an associated condition previously listed.

Burton JL: Livedo reticularis, porcelain-white scars, and cerebral thromboses. Lancet 1988;1:1263.

ACROCYANOSIS

Acrocyanosis is a condition characterized by continuous bluish discoloration of the lower legs and feet. Patients complain of the sensation of coolness in the affected areas. There is a symmetric distribution to this disorder as well, and it is encountered almost exclusively in women. It may be found in up to 20% of women with anorexia nervosa. The discoloration and coolness are worse in cold weather but are present even in warm weather. Arterial pulses are present, and episodic color changes do not occur. Symptoms are al-

ways worse in cold weather. The cause of acrocyanosis is unknown, but it is probably related to dysfunction of the sympathetic nervous system with resultant abnormal and continuous cutaneous arteriolar spasm. The condition is usually benign and skin ulceration is extremely rare. Treatment consists in avoidance of exposure to cold. Sympatholytic agents such as those used in the treatment of Raynaud's syndrome may occasionally be necessary to produce symptomatic relief.

Bhanj S, Mattingly D: Acrocyanosis in anorexia nervosa. Postgrad Med J 1991;67:33

POSTTRAUMATIC PAIN SYNDROMES

Posttraumatic pain syndromes—causalgia and mimo-causalgia—are 2 of the most poorly understood conditions in medicine. This is particularly surprising, since it was described over 100 years ago. Failure to recognize these entities creates a disturbing delay in diagnosis and proper treatment. Confusion arises from the presence of over 30 terms in the literature describing minor variations of the same symptom complex.

These are listed in Table 14–3. All these terms describe situations that have several factors in common, namely, pain, sympathetic dysfunction, delayed functional recovery, and trophic changes.

In 1973, Patman presented a classification of these posttraumatic pain syndromes in an effort to simplify and standardize the terms, but historically preserve the original description of classic causalgia. Patman provided the 2 major categories of posttraumatic pain syndromes (causalgia and mimo-causalgia), which have the aforementioned characteristics. This simple classification has been adopted in an effort to standardize the literature and create a better understanding of this important entity.

CAUSALGIA

Essentials of Diagnosis

- Delayed resolution of pain in an extremity after a traumatic event to that limb with a disparity between the severity and duration of pain and the apparent injury.
- Signs of sympathetic nervous system hyperactivity: hyperhidrosis and decreased skin temperature.
- Possible peripheral nerve injury or deficit.
- Trophic changes (pale shiny skin, muscle atrophy, bone demineralization) in advanced cases.

General Considerations

After trauma of almost any variety and severity in an extremity, orderly and predictable healing of the wound, return of function, return of circulatory dynamics, and a gradual cessation of pain are expected. This usually occurs within a certain period of time based on the type and extent of injury. Occasionally, this predictable physiologic response to injury reacts in a most bizarre fashion despite adequate treatment and in the absence of obvious factors detrimental to prompt healing. Pain may become severe and unrelenting, but may be of any gradation. Often a marked disparity exists between the severity of pain and the apparent injury. Sympathetic dysfunction, usually overactivity, is evident, but it may be mild or severe. These symptoms, if prolonged, eventually delay functional recovery and become a predominant feature of the syndrome. Trophic changes in the distal portion of the extremity appear and may become irreversible if the process is left unattended. This sequence of events should alert the clinician to the possible presence of a posttraumatic pain syndrome. Early recognition and proper therapy of these syndromes can obviate most irreversible changes and relieve pain completely.

In 1864, Mitchell, Morehouse, and Keen described a syndrome of burning pain in the extremities of Union Army soldiers with gunshot wounds of the peripheral nerves. In an article published in 1867, Mitchell wrote:

> Causalgia—there is, however, one species of pain arising out of nerve wounds which have never been described except by my colleagues and myself, although the state of skin which is usually found with it had been spoken of by Mr. Paget, who seems to have seen it only in association with common neurologic pain. In writing of this peculiar kind of suffering, I felt that it would be well to give it some more convenient name than merely "burning pain," and I have therefore adopted the term causalgia as being both descriptive and convenient. (page 164.)

The term **causalgia** was derived from the Greek words *kausos,* meaning heat, and *algos,* meaning pain. In its strictest sense, causalgia is taken to mean a painful syndrome that may follow injury to a main nerve, the pain being of a burning nature.

Clinical Findings
A. Signs and Symptoms: In most cases of causalgia, pain nearly always appears soon after the time of injury. A sensation of burning pain involves the peripheral portions of the extremity. The pain and dysesthesias are not restricted to the area supplied by the nerve that is injured. The cutaneous dysesthesias may be so intense that the patient will not tolerate contact with clothing. Any form of stimulus to the limb can precipitate agonizing pain.

Table 14–3. Terms found in the literature for posttraumatic states.

Posttraumatic sympathetic dystrophy	Mitchell's causalgia
Posttraumatic pain syndromes	Causalgia
Sympathetic neurovascular dystrophy	Major causalgia
Reflex nervous dystrophy	Minor causalgia
Posttraumatic sympathetic dysfunction	Homan's minor causalgia
Reflex dystrophy of the extremities	Causalgia-like states
Posttraumatic painful osteoporosis	Sudeck's atrophy
Posttraumatic spreading neuralgia	Sudeck's syndrome
Posttraumatic vasomotor disorders	Traumatic angiospasm
Steinbroker's shoulder-hand syndrome	Shoulder-hand syndrome
Reflex sympathetic dystrophy	Reflex dystrophy
Posttraumatic dystrophy	Sympathalgia
Traumatic edema	Chronic traumatic edema
Traumatic neuralgia	Peripheral trophoneurosis
Acute atrophy of bones	Painful osteoporosis

The extremity is protected in a posture that prevents venous congestion. Affected arms are usually held flexed and abducted in close approximation to the trunk. Vasomotor dysfunction is invariably present but may be severe or mild. Two principal variations may be observed: vasodilatation or vasoconstriction. **Vasoconstriction** is most common, and the skin of the palms or soles of the feet becomes shiny, moist, cyanotic, and cold to the touch. Immobilization by the patient eventually causes functional loss and atrophy of the distal portion of the involved extremity. The trophic changes are almost always present in varying degrees, and if the process is left unattended, they may become irreversible (Figs 14–4 and 14–5).

B. Imaging Studies: X-rays of the affected limb may show bony demineralization. Increased activity can be seen on bone scans os the involved limb as well.

MIMO-CAUSALGIA

Essentials of Diagnosis

- Absence of peripheral nerve injury.
- Delayed resolution of pain in an extremity after a traumatic event to that limb with a disparity between the severity and duration of pain and the apparent injury.
- Hyperhidrosis and decreased skin temperature.
- Trophic changes (pale shiny skin, muscle atrophy, bone demineralization) in advanced cases.

General Considerations

The major difference between causalgia and mimo-causalgia is that in the latter there is no evidence of a major peripheral nerve injury. Mimo-causalgia may occur after extremity trauma of almost any variety and severity. Undoubtedly, this occurs secondary to some form of injury to minor nerves in a variety of clinical settings—hence, the more than 30 aforementioned terms used to describe the varied manifestations. Mimo-causalgia may also occur after cervical, head, or truncal injury but much less frequently. These confusing terms all relate to similar syndromes that constitute one large category similar to but distinct from true causalgia. The terms have been grouped together under a single designation: "mimo-causalgia states." *Mimo* in Greek means an attempt to recreate or imitate. The term mimo-causalgia, therefore, is used to designate all of the posttraumatic pain syndromes that have no demonstrable major peripheral nerve injury.

Clinical Findings

A. Signs and Symptoms: The primary symptoms of mimo-causalgia are pain, sympathetic dysfunction, abnormal functional recovery, and trophic changes (Fig 14–6). The pain is most often described as burning, stinging, throbbing, aching, bursting, lancinating, or knife-like. Pain may be present at rest or only with motion and is almost always aggravated by motion. Like patients with causalgia, patients with mimo-causalgia also assume a protective posture. Pain

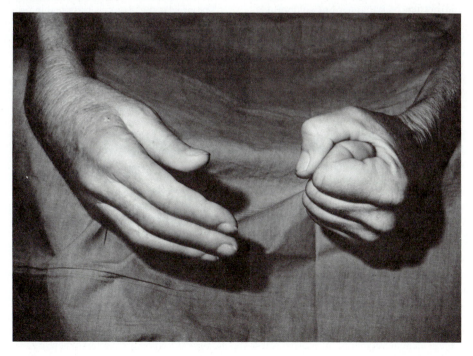

Figure 14–4. Patient with longstanding causalgia of the right upper extremity following incomplete peripheral nerve severance. Following sympathectomy, the causalgic pain was relieved but patient continued to have severe trophic changes with limitations of joint motion.

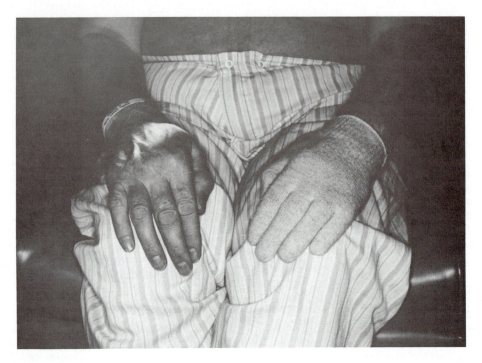

Figure 14–5. Patient with causalgia in its extreme form. He kept left hand protected in a glove at all times. Before treatment, patient stated that all forms of stimuli such as touching, drafty rooms, even loud music aggravated the pain.

may be of the same intensity and constant, or it may be aggravated by external stimuli. It is relieved slightly by the administration of narcotics but seldom adequately controlled for any length of time. The pain is almost always more severe in the periphery of the extremity, although notable exceptions occur.

Nearly all patients demonstrate vasomotor alteration as evidenced by edema, cyanosis, coldness, and hyperhidrosis (Fig 14–4). A significant number exhibit one of these changes out of proportion to the others.

Alterations in cutaneous sensation are most common in those with mimo-causalgia. Simply touching or slight pressure to the involved area may be intolerable. Motion is limited because pain and stiffness are commonly aggravated in the fingers, hand, wrist, elbow, shoulder, and ankle. Muscle atrophy is always present from disuse.

If affected patients are allowed to go untreated for any length of time, the trophic changes may continue despite relief of pain after treatment. The mimo-causalgia states are often not as dramatic and clearly defined as classic causalgia. They may result in significant permanent incapacitation and therefore are most important to recognize early.

B. Imaging Studies: X-rays of the affected limb may show bony demineralization. Increased activity can be seen on bone scans of the involved limb as well.

Causes of Posttraumatic Pain Syndromes

The precise mechanisms responsible for the development of causalgia and mimo-causalgia remain unclear. Several theories have been proposed, but none has been able to explain why some develop the syndrome and others do not. A simple explanation is that the sympathetic nerve fibers themselves transmit the pain impulses to the central nervous system. Unfortunately, there is no strong evidence that there are afferent fibers in the sympathetic pathways to the extremities. White and Sweet (1967) state that the responses of some of their patients accompanied by the observations on patients recorded by Echlin (1949) and Ellonen (1946) forced them to concede that there may be exceptions to the theory that pain fibers from the arm and leg do not traverse the sympathetic plexuses. Doupe and associates (1944) suggested that artificial synapses occur at the site of injury.

Livingston (1943) suggested a cycle of reflexes to explain the pain, with 3 main components consisting of (1) increased production and release of afferent impulses into a peripheral sensory nerve after injury or irritation from any cause, (2) abnormal activity or increased stimulation in the internuncial pool located in the anterior horn of the spinal cord, and (3) subsequent increase in sympathetic efferent activity.

Melzak and Wall (1963) suggested a theory similar to Livingston's to explain pain transmission. They

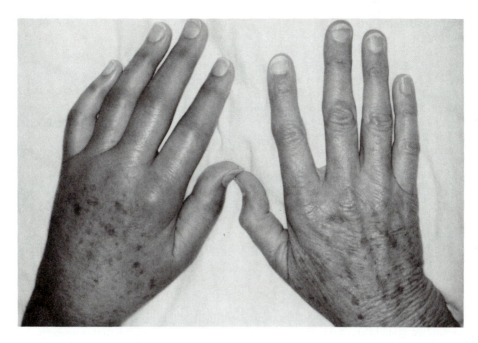

Figure 14–6. Patient with mimo-causalgia. Left hand displays shiny skin, edema, and vasomotor imbalance with hyperhidrosis.

contend that certain cells in the substantia gelatinosa of the dorsal horn of the spinal cord act as a computer or gate control system that directs the incoming afferent sensory impulses. These cells, in a highly sophisticated manner, interpret the type, number, and frequency of afferent sensory impulses, and then relay these impulses to the brain for perception of pain.

Another theory proposes that impulses along large myelinated fibers inhibit this control system or "gate," and impulses transmitted along small fibers, perhaps afferent sympathetic, tend to stimulate or "open the gate" and thus increase the impulses transmitted centrally via the neurons in the spinal center. Regardless of the cause, causalgia is produced by sympathetic stimulation. When no effective treatment was known, causalgia frequently resulted in invalidism, mental deterioration, drug addiction, and suicide.

Differential Diagnosis

It can be challenging and difficult to differentiate a posttraumatic pain syndrome from the other conditions that cause obscure extremity pain. Nerve entrapment, peripheral neuritis, disk disease and residual underlying inflammation (the myofascial pain syndromes) are the main entities to consider. Trigger points are discrete locations at which externally applied pressure precisely reproduces the patient's pain often in a sharp and radiating manner and an entrapped

nerve will be associated with this finding. If local anesthetic is injected into this area prompt, although temporary, relief occurs.

The symptoms of peripheral neuritis are similar to those of the posttraumatic pain syndromes. Generally, however, a traumatic history, trophic changes and signs of sympathetic dysfunction are absent. Obviously spinal disk disease with nerve root compression causes extremity pain and sensory abnormalities, but these are frequently positionally related and present in a radicular pattern.

Many patients with previous injuries can have persistent underlying inflammation in the involved area. This is commonly referred to as myofascial pain syndrome and is characterized by pain and restricted movement of the extremity. It responds to treatment with anti-inflammatory agents, muscle relaxants, and physiotherapy.

It is important to realize that these conditions can coexist with the posttraumatic pain syndromes. The presence of posttraumatic pain syndrome can be easily verified by its response to sympathetic blockade. An incomplete response to this suggests the additional presence of one of these other disorders and a complete lack of response to a sympathetic block implies that one of these disorders is the sole cause of the patient's pain. Because of this complexity, it is essential that the clinician treating such patients have a thorough understanding of these other disease processes.

Treatment of Posttraumatic Pain Syndromes

A number of various procedures have been researched but none of them gave consistently good results. Neurolysis was invariably ineffective. It was recommended that resection and suture be performed in cases of classic causalgia. This procedure amounted to a destructive operation in many cases because the nerve injury was seldom complete and the neurologic deficit often minimal prior to nerve resection. Sicard (1918) and Lewis and Gatewood (1920) recommended the injection of 60% alcohol into the nerve proximal to the site of injury on the basis that it interrupted sensory fibers but did not cause motor paralysis. This procedure was unsuccessful in most cases, however.

Unquestionably, the most definitive therapy in posttraumatic pain syndrome is sympathectomy, either chemical or surgical. There are many treatment methods that have varying degrees of success but most generally focus on decreasing or eliminating sympathetic influences. Other reported treatments include physical therapy, thermal biofeedback, low dose ultrasound, transcutaneous nerve stimulation, systemic steroids, regional intravenous reserpine, various peripheral vasodilator drugs, and thalamic stimulation. A physical therapy program emphasizing use of the extremity and increasing the range of motion is invariably helpful, particularly in the longstanding cases, but not to the exclusion of sympathetic blockade.

When a patient suspected of having true causalgia or mimo-causalgia is first seen, the initial step in diagnosis and therapy should be a sympathetic nerve block. This remains the most reliable test for mimo-causalgia. Both forms (causalgia and mimo-causalgia) should have a salutary response to an effective block.

Patients with true causalgia seldom have longlasting relief of pain from sympathetic blocks. In general, most patients with causalgia ultimately require surgical sympathectomy.

Patients with mimo-causalgia may often respond to sympathetic blocks. In over 300 cases, about 40% of the mimo-causalgia states have responded to multiple sympathetic blocks. If treatment is instituted early, relief of pain may last beyond the duration of the block and may even be curative. Repeated blocks should be performed until the pain is controlled. If the results of sympathetic block are equivocal, a control block with normal saline may be performed. If relief from repeated sympathetic blocks becomes less effective or static and the initial response is dramatic but of short duration, surgical sympathectomy should be performed.

Only rarely is a definitive cure seen if the patient requires over 5 sympathetic blocks. If this circumstance prevails, it is more propitious to proceed with surgical sympathectomy. Early surgical sympathectomy will prevent the occurrence of irreversible trophic changes and obviate the establishment of fixed pain patterns, which may become refractory even to sympathectomy if the syndrome is allowed to be prolonged without definitive therapy.

Prognosis

Surgical sympathectomy offers excellent relief of pain in causalgia and mimo-causalgia, but residual somatic pain may persist. Some of these residual symptoms are due to the original injury in which soft tissue, muscles, nerve bone, or joint loss occurs. In some instances of mimo-causalgia, there is no major tissue loss and residual symptoms result from stiffness of joints and limitations of motion. Irreversible changes occur from pain and trophic changes that stem from the prolonged mimo-causalgia state itself. Accurate diagnosis and early sympathectomy yield predictably good results. Sympathectomy is so specific for these disorders that there is seldom an indication to delay sympathectomy in lieu of other forms of treatment previously mentioned. In delayed cases of posttraumatic pain syndrome, sympathectomy should not be held in disfavor if it does not result in complete resolution of all forms of pain and all trophic changes. Patients with posttraumatic pain syndromes also may have prominent myofascial pain. Sympathectomy does not preclude careful scrutiny and treatment of other causes of residual pain and disability.

Barowski EI, Zewig JB, Moskowitz J: Thermal biofeedback in the treatment of symptoms associated with reflex sympathetic dystrophy. J Child Neurol 1987;2:229.

Bingham JAW: Some problems of causalgic pain: A clinical and experimental study. Br Med J 1948;64:334.

Doupe J, Cullen CH, Chance GQ: Post-traumatic pain and the causalgia syndrome. J Neurol Psychiatr 1944; 7:33.

Echlin F: Pain responses on stimulation of the lumbar sympathetic chain under local anesthesia: A case report. J Neurosurg 1949;6:530.

Ellonen A: L'effet de la sympathectomie sur le fantome douloureux d'un amputé. Acta Chir Scand 1946;93:131.

Kwan ST: The treatment of causalgia by thoracic sympathetic ganglionectomy. Ann Surg 1935;101:222.

Lewis D, Gatewood W: Treatment of causalgia: Results of intraneural injection of 60% alcohol. JAMA 1920; 74:1.

Livingston WK: *Pain Mechanisms: A Physiological Interpretation of Causalgia and Its Related States.* Macmillan, 1943.

Melzak R, Wall PD: Gate control theory of pain. In: *Pain.* Soulairoc A, Cohn J, Carpentier J (editors). Academic Press, 1968:11.

Mitchell SW: *On the Diseases of Nerves, Resulting from Injuries in Contributions Relating to the Causation and Prevention of Disease, and to Camp Diseases.* In: US Sanitary Commission Memoirs. Flint A (editor). 1867.

Mitchell SW: *Injuries of Nerves and Their Consequences.* JB Lippincott, 1872.

Mitchell SW, Morehouse GR, Keen WW: *Gunshot Wounds and Other Injuries of Nerves.* JB Lippincott, 1864.

Patman RD: Management of post-traumatic pain syndromes. In: *Traumatic Medicine and Surgery for the Attorney,* vol. 4, Release No. 23 and 24, pages 193–210. Matthew Bender, 1975.

Patman RD: Posttraumatic pain syndromes. Compr Ther 1977;3:44.

Patman RD, Thompson JE, Persson AV: Management of posttraumatic pain syndromes: Report of 113 cases. Ann Surg 1973;177:780.

Platt H, Bristow WR: Remote results of operations for injuries of peripheral nerves. Br J Surg 1924;11:535.

Richards RL: The term "causalgia." Med Hist 1967;2:97.

Schwartzman RJ: Reflex sympathetic dystrophy and causalgia. Neurol Clin 1992;10:953.

Sicard JA: Painful neuritis resulting from wounds of war: Treatment by inner truncal alcoholization of the nerves. Lancet 1918;1:213.

Spurling RG: Causalgia of the upper extremity: Treatment by dorsal sympathetic ganglionectomy. Arch Neurol Psychiatr (Chir) 1930;23:704.

Turnbull IM, Shulman R, Woodhurst WB: Thalamic stimulation for neuropathic pain. J Neurosurg 1980;52:486.

Walker AE, Nielson S: Electric stimulation of the upper thoracic portion of the sympathetic chain in man. Arch Neurol Psychiatr 1947;59:559.

White JC, Sweet WH: Other varieties of peripheral neuralgia. In: *Pain and the Neurosurgeon.* White JC (editor). Charles C Thomas, 1967.

Nonatherosclerotic Vascular Diseases & Conditions

R. Donald Patman, MD, & William P. Shutze, MD

Atherosclerosis is the primary underlying disease in over 90% of those with peripheral vascular disease; however, a significant number of vascular patients are affected by illnesses or conditions dissimilar from arteriosclerosis. Nonatherosclerotic diseases can be divided into 2 categories: inflammatory and noninflammatory (Table 15–1).

I. INFLAMMATORY NONATHEROSCLEROTIC DISEASE

ARTERITIS

Arteritis refers to a group of diseases characterized by vascular inflammatory changes, usually of the transmural necrotizing variety, but often the causes are unknown. The term "vasculitis" is used interchangeably with arteritis, but it should apply only to disease processes that occur in association with a variety of syndromes that have accompanying necrosis and occlusive changes of blood vessels (arteries and veins). Precise pathogenic mechanisms for these disorders are poorly understood, but a multiplicity of different immune or hypersensitivity reactions may form a common pathway.

TAKAYASU'S ARTERITIS

Essentials of Diagnosis

- Onset of claudication, bruits, pulse deficits, limb blood pressure discrepancies or hypertension on patient less than 35 years of age.
- Arterial stenosis limited to the aorta or its major branches sparing the distal and parenchymal portions of these branch vessels.

General Considerations

Takayasu's arteritis consists primarily of stenosing inflammation of the aorta and its branches. It predominates in young women (less than 35 years of age) by a margin of 3 to 1. Takayasu's arteritis is also referred to as pulseless disease, nonspecific aortoarteritis, arteritis of young women, atypical aortic coarctation, and middle aorta syndrome.

Takayasu's arteritis is more prevalent in Asian countries but may be found anywhere in the world. Its incidence in the USA is 2.6 per million. The exact cause of the disease process is unknown but is thought to be an autoimmune phenomenon targeting the involved vessels. The triggering mechanism may be a chronic infection. The aortic arch and its branches are involved most frequently (Fig 15–1*A* and *B*). The second most common site is the proximal abdominal aorta and its branches, followed by the visceral/renal arteries; however, any branch of the aorta can be affected. Pulmonary artery involvement is rarely symptomatic but is identified radiographically in up to 50%. It's presence helps establish the diagnosis of Takayasu's arteritis. The coronary arteries are rarely affected. Note that the intraparenchymal portions of the vessels remain unaffected by Takayasu's arteritis.

The diseased vessels show granulomatous inflammation in the adventitia, vasa vasorum, and media with loss of elastic elements, resulting in a subsequent panarteritis. Reactive hypertrophic intimal and adventitial proliferation develop with medial thinning as the inflammatory infiltrate subsides. As this progresses, the vessels sclerose, and calcification may occur. Occasionally, aneurysms, dilatation, or occlusion are produced.

Clinical Findings

A. Signs and Symptoms: The symptoms in the chronic phase of Takayasu's arteritis depend on the vessels affected, but hypertension, cerebrovascular symptoms, congestive heart failure, claudication, impotence, and angina have been noted. If extensive aortic arch involvement is present and the patient has hypertension from coarctation or renal artery involvement, the hypertension may not be detected by periph-

Table 15–1. Nonatherosclerotic vascular conditions.

Inflammatory Conditions
  Arteritis
    Takayasu's arteritis
    Giant cell arteritis
    Polyarteritis nodosa
    Hypersensitivity vasculitis
    Kawasaki disease
  Behçet's disease
  Buerger's disease
Noninflammatory Conditons
  Fibromuscular dysplasia
  Inherited angiopathy
    Marfan syndrome
    Ehlers-Danlos syndrome
    Pseudoxanthoma elasticum
  Congenital and developmental disease
    Abdominal aortic coarctation
    Persistent sciatic artery
    Adventitial cystic disease
    Popliteal artery entrapment

eral blood pressure measurement and secondary signs of its presence should be sought.

Nonspecific complaints such as fever, malaise, anorexia, weight loss, arthralgias, and myalgias represent the acute phase of Takayasu's arteritis. These flu-like symptoms are transient. Because the vasculitis takes time to produce arterial stenosis, several years may elapse before the patient presents with symptoms of arterial insufficiency.

In the advanced stage, diminished or absent peripheral pulses, bruits, systolic murmurs, atrophy, blood pressure asymmetry, retinal arteriovenous anastomoses, visual field deficits, headache, cardiomegaly, and tachycardia may be present, depending on the location and extent of the disease.

B. Laboratory Findings: In addition to the usual laboratory tests (cbc, serum chemistries, urinalysis), an electrocardiogram (ECG), chest radiograph, and a sedimentation rate (sed rate) should be performed. Anemia is seen in 50% of cases, and an elevated sed rate is a common and useful marker for ongoing inflammation. Left ventricular hypertrophy and left atrial enlargement reflect the presence of hypertension. Chest x-ray abnormalities, seen in over 50% of patients with Takayasu's arteritis, include cardiomegaly and an abnormal aortic contour.

C. Imaging Studies: The key to diagnosis is angiography (Figure 15–1C) to delineate to extent of disease as the pattern of involvement does not usually allow diagnostic biopsy (see Fig 15–1C). Angiography shows the characteristic pattern of stenosis as being limited to the aorta and its branches in a young person. This pattern, in combination with pulmonary artery abnormalities, is enough to presume the diagnosis.

Treatment

The Takayasu's arteritis may be treated with nonsteroidal anti-inflammatory agents, steroids, cyclophosphamide, or cyclosporine. If signs of active disease are present, steroids should be administered and, if necessary, cyclophosphamide added. The sed rate can be used to monitor the patient's response to this treatment. In contrast to that which occurs in giant cell arteritis, the lesions in Takayasu's arteritis do not usually disappear with immunosuppressant therapy.

Hypertension and lesions that produce symptoms of end-organ ischemia indicate the need for reconstructive surgery. Although endarterectomy and balloon angioplasty are options, **bypasses** are the preferred surgical procedure. Generally, bypasses should begin and end in disease-free areas. Inflammation should be suppressed before any surgery to achieve optimal results.

Prognosis

Reconstructive surgery for Takayasu's arteritis is generally successful. When all patients are considered those with stable nonprogressive disease have a 6 year survival rate of 98%, but those with severe complications and progression have a mortality rate of 45% after 6 years. Although the long-term prognosis remains unclear because of limited experience with this disease, current drug therapies and surgery appear to be beneficial.

Arend WP et al: The American College of Rheumatology 1990 criteria for the classification of Takayasu arteritis. Arthritis Rheum 1990;33:1129.

Hall S, Buchbinder R: Takayasu's arteritis. Rheum Dis Clin North Am 1990;16:411.

Ishikawa K: Diagnostic approach and proposed criteria for the clinical diagnosis of Takayasu's arteriopathy. J Am Coll Cardiol 1988;12:964.

Robbs JV, Human RR, Rajaruthnam P: Operative treatment of nonspecific aortoarteritis (Takayasu's arteritis). J Vasc Surg 1986;3:605.

Scott D et al: Surgical repair of visceral artery occlusions in Takayasu's disease. J Vasc Surg 1986;3:904.

Takayasu U: A case with unusual changes of the central vessels of the retina. Acta Soc Ophthalmol Jap 1908;12:554.

Weaver FA et al: Surgical procedures in the management of Takayasu's arteritis. J Vasc Surg 1990;12:429.

GIANT CELL ARTERITIS

Essentials of Diagnosis

- Systemic symptoms of fever, myalgias, and weight loss.
- Commonly associated with polymyalgia rheumatica and mainly in females 55 and older.
- The temporal arteries may be abnormal by palpation.
- Diminished pulses with claudication in extremity involvement.
- Erythrocyte sed rate greater than 50 mm/hr.
- Angiographic findings of bilaterally symmetric tapering stenoses with collateralization and poststenotic dilatation.

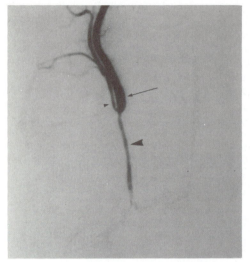

A

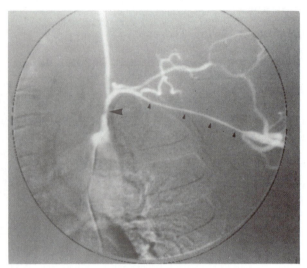

B

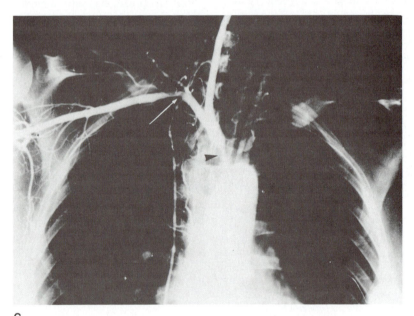

C

Figure 15–1. Arteriograms of a 20-year-old Hispanic female with Takayasu's arteritis, who had absent left carotid and left arm pulses. **A:** The left common carotid artery is diffusely narrowed (*larger arrowhead*). Note the characteristic sparing of the internal carotid artery (*arrow*) and the external carotid artery (*small arrowhead*). **B:** The left subclavian artery is stenosed in the prevertebral portion (*large arrowhead*), and the distal subclavian and axillary arteries (*small arrowheads*) demonstrate a long segment stenosis. **C:** This angiogram is of another patient with Takayasu's arteritis who had absent right arm pulses. The arteriogram shows the proximal innominate artery obstruction (*black arrow*) and the subclavian and vertebral artery (*arrow*) stenoses as well.

General Considerations

Ten times more common than Takayasu's arteritis, **giant cell arteritis** (GCA) is a systemic granulomatous panarteritis that occurs mainly in females above the age of 55 years. The most common form of this illness is temporal arteritis, which affects the branches of the carotid arterial system. In 10% of cases, other peripheral vascular involvement occurs, and classically the axillobrachial arteries are afflicted. The subclavian arteries may also be diseased, and this upper limb involvement is more common than that of the superficial femoral and profunda femoral vessels. The pattern is usually bilateral, and there is a striking association of GCA with polymyalgia rheumatica. Other potentially affected sites include the aorta and the visceral, renal, vertebral, and coronary arteries.

The focal and segmental inflammation yields stenoses and occlusions but aneurysms and dissections have been noted in the larger vessels. Vascular biopsies show an infiltrate of mononuclear and multinucleated giant cells (Fig 15–2). Elastic fiber fragmentation is present, and the giant cells, which are often in direct contact with the elastic lamina, may contain fragments of elastin.

The incidence of GCA varies worldwide but may be as high as 1 in 500 in the USA. Also, the overall incidence is increasing annually mostly because of an increase of GCA in females. No specific causes have been identified, but there may be a relationship between existing vascular disease or smoking and GCA. Recently, attention has been focused on the HLA (human leukocyte antigen)-DR histocompatibility antigens as well as abnormalities in lymphocyte subtype ratios as possible etiologic factors.

Clinical Findings

A. Signs and Symptoms: Nonspecific symptoms of GCA—fever, headache, myalgias, and weight loss—manifest first. After a prodromal period of several weeks, other symptoms arise. Temporal arteritis can lead to masticatory claudication and visual symptoms, which can be catastrophic. The visual symptoms consist of blindness, amaurosis fugax, or extraocular muscle palsies; they occur in up to 50% of GCA patients. These conditions are secondary to any of the following: ischemic optic neuritis, retrobulbar neuritis, ophthalmic arteritis, and occlusion of the central retinal vessels. Involvement of the limb circulation causes characteristic claudication. Polymyalgia rheumatica is present in about 50% of the patients.

About 50% of GCA patients with temporal arteritis have indurated or tender temporal arteries, an erythematous periarterial dermis, or abnormal pulses in this location. In the systemic form of the disease, diminished or absent distal pulses are identified.

B. Laboratory Findings: An elevated erythrocyte sed rate (>40 mm/hr) indicates temporal arteritis; however, GCA cases have been documented in which sed rate is normal. Biopsy of the temporal artery usually reveals the characteristic pathologic changes.

C. Imaging Studies: Angiography is performed to evaluate patients presenting with claudication or visual abnormalities. The multiple stenoses may vary in length, may taper at each end, and may have intervening segments of normal vessel. Numerous collateral arteries are seen, poststenotic dilatation may be present, and arteries usually are bilaterally (and sometimes symmetrically) involved with the remaining vascular system free of disease (Fig 15–3). In patients demonstrating peripheral involvement, a characteristic angiogram, elevated sed rate, and an appropriate history

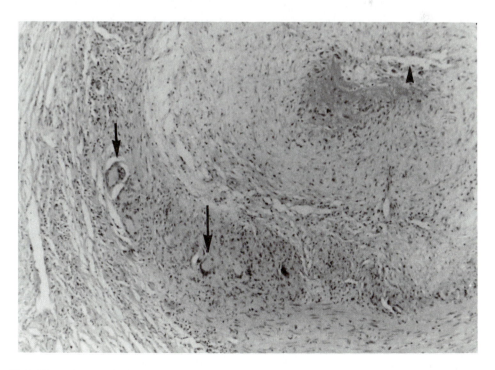

Figure 15–2. Photomicrograph of a section of temporal artery from a 72-year-old woman with giant cell arteritis. Intimal thickening, focal medial necrosis, granuloma formation, and multinucleated giant cells (*arrows*) are present.

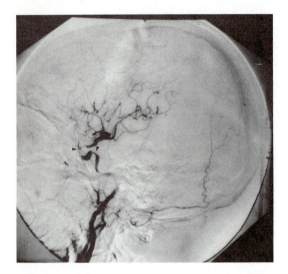

Figure 15–3. Cerebral angiogram of a 73-year-old woman with biopsy-proven giant cell arteritis. Severe tapering stenoses (*arrowheads*) are seen in the intracranial internal carotid artery, and mirror image stenoses were also present in the contralateral side.

are sufficient for the diagnosis if an appropriate biopsy site is unavailable.

Treatment

Steroid therapy is the mainstay of treatment for GCA. Once the diagnosis is suspected, high-dose therapy should be instituted without delay, because the ocular complications can be devastating, even if the diagnostic biopsy has not been performed. Steroids are tapered slowly after the systemic symptoms are resolved and sed rate normalizes. The sed rate is monitored frequently during the tapering process to ensure adequate disease suppression, and it must be kept in a normal range. Although up to 2 years may be required for weaning from steroids, nearly all patients can become steroid independent.

Surgical intervention is limited to diagnostic biopsy in patients with temporal arteritis. Patients presenting with pulse deficits and claudication may return to their premorbid state with appropriate immunosuppressive treatment. As such, revascularization is usually unnecessary. Although it may be tempting to operate on these patients, the distal ischemia is rarely severe, and bypass failure rates are high in the active illness. The occasional complications of GCA such as aortic valve incompetence, dissection, or aneurysms should not be overlooked.

Prognosis

Early recognition of GCA is essential because the initial management is nonsurgical and the ocular complications can be devastating. The mortality rate in patients with GCA is identical with that of the general population however with appropriate care the incidence of blindness has decreased from almost 50% to less than 20%.

Henret J-P et al: The history of temporal arteritis or ten centuries of fascinating adventure J Mal Vasc 1989;14:93.

Hunder GG et al: The American College of Rheumatology 1990 criteria for the classification of giant cell arteritis. Arthritis Rheum 1990;33:1122.

Hunder GG et al: Pathogenesis of giant cell arteritis. Arthritis Rheum 1993;36:757.

Joyce JW: The giant cell arteritides: Diagnosis and the role of surgery. J Vasc Surg 1986;3:827.

Lie JT: Diagnostic histopathology of major systemic and pulmonary vasculitis syndromes. Rheum Dis Clin North Am 1990;16:269.

Machioni P et al: Lymphocyte subpopulations analysis in peripheral blood in polymyalgia rheumatica/giant cell arteritis. Br J Rheumatol 1993;32:666.

POLYARTERITIS NODOSA

Essentials of Diagnosis

- Presence of multisystem disease with symptoms and signs of generalized inflammation including any of the following: weight loss, livedo reticularis, myalgias, diastolic hypertension, elevated BUN and creatinine, testicular pain or tenderness, purpura, or subcutaneous tender nodules.
- Any combination of renal, gastrointestinal, central nervous system, peripheral nervous system, and skin lesions.
- Visceral (including renal) angiography showing small vessel aneurysms.
- Biopsy of involved tissue showing a necrotizing vasculitis of the medium and small vessels.

General Considerations

Polyarteritis nodosa (PAN) is a focal necrotizing vasculitis caused by immune complex-induced injury that involves the medium and small arteries in a disseminated pattern. First extensively described by Kussmaul in 1866, the disease process affects various vessels at different times while it proceeds through a pattern of inflammation, fibrinoid necrosis, and finally fibrous occlusion or aneurysm development. A focal and segmental polymorphonuclear cell inflammatory infiltrate is present in all layers, and a fibrointimal proliferative reaction occurs that can lead to vessel occlusion. The aneurysms result from the necrosis in the medial layer (Fig 15–4A). In contrast to giant cell and Takayasu's arteritides, PAN is twice as common in males. PAN can develop in a person of any age with the mean being 45 years old. Its incidence is about 5–10 per million.

Clinical Findings

A. Signs and Symptoms: Systemic complaints of fever, weight loss, fatigue, myalgias, and arthralgias

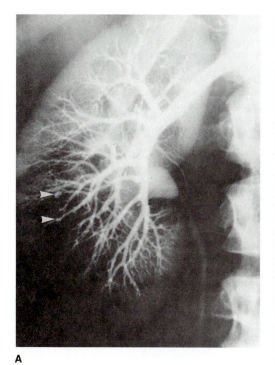
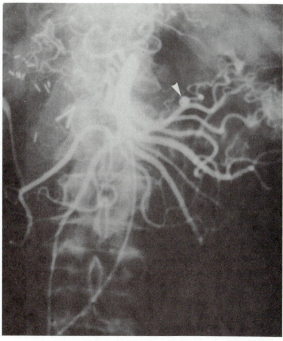

A   B

Figure 15–4. **A:** Right renal angiogram in a patient with polyarteritis nodosa (PAN). Multiple microaneurysms (*arrowheads*) are present and chiefly affect the vessel branch points. **B:** Visceral angiogram in a patient with PAN reveals a significant aneurysm at a branch point (*arrowhead*) in one of the superior mesenteric artery branches to the jejunum. Such aneurysms can produce life-threatening hemorrhage, and their identification calls for aggressive cytotoxic treatment.

may be present in PAN patients. Other complaints depend on the pattern and sequence of organ involvement. Skin lesions (purpura, livedo reticularis, nodules) and digital cutaneous ischemic changes develop in 20–40% of patients. Renal disease is present in 70%, with manifestations including hypertension, glomerulonephritis, and microhematuria. Peripheral nerve damage appears as mononeuritis multiplex, and central nervous system involvement occurs in 25%. Inflammation can also be found in the vertebral, carotid, meningeal and cerebral vessels. Cardiac involvement is commonly seen at autopsy with coronary arteritis, pericarditis, hypertrophy, and infarction.

The gastrointestinal lesions in PAN patients can be vague, varied, and difficult to treat. Vasculitis in the splanchnic circulation causes cholecystitis, visceral infarction, hemorrhage, gut perforation, and delayed stricture. Mesenteric venous thrombosis is also possible. Interventions directed at these secondary events will not succeed unless the underlying cause is recognized and treated.

B. Laboratory Findings: The laboratory findings in PAN are generally not helpful. Anemia, leukocytosis, thrombocytosis, decreased complement levels, elevated sed rate, and C-reactive protein levels may be identified. About 30% have hepatitis B surface antigenemia. Factor VIII-related antigen levels are elevated in PAN patients but are also elevated in many

noninflammatory vascular injuries. Nonetheless, factor VIII-related antigen levels may be a useful marker to guide medical therapy.

Biopsy is an accurate diagnosing tool that identifies the presence and extent of PAN. Biopsy of involved tissue that demonstrates a necrotizing vasculitis supports the diagnosis in the correct clinical setting. Appropriate biopsy sites are sural nerve, skin, muscle, kidney, rectum, and testis. Site selection should be based on involvement.

C. Imaging Studies: In combination with biopsy, angiography plays an important role in diagnosing the presence and extent of PAN. Visceral arteriography demonstrates small vessel aneurysms in 80% of patients (see Fig 15–4*B*); however, these aneurysms can be seen in other diseases as well. Aneurysms have also been found in the cerebral, pulmonary, lumbar, intercostal, inferior phrenic, epigastric, and gastroduodenal arteries. Patients with hepatitis B surface antigenemia should undergo visceral angiography because of the almost uniform presence of mesenteric aneurysms in those affected.

Differential Diagnosis

The diagnosis of PAN is often one of exclusion and includes any multisystem necrotizing arteritis that does not conform to any other recognized vasculitic syndrome. Other systemic vasculitides that may have similar signs and symptoms to those of PAN but are distinct either because of their pattern of involvement or their mechanism are allergic angiitis and granulomatosis (Churg-Strauss syndrome), overlap syndrome, Wegener's granulomatosis, and lymphomatoid granulomatosis. PAN spares the pulmonary system; thus, involvement of this system is more likely to be allergic angiitis and granulomatosis. This disease is also differentiated from PAN by the presence of peripheral and tissue eosinophilia; by its predilection for patients with bronchial asthma, respiratory allergy or chronic sinusitis; and by findings of intravascular and extravascular granuloma consisting of pleomorphic cells and eosinophilic inflammatory cells. A condition in which characteristics of PAN and Churg-Strauss syndrome occur together is called **overlap syndrome,** which implies that these 2 illnesses are part of a disease spectrum. Therapy is the same as that for PAN.

Wegener's granulomatosis is described as a triad of granulomatous vasculitis affecting the respiratory system, glomerulonephritis, and small vessel hypersensitivity vasculitis. Its characteristics are similar to those of PAN, with a peak incidence in the fourth and fifth decades of life. Antineutrophil cytoplasmic antibodies are found in 60–70% of cases and are highly specific to Wegener's granulomatosis. A lung biopsy revealing vasculitis and necrotizing granulomas is diagnostic. Treatment for Wegener's granulomatosis is the same as that for PAN. Cures are rare, but improvement occurs in 75–90%. The mean survival of untreated persons is 5 months.

Lymphomatoid granulomatosis is characterized by angiotropic infiltration with destruction of various tissues, especially lung, with atypical lymphocytoid and plasmacytoid cells. Skin (45%), kidney (45%), and central nervous system (20%) manifestations are present, and lymphomas evolve in 13%. Without treatment, death occurs rapidly.

Treatment

Steroids, cyclophosphamide, and azathioprine are used to control the inflammatory process of PAN. Other than treating the complications of PAN, there is no role for surgical therapy and because of the size of vessels affected, revascularization is not reasonable. With the advent of effective immunosuppressive therapy, the mortality rate has decreased from about 90% to 40%. Fifty percent of the deaths are secondary to the renal disease, and central nervous system disorders are the second most common cause of death. Rupture of intra-abdominal PAN aneurysms has been described, which may lead to death. These aneurysms have been documented to regress after vigorous steroid and cytotoxic therapy. This therapy is recommended for all asymptomatic visceral aneurysms.

Conn DL: Polyarteritis. Rheum Dis Clin North Am 1990;16:341.

Falk RJ, Jennette JC: Anti-neutrophil cytoplasmic autoantibodies with specificity for myeloperoxidase in patients with systemic vasculitis and idiopathic necrotizing and crescentic glomerulonephritis. N Engl J Med 1988;318: 1651.

Ferraro G et al: Anti-endothelial cell antibodies in patients with Wegener's granulomatosis and micropolyarteritis. Clin Exp Immunol 1990;79:47.

Kussmaul A, Maier K: Über eine bischer nicht beschreibene eigenthümliche arterinerkrankung die mit morbus brightii und rapid fortschreitender allgemeiner muskellähmung eithergeht. Dtsch Arch Klin Med 1866;1:484.

Ledford DK: Immunologic aspects of cardiovascular disease. JAMA 1992;268:2923

Lightfoot RW et al: The American College of Rheumatology 1990 criteria for the classification of polyarteritis nodosa. Arthritis Rheum 1990;33:1088.

Michet CJ: Epidemiology of vasculitis. Rheum Dis Clin North Am 1990;16:261.

Selke FW et al: Management of intraabdominal aneurysms associated with periarteritis nodosa. J Vasc Surg 1986;4: 294.

HYPERSENSITIVITY VASCULITIS

Essentials of Diagnosis

- Patient over 16 years of age with palpable purpura or maculopapular rash.
- History of antigenic exposure, such as medication, connective tissue disease, cryoglobulins, or malignancy.
- Biopsy showing polymorphonuclear cells or eosinophils in vessel wall.

General Considerations

Hypersensitivity vasculitis is an immune complex disease with deposition of these antigen-antibody complexes into the small blood vessels (capillaries, venules, arterioles), usually of the dermis. A leukocytoclastic vasculitis is produced with blood vessel necrosis, fibrin deposition, pleomorphic cellular infiltrate, nuclear dust, and erythrocyte extravasation. Any disease or condition which is accompanied by circulating antigens can lead to hypersensitivity vasculitis. Hypersensitivity vasculitis accounts for about 25% of vasculitis cases. The primary diseases associated with hypersensitivity vasculitis are listed in Table 15–2.

Clinical Findings

A. Signs and Symptoms: More than 95% of hypersensitivity vasculitis patients have demonstrable purpura or other dermatologic findings such as petechiae, ulcerations, bullae, urticaria, erythema multiforme, and livedo reticularis. The buttocks and legs are most commonly affected. Other organ systems may be involved producing arthritis/arthralgias, glomerulonephritis, pulmonary infiltrates, and neuropathy. Vasculitis of the mesenteric circulation can give way to ischemia of the gut with infarction, ischemic perforation, or hemorrhage.

Table 15–2. Disorders associated
with hypersensitivity vasculitis.

Collagen and vascular related
  Systemic lupus erythematosus, rheumatoid arthritis,
    relapsing polychondritis, Reiter's syndrome, ankylosing
    spondylitis
Serum sickness
Infection
Drug-related disorders (due to methyldopa, phenytoin,
    hydralazine)
Henoch-Schönlein purpura
Cryoglobulinemia
Malignancy
  Chronic lymphocytic leukemia, lymphoma, Hodgkin's
    disease, multiple myeloma

Some of the rheumatic diseases have been found in association with aneurysms of the aorta or aortitis. Although the role of aneurysm screening is not clear, it is recommended if any of these conditions are suspected. Aortic valve incompetence has been noted as well.

B. Laboratory Findings: The sed rate and acute phase reactants are elevated in patients with hypersensitivity vasculitis. A leukocytosis and decreased serum complement levels may be present, but no specific test is available for this condition. The most informative test is a biopsy of the involved dermis to demonstrate the leukocytoclastic vasculitis if the lesions persist or recur.

Treatment

Nonsteroidal and antihistamine therapy may suffice for treatment of hypersensitivity vasculitis. For more persistent cases or those associated with chronic rheumatologic disease or life-threatening complications such as mesenteric or renal involvement, immunosuppressive therapy should be administered.

Prognosis

Prognosis for hypersensitivity vasculitis patients is generally good, especially if the initiating antigen can be removed and the disease does not involve major viscera.

Calabrese LH et al: The American College of Rheumatology 1990 criteria for the classification of hypersensitivity vasculitis. Arthritis Rheum 1990;33:1108.

Fauci AS, Haynes BF, Katz P: The spectrum of vasculitis: Clinical, pathological, immunologic and therapeutic considerations. Ann Intern Med 1978;89:660.

Gravallese EM et al: Rheumatoid aortitis: A rarely recognized but clinically significant entity. Medicine 1989; 68:95.

Ledford DK, Espinoza LR: Immunologic aspects of cardiovascular disease. JAMA 1987;258:2974

Montanaro A: Vasculitis in older patients: Presentations and significance. Geriatrics 1988;43(Mar):75.

Vollertsen RS, Conn DL: Vasculitis associated with rheumatoid arthritis. Rheum Dis Clin North Am 1990;16:445.

KAWASAKI DISEASE
(Mucocutaneous Lymph
Node Syndrome)

Kawasaki disease is an acute inflammatory process that primarily affects infants and small children with a peak incidence between 1 and 2 years of age. It is more common in Asians, but it may occur in any race or culture. The causative agent is unknown, but epidemiologically it behaves like an infectious disease. The diagnosis of Kawasaki disease is made according to the criteria in Table 15–3. The cardiac manifestations (pericardial effusion, myocarditis, and coronary artery aneurysms) are the most important features of this illness and constitute the main cause of morbidity and mortality. Coronary arteritis may progress with the development of stenotic lesions and ischemic symptoms. Of concern to the vascular surgeon is that in patients with coronary artery abnormalities aneurysms of the renal, axillary, brachial, iliac, and femoral arteries can develop. Rare cases of peripheral gangrene have been reported. Aspirin therapy is recommended for patients with Kawasaki disease, and the addition of intravenous γ-globulin decreases the incidence of coronary artery abnormalities.

Dajani AS et al: Diagnosis and therapy of Kawasaki disease in children. Circulation 1993;87:1776.

Kato H, Inoue O, Akagi T: Kawasaki disease: Cardiac problems and management. Pediatr Rev 1988;9:209.

Newberger JW et al: The treatment of Kawasaki syndrome with intravenous gamma globulin. N Engl J Med 1986; 315:341.

BEHÇET'S DISEASE

Essentials of Diagnosis

* Oral ulcerations that recur at least 3 times a year.
* At least 2 of the following: recurrent genital ulceration, uveitis, skin lesions, positive pathergy test.
* Vascular complications, such as venous thrombosis, arterial occlusion, or aneurysm formation.

General Considerations

Behçet's disease is a vasculitis typified by intimal hyperplasia, internal elastic membrane disruption with

Table 15–3. Diagnosis of Kawasaki disease.

Fever persisting at least 5 days plus at least 4 additional features:
  1. Changes in extremities
     Acute: erythema and edema of hands and feet
     Convalescent: membranous desquamation of fingertips
  2. Polymorphous exanthem
  3. Bilateral painless bulbar conjuctival injection without exudate
  4. Changes in lips, strawberry tongue, diffuse injection of oral and pharyngeal mucosa
  5. Acute, nonpurulent cervical lymphadenopathy (>1.5 cm. in diameter), usually unilateral

medial thinning, and an adventitial/perivascular infiltrate of plasma cells and neutrophils. It is more common in Japan and the Mediterranean and is seen slightly more often in males. The incidence of Behçet's disease in the USA is about 1 in 20,000. Etiologic possibilities are infectious, autoimmune, and possibly genetic; HLA-B51 and HLA-DRw52 histocompatibility antigens have an association with this illness in the Japanese. Endothelial cell dysfunction may contribute to the thrombotic vascular complications.

Clinical Findings

A. Signs and Symptoms: This multisystem vasculitis is characterized by a clinical triad of ulcerations of the oral cavity and genitalia, and uveitis or hypopyon. The articular, gastrointestinal, vascular, and nervous systems can be affected as well.

Vasculo-Behçet's disease affects veins more often than arteries; arterial complications occur in about 10% of those affected, and venous thrombosis occurs in about 30%. Superficial thrombophlebitis and venous occlusions of the extremities are the most frequently encountered vascular lesions. The second most common complication is thrombosis of either vena cava, followed by aneurysms or occlusions of the limb arteries. The renal, hepatic, dural, and jugular veins can be affected. Occlusions and aneurysms may form metachronously and sometimes rapidly in various arteries including the aorta and the subclavian, carotid, renal, splenic, iliofemoral, and pulmonary arteries.

Gastrointestinal symptoms such as vomiting, abdominal pain, flatulence, diarrhea, and constipation are present in 50% of those with Behçet's disease (entero-Behçet's disease). This leads to ulcerations in the ileocecal area in 75%, perforation occurs in 40%, and bleeding in 20%. About 10% will develop neuro-Behçet's syndrome with meningoencephalitis, sensory, motor, and psychiatric symptoms. Lung infiltrates with hemoptysis herald the presence of pulmonary vasculitis.

Other manifestations of Behçet's disease may be exist alone or in combination with the above system subtypes of Behçet's disease. Skin lesions such as erythema nodosum, pseudofolliculitis, papulopustules, or acneiform eruption may be present in up to 84% of patients. Synovitis, arthralgias, and effusions are characteristic of joint involvement (seen in 50%), with the knee being the most common site.

B. Laboratory Findings: The **pathergy test** determines whether an organ system is involved in Behçet's disease. In this test, the subject's skin is pricked with a needle, which provokes a sterile pustule to form within 24 hours. A positive pathergy test can replace one organ system involvement to meet the diagnostic criteria. Occasionally, the vascular, enteric, or neural system disease dominates the picture, and the actual diagnosis can be overlooked.

C. Imaging Studies: The evaluation of the vascular complications obviously depends on their nature and location. Because of the increased risk of pseudoaneurysm or thrombosis during an angiogram, noninvasive imaging is preferred for surveillance and evaluation of the associated vascular problems in these patients.

Diagnosis

The diagnosis of Behçet's disease is a clinical one with the patient showing recurrent oral ulcerations and involvement of 2 other systems (skin, eye, or genital). In the pathergy test the subject's skin is pricked with a needle and a sterile pustule forms within 24 hours. A positive pathergy test can replace one organ system involvement to meet the diagnostic criteria. Occasionally the vascular, enteric and neural system disease dominates the picture and the actual diagnosis can be overlooked.

Treatment

Immunosuppressive therapy is recommended for the ulcerations and ocular and meningeal symptoms. Glucocorticosteroids, chlorambucil, cyclophosphamide, azathioprine, and cyclosporine all have been used for patients with Behçet's disease, and FK 506 has recently been used but blindness is still a 50–80% risk.

Revascularization of the arterial system is fraught with difficulties. There is a high rate of anastomotic disruption, and patency rates are substandard. Because Behçet's disease affects vessels in a focal but random manner extra-anatomic grafting may provide better results if the inflow and outflow vessels are uninvolved.

Anticoagulation is necessary to treat the thrombotic complications of Behçet's disease. Although it is unknown, the duration of anticoagulation probably should be indefinite. Anticoagulation, however, is to be avoided if pulmonary disease is present. Prophylactic treatment also may be prudent when superficial thrombophlebitis has occurred.

Prognosis

The overall mortality rate for persons with Behçet's disease is 3–4% and is usually the result of aneurysm rupture, intestinal perforation, or severe central nervous system disease.

Behçet HH: Uber Rezidivierende, Apthose, durch ein Virus verursachte geschwure am mund, am Auge unde under Genitalen. Dermatol Wochenshr 1937;105:1152.

Bartlett ST et al: Multiple aneurysms in Behçet's disease. Arch Surg 1988;123:1004.

International Study Group for Behçet's disease: Criteria for diagnosis of Behçet's disease. Lancet 1990;335:1078.

Katoh K et al: Pathologically defined neuro-, vasculo-, entero-Behçet's disease. J Rheumatol 1985;12:1186.

Koç Y et al: Vascular involvement in Behçet's disease. J Rheumatol 1992;19:402.

Matsumoto T, Uekasa T, Fukuda Y: Vasculo-Behçet's disease: A pathologic study of eight cases. Hum Pathol 1991; 22:45.

Yamana K et al: Vasculo-Behçet's disease: Immunologic study of the formation of aneurysm. J Cardiovasc Surg 1988;29:751.

Yazici H et al: A controlled trial of azathioprine in Behçet's syndrome. N Engl J Med 1990;322:281.

BUERGER'S DISEASE
(Thromboangiitis Obliterans)

Essentials of Diagnosis
- Ischemic signs and symptoms of the distal upper or lower extremities in a smoker, usually a male.
- Commonly associated with Raynaud's syndrome.
- Absent distal pulses with preserved proximal pulses.
- Migratory superficial phlebitis.
- Absence of atherosclerosis or its non-tobacco-related risk factors.
- Absence of any other vasculopathy, arteritis, or hypercoagulable state.
- Onset of disease before 45–50 years of age.

General Considerations
Buerger's disease is an inflammatory process involving the medium and small arteries of the extremities, although the accompanying veins can be affected as well. The age of onset is usually between 35 and 50 years, and it tends to occur more frequently in males. Buerger's disease is a disease of smokers only and is seen more often in people from the Middle and Far East. Smoking is a permissive or accelerating factor, and although the actual cause is unknown it is thought to be immunologically related.

Histologically, the acutely affected vessel is filled with unorganized thrombus associated with multi-nucleated giant cells. The thrombi contain micro-abscesses consisting of neutrophils encircled by mononuclear epithelioid cells. Vascular wall necrosis is absent and notably the internal elastic lamina is preserved. The subacute lesions in Buerger's disease are not as distinctive, but the organizing thrombi may still contain some mild inflammation that is not routinely seen in clot. Chronically, there is intraluminal and perivascular fibrous transformation, but the vessel wall structures are mostly preserved.

Clinical Findings
A. Signs and Symptoms: The earliest complaints of persons with Buerger's disease are rest pain involving the feet or hands, painful digital ulcerations, or gangrene because the vascular involvement is distally located. If claudication is present, it is usually limited to the foot. Patients may also complain of Raynaud's symptoms or paresthesias. Usually 2 or more extremities are involved, and the lower limbs are predominantly affected. The arms can be diseased in up to 50% of patients, and the upper extremity is the presenting symptomatic limb in 20% of patients.

The digits are cold and moist with a mottled but ruborous appearance of the skin. Shallow dry ulcers may be located on the tips of the toes or fingers. These ulcers are usually tender. An acutely inflamed artery or vein is detected by the erythematous overlying dermis. Superficial phlebitis occurs in 30% of affected patients and may be recurrent. The proximal pulses (femoral and axillary) are usually normal, and the distal pulses (radial, ulnar, posterior tibial, and dorsalis pedis) in the involved limbs are absent. The pulses at the knee and elbow may be normal, depending on the proximal extent of thromboangiitis.

B. Laboratory Findings: Laboratory studies are directed at excluding atherosclerosis, vasculopathy, and hypercoagulability. A complete blood count (CBC), blood urea nitrogen, fasting glucose (glucose tolerance test, if necessary), and lipid profile are the basic tests.

If rheumatic disease or vasculitis is suspected, a sed rate, antinuclear antibody, and rheumatoid factor can be obtained. To rule out hypercoagulable states, the evaluation of protein C and S levels, antithrombin III levels, lupus anticoagulant, and anticardiolipin antibodies should be considered. If dysfibrinogenemia is suspected, more elaborate tests can be done.

C. Imaging Studies: Arteriograms demonstrate distal occlusive disease with sparing of the proximal segments. Vessel tortuosity, abrupt occlusions, and skip areas with intervening normal arteries are present. Frequently, a single distal artery remains unaffected. The collateral arteries tend to have a "tree root" or "corkscrew" appearance.

Diagnosis
The diagnosis of Buerger's disease is made chiefly by history and physical examination with supporting information obtained from peripheral arterial pressures and arteriography. The criteria to diagnose this condition generally consist of an early age of onset (before 45–50 years), a positive smoking history with no other risk factor for atherosclerosis (eg, diabetes mellitus, hyperlipidemia, hypertension), no other vasculopathy, and distal occlusive disease only (beyond the knee or elbow), as documented by segmental arterial Doppler pressures or arteriography. Superficial phlebitis is a helpful but not absolute criterion.

Treatment
Buerger's disease begins distally and propagates proximally. Usually when patients are first seen, extensive distal disease may be present, but the digits and limbs are viable. If the patient successfully quits smoking, disease progression and major limb loss are unlikely. If the patient continues to smoke, however, the inflammatory process will continue unabated, disease progression is assured, and the chance of limb loss increases. Neither ulceration nor gangrene will occur in about 25% of those affected, whereas 45% will suffer from recurrent ulcerations. Buerger's disease tends to abate a little with age, and tissue necrosis is not seen in a person over 60 years of age.

Prognosis

The survival rate of Buerger's disease patients equals that of aged-matched controls. This is because of the limited nature of the occlusive process, which spares the coronary, cerebral, and viscerorenal vasculature. If these vessels are affected by occlusive disease, it is usually secondary to smoking-induced atherosclerosis and not to thromboangiitis.

Treatment

Besides quitting smoking, treatment for Buerger's disease is limited to local wound care for ischemic ulcers and tissue loss, antibiotics for infections, and avoidance of trauma. Many medications have been tried unsuccessfully, including prostaglandins, vasodilators, antiplatelet drugs, hemorrheologic agents, and anticoagulants.

Sympathectomy may help to heal refractory ulcers or to alleviate rest pain. Surgical revascularization is possible in less than 10% of patients because of the lack of available outflow vessels. Bypass grafts have a higher failure rate in Buerger's disease than in atherosclerotic patients.

Twenty percent of patients with leg involvement can be expected to need toe or forefoot amputation, and another 20% will eventually undergo a major lower limb amputation. With upper extremity involvement, major amputation is rare because the disease infrequently spreads into the brachial artery and less than 10% require a digital amputation.

Buerger L: Thromboangiitis obliterans: A study of the vascular lesions leading to presenile spontaneous gangrene. Am J Med Sci 1908;136:567.

Matsushita M, Shionoya S, Matsumoto T: Urinary cotinine measurements in patients with Buerger's disease: Effects of active and passive smoking on the disease process. J Vasc Surg 1991;14:53.

McKusick VA et al: Buerger's disease: A distinct clinical and pathological entity. JAMA 1962;181:93.

Mills JL, Porter JM: Buerger's disease. Semin Vasc Surg 1993;6(1):14.

Ohta T, Shionoya: Fate of the ischemic limb in Buerger's disease. Br J Surg 1988;75:259.

Stanson AW: Roentgenographic findings in major vasculitic syndromes. Rheum Dis Clin North Am 1990;16:293.

II. NONINFLAMMATORY ATHEROSCLEROTIC DISEASES

FIBROMUSCULAR DYSPLASIA

Essentials of Diagnosis

- Typical angiographic appearance affecting the muscular medium-sized vessels usually in young and middle aged caucasian females.
- Involvement of renal and distal cervical internal carotid arteries most frequently.
- Lesions asymptomatic or producing hypertension or cerebrovascular symptoms.
- "String of beads" most frequent arteriographic finding.

General Considerations

Fibromuscular dysplasia (FMD) Fibromuscular dysplasia is an unusual vaculopathy in which abnormal growth and organization in one of the three arterial wall layers occurs. This leads to stenosis or aneurysm formation in the affected arterial segment. This intriguing arteriopathy is most prone to affect white females and is usually discovered when they are young or middle aged. Although FMD is found most frequently in the distal internal carotid and renal arteries, other arteries can be also affected, such as the vertebral, subclavian, axillary, external iliac, visceral, and femorocrural arteries, and rarely, the coronary arteries. Chapter 10 discusses cerebrovascular FMD more thoroughly. There are three main types of fibromuscular dysplasia (FMD) recongnized: intimal, medial, and periadventitial fibroplasia. Medial FMD has 3 subtypes: medial fibroplasia, perimedial fibroplasia, and medial hyperplasia. These can be differentiated histologically, but they also have characteristic angiographic patterns. Medial fibroplasia is the most common type and has a typical "string of beads" arteriographic appearance (Fig 15–5A).

The etiology of this arteriopathy is unknown but proposed causes include neonatal infection, developmental, posttraumatic and hormonal. Because of its propensity to limit itself to medium-sized muscular arteries without branches (internal carotid, renal, and external iliac arteries), FMD may be secondary to intramural ischemia and fibrosis with secondary microaneurysm formation. The vasa vasora take their origin from branch points, and vessels without branches would have a relative deficiency of nutrient vessels that could lead to such vessel wall ischemia. The overwhelming female preponderance suggests that hormonal influences may be active.

Clinical Findings

A. Signs and Symptoms: Many persons with FMD are asymptomatic, but the actual percentage is unknown because this group usually remains undiagnosed. Symptoms attributed to FMD are obviously related to the location of disease. The renal arteries are the most commonly affected, and FMD is the second leading cause of renovascular hypertension. These patients are usually young females with a rather brief duration of hypertension, which is frequently the only symptom; a perinephric bruit may be present. Patients with cervical (carotid and vertebral) FMD make up the second largest group, and symptoms may be nonspecific such as headaches, dizziness, tinnitus, or vertigo. Symptoms may also be those of classic transient

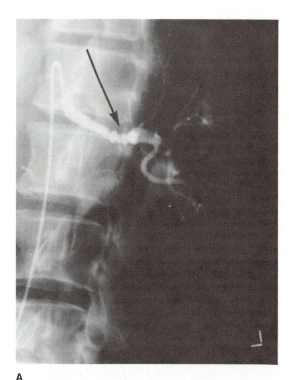

A

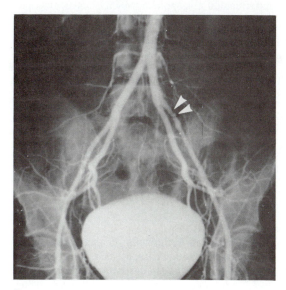

B

Figure 15–5. *A:* Left renal arteriogram in a young hypertensive female with bilateral fibromuscular dysplasia (FMD). The classic "string of beads" appearance (*arrow*) of the medial fibroplasia subtype can be seen. This subtype responded nicely to percutaneous transluminal angioplasty with resolution of the woman's hypertension. ***B:*** Aortogram showing left external iliac artery FMD (*arrowheads*) in a young woman with carotid and renal FMD as well.

ischemic attacks, amaurosis fugax, and stroke. Carotid dissections may occur as a complication of FMD, and patients present with a sudden cerebral catastrophe.

Visceral involvement may lead to abdominal angina, food fear, and weight loss, or the disease may remain quiescent. Extremity FMD may produce claudication, bruits, diminished pulses, "blue toe" syndrome, or sudden ischemia from dissection or thrombosis. Most patients with external iliac FMD have associated renal FMD as well (see Fig 15–5*B*).

B. Laboratory Findings: Arteriography for the appropriate symptoms is the only definitive way to diagnose FMD as well as to define its extent (see Fig 15–5*A* and *B*).

Duplex scanning has not been a reliable method of diagnosing FMD because of the locations involved.

Treatment

Regardless of the location of FMD, 2 basic tenets apply. Asymptomatic patients should be observed only, and symptomatic patients can be treated medically or surgically or with balloon angioplasty. For renal FMD, many new and potent antihypertensive medications are now available including the angiotensin-converting enzyme inhibitors. These drugs make it possible to control the renovascular hypertension to prevent the secondary complications of long-standing high blood pressure. However, no longitudinal studies have been performed to date to assess the outcome of such an approach, and when symptomatic renal FMD is encountered it is usually corrected.

Because of the distal arterial location of the renal FMD, graduated internal dilatation has been the preferred surgical approach when possible. However, bypasses are sometimes required, and ex vivo reconstruction may be needed.

Nephrectomy is almost never required for renal FMD. The lesions of FMD are amenable to balloon angioplasty, and enough experience has accrued to demonstrate that the results with balloon angioplasty compare favorably with the surgical results. This modality is now preferred not only for renal FMD but for all other sites of FMD except cerebrovascular. (See Chapter 10 for a discussion of the treatment of cerebrovascular FMD.)

The options for FMD of the limb vessels mirror those of renal FMD, although experience with the various clinical FMD entities is very limited. If distal embolization is occurring, it has been recommended to resect the diseased area. However, either surgical or percutaneous dilatation is usually sufficient because of the way this illness responds to such intervention. Symptoms from visceral FMD are unusual because of the redundancy of the mesenteric circulation, but this has been reported and treated by either surgical or interventional dilatation.

Prognosis

The natural history of FMD is difficult to define because of the suspected large number of patients with occult disease. Studies of patients with renal FMD show that the disease tends to progress anatomically in about 35% of persons, but arterial occlusion and renal insufficiency are rare sequelae. Many patients with FMD smoke, which may affect the course of their disease.

Progression is less likely in cerebrovascular FMD. In this subset of patients, there are those who are asymptomatic and will remain so and those who are symptomatic at the time of presentation and will remain so unless intervention is carried out. Insufficient information is available on FMD in other locations to make any statements regarding the course of disease in these cases.

Generally, about 50% of those with renal FMD are cured of hypertension following surgical or interventional treatment and another 25% will improve. These figures are much more gratifying than those associated with atherosclerotic renovascular disease. Experience with the extrarenal and noncerebrovascular forms of FMD is limited and anecdotal, but results have been favorable making this is really a rewarding disease to treat. Limb loss from extremity FMD, although rare, has occurred. The life expectancy of FMD patients is more likely to be related to their overall health and the existence of comorbid conditions.

Iwai T, Konno S, Hiejima K: Fibromuscular dysplasia in the extremities. J Cardiovasc Surg 1985;26:296.

Lüscher TF et al: Arterial fibromuscular dysplasia. Mayo Clin Proc 1987;62:931.

Parnell AP, Loose HW, Chamberlain J: Fibromuscular dysplasia of the external iliac artery: Treatment by percutaneous transluminal angioplasty. Br J Radiol 1988;61: 1080.

Sauer L et al: Clinical spectrum of symptomatic external iliac fibromuscular dysplasia. J Vasc Surg 1990;12:488.

Stanley JC, Wakefield TW: Arterial fibrodysplasia. In: *Vascular Surgery.* Rutherford RB (editor). 1989. Saunders.

Stewart MT et al: The natural history of carotid fibromuscular dysplasia. J Vasc Surg 1986;3:305.

Wessen CA, Elliott BM: Fibromuscular dysplasia of the carotid arteries. Am J Surg 1986;151:448.

INHERITED ANGIOPATHIES

MARFAN SYNDROME

Essentials of Diagnosis

- Major manifestations: aortic dissection, aortic root dilatation, ectopia lentis, dural ectasia.
- Minor manifestations found in numerous systems: cardiovascular, ocular, skeletal, pulmonary, dermal, and central nervous system (Table 15–4).

General Considerations

Marfan syndrome is an autosomal dominant disease of connective tissue, which is inherited with

Table 15–4. Minor manifestations of Marfan syndrome.

Cardiovascular
 Aortic regurgitation, mitral valve prolapse, mitral regurgitation, dysrhythmia, endocarditis
Ocular
 Myopia, retinal detachment
Skeletal
 Tall stature, arachnodactyly, dolichostenomelia, vertebral column deformity, pectus excavatum, flat feet, highly arched palate, joint hypermobility or contractures
Pulmonary
 Spontaneous pneumothorax, apical bleb, restrictive lung disease due to thoracic cage deformity
Dermal
 Striae distensae, hernias
CNS
 Learning disability, hyperactivity

widely variable penetrance. The incidence of Marfan syndrome is about 1 in 10,000. The major manifestations of this inherited connective tissue disorder are in the skeletal, ocular, and cardiovascular systems, and the discovery of its genetic basis has finally explained the unusual association of such widely disparate areas.

Over 95% of cases of Marfan's syndrome are caused by mutations in the fibrillin gene, which is found on chromosome 15. **Fibrillin** is a newly discovered structural glycoprotein, which is a major component of elastic microfibrils. This complex extracellular matrix is a significant part of the connective tissue in many different tissues in the body including blood vessels, periosteum, and the ciliary zonules of the eye that hold the lens in place.

The overriding concerns in patients with Marfan syndrome are the cardiovascular sequelae. Dilatation of the ascending aorta, which leads to aneurysms, rupture, or dissection, is the most common and most feared sequela (Fig 15–6). However, other arteries can develop aneurysms including the descending thoracic aorta, the abdominal aorta, and the pulmonary, coronary, carotid, and splenic arteries. Valvular disease and congestive heart failure are similarly possible.

Clinical Findings

A. Signs and Symptoms: Patients with Marfan syndrome may complain of chest pain (from aortic dissection or pneumothorax), dyspnea (secondary to congestive heart failure or restrictive lung disease), palpitations (dysrhythmias), or dizziness and syncope. In about 25% of cases, there is no family history of Marfan syndrome, which indicates a spontaneous mutation has occured. Ectopia lentis is present in about 50%. Cardiac murmurs or clicks may be noted.

B. Imaging Studies: Slit-lamp examination can be used to detect the ophthalmic abnormalities of Marfan syndrome. However, the most important maneuver is to assess the proximal aorta and heart. Echocardiography and transesophageal echocardiography can be diagnostic. In patients without serious cardiovascular complications, serial echocardiograms are performed

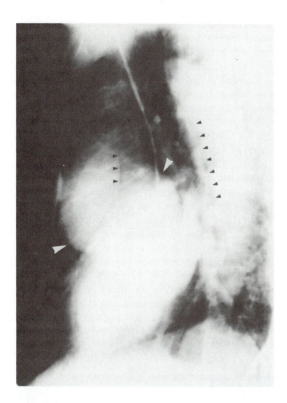

Figure 15–6. Arch aortogram in a 32-year-old male with Marfan syndrome demonstrates an ascending aortic aneurysm complicated by dissection. Small arrowheads outline the intimal flap; large arrowheads define the dilated aortic root.

to monitor this system so that intervention can be carried out before a catastrophe strikes. The evaluation and management of acute aortic dissections are described in Chapter 11.

Diagnosis

The diagnosis of Marfan syndrome is still a clinical one based upon the presence of major and minor criteria. The major criteria are aortic dissection, aortic root dilation, ectopia lentis, and dural ectasia. The minor criteria are listed in Table 15–4. If a first degree relative of the subject has Marfan syndrome then 2 systems must be involved and there must be at least one major characteristic present. If there is not a first degree relative affected the subject must have: skeletal involvement, at least two other systems involved and at least one other major manifestation.

Treatment

After a patient is diagnosed with Marfan syndrome, physical activity should be limited with avoidance of contact sports and heavily exertional activities. Institution of β-blockade will slow the progression of aortic root dilation and delay or hopefully avert aortic replacement. However, when the proximal aorta expands to 5–6 cm or greater, it should be replaced because the risk of dissection increases at this juncture. Note that those with a family history of dissection are at even greater risk for this complication than other Marfan syndrome patients.

Prognosis

The prognosis for patients with Marfan syndrome is not positive. Patients afflicted have a shortened life span with an average age of death around 40 years. Over 90% patients die from cardiovascular complications, the most common of which is aortic dissection.

El Habbal MH: Cardiovascular manifestations of Marfan's syndrome in the young. Am Heart J 1992;123:752.

Gerry JL, Morris L, Pyeritz RE: Clinical management of the cardiovascular complications of the Marfan syndrome. J La State Med Soc 1991;143:43.

Hirata K et al: The Marfan syndrome: Cardiovascular physical findings and diagnostic correlates. Am Heart J 1992; 123:743.

Marfan AB: Un cas de déformation congénitale des quatre membres, plus prononcée aux extrémités caractérisée par l'allongengement des os avec un certain degré d'amincissement. Bull Mem Soc Méd Hôp (Paris) 1896;13:220.

Pyeritz RE: Marfan syndrome: Current and future clinical and genetic management of cardiovascular manifestations. Semin Thor Cardiovasc Surg 1993;5:11.

Reed CM, Fox ME, Alpert BS: Aortic biomechanical properties in pediatric patients with the Marfan syndrome, and the effects of atenolol. Am J Cardiol 1993;71:606.

Tahernia AC: Cardiovascular anomalies in Marfan's syndrome: The role of echocardiography and ß-blockers. South Med J 1993;86:305.

Tsipouras P et al: Genetic linkage of the Marfan syndrome, ectopia lentis, and congenital contractural arachnodactyly to the fibrillin genes on chromosome 15 and 5. N Engl J Med 1992;326:905.

EHLERS-DANLOS SYNDROME

Essentials of Diagnosis

- Cutaneous laxity and joint hypermobility.
- Collagen abnormality.
- Poor wound healing.
- Cardiovascular, gastrointestinal, orthopedic, and ocular defects.

General Considerations

Ehlers-Danlos syndrome (EDS) is a group of disorders of collagen synthesis or structure with predominant clinical characteristics of skin and joint laxity and tissue frailty. Eleven types have been described, but 2 are known not to be secondary to collagen abnormalities and have been reclassified under other illnesses so that only 9 types are now recognized. About 50% of patients with EDS cannot be classified into only one of these categories. The genetic mutation responsible for many of these has not been elucidated.

Although the vascular surgeon may encounter any of these, type IV EDS is the most threatening form of this group of mutations and the most likely to need vascular intervention. It is referred to as the **arterial-ecchymotic type** or the **Sack-Barabas type**. Type IV EDS affects mainly the blood vessels and the bowel. Patients present acutely and without warning with either a life-threatening hemorrhage from vascular disruption or peritonitis from a ruptured viscus. Although not due to a single defect, type IV EDS is actually a cohort of genetic alterations that lead to a deficiency or an abnormal structure of type III collagen. Of the 19 different collagens discovered thus far, type III collagen provides structural support for the blood vessels and the intestinal tract. About 20 different mutations have been characterized, which explains why inheritance of type IV EDS can be autosomal recessive or dominant.

Clinical Findings

A. Signs and Symptoms: Patients with type IV EDS (4% of EDS cases) have thin and fragile skin, premature dermal aging, bruising, and scarring. The cutaneous laxity and joint hypermobility are much more subtle in these patients compared with those found in other EDS patients. The facial appearance of patients with type IV EDS is characteristic of EDS patients demonstrating large eyes, a thin nose, and lobeless ears. **Meischer's elastoma**, a circinate rash with histologic extrusion of elastic fibers, may affect the skin of these patients. Also present may be acro-osteolysis of the terminal phalanges, arthropathy mainly affecting the small joints of the foot and hand (pes planus, genu recurvatum, temporomandibular joint), keloids, fibrotic contractures, recurrent pneumothoraces, varicose veins, mitral valve prolapse, and myopia.

The important complications of type IV EDS are rupture of blood vessels and rupture of bowel. Almost every major blood vessel has ruptured or developed aneurysms in type IV EDS. These present in a catastrophic manner without warning, and the vascular disruptions are highly frustrating to manage.

B. Imaging Studies: Arteriography may be a diagnostic essential but there is a much higher incidence of morbidity and mortality in type IV EDS patients because of the risk of local or remote arterial perforation.

Diagnosis

The diagnosis of EDS is made clinically, but misdiagnosis and missed diagnosis rates are as high as 25%. Patients with type IV EDS have more subtle dermal and articular changes, and the diagnosis is frequently overlooked. Therefore, they are usually initially seen with a sudden catastrophe and a diagnostic workup is not possible.

Treatment

Because of the tenuous and frail nature of the blood vessels in EDS patients, perforated blood vessels should be treated by ligation. If repair is necessary then it should be tension free. Extreme care must be used in handling the tissues, and reinforcement of suture lines is a must. Autogenous reconstruction is to be avoided (Fig 15–7). Ruptured extremity vessels should be managed with compression and transfusion initially. Desmopressin acetate may be useful since EDS patients' platelets aggregate poorly in the absence of normal collagen. Asymptomatic EDS patients must avoid trauma and injury.

Prognosis

The limited number of type IV EDS patients causes little to be known about the life span, although some patients have lived for a long time. Most patients have recurrent episodes of bleeding with a mortality rate of 64%.

The ruptured vessels respond poorly to the standard vascular techniques, and operative mortality from acute hemorrhage is 19%. Another 44% with bleeding expire before intervention can take place.

Cikrit DF, Miles JH, Silver D: Spontaneous arterial perforation: The Ehlers-Danlos specter. J Vasc Surg 1987;5:248.

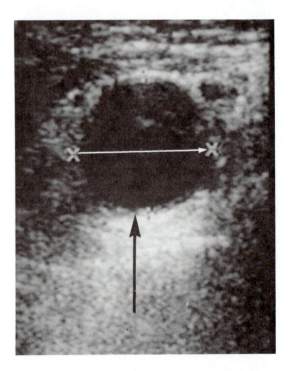

Figure 15–7. Cross-sectional view on duplex scan of a reverse saphenous vein graft (*black arrow*) in the femoral position in a young female with Ehlers-Danlos syndrome (EDS). This graft originally measured 5 mm in diameter and was placed because of a traumatic injury prior to diagnosis of EDS. Two years later, the graft has become aneurysmal (white arrow measures a diameter distance of 2 cm). This is an example of why autogenous grafts are to be avoided in EDS patients.

Danlos M: Un cas de cutis laxa avec tumeurs par contusion chronique des condes et des mace des genoux (xanthome juvenile pseudodiabétique de M.M. Mace de Lepinay). Bull Soc Fr Dermatol Syph 1908;19:70.

Ehlers E: Cutis laxa, neigung zu Hemorrhagien in der haut, lockerung mehrerer Artikulationen. Dermatol Z 1901;8: 173.

Hunter GC et al: Vascular manifestations in patients with Ehlers-Danlos syndrome. Arch Surg 1982;117:495.

Kivirikko KI: Collagens and their abnormalities in a wide spectrum of diseases. Ann Med 1993;25:113.

Thomas IT, Frias JL: The cardiovascular manifestations of genetic disorders of collagen metabolism. Ann Clin Lab Sci 1987;17:377.

PSEUDOXANTHOMA ELASTICUM

Essentials of Diagnosis

- Angioid retinal streaks, dermal pseudoxanthomas of neck or axillae.
- Premature cardiovascular disease with medial calcification.

General Considerations

Pseudoxanthoma elasticum (PXE) is an elastic tissue disease and is typified by angioid retinal streaks (secondary to Bruch's membrane disruption) and small localized yellowish skin plaques (pseudoxanthomas) in flexural areas of high movement such as the neck and axillae and also the antecubital fossae, nasolabial folds, and even some mucosal surfaces. An incidence of only 1 in 100,000 makes PXE a rare disorder.

PXE patients have a propensity to develop premature cardiovascular disease. The vascular elastin degenerates and becomes calcified, affecting mainly the medium-sized vessels and giving them an appearance similar to that of Mönckeberg's medial calcification. The current and much criticized classification includes Type 1 and Type 2 PXE. Each type consists of an autosomal recessive subtype and an autosomal dominant subtype. The type I autosomal dominant form has the most severe vascular disease.

Clinical Findings

Other symptoms of PXE affecting the eye include a *peau d'orange* mottling of the fundus, retinal hemorrhage, choroiditis, and visual deficiencies. In addition to the ocular findings, PXE patients usually have the characteristic skin lesions, although an occult form has been identified in which pseudoxanthomas are absent. Gastrointestinal bleeding affects up to 12% of patients with PXE. The cardiovascular symptoms include intermittent claudication, hypertension, angina, and mitral valve prolapse. Peripheral pulses may be diminished, but advanced ischemia is unusual. Myocardial infarction has been reported.

Diagnosis

Skin biopsy is diagnostic of PXE and can be performed on normal skin or scar in the occult form. The elastic fibers are calcified, and in advanced lesions the fibers look twisted, bent, and broken.

Treatment

No specific treatment is available for patients with PXE. It is suggested that the dietary calcium intake be kept under 800 mg/day because, high intake may aggravate the disease. Affected patients should avoid heavy exertion and contact sports. Because advanced peripheral ischemia is unusual, the need for vascular surgery is unlikely and the role is one of diagnosis, institution of nonoperative therapy, and monitoring. If revascularization is needed, conventional methods have been successful in PXE patients. Patients should be genetically counseled and followed up by an ophthalmologist.

Prognosis

Life expectancy of PXE patients is reduced with early deaths beginning in the fifth decade.

Fann JL, Dalman RL, Harris EJ: Genetic and metabolic causes of arterial disease. Ann Vasc Surg 1993;7:594.

Hacker SM et al: Juvenile pseudoxanthoma elasticum: Recognition and management. Pediatr Dermatol 1993; 10:19.

Jacyk WK, Lodder JV, Dreyer L: Pseudoxanthoma elasticum in South African black patients. S Afr Med J 1988;74:184.

Lebwohl M, Halperin J, Phelps RG: Brief report: Occult pseudoxanthoma elasticum in patients with premature cardiovascular disease. N Engl J Med 1993;329:1237.

Rosenzweig BP, Guarneri E, Kronzon I: Echocardiographic manifestations in a patient with pseudoxanthoma elasticum. Ann Intern Med 1993;119:487.

CONGENITAL AND DEVELOPMENTAL VASCULAR DISEASE

ABDOMINAL COARCTATION

Essentials of Diagnosis

- Hypertension associated with diminished or absent lower extremity pulses in pediatric patients or young adults.
- Brachial blood pressures equal and higher than thigh blood pressures.
- Narrowed abdominal aorta, usually in the proximal visceral portion and often with renal artery orifice stenosis.

General Considerations

Abdominal coarctation (stricture) usually affects the aorta in the visceral area; several subtypes have been noted, depending on the location of involvement (suprarenal, interrenal, infrarenal, and diffuse). This has led to several classification attempts but none is entirely satisfactory. Stenosis of the visceral branches is present in 26%, multiple renal arteries are found in 70%, and renal artery stenosis is identified in 84%.

Coarctation of the abdominal aorta is an uncommon finding. It represents less than 2% of all coarctations, and only 150 cases have been reported. In the absence of inflammatory changes, this is most likely due to congenital hypoplasia or a developmental anomaly resulting from improper fusion and maturation of the paired embryonic dorsal aortas. Although the terminology is inexact, **middle aorta syndrome** has been the term used to describe any stenosis of the visceral aorta; the term *abdominal coarctation* has been reserved to describe congenital stenosis.

Neurofibromatosis has often been found in patients with abdominal coarctation, who usually have associated renal ostial narrowing as well. In fact, 10% of those with neurofibromatosis have vasculopathy that can affect the visceral, coronary, and cerebrovascular circulation. Stenoses have also been seen in the thoracic aorta and the subclavian and innominate arteries. The large vessel lesions are secondary to adventitial neurofibromas, and small vessel obstructions are from spindle cell proliferation in the arterial wall.

Clinical Findings

A. Signs and Symptoms: Patients with abdominal coarctation usually present in their teens or in early adulthood (average 20 years of age) but may be seen at any age. The main symptom is hypertension and the symptoms that longstanding uncontrolled hypertension produces. Intermittent claudication is common and affected patients have diminished leg pulses; advanced limb ischemia and renal failure are uncommon. Mesenteric insufficiency can develop with its classic symptoms.

B. Imaging Studies: Angiography with biplanar views is essential to document the location and extent of the coarctation as well as to evaluate the aortic branches for involvement (Fig 15–8).

C. Laboratory Findings: A normal sed rate essentially rules out active inflammation, for which treatment would be necessary if the stenosis were from an aortitis.

Treatment

Hypertension should be controlled medically when possible prior to surgery. For suprarenal and infrarenal coarctations aorta-to-aorta bypass is recommended. When the stenosis is diffuse or interrenal, aorta-to-aorta bypass and grafting to ischemic visceral and renal arteries are needed. Extra-anatomic bypass to the renal arteries has been recommended as sufficient to treat the hypertension, since the claudication is not a severe problem. Balloon angioplasty and endarterectomy are not appropriate for this type of lesion.

Prognosis

Most hypertensive patients (70–80%) are improved or cured after surgery. The operative mortality rate is 4–8%, and the impact of revascularization on longevity is unknown but is expected to be considerably improved.

The hypertension that patients with abdominal coarctation frequently have limits their life expectancy to 30 or 40 years. Although 26 of the 150 patients reported in the literature have been over 40, only 1 has been over 60 years.

Cohen JR, Birnbaum E: Coarctation of the abdominal aorta. J Vasc Surg 1988;8:160.

Graham LM et al: Abdominal aortic coarctation and segmental hypoplasia. Surgery 1979;86:519.

Hallett JW Jr et al: Coarctation of the abdominal aorta: Current opinions in surgical management. Ann Surg 1980; 191:430.

Lie JT: Vasculitis simulators and vasculitis look-alikes. Curr Opin Rheumatol 1992;4:47.

Messina LM et al: Middle aorta syndrome: Effectiveness and durability of complex arterial revascularization techniques. Ann Surg 1986;204:331.

Stanley JC et al: Developmental occlusive disease of the abdominal aorta and the splanchnic and renal arteries. Am J Surg 1981;142:190.

Zochodne D: Von Recklinghausen's vasculopathy. Am J Med Sci 1984;287:64.

PERSISTENT SCIATIC ARTERY

Essentials of Diagnosis

- Pulsating gluteal mass, claudication, limb pain, gangrene, or buttock pain.
- Pulses felt at the sciatic foramen.
- A large posteriorly coursing artery arising from the hypogastric artery and extending from the pelvis to the thigh or knee.

General Considerations

A **persistent sciatic artery** (PSA) is an interesting congenital anomaly in which the sciatic artery fails to obliterate in fetal development. The initial vascular supply to the lower limb in the early embryo is the sciatic artery. This vessel is a continuation of the internal iliac artery and courses posteriorly through the pelvis and down the posterior thigh before joining the popliteal artery. In early fetal development, the sciatic artery obliterates as the iliofemoral vessels develop and become the principal blood supply to the leg. Failure to obliterate leads to 1 of 4 situations. The PSA can be completely developed and proceed all the way to the popliteal artery with the iliofemoral system being either normal or hypoplastic. In the 2 other situations, the PSA terminates before reaching the popliteal fossa, and the iliofemoral system again is either normal or hypoplastic. The condition is bilateral, but not necessarily symmetric, in 20%. PSA can be encountered at any age and occurs equally in men and women.

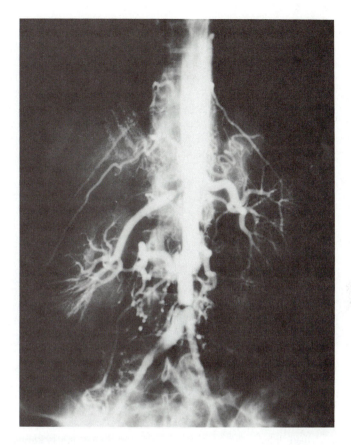

Figure 15–8. Angiography shows occlusion of the celiac, superior, and inferior mesenteric arteries as well as aortic bifurcation stenosis in 33-year-old woman who had abdominal angina when walking. The differential diagnosis included Takayasu's arteritis, but at surgery hypoplasia was found.

Clinical Findings

A. Signs and Symptoms: Ninety percent of patients with PSA have symptoms such as a pulsating gluteal mass, limb pain, gangrene, or buttock pain. These patients have pulses over the PSA at the sciatic foramen. If an aneurysm is present, there is a pulsatile mass. Aneurysm formation occurs in about 50% of those affected and may lead to limb loss from thrombosis or distal embolization in about 16%. The incidence of aneurysm formation is higher in those with incomplete development of the superficial femoral artery.

If the iliofemoral system is inadequate, patients can have absent femoral pulses and palpable pedal pulses. Claudication can be present when both the PSA and the iliofemoral system are incompletely developed.

B. Imaging Studies: Angiography demonstrates a large posteriorly coursing artery arising from the hypogastric artery and extending from the pelvis to the thigh or knee (Fig 15–9).

Treatment

Aneurysms in PSA should be repaired when encountered because of the high risk of limb loss, and asymptomatic PSA patients should be followed up closely for aneurysmal development. Vascular bypasses are recommended according to standard technique with reported good results.

Shutze WP et al: Persistent sciatic artery: Collective review and management. Ann Vasc Surg 1993;7:303.

ADVENTITIAL CYSTIC DISEASE

Essentials of Diagnosis

- Usually abrupt onset of intermittent claudication in middle-aged, nonsmoking males.
- Normal pedal pulses that disappear when knee flexed with popliteal adventitial cysts.
- Hourglass or scimitar deformity of involved vessel.

General Considerations

Adventitial cystic disease is an uncommon and unique vasculopathic entity characterized by a highly viscous and mucinous cyst located in the adventitia of the artery and whose contents resemble that of a gan-

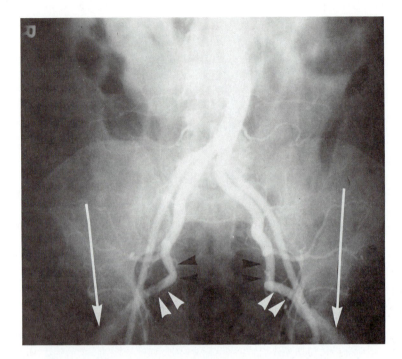

Figure 15–9. Bilateral persistent sciatic arteries are seen as continuations of the hypogastric arteries (*arrowheads*). Bilateral aneurysms (*arrows*) are also present at the level of the greater trochanter.

glion. Although first described in the external iliac artery, the disease is described more often in the popliteal artery. Other vessels that can be involved are the femoral artery, the external iliac vein, and the femoral vein. As the cyst enlarges, it leads to vascular compression with stenosis or occlusion. The origins of adventitial cysts are unknown, but connections to the most adjacent synovial space have been identified, suggesting that the cyst is a ganglion variant.

Clinical Findings

A. Signs and Symptoms: Patients with adventitial cystic disease are generally young or middle-aged and without risk factors for atherosclerosis. The earliest symptom is the abrupt onset of intermittent claudication, which can be very limiting. The pedal pulses are normal, but with knee flexion a popliteal adventitial cyst can compress the artery and cause loss of these pulses. A bruit may be heard over the popliteal space, but the cyst itself is nonpalpable. In one-third of cases, the artery is occluded and the clinical findings are consistent with a popliteal artery occlusion.

B. Imaging Studies: In the absence of arterial occlusion, the resting ankle pressures are normal but drop with exercise. A duplex scan shows the arterial abnormality and flow disturbance. Computed tomography (CT) or magnetic resonance imaging (MRI) can also document the abnormal structure as well as exclude popliteal entrapment. Angiography is the best evaluation (Fig 15–10). If the artery is patent, it has

either an "hourglass" or eccentric deformity. The latter is curvilinear and is known as the **scimitar sign** (Fig 15–10).

Treatment

Adventitial cystic disease is a focal process and does not make an impact on other arteries or the general health of the patient. All patients discovered to date have undergone surgery, but it is unlikely that the process would abate or resolve spontaneously. Most non-surgically-treated patients would be expected to develop arterial occlusions in time.

If an artery is occluded, resection and interposition grafting are performed. For stenotic arteries, cyst unroofing and evacuation are recommended over enucleation, although both methods are acceptable (see Fig 15–10*B* and *C*). Any synovial connection must be obliterated. Cyst aspiration has been performed, but the consistency of the cyst contents makes this difficult to accomplish and recurrence is likely because the cyst is still intact. With appropriate treatment, the results have been excellent. Patency rates are high and no amputations have been reported.

Atkins HJB, Key JA: A case of myxomatous tumor arising in the adventitia of the left external iliac artery. Br J Surg 1947;34:426.

Jasinski RW et al: Adventitial cystic disease of the popliteal artery. Radiology 1987;163:153.

Macfarlane R et al: Cystic adventitial arterial disease. Br J Surg 1987;74:89.

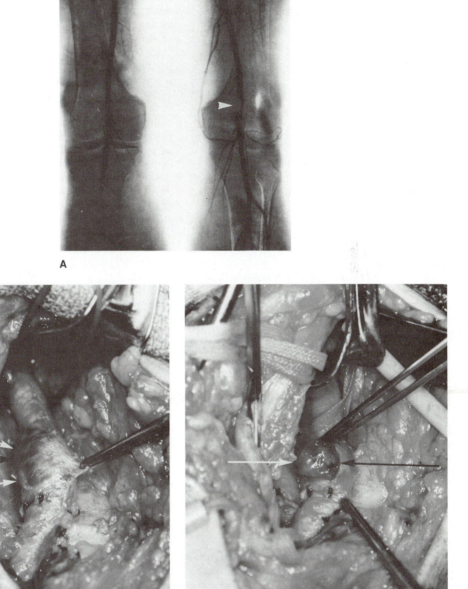

Figure 15–10. **A:** The left popliteal artery shows the characteristic scimitar sign (*arrowhead*) of popliteal adventitial cystic disease. **B:** At exploration via a posterior approach, the cyst is easily seen. **C:** These adventitial cysts (*arrow*) contain gelatinous material that can be enucleated from within the cyst itself.

Melliere D et al: Adventitial cystic disease of the popliteal artery: Treatment by cyst removal. J Vasc Surg 1988;8:638.

Sieunarine K et al: Adventitial cystic disease of the popliteal artery: Early recurrence after CT guided percutaneous aspiration. J Cardiovasc Surg 1991;32:702.

POPLITEAL ARTERY ENTRAPMENT

Essentials of Diagnosis

- Claudication in child or young adult without atherosclerosis.
- Decreased pulses with active plantar flexion or passive dorsiflexion.
- Abnormal anatomy in popliteal space with compression of popliteal artery.

General Considerations

In **popliteal artery entrapment**, the popliteal artery is extrinsically compressed or occluded. This rare syndrome (incidence > 0.2%), first anatomically described by a medical student, was found on an amputated and gangrenous limb. Entrapment usually arises when the popliteal artery courses medially around the medial head of the gastrocnemius rather than between the 2 heads of this muscle. The artery then becomes compressed by the muscle during flexion leading to decreased flow during this maneuver. In chronic entrapment, the artery can become aneurysmal or thrombosed. Entrapment can also occur with a normally coursing artery but with a more laterally positioned insertion of the medial gastrocnemius head onto the femur, or it can occur when an accessory muscle slip is present. Anomalous fibrous bands arising from the popliteus and semitendinosus muscles have also been implicated. Thirty percent of cases of popliteal artery entrapment are bilateral, and in 10% the popliteal vein is involved.

Clinical Findings

A. Signs and Symptoms: The most common presenting complaint in patients with popliteal artery entrapment is that of slowly progressive claudication, which paradoxically has occasionally been more severe with walking than with running. Positional ischemic symptoms have been noted as well.

The perigeniculate area is hyperthermic from increased collateral flow, and pedal pulses are normal if the artery is still patent. In the latter case, active plantar flexion or vigorous passive dorsiflexion diminish or obliterate the distal pulses.

B. Age and Gender: Popliteal artery entrapment is 10 times more common in men than in women and is generally diagnosed in persons between the ages of 17 and 48 years.

C. Imaging Studies: Continuous Doppler wave or duplex examination of the popliteal artery and foot pulses during the previously mentioned maneuvers may be helpful but can also be abnormal without entrapment. A CT scan or MRI of the knee nicely demonstrates the abnormal anatomy and aids the operative planning. Angiography verifies the absence of atherosclerosis and delineates the runoff vessels if occlusion is present (about 50%). Prior to occlusion, a stress arteriogram with the above pedal positioning shows the induced extrinsic compression of an otherwise unobstructed vessel.

Treatment

Surgical correction for popliteal artery entrapment is recommended for those with symptoms. Prior to occlusion of the popliteal artery, division of the medial gastrocnemius head or other offending structure is curative. If the artery is thrombosed or aneurysmal, resection and grafting are performed; results with have been good in about 90% of cases. However, thromboendarterectomy results have been suboptimal. Popliteal entrapment is one condition in which the posterior popliteal approach is more helpful than the usual medial approach. Asymptomatic entrapped arteries, such as those discovered opposite a symptomatic lesion, can probably be followed up as long as no secondary arterial damage is seen and no symptoms develop.

diMarzo L et al: Surgical treatment of popliteal artery entrapment syndrome: A ten year experience. Eur J Vasc Surg 1991;5:59.

Murray A, Halliday M, Croft RJ: Popliteal artery entrapment syndrome. Br J Surg 1991;78:1414.

Persky JM, Kempczinski RF, Fowl RJ: Entrapment of the popliteal artery. Surg Gynecol Obstet 1991;173:84.

Stuart TPA: A note on the variation in the course of the popliteal artery. J Anat Physiol 1879;13:162.

Aortoiliac Occlusive Disease

16

David C. Brewster, MD

Arteriosclerotic occlusive disease involving the infrarenal abdominal aorta and iliac arteries is a common cause of symptomatic arterial insufficiency of the lower extremities. Because arteriosclerosis is usually a generalized process, obliterative disease in the aortoiliac segment frequently coexists with disease in the infrainguinal vessels. Nonetheless, correction of hemodynamic problems in the inflow system frequently provides good clinical relief of leg ischemic symptoms. In addition, careful evaluation of the adequacy of arterial inflow is important even in patients whose primary difficulty lies in the femoropopliteal outflow segment. Despite its generalized nature, chronic arteriosclerotic disease is usually segmental in distribution, thereby making the disease process amenable to effective surgical treatment.

During the 4 decades since the introduction of surgical methods of arterial reconstruction for aortoiliac disease, great progress has been achieved. Accurate physiologic assessment of the severity of the disease process is currently possible, whereas advances in arteriography and other imaging techniques allow precise demonstration of the extent and distribution of occlusive lesions, thereby enabling appropriate intervention to be planned. Development of methods to better evaluate patient risk in terms of coronary artery disease and other comorbid medical conditions commonly associated with arteriosclerotic vascular disease have led to improved patient selection and safety of revascularization procedures. Improvements in prosthetic materials, simplification of surgical techniques, and refinements in perioperative care all have contributed to a steady reduction of operative morbidity and mortality and excellent long-term results. A variety of methods of revascularization are available for use, depending on the extent of disease, the patient's risk factors, and other clinical variables. With proper selection of the most appropriate procedure for a specific individual patient, safe and effective treatment of aortoiliac disease is possible in almost all patients.

Essentials of Diagnosis

- Claudication.
- Sexual impotence.
- Ischemic rest pain.
- Ischemic tissue necrosis.

General Considerations

A. Anatomic Relationships: The abdominal aorta begins at the aortic hiatus of the diaphragm in front of the lower border of the last thoracic vertebra and descends in front of the vertebral column slightly to the left of midline. As it courses distally, it diminishes in size as a consequence of the many large visceral and parietal branches that arise from this conduit vessel. The most important of these branches are the celiac trunk, the superior mesenteric artery, the right and left renal arteries, the inferior mesenteric artery, and about 4 sets of paired lumbar arteries. The abdominal aorta generally terminates at the level of the 4th lumbar vertebra by bifurcating into the common iliac arteries. Topographically, this usually corresponds to the approximate level of the umbilicus on the abdominal wall.

Because of its deep posterior retroperitoneal location, surgical exposure of the abdominal aorta is often difficult. This is particularly true of its upper aspect, the suprarenal aortic segment from the diaphragm to the renal artery level. Here, the aorta is enveloped by the muscular crura of the diaphragm as they insert onto the lumbar vertebrae and is covered anteriorly by the lesser omentum, stomach, pancreas, and left renal vein, which generally crosses the aorta anteriorly. Mobilization of the suprarenal aorta is further complicated by the origin of the celiac axis and superior mesenteric artery from the anterior wall of the aorta. Exposure of the infrarenal aorta requires opening of the overlying retroperitoneal tissue and displacement of the inferior aspect of the duodenum and overlying small bowel mesentery. The inferior vena cava is often closely approximated to the right side of the infrarenal aorta.

It is distinctly unusual for clinically significant occlusive disease to involve the suprarenal aorta. Similarly, the aorta immediately distal to the renal arteries is usually relatively spared from advanced occlusive disease, an important feature that is exploited in aortic reconstructive surgery.

The common iliac arteries diverge from the aortic bifurcation and pass downward and laterally. They are usually about 5 cm long before dividing into the internal (hypogastric) and external iliac arteries. The former supplies the viscera and parietes of the pelvis, and the latter the lower extremity. The femoral artery is the direct continuation of the external iliac artery beginning at the level of the inguinal ligament. About 4–5 cm below the inguinal ligament, the common femoral artery divides into its superficial and deep (profunda) branches. Because of the high incidence of associated obliterative disease of the superficial femoral artery (50–65%) in patients with aortoiliac occlusive disease, the deep femoral artery is often very important in arterial reconstructive procedures for proximal (inflow) disease.

B. Collateral Pathways: Potential pathways of collateral circulation to compensate for aortoiliac disease include both visceral and parietal routes, such as internal mammary to inferior epigastric, intercostal and lumbar arteries to circumflex iliac and hypogastric networks, hypogastric and gluteal branches to common femoral and profunda femoral arteries, and superior mesenteric to inferior mesenteric and superior hemorrhoidal pathways via the marginal artery of Drummond (meandering mesenteric artery) and arch of Riolan.

Because of the abundant potential for collateral circulation, distal blood flow to the lower extremities is rarely critically reduced as long as the occlusive process is restricted to the intra-abdominal aortoiliac segment. Claudication or sexual impotence is commonly present; the blood flow at rest remains adequate; and viability of the extremity is rarely threatened. More advanced ischemic symptoms nearly always indicate additional distal disease.

C. Pathophysiology: Arteriosclerosis may produce partial or complete occlusion of the aorta and iliac arteries. As progressive narrowing of these vessels reduces blood flow to the pelvic viscera and lower extremities, characteristic symptom complexes develop (described in the following text). The disease process is commonly centered around the aortic bifurcation; hence, disease is usually maximal in the lower infrarenal aorta, aortic bifurcation, and common iliac arteries (Fig 16–1). As is typical of arteriosclerotic disease, the occlusive process is often most pronounced at arterial bifurcations. Plaque is also generally more extensive on the posterior arterial wall, often causing the distal lumbar arteries and median sacral vessel to be occluded at an earlier stage of disease.

Symptoms result when progressive narrowing of the vessel lumen and consequent reduction of distal tissue perfusion outpace the ability of collateral circulation to adequately compensate. Claudication discomfort with exercise is almost always the earliest manifestation of aortoiliac occlusive disease, a logical consequence of the fact that collateral blood flow may be sufficient for tissue nutrition at rest but insufficient to accommodate the 5- to 10-fold increase in blood flow associated with maximal exercise in the normal leg. More advanced ischemic systems, such as ischemic pain at rest of ischemic tissue necrosis (ulceration or digital gangrene), occur when resting blood flow is insufficient to satisfy basic metabolic requirements for nonexercising tissue (Fig 16–2).

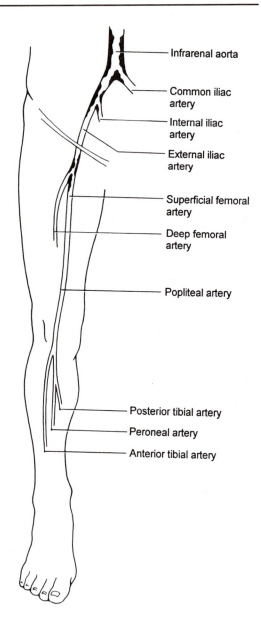

Figure 16–1. Common sites of arteriosclerotic lesions in aortoiliofemoral occlusive disease. Although often a generalized process, partially segmental distribution of major disease, most prominent at arterial bifurcations, usually allows surgical revascularization.

With progressive stenosis of a diseased vessel, blood flow may be reduced to a point at which total thrombosis of the diseased segment occurs, often accounting for a sudden worsening in symptomatology in a patient with previously mild ischemic manifestations. Similarly, degeneration or ulceration of plaques may lead to distal embolization of thrombin/platelet aggregations that have accumulated on its irregular surface or to dislodgment of actual atherosclerotic de-

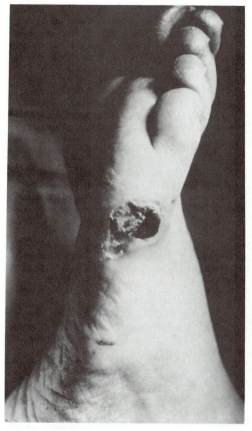 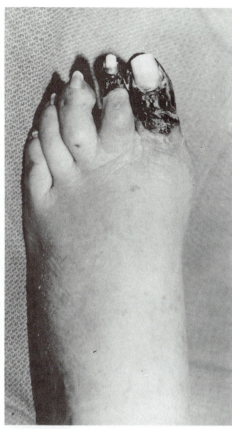

A   **B**

Figure 16–2. Examples of ischemic tissue necrosis. **A:** Ischemic ulcerations; **B:** Digital gangrene.

bris from the plaque itself, a process referred to as **atheromatous embolization** (Fig 16–3).

Clinical Presentation

A. Patterns of Disease: The symptoms, natural history, and choice of optimal method of surgical reconstruction are strongly influenced by the extent and distribution of occlusive disease (Fig 16–4). Disease truly confined to the distal aorta and proximal iliac vessels (type I) is relatively uncommon, noted in about 10% of surgical candidates. It should be recognized that such data are derived from arteriographic findings in patients with sufficiently severe symptoms to warrant surgical intervention. Localized disease is much more likely to be present earlier in the disease process when symptoms are few, if any, and when invasive investigation is often not undertaken.

B. Localized Disease: In localized aortoiliac disease, patients typically present with claudication alone, often involving primarily the proximal musculature of the thigh, hip, or buttock area. More advanced ischemic complaints are absent unless distal atherosclerotic disease is also present or atheroembolic com-

plications have occurred. In males, impotence is often an associated complaint, present in varying degrees of severity in at least 30–50% of males with aortoiliac disease.

Patients with a type I disease pattern are characteristically younger, with a relatively low incidence of hypertension or diabetes, and frequently noted to have abnormal blood lipids. In contrast to the usual male predominance in chronic peripheral vascular disease, almost 50% of patients with localized aortoiliac disease are women, often with small aortic, iliac, and femoral vessels. Such a characteristic clinical picture is often termed the **hypoplastic aorta syndrome.**

C. Disease Progression: Progression of localized disease initially located in the region of the aortic bifurcation commonly advances to cause occlusion of 1 iliac artery or extends to involve the external iliac or femoral vessels, usually by a posterior tongue of atheroma. Although circulation to both lower extremities may be maintained by hypogastric collateral networks of the stenotic limb, this pattern of disease is relatively unstable. Occlusion of the remaining common iliac artery may result in thrombus propagating to the

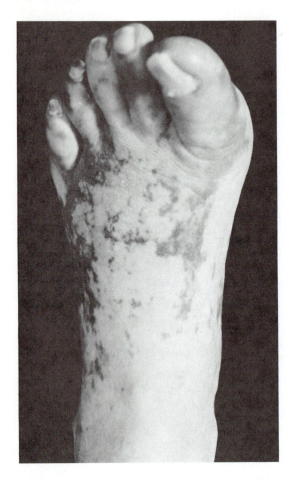

Figure 16–3. Typical appearance of the foot in a patient with distal atheroembolism.

occlusive disease still confined largely to the abdominal vessels but also involving the external iliac and perhaps common femoral arteries. Most frequently, occlusive disease involving both inflow and infrainguinal outflow arterial segments (type III) is noted. Such diffuse disease has been found to affect up to two-thirds of patients in our experience and accounts for at least 50% in other major surgical series. Patients with such multilevel disease (also frequently referred to as "combined segment" or "tandem" disease) are typically older, male (about 6:1 ratio), and much more likely to have diabetes, hypertension, and associated atherosclerotic disease involving the coronary, cerebral, or visceral arteries. Most patients with multilevel disease manifest symptoms of more advanced ischemia, such as ischemic pain at rest or varying degrees of actual tissue necrosis, and operation is more often undertaken for limb salvage rather than simply for relief of claudication.

As would be expected, the higher incidence of associated systemic arteriosclerotic disease and other comorbid medical problems in patients with multilevel disease increases the morbidity and morality risk of intervention in such patients. Also, these features lead to a decrease in life expectancy of 10 or more years in contrast to patients with localized aortoiliac disease, who have a long-term survival that is nearly equivalent to age and sex-matched controls.

Clinical Findings

A. Signs and Symptoms: In most instances, an accurate history and carefully performed physical examination can unequivocally establish the diagnosis of aortoiliac disease. A reliable description of claudication in one or both legs, possible decreased sexual potency in the male, and diminished or absent femoral pulses define the characteristic triad often referred to as the **Leriche syndrome**.

Claudication symptoms are exercise-related crampy pain or fatigue in major muscle groups of the lower extremity. Typically, such symptoms are absent when the patient first begins walking, then develop after a certain distance and become progressively more severe until the patient must stop walking. Characteristically, the discomfort disappears within several minutes of walking cessation and simply standing still. Symptoms occur more quickly or are more severe when the patient walks up an incline or walks at a faster pace. The distance walked before onset of discomfort is usually constant from day to day, although disease progression over longer time periods may reduce tolerated distances.

Although proximal claudication symptoms in the distribution of thigh, hip, and buttock musculature are usually a reliable indicator of clinically important inflow disease, a significant number of patients with aortoiliac disease will nonetheless complain only of calf claudication, particularly those with multilevel disease. Therefore, the location of claudication symptoms

groin, causing severe ischemia of both lower extremities and precipitating the need for emergency intervention, which is otherwise rarely necessary in chronic aortoiliac disease.

Bilateral occlusion of the common iliac arteries leads to propagation of thrombus and total occlusion of the infrarenal aorta. Complete aortic occlusion extends to the level of the inferior mesenteric artery (Fig 16–5A); or, if this vessel has undergone prior obliteration, superimposed thrombus extends proximally to a juxtarenal level (see Fig 16–5B), with the renal vessels themselves acting as an outflow tract for the proximal aorta. Rarely, further proximal extension of clot may compromise the renal arteries or superior mesenteric artery, but this is quite unusual unless these vessels themselves are stenotic secondary to associated occlusive disease. About 5–10% of patients undergoing aortoiliac surgery for occlusive disease have been found to have a totally occluded aorta.

D. Multilevel Disease: Most patients who are candidates for aortoiliac operations have diffuse disease. About 20–25% will have a type II pattern, with

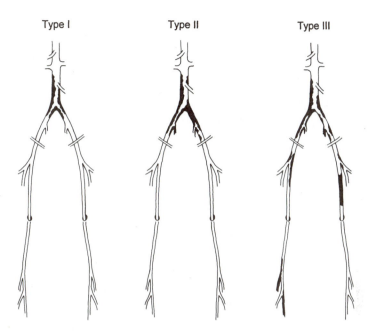

Figure 16–4. Patterns of aortoiliac disease. In Type I, localized disease is confined to the distal aorta and common iliac arteries. More widespread intra-abdominal disease is present in Type II, whereas a Type III pattern signifies multilevel disease with associated infra-inguinal occlusive lesions.

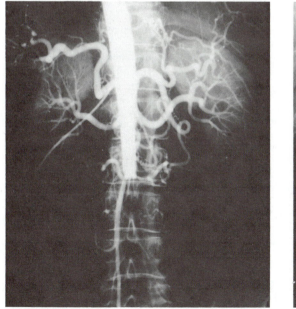

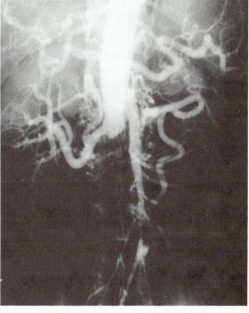

A   B

Figure 16–5. Arteriographic examples of total aortic occlusion. **A:** Occlusion to midinfrarenal aorta, with patency of upper infrarenal aortic segment maintained by inferior mesenteric and lumbar artery runoff. **B:** Complete juxtarenal aortic occlusion with retrograde thrombosis to the level of renal artery runoff.

may not be a reliable indication that clinically significant aortoiliac disease is present.

Diminished or absent femoral pulses are the characteristic finding on physical examination of patients with aortoiliac disease. However, it is well recognized that clinical grading of femoral pulses may sometimes be inaccurate, particularly in obese patients or those with scarred groins from prior operations. Also, patients with iliac stenosis may have fairly normal femoral pulses at rest, but physiologic impairment of lower extremity pressure and flow with exercise because of being unable to augment distal blood flow sufficiently. In addition to pulse palpation, the examiner should listen over the lower abdomen and femoral region with a stethoscope. Frequently, audible bruits may be appreciated over the lower abdomen or femoral vessels, particularly after exercise, and lend additional clues to the presence of occlusive disease. Elevation pallor, rubor on dependency, shiny atrophic skin in the distal limbs and feet, and possible areas of ulceration or ischemic necrosis or gangrene may be noted, depending on the extent of atherosclerotic impairment.

B. Imaging Studies: A variety of noninvasive physiologic studies (see Chapter 2) are available to assist in assessment of the presence and severity of lower extremity occlusive disease. Segmental limb Doppler pressures and pulse-volume recordings (plethysmography) are most widely used, with determinations both before and after exercise. In recent years, duplex scanning has also been used more frequently. Such studies are helpful in confirming the diagnosis of occlusive disease suspected on the basis of history and physical examination and very valuable in evaluating and quantifying its severity. Noninvasive testing is particularly useful in differentiating other possible causes of lower extremity pain described previously. Such studies may also contribute substantially to clinical decision making, such as helping to predict the likelihood of healing of foot or toe lesions without revascularization or differentiating diabetic neuropathic pain from ischemic rest pain. Finally, the objective data provided by noninvasive tests provide a reliable baseline by which a patient's course may be followed.

C. Arteriography: If clinical evaluation suggests that the patient is a likely candidate for arterial reconstructive surgery, arteriography is performed to obtain the anatomic information necessary for the surgeon to select the best method of revascularization and properly plan an operative procedure. In addition to noting the actual anatomic distribution of occlusive disease in the aortoiliac segment and distal vessels, the surgeon should examine the films for potentially important or, in some instances, critical anatomic variations or associated occlusive lesions in the renal, visceral, or run-off vessels. For example, an enlarged meandering left colic artery may often be an indicator of associated occlusive disease in the superior mesenteric artery, which can usually be appreciated only on a lateral view. Failure to recognize this may lead to catastrophic bowel infarction if the inferior mesenteric artery is ligated at the time of aortic reconstruction.

For most patients, a full and complete arteriographic survey of the entire intra-abdominal aortoiliac segment and infrainguinal run-off vessels is advisable. In general, run-off views are obtained to at least the level of the midcalf. In selected patients with advanced distal disease and threatened limbs, more distal views including those of the distal leg, ankle, and even foot itself may be advisable if the possibility of very distal infrapopliteal bypass grafting is considered likely.

The major risk of conventional contrast angiography is contrast-induced renal dysfunction. Although the incidence of this difficulty may be minimized by adequate hydration and limitation of contrast volume, certain high-risk patients such as diabetics with preexistent chronic renal insufficiency may represent a significant hazard. In such instances, alternative imaging modalities may be considered. Development of magnetic resonance angiography (MRA) in recent years has substantial promise as a satisfactory substitute for conventional arteriography, both for diagnosis and planning of therapy. In the near future, progress with this technique as well as other new imaging modalities such as spiral CT scanning is likely to lead to more frequent use.

D. Pressure Measurements: Although an accurate assessment of occlusive disease is possible by traditional clinical evaluation and good quality arteriography in most patients, difficulty may exist in patients with multilevel occlusive disease. Assessment of the hemodynamic significance of occlusive disease at each segmental level is obviously of critical importance in selection of an appropriate reconstructive procedure.

For this purpose, actual measurement of femoral artery pressure (FAP) may often be of considerable value. Peak systolic pressure in the femoral artery is compared with distal aortic or brachial systolic pressure. A resting systolic pressure difference greater than 5 mmHg or a fall in FAP greater than 15% with reactive hyperemia induced pharmacologically by intra-arterial injection of a vasodilating drug, such as papaverine or tolazoline (Priscoline), or by inflation of an occluding thigh cuff for 3–5 minutes implies hemodynamically significant inflow disease (Fig 16–6). If revascularization is indicated in such patients, attention should first be directed at correction of the inflow lesions. With a negative study, the surgeon may more confidently proceed directly with distal revascularization without fear of premature compromise or closure of the distal graft and without subjecting the patient to an unnecessary inflow operation.

Differential Diagnosis

In some instances, the diagnosis of aortoiliac occlusive disease may not be readily apparent, and pitfalls may exist in terms of certain complaints that may

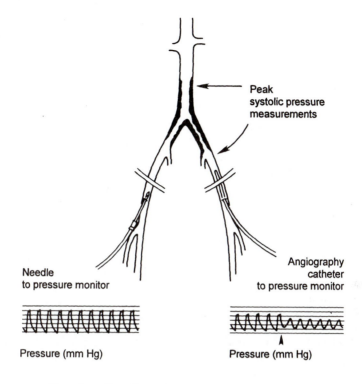

Figure 16–6. Femoral artery pressure measurement to assess hemodynamic significance of aortoiliac disease. A significant decrease in peak systolic pressure is recorded on left (*arrowhead*) as catheter is withdrawn across diseased segment in left iliac arterial system.

cause diagnostic confusion. In some patients, pulse evaluation and appearance of the feet may be judged to be entirely normal at rest, despite the presence of proximal stenoses that are physiologically significant with exercise. This is often the case in patients presenting with distal microemboli secondary to atheroembolism. In other instances, complaints of exercise-related pain in the leg, hip, buttock, or even low back may be mistaken for symptoms of degenerative hip or spine disease, nerve root irritation caused by lumbar disk herniation or spinal stenosis, diabetic neuropathy, or other neuromuscular problems. Many such patients may be distinguished from patients with true claudication by the fact that their discomfort is often relieved only when they sit or lie down, not when they stop walking.

In addition, the typical sciatic distribution of the pain and the fact that often the complaints are brought on simply by standing, rather than by walking a certain distance, suggest nonvascular causes. Other features suggestive of such neuro-orthopaedic causes of exercise-related lower extremity pain are that tolerable walking distance often varies from day to day and that pain is often noted immediately when walking is

begun and may actually lessen as the patient continues. In many such circumstances, use of noninvasive vascular laboratory testing modalities, including treadmill exercise, may be extremely valuable.

Treatment

A. Medical Treatment: No truly effective medical treatment for aortoiliac occlusive disease is currently available. Nonoperative care is aimed at limiting disease progression, encouraging development of collateral circulation, and preventing local tissue trauma or infection in the foot. With such care, spontaneous improvement may be noted in a few patients, although in most instances slow progression of symptoms may be anticipated. Progression of the atheromatous process may sometimes be slowed by altering the patient's risk factors.

Complete cessation of cigarette smoking is of paramount importance and cannot be overemphasized to the patient with vascular disease. Weight reduction, treatment of hypertension, correction of abnormal serum lipids, and regulation of diabetes all seem desirable and logical, although definite benefit in terms of stabilization or improvement of occlusive symptoms is less well established. A regular exercise program, often involving no more than regular walking of a specific distance on a daily basis, seems the best stimulant to collateral circulation. Good local foot care is extremely important because trauma and digital infection are often the precipitating causes of gangrene and amputation, particularly in the diabetic patient.

Although numerous vasodilator drugs exist, none is of established benefit in patients with chronic occlusive disease. None of these drugs has been shown to increase the exercising muscle blood flow in the claudicating extremity, the critical requirement for an effective agent in the treatment of claudication. A multiinstitution, double-blind, placebo-controlled trial of pentoxifylline (Trental) in treatment of patients with claudication showed a significant increase in walking distance of pentoxifylline-treated patients compared with the placebo-controlled group, and the drug has been approved by the Food and Drug Administration for the treatment of claudication. About 25% of patients have been found to show some improvement in claudication symptoms. It is often difficult to know whether this improvement is attributable to the drug or to other lifestyle modifications including weight loss and regular exercise. Although pentoxifylline may be used in patients with moderate claudication, it does not appear to have changed the eventual need for surgical revascularization in patients with severe claudication, resting ischemia, or more advanced symptoms.

The role of percutaneous transluminal angioplasty (PTA) and other forms of endovascular intervention such as atherectomy is discussed more fully in Chapter 4. PTA may be a valuable treatment modality in properly selected patients with aortoiliac occlusive disease. However, patient selection is of paramount importance. To be appropriate for PTA, the lesion should be relatively localized and preferably a stenosis rather than a total occlusion. A localized stenosis of the common iliac artery less than 5 cm long is the most favorable situation for PTA, with excellent early and late patency rates. Such a situation may exist in possibly 10–15% of patients with aortoiliac disease and symptoms severe enough to warrant arteriographic study and possible interventional treatment. PTA is generally not recommended for patients with diffuse iliac disease, unless they are extraordinarily poor surgical candidates, or for those with totally occluded iliac arteries because of the higher risk of complications or recurrent occlusion. Whether or not use of intraluminal stents will enable more extensive disease to be reliably treated by endoluminal methods remains to be established. Alternatives for surgical revascularization in high-risk patients with such situations unfavorable to PTA or other endovascular therapies almost always exist.

B. Surgical Treatment:

1. Indications—Ischemic pain at rest or actual tissue necrosis, including ischemic ulcerations or frank digital gangrene, are well accepted as indicative of advanced ischemia and threatened limb loss. True ischemic rest pain or ulceration may occasionally resolve because of collateral development, but this is infrequent. An exception is ischemia that occurs after an acute thrombotic event, such as terminal thrombosis of a previously stenotic artery. Improvement of collateral circulation over a period of days to a few weeks may result in diminished ischemia and only claudication symptoms.

It is generally accepted that most untreated patients with limb-threatening ischemic symptoms eventually require a major amputation. Because of this, all surgeons agree that these symptoms are clear-cut indications for arterial reconstruction, if anatomically feasible. Age, per se, is rarely an important consideration in the decision whether to surgically treat patients with aortoiliac occlusive disease. Even elderly or frail patients or patients at high risk from multiple associated medical problems may generally be revascularized by alternative surgical methods if direct aortoiliac reconstruction is deemed inadvisable.

Some controversy remains concerning operation for claudication symptoms alone. In each patient, such decisions must be individualized, with consideration of age, associated medical disease, employment requirements, and lifestyle preferences. In general, claudication that jeopardizes the livelihood of a patient or significantly impairs the desired lifestyle of an otherwise low-risk patient may be considered to be a reasonable indication for surgical correction, assuming that a favorable anatomic situation for operation exists. In general, most surgeons are more liberal in recommending surgical operations for patients with claudication alone if symptoms can be attributed to isolated proximal inflow disease rather than the more distal disease in the femoropopliteal arterial segment. This seems logical and appropriate because of the generally excellent and long-lasting results currently achieved by aortoiliac reconstruction at low risk to the patient.

A less common but recognized indication for surgical intervention is distal atheromatous embolization from proximal aortoiliac disease. If the clinical presentation is consistent with this diagnosis and arteriography demonstrates shaggy or ulcerated atherosclerotic plaques in the aortoiliac system as being the likely source of such embolic debris, treatment by means of endarterectomy or grafting with exclusion of the segment may be advisable.

2. Procedure selection—A variety of operative approaches and methods are available for the management of patients with aortoiliac disease. In each instance, the decision of the best procedure in a particular patient is based on the general condition of the patient, the extent and distribution of occlusive disease, and the experience and training of the surgeon. Currently, the methods of direct bilateral aortoiliac reconstruction, usually using prosthetic bypass grafts, offer the most successful and durable results. Remote or extra-anatomic procedures are generally reserved for the relatively small group of patients with concomitant serious medical problems, most often advanced coronary disease, which places them at high risk for conventional anatomic reconstruction, or for patients with infection or other technical problems that create a "hostile abdomen," which may hamper standard direct operation. Finally, more limited procedures may be used for truly unilateral iliac disease if clinical considerations or patient condition suggest that such an approach may be the most prudent.

In addition to the anatomic distribution and extent of occlusive disease, careful assessment of patient risk is generally the most important consideration in selecting the most appropriate operative procedure. Routine preoperative evaluation of pulmonary and renal function may reveal abnormalities that suggest that direct aortic operation would probably carry a risk of considerably greater magnitude than that in the average patient with aortoiliac disease. Most important is evaluation of cardiac status, particularly ischemic heart disease secondary to associated atherosclerotic coronary artery disease (CAD). It is well known that CAD is the cause of most early and late deaths following aortic revascularization operations. The incidence of CAD exceeds 50% in patients with aortoiliac disease and may be asymptomatic in 10–20% of patients.

A variety of methods are available for evaluation of the extent and physiologic compensation of CAD preoperatively. However, most available screening methods suffer from a lack of sensitivity and specificity in predicting postoperative cardiac complications. The extent to which preoperative patients should be screened (routine versus selective versus none) also remains controversial. Many have found the use of preoperative dipyridamole-thallium-201 imaging to be valuable in identifying a subset of patients at risk who may warrant more invasive investigation preoperatively, such as coronary angiography. Consideration of clinical markers of CAD is also useful. Patients with no clinical evidence of CAD probably require no further screening tests.

Procedures

A. Aortoiliac Endarterectomy: Although aortoiliac endarterectomy was frequently used in the early years of aortic reconstruction, it is rarely used by most vascular surgeons in current practice (Fig 16–7). The principal potential benefit of endarterectomy is avoidance of use of prosthetic grafts, with their possible complications of dilatation, infection, anastomotic aneurysm, and other degenerative problems. However, these are all unusual problems, especially with the improved quality of modern vascular grafts. Endarterectomy is also advocated by some proponents as being more likely to improve sexual potency in male patients

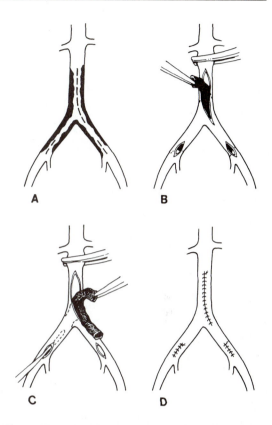

Figure 16–7. Aortoiliac endarterectomy. **A:** Endarterectomy may be considered if disease is localized to the distal abdominal aorta and common iliac arteries. **B:** A proper endarterectomy plane is established, and atheromatous disease is removed from the level of the aortic clamp proximally to the aortic bifurcation. **C:** Satisfactory end-point of endarterectomy at the iliac bifurcation is essential, with tacking sutures occasionally necessary. Atheromatous core is then mobilized proximally. **D:** Primary closure of the arteriotomies is usually feasible, with patch closure occasionally employed.

by more directly improving hypogastric artery blood flow. However, this has not been demonstrated in any study, and the more extensive dissection in the region of the aortic bifurcation required in endarterectomy seems likely to result in a higher incidence of neurogenic problems and retrograde ejaculation.

Endarterectomy may be used for patients with localized disease confined to the distal aorta, aortic bifurcation, and common iliac arteries. In patients with such a disease pattern, the long-term patency is excellent and equivalent to that which is brought about by graft procedures. However, it has been well documented that more extensive endarterectomy extending into the external iliac arteries or beyond does not have the same durability and patency of bypass grafting. Because localized aortoiliac disease truly suitable for possible endarterectomy is encountered in

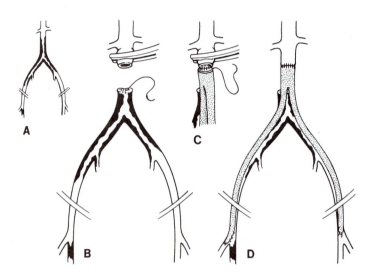

Figure 16–8. Basic principles of aortofemoral graft reconstruction. **A:** Schematic representation of typical arteriographic distribution of disease. **B:** The proximal anastomosis is placed high in the infrarenal aorta, at the level of the left renal vein. A short segment of the diseased aorta below the clamp is resected and the distal aorta is closed. **C:** End-to-end anastomosis is constructed, with limited endarterectomy of the cuff of the aorta as required. **D:** Completed graft implantation. The body of the prosthesis is short, allowing it to be placed in the anatomic bed of the resected section of native aorta, thereby facilitating soft tissue coverage of the graft.

only 5–10% of patients requiring aortic reconstruction, most patients with more extensive disease are not amenable to endarterectomy and will be better treated by graft insertion.

Endarterectomy is also contraindicated in several other circumstances. Any evidence of aneurysmal change in the aorta makes endarterectomy ill advised because of possible continued aneurysmal degeneration of the endarterectomized segment in the future. Second, if extensive occlusive disease extends superiorly close to the level of the renal arteries, transection of the aorta close to the renal vessels with thromboendarterectomy of the aortic cuff below the clamp followed by graft insertion is easier, faster, and more definitive.

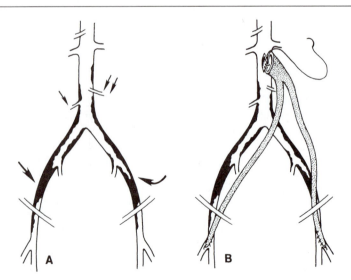

Figure 16–9. A: Anatomic circumstances favoring end-to-side aortic anastomosis include large accessory renal arteries arising from the lower aorta (*arrow*), a patent inferior mesenteric artery—believed important for colonic blood supply (*double arrow*), or severe occlusive disease confined largely to external iliac arteries that precludes retrograde pelvic perfusion (*bold curved arrows*). **B:** In such patterns of disease, end-to-side proximal graft anastomosis can be used to avoid the need to reimplant visceral vessels and minimize pelvic devascularization.

In addition, in the last decade PTA, atherectomy, stent insertion, and other endovascular less invasive procedures have increasingly replaced surgical correction of such localized disease. Finally, endarterectomy is acknowledged to be a technically demanding procedure. Most vascular surgeons trained within the past 15–20 years have little to no training and experience with this technique.

For reasons, bypass grafting has become the standard method of direct surgical repair for occlusive disease in almost all patients, offering the most durable and expeditious reconstruction available. Endarterectomy remains useful for a small number of patients with localized disease, particularly very young patients with an expected life span of 20–30 years in whom a higher incidence of possible graft-related problems might be anticipated and patients who may have an increased risk of infection with a nonautogenous reconstruction. Finally, endarterectomy may be considered for patients with atheromatous emboli originating from fairly discrete ulcerated plaques in the aorta or iliac arteries.

B. Aortobifemoral Bypass Grafts: Prosthetic bypass grafting from the infrarenal aorta to femoral arteries (Fig 16–8) is the most frequently used reconstructive procedure for aortoiliac occlusive disease and offers the most effective and durable method of revascularization currently available.

The proximal aortic anastomosis may be either end-to-end or end-to-side aorta. End-to-end anastomosis is clearly indicated in patients with coexisting aneurysmal disease or complete aortic occlusion up to the renal arteries. It is also preferred by many vascular surgeons for routine use in most cases because of apparent better long-term patency, although no randomized or controlled series have definitively established this.

Several potential explanations of superior long-term patency of end-to-end grafts have been suggested by advocates. These include superior hemodynamic characteristics, with high-volume direct in-line flow through the graft and less chance of competitive flow with diseased but still patent native vessels, which may promote sluggish graft flow and deposition of laminar thrombus in the prostheses. End-to-side proximal anastomosis may be advantageous if the surgeon wished to preserve a patent inferior mesenteric artery or sizable accessory renal artery, or if the anatomic pattern of disease suggests that end-to-end bypass is likely to devascularize both hypogastric arteries and hence the pelvic region (Fig 16–9).

Regardless of the technique used, the important principle is to place the proximal anastomosis as high as possible in the infrarenal aorta, where there is almost always a lesser amount of occlusive disease, to minimize the incidence of recurrent difficulties.

Although the distal anastomosis of the graft may sometimes by placed in the external iliac artery in the pelvis, it is almost always preferable in patients with aortoiliac occlusive disease to carry the graft to the femoral level. The fear of a higher incidence of infection if grafts were carried below the inguinal ligament has not been substantiated by extensive experience. At the femoral level, exposure is usually much better, the anastomosis technically easier, and most important, assessment and correction of any associated profunda origin disease most expediently accomplished. Because such a high percentage of patients have associated occlusive disease of the femoropopliteal segment, establishment of adequate graft outflow via the profunda femoris artery is of paramount importance in both early and late results (Fig 16–10).

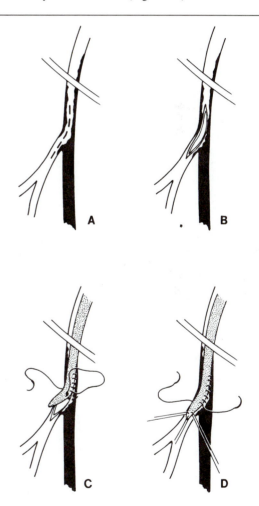

Figure 16–10. Femoral anastomosis of inflow graft. **A** & **B:** In patients with coexistent superficial femoral artery occlusion, runoff via the profunda femoris artery is essential. Any stenosis at the origin of the profunda must be corrected by extension of the common femoral arteriotomy into the profunda and profunda origin endarterectomy. **C:** The arteriotomy is patched by the beveled tip of the graft limb. The anastomosis is begun at the heel of the graft hood and run down both sides. **D:** Three to five interrupted sutures are placed at the tip of the anastomosis to facilitate good visualization and accurate placement without constriction, and anastomosis then completed.

C. Iliofemoral Grafts: Although aortoiliac disease is generally a diffuse process eventually involving both iliac arteries, it is not uncommon for patients to initially present with largely unilateral symptoms. If arteriography confirms largely unilateral iliac disease, more limited arterial reconstruction by means of an iliofemoral bypass may be considered.

Ipsilateral iliofemoral grafts are useful principally for patients with disease confined to the external iliac artery of the symptomatic extremity, with a fairly good common iliac artery that can be used for proximal graft anastomosis. A retroperitoneal approach by means of an oblique lower abdominal incision provides good exposure and may be carried out with low patient morbidity (Fig 16–11). The advantages of iliofemoral grafts are that they provide a direct in-line reconstruction with potentially better late patency rates than indirect extra-anatomic (femorofemoral) grafts, they do not involve procedures on the asymptomatic contralateral iliofemoral systems, and they carry less morbidity and mortality risk than conventional aortobifemoral grafts. As such, iliofemoral grafts are a useful and effective alternative in appropriate patients.

Concern about the possible progression of disease in the contralateral untreated iliac system to necessitate later reoperation on that side has led many authorities to regard aortobifemoral grafts as the most definitive reconstruction option even in patients with mostly unilateral iliac disease, particularly in younger low-risk patients. The incidence of such progression requiring reoperation has been cited to be as high as 30–40%, but recent reports suggest that this occurs in only about 10% of patients.

D. Indirect Methods of Revascularization: Bypass grafts that use significantly different anatomic pathways than the native vessels that they are meant to replace were originally devised as a compromise procedure for unusual or frequently desperate clinical problems, such as infection or serious complications of aortoiliac reconstruction. Within a short time, however, their potential application for revascularization in patients at potentially high risk for conventional procedures due to associated medical diseases became apparent. Indeed, growing acceptance of such procedures has led to more widespread use in recent years.

Such "extra-anatomic" bypass grafts generally are routed in remote subcutaneous tissue planes, deliberately avoiding the natural location of the blood supply because of hostile pathologic conditions in that area (eg, infection, prior irradiation, multiple previous operations, abdominal stomas) or because entering the area would likely increase the risk of operation (as in the transabdominal direct aortic approach). Although a large number of ingenious routes and methods have been described for different clinical problems, by far the most frequently used extra-anatomic grafts are the axillofemoral and femorofemoral bypass or their frequently used combination, the so-called **axillobifemoral bypass** (Fig 16–12).

Axillobifemoral grafts are chosen whenever bilateral iliac disease requires an extra-anatomic means of inflow restoration, whereas femorofemoral grafts are used for unilateral iliac disease if the contralateral iliac artery is free of hemodynamically significant disease and can adequately serve as a donor inflow source. If disease in the contralateral iliac artery is focal, PTA on this side may be carried out to establish adequate inflow for a femorofemoral graft. Femorofemoral grafts are also felt by many vascular surgeons to be a most expedient and successful method of management for occlusion of one limb of an aortobifemoral graft that cannot be successfully reopened by thrombectomy.

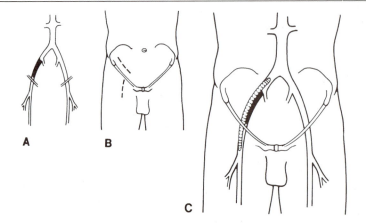

Figure 16–11. Iliofemoral bypass graft, applicable for unilateral iliac disease confined principally to ipsilateral external iliac artery. **A:** Typical pattern of disease appropriate for iliofemoral bypass. The common iliac artery is suitable for proximal graft anastomosis. **B:** The diseased iliac system is exposed via a lower quadrant oblique incision and retroperitoneal approach, with a separate standard vertical groin incision. **C:** Completed iliofemoral graft.

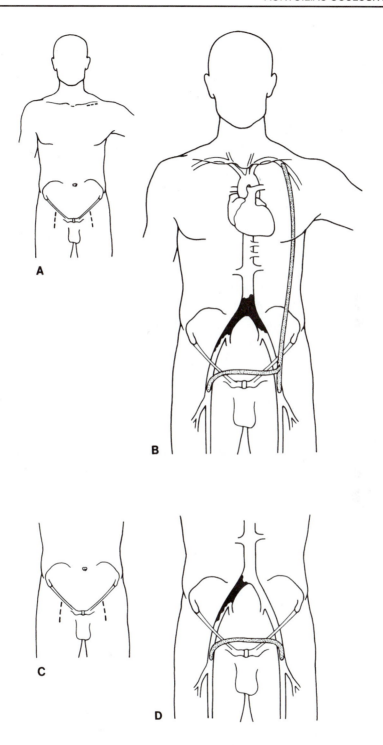

Figure 16–12. Extra-anatomic methods of revascularization in aortoiliac disease. **A:** Axillo-bifemoral bypass. **B:** Femorofemoral bypass.

Such extra-anatomic grafts useful in the management of aortoiliac disease in certain patients are discussed in more detail in Chapter 28.

Prognosis

Excellent early and late results of anatomic aortoiliofemoral operations can be anticipated, achievable at very acceptable levels of patient morbidity and mortality. A consensus of important large series in the modern era clearly documents this. Based on such data, it is reasonable to expect about 85–90% graft patency rates at 5 years and 70–75% at 10 years. Perioperative mortality rates well below 5% are now uniformly achieved, with many experienced centers reporting operative mortality rate of only 1–2%. Mortality risks for direct reconstruction in patients with relatively localized aortoiliac disease can be expected to be extremely low, whereas patients with more widespread multilevel disease have a somewhat higher mortality risk, as expected from their greater age and more frequent associated atherosclerotic disease in coronary, carotid, and visceral vessels.

Successful direct reconstructive procedures affords relief of symptoms that led to operation in nearly all patients with relatively localized disease. However, because most operative candidates have more diffuse multilevel disease, symptom relief may be incomplete in 25–30% of patients.

Major early complications of direct aortic operation occur in 5–10% of patients. Many are largely technical in nature and therefore uncommon with an experienced surgeon and operating team. Bleeding that requires reoperation or acute limb ischemia secondary to graft thrombosis or distal thromboembolism each are encountered in 1–2% of patients. Acute renal failure is currently infrequent with recognition of the importance of adequate fluid volume during surgery, optimization of cardiac function intraoperatively and avoidance of declamping hypotension. Spinal cord and bowel ischemia are much more difficult to predict but fortunately are rare occurrences. Nonfatal myocardial infarction is noted in about 3–5% of patients, often with little hemodynamic compromise. Significant pulmonary insufficiency is unusual today in the absence of severe preoperative chronic lung disease.

The prevalence of late complications in patients with aortic grafts largely depends on the length of follow-up. Over a 10-year period, 10–20% of patients may experience occlusion of a graft limb. Anastomotic aneurysm is the second most common late complication of aortic graft insertion, seen in 3–5% of patients and almost always at the femoral anastomosis. Graft infection and enteric fistula remain dreaded and difficult to manage late problems but fortunately are uncommon.

Long-term survival of patients undergoing aortoiliac reconstruction continues to be compromised. The cumulative long-term survival rate remains about 10–15 years less than that which might be anticipated for a normal age- and sex-matched population. Overall, about 20–30% of patients will be dead within 5 years and 50–60% within 10 years of reconstruction. Most late deaths are attributable to coronary artery disease and its sequelae.

REFERENCES

Baird RJ et al: Subsequent downstream repair after aorta-iliac and aorta-femoral bypass operations. Surgery 1977; 82:785.

Bernhard BM, Ray LI, Militello JP: The role of angioplasty of the profunda femoris artery in revascularization of the ischemic limb. Surg Gynecol Obstet 1976;142:840.

Brewster DC: Clinical and anatomic considerations for surgery in aortoiliac disease and results of surgical treatment. Circulation 1991;83(Suppl I):I-42.

Brewster DC: Complications of aortic and lower extremity procedures. In: *Vascular Diseases: Surgical and Intervention Therapy.* Strandness DE, Van Breda A (editors). Churchill Livingstone, 1994:1151.

Brewster DC, Cooke, JC: Longevity of aortofemoral bypass grafts. In: *Long-term Results in Vascular Surgery.* Yao JST, Pearce WH (editors). Appleton & Lange, 1992: 149.

Brewster DC, Darling RC: Optimal methods of aortoiliac reconstruction. Surgery 1978;84:739.

Brewster DC, Edwards JP: Cardiopulmonary complications related to vascular surgery. In: *Complications in Vascular Surgery.* Bernhard VM, Towne JB (editors). Quality Medical Publishing, 1991:23.

Brewster DC et al: Aortofemoral graft for multilevel occlusive disease: Predictors of success and need for distal bypass. Arch Surg 1982;117:1593.

Brewster DC et al: Femoral artery pressure measurement during aortography. Circulation 1979;60(Suppl I):120.

Brewster DC et al: Long-term results of combined iliac balloon angioplasty and distal surgical revascularization. Ann Surg 1989;210:324.

Brewster DC et al: Reoperation for aortofemoral graft limb occlusion: Optimal methods and long-term results. J Vasc Surg 1987;5:363.

Brewster DC et al: Selection of patients for preoperative coronary angiography: Use of dipyridamole-stress thallium myocardial imaging. J Vasc Surg 1985;2:504.

Cambria RP et al: The impact of selective use of dipyridamole-thallium scans and surgical factors on the current morbidity of aortic surgery. J Vasc Surg 1992;15:43.

Cambria RP et al: The potential for lower extremity revascularization without contrast arteriography. J Vasc Surg 1993;17:1050.

Coffman JD: Vasodilator drugs in peripheral vascular disease. N Engl J Med 1979;300.

Corson JD, Brewster DC, Darling RC: The surgical management of infrarenal aortic occlusion. Surg Gynecol Obstet 1982;155:369.

Crawford ES et al: Aortoiliac occlusive disease: Factors influencing survival and function following reconstructive operation over a twenty-five year period. Surgery 1981; 90:1555.

Cronenwett JL et al: Aortoiliac occlusive disease in women. Surgery 1980;88:775.

Dalman RL et al: Simultaneous operative repair of multilevel lower extremity occlusive disease. J Vasc Surg 1991;13: 211.

Dunn DA, Downs, AR, Lye CR: Aortoiliac reconstruction for occlusive disease: Comparison of end-to-end and end-to-side proximal anastomoses. Can J Surg 1982;25:382.

Eagle KA et al: Combining clinical and thallium data optimizes preoperative assessment of cardiac risk before major vascular surgery. Ann Intern Med 1989;110:859.

Flanigan DP et al: Hemodynamic evaluation of the aortoiliac system based on pharmacologic vasodilatation. Surgery 1983;93:709.

Goodreau JJ et al: Rational approach to the differentiation of vascular and neurogenic claudication. Surgery 1978;84: 749.

Harris PL, Cave Bigley DJ, McSweeney l: Aortofemoral bypass and the role of concomitant femorodistal reconstruction. Br J Surg 1985;72:317.

Hertzer NR et al: Coronary artery disease in peripheral vascular patients: A classification of 1000 coronary angiograms and results of surgical management. Ann Surg 1984;199:223.

Inahara T: Evaluation of endarterectomy for aortoiliac and aortoiliofemoral occlusive disease. Arch Surg 1985;110: 1458.

Johnston KW et al: Five-year results of a prospective study of percutaneous transluminal angioplasty. Ann Surg 1987;206:403.

Kalman PG et al: Unilateral iliac disease: The role of iliofemoral graft. J Vasc Surg 1987;6:139.

Karmody AM et al: "Blue toe" syndrome: An indication for limb salvage surgery. Arch Surg 1976;111:1263.

Kempczinski RF: Lower extremity arterial emboli from ulceration atherosclerotic plaques. JAMA 1979;241:807.

Kohler TR et al: Duplex scanning for diagnosis of aortoiliac and femoropopliteal disease: A prospective study. Circulation 1987;76:1074.

Malone JM, Moore WS, Goldstone J: The natural history of bilateral aortofemoral bypass grafts for ischemia of the lower extremities. Arch Surg 1975;110:1300.

Malone JM, Moore WS, Goldstone J: Life expectancy following aortofemoral arterial grafting. Surgery 1977;81: 551.

Martinez BD, Hertzer NR, Beven EG: Influence of distal arterial occlusive disease on prognosis following aorto-bifemoral bypass. Surgery 1980;88:795.

Mortin JF et al: Factors that determine the long-term results of percutaneous transluminal dilatation for peripheral arterial occlusive disease. J Vasc Surg 1986;4:68.

Nevelsteen A, Wouters L, Suy R: Aortofemoral Dacron reconstruction for aortoiliac occlusive disease: A 25-year survey. Eur J Vasc Surg 1991;5:179.

Pierce HE et al: Evaluation of end-to-side v. end-to-end proximal anastomosis in aortobifemoral bypass. Arch Surg 1982;117:1580.

Piotrowski JJ et al: Aortobifemoral bypass: The operation of choice for unilateral iliac occlusion? J Vasc Surg 1988; 8:211.

Porter JM et al: Pentoxifylline efficacy in the treatment of intermittent claudication: Multicenter controlled double-blind trial with objective assessment of chronic occlusive arterial disease patients. Am Heart J 1982;104:66.

Queral LA et al: Pelvic hemodynamics after aortoiliac reconstruction. Surgery 1979;86:799.

Ricco J-B: Unilateral iliac artery occlusive disease: A randomized multicenter trial examining direct revascularization versus crossover bypass. Ann Vasc Surg 1992;6:209.

Rutherford RB, Patt A, Pearce WH: Extra-anatomic bypass: A closer view. J Vasc Surg 1987;6:437.

Rutherford RB et al: Serial hemodynamic assessment of aortobifemoral bypass. J Vasc Surg 1986;4:428.

Szilagyi DE et al: A thirty-year survey of the reconstructive surgical treatment of aortoiliac occlusive disease. J Vasc Surg 1986;3:421.

van der Akker PJ et al: Long-term results of prosthetic and non-prosthetic reconstruction for obstructive aortoiliac disease. Eur J Vasc Surg 1992;6:53.

Yeager RA, Moneta GL: Assessing cardiac risk in vascular surgical patients: Current status. Perspect Vasc Surg 1989;2:18.

17

Complications of Aortic Grafts

Richard M. Green, MD

Operations on the abdominal aorta are highly successful both in prolonging life, as in patients with aneurysmal disease, and in reducing ischemia, as in patients with occlusive disease. Careful attention to details is essential to prevent the many complications that can occur during the course of aortic graft procedures. Although advances in fabric design have eliminated the need for biologic material, and with it the problem of aneurysmal deterioration, other complications of aortic grafts remain (Table 17–1). Following is a discussion of the major complications that can occur after graft replacement of the abdominal aorta: hemorrhage, thrombosis, embolization, infection, ureteral injury, ischemic colitis, paraplegia, and false aneurysm formation. In every instance, prevention is the best treatment available since each complication has dire consequences to both limb and life.

HEMORRHAGE

General Considerations

Hemorrhage is an infrequent complication (1–2%) of aortic operations. Most hemorrhage occurs because of faulty operative techniques or a defect in the coagulation system. The coagulopathy may be due to a preexisting disorder or from dilution due to the transfusion of large volumes of stored blood without concomitant administration of appropriate coagulation factors and platelets.

Patients should be screened for bleeding tendencies prior to operation. A history of prolonged bleeding after minor injuries or a family history of bleeding could be significant and should be investigated. If there is no such history, a platelet count, blood smear, and a partial thromboplastin time (PTT) are sufficient to identify platelet abnormalities, a circulating anticoagulant, or intravascular coagulation. When a positive history of bleeding is present, a platelet count and a bleeding time should be performed to assess platelet function, a prothrombin time and PTT used to assess coagulation, and the fibrin clot analyzed to detect abnormal fibrinolysis. Patients with abnormal screening tests should be seen by a hematologist for more specific tests of platelet aggregation and coagulation.

Treatment

Most intraoperative bleeding is due to local problems of hemostasis. Note that the aorta should be dissected in as normal an area as possible. This not only prevents unwanted bleeding, but also reduces the risks of atheroembolization. In procedures on the abdominal aorta, excessive dissection, particularly around the bifurcation, is both dangerous and unnecessary. The proximity of the iliac veins to the aortic bifurcation makes dissection very treacherous; because this is usually the site of the severest occlusive process, the dissection is more difficult.

Suture line bleeding can result in severe postoperative hemorrhage and require return to the operating room. Liberal use of pledgeted sutures to repair any anastomotic defect is critical. These additional sutures should be placed with the proximal aorta clamped. It is much easier to repair the posterior wall of the proximal anastomosis before beginning the distal anastomosis, and this should be done whenever a significant defect exists.

Patients may develop a dilutional coagulopathy after massive transfusions. This may occur in the setting of a ruptured aortic aneurysm or after large amounts of bleeding are encountered in an elective procedure. The exchange of 1 blood volume (11 units in a 75-kg man) decreases the platelet count from 250,000/mm^3 to 80,000/mm^3. Spontaneous bleeding should not occur with platelets counts greater than 50,000/mm^3, but higher levels are required to ensure hemostasis during surgery. Concentrated platelet pack transfusions can temporarily raise the platelet count by 10,000/mm^3 per unit. Patients with chronic renal failure may have a functional platelet abnormality that can be treated with vasopressin. Other coagulation factors should be replaced with fresh frozen plasma and cryoprecipitate. If defibrination occurs (fibrinogen < 100 mg/dL), fibrinolytic inhibitors such as ϵ-aminocaproic acid (EACA) can be used in conjunction with heparin. This is rarely indicated in aortic procedures.

GRAFT OCCLUSION

Essentials of Diagnosis
- Nonpalpable pulses.
- No increase in ankle-to-brachial pressure following surgery.
- Return or exasercation of ischemic symptoms.

Table 17–1. Complications of aortic grafts.

Condition	Incidence	Key Factors
Hemorrhage	1–2%	Avoid excessive dissection; use pledgeted sutures for anastomotic bleeding; be aware of coagulopathy.
Thrombosis		
Immediate	1–2%	Ensure that all kinks and residual thrombi are removed; early diagnosis important.
Postoperative	10–15% at 5-yr follow-up	Use special extraction catheter and provide new outflow.
Embolization	2–5%	Excessive manipulation of diseased areas or residual thrombus in limb of graft; may be very minor or limb threatening.
Infection	0.5–3%	Increased incidence with groin incision; treatment requires removal of infected prosthesis and revascularization through an uninfected site; mortality rate 50–75% with aortic involvement.
Ureteral injury	Rare but postoperative hydronephrosis in up to 20% of cases	Very serious because urinary leakage or obstruction can result in an infected graft; usually mandates nephrectomy.
Ischemic colitis	0.5–6% depending on diagnostic criteria	Early diagnosis by sigmoidoscopy and aggressive treatment with colostomy and resection for transmural involvement.
Paraplegia	Rare	Usually due to pelvic devascularization and associated with colonic and buttock ischemia.
Pseudoaneurysm	3–15% after aorto-femoral bypass	Aortic pseudoaneurysms hard to diagnose until symptomatic. Due to degeneration of the arterial wall; dangerous and should be repaired.

1. IMMEDIATE OCCLUSION

General Considerations

Graft occlusion may occur from kinking, anastomotic errors, inadequate outflow, residual thrombus in the graft, or coagulopathy. It is important to define the cause because treatment varies. Immediate graft occlusion may be difficult to diagnose.

Clinical Findings

A. Signs and Symptoms: The patient often arrives in the recovery room with relative hypothermia. Pulses may not be palpable because of concomitant superficial femoral artery occlusion. Therefore, goals for the aortic reconstruction must be established preoperatively, and some objective measurement of arterial perfusion must be obtained prior to the surgeon's leaving the operating room to ensure that these goals have been met.

B. Imaging Studies: The simplest objective test that can be done at the bedside is the Doppler-derived, ankle-to-brachial pressure index. An increase in pressure of greater than 0.15 is necessary to show an improvement following operation. Failing that, a cause must be considered, one of which is graft occlusion.

Treatment

Immediate graft occlusions can usually be treated with catheter thrombectomy and examination of the distal anastomosis for technical defects. The entire abdomen and both legs are prepped. Thrombectomy of the limb is performed. If this is not possible, a kink may be present and the abdominal incision must be reopened and the graft explored. The arteriogram shown in Figure 17–1 shows the site of the typical kink, which occurs at the graft bifurcation. This is usually the site at which the presence of the ligated aortic stump pushes the graft limb anteriorly. This complication can be eliminated by keeping the body of the graft as short as possible. If adequate flow can be obtained in the graft limb, the distal anastomosis is inspected. If satisfactory, an arteriogram is performed to assess the outflow, and corrective actions are taken as necessary. This may include catheter embolectomy of the popliteal artery. If no technical error is identified, flow is restored and the presumptive diagnosis of residual thrombus within the graft due to inadequate flushing or heparinization is made.

2. LATE OCCLUSION

General Considerations

Aortic grafts have patency rates ranging from 85% to 90% at 5 years. Occlusions are the result of neointimal hyperplasia, progression of atherosclerosis, or false aneurysm. Again, the treatment varies according to the cause. Occlusion is usually associated with ischemia more severe than the original operative indication, and urgent intervention is required. Figure 17–2 shows an occlusion of the right limb of an aorto-femoral graft placed 8 years previously for occlusive disease. The occlusion occurred 30 days prior to admission. At operation, there was organized thrombus in the graft limb and an anastomotic narrowing, which caused the occlusion. Although standard balloon catheters can remove the thrombus from an acutely occluded graft limb, an adherent fibrin layer often cannot be removed in this fashion. Thrombectomy was performed on this graft with a Fogarty Graft Thrombectomy Catheter (Baxter Healthcare Corporation, Santa Ana, CA). This catheter has a wire stripper rather than an inflatable balloon; it is designed specifically for use with occluded prosthetic grafts and is helpful in extracting the adherent fibrin layer.

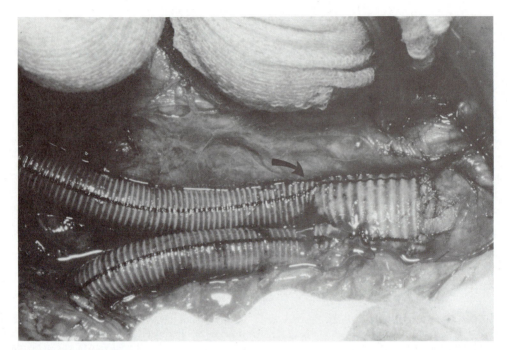

Figure 17–1. Operative photograph of an aortobifemoral graft. It is important to keep the body as short as possible. Kinks tend to occur at the site of the arrow, where the residual aortic stump pushes the graft anteriorly. A shorter body reduces this effect.

Treatment

Some form of distal reconstruction is necessary after flow is restored in the graft limb. Most of these occluded grafts can be repaired with a short graft extension or a patch angioplasty. Outflow stenoses in the setting of a small or very diseased deep femoral artery require a femoropopliteal or crural bypass graft.

If satisfactory inflow cannot be restored in the occluded limb, a femorofemoral bypass from the opposite side is the next best option. Replacement of the limb by means of a retroperitoneal or intra-abdominal procedure is usually not necessary for a unilateral occlusion unless the problem is related to kinking at the prosthetic bifurcation. If proximal or aortic problems occur, the entire prosthesis will require replacement. A variety of secondary inflow choices are available in this setting, namely, the infrarenal aorta, the descending thoracic aorta, the supraceliac aorta, the ascending aorta, or the axillary arteries, depending on the condition of the patient.

EMBOLIZATION

Essentials of Diagnosis
- Post-Operative renal failure.
- Cadaveric extremity.
- Loss of pulses.
- Excessive dissection of diseased vessels.

Atherosclerotic debris may undergo embolization caused by excessive manipulation of diseased arterial segments, clamping in an area of disease, or inadequate evacuation of thrombus lining the graft during

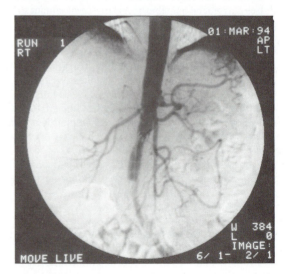

Figure 17–2. Arteriogram showing an occlusion of the right limb of an 8-year-old aortobifemoral bypass graft. The occlusion occurred 30 days prior to admission and was successfully treated by catheter extraction of the clot and profundoplasty. Chronic occlusion is almost always due to outflow problems.

implantation. The emboli may lodge in the renal vessels when juxtarenal atherosclerosis is present and not recognized prior to placement of the proximal clamp. If debris is suspected at the site of the proximal clamp, the renal arteries should be clamped prior to clamping the aorta. The juxtarenal aortic debris can then be removed without risking embolization to the kidneys and postoperative renal failure. Emboli can also traverse a patent inferior mesenteric artery and cause intestinal ischemia. The distal spinal cord can be damaged by emboli via the hypogastric arteries. Emboli most commonly affect the lower extremities. Only the lower extremities can be treated, and careful inspection of the patient's lower extremities by the surgeon (Feet which have been "trashed" are initially cadaveric in appearance. With time mottling appears. Pedal pulses may return even if the digital arteries are involved. In this situation no intervention will help. If pedal pulses are absent catheter thrombectomy can restore flow and should be attempted.) prior to leaving the operating room is necessary to ensure that the patient will not be required to return to have thrombus extracted from the legs. In general, emboli can be avoided by careful handling of the aorta and clamping of the outflow vessels prior to aortic manipulation.

GRAFT INFECTION

Essentials of Diagnosis
- Systemic sepsis.
- Gastrointestinal bleeding, even minor.
- Fever, malaise, leukocytosis.
- Drainage of wound abscess, persistent sinus tract over graft with possible exposure of prosthesis.
- False aneurysm.
- Bleeding or hemorrhage retroperitoneally.
- Possible abdominal or back pain.

General Considerations
An **infected graft** is defined as one with established bacterial colonization and growth. Graft infection is one of the most serious complications of aortic grafting procedures, with an incidence ranging from 0.5% to 3%, depending on whether the graft is extended into the groin. The incidence of infection is 2 to 3 times higher when an inguinal incision is made. The mortality rates range from 20% to 75%, with the latter associated with involvement of an aortic anastomosis. The 3 main mechanisms for aortic graft infection are intraoperative contamination, erosion into adjacent viscera, and septicemia.

Pathophysiology
A number of infecting sources are possible at the time of operation:

- Skin flora
- Bacteria in the fluid in the intestinal bag

- Bacteria in the aneurysm thrombus
- Technical errors resulting in breaks in aseptic techniques
- Contamination from concomitant nonvascular procedures

Intraoperative contamination is the most common cause of aortic graft infection. Contamination from skin flora is more common when the procedure is extended into the groin where the bacterial skin counts are higher. This is particularly true in the obese patient in whom the panniculus hangs down over the inguinal crease. Delaying skin shaving from the night preceding to immediately before the operation can reduce the incidence of infection significantly. Finally, the issue of performing nonvascular procedures during an aortic resection is controversial. The data suggest, however, that a higher incidence of graft infection is present even with elective cholecystectomy and interval appendectomy, and these procedures should not be routinely performed in the setting of an aortic graft placement.

Mechanical erosion of the graft into adjacent intestine with subsequent aortoenteric fistula is another mechanism of aortic graft infection. This may be a direct erosive effect due to mechanical forces, or it may secondary to a false aneurysm. Note that there is a significant number of enteric fistulas whose culture shows gram-positive cocci not normally found in the intestinal flora. This suggests that a false aneurysm due to a gram-positive microorganism preceded the enteric fistula. A viable layer of tissue must be placed to separate the graft from the intestine at the original operation. If sufficient peritoneum or aneurysm wall is not present, an omental flap should be used. Adequate coverage should prevent the development of erosion.

Finally, aortic grafts can become infected as a result of a **bacteremia**. The precise incidence of this phenomenon is unknown because the bacteremic event may be hard to document. The susceptibility of a graft to a bacteremic episode depends on the degree of neointima formation. Experimentally, grafts with a complete neointima are resistant to infection, whereas those without are highly susceptible. This is a compelling reason for prophylactic antibiotic use against *Staphylococcus aureus* and common gram-negative pathogens in the immediate postoperative period during which indwelling catheters are likely to produce a bacteremic episode. Antibiotics may also be useful whenever the patient is subjected to a stress likely to produce a bacteremia, such as dental prophylaxis.

Clinical Findings
A. Signs and Symptoms: The inguinal incision is the site of most graft infections (57–77%). The typical sequence of events is the draining of a wound abscess with the development of a persistent sinus tract over the graft with or without exposure of the prosthesis. Development of a false aneurysm and hemorrhage

is likely if the anastomosis is involved. Abdominal graft infections are more difficult to diagnose, and patients may initially present with fever, malaise, and leukocytosis. Abdominal or back pain may follow. Bleeding is usually a late manifestation of graft infection and may occur either retroperitoneally or through the gastrointestinal tract in the form of an aortoenteric fistula. Infection should be considered as being present in any patient with an aortic graft who presents with signs of systemic sepsis or gastrointestinal bleeding.

B. Imaging Studies: Computed tomography (CT) or magnetic resonance imaging (MRI) may reveal perigraft gas or fluid that can be aspirated under imaging CT or ultrasound control. MRI is more accurate than CT scanning (89% compared with 42%) largely because T_2-weighted images distinguish blood-based rather than non-blood-based fluids. Gastrointestinal bleeding (even minor) should be investigated with upper tract endoscopy. Arteriography is helpful in defining the presence of a pseudoaneurysm but not in defining infection per se. The arteriogram in Figure 17–3 shows a pseudoaneurysm at the distal anastomosis of a previously placed aortic graft. Isotope scanning using ^{111}In or ^{99m}Tc-hexametazime-labeled leukocytes has a high sensitivity and negative predictive value when used in patients with possible graft infections. Some caution must be exercised in the immediate postoperative period in using the indium test since 53% of patients will have positive scans at the time of hospital discharge.

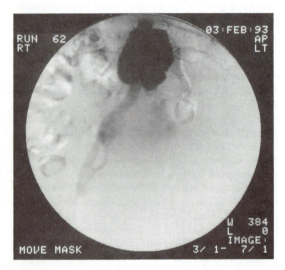

Figure 17–3. Arteriogram showing a false aneurysm at the distal end of a straight aortic prosthesis. This graft was secondarily infected after urinary tract sepsis. Treatment included control of the aorta at the diaphragm, removal of the entire graft, and closure of both stumps with monofilament sutures. Cultures grew a *Pseudomonas* sp. Revascularization was accomplished by an axillobifemoral bypass graft.

C. Laboratory Findings: The most common organism seen in prosthetic graft infections is *S aureus*. Around 50% are infected with organisms of low virulence (eg, *Staphylococcus epidermidis*), which can exist quiescently for long periods of time in a perigraft slime. The remaining organisms are a mixture of gram-negative enteric bacteria. Improved culture methods have increased the yield of low-virulence organisms. A yield of greater than 90% can be obtained when pieces of graft material are explanted and subjected to sonication. *S epidermidis* has been shown to lay down a surface biofilm (glycocalyx) that isolates the bacteria from the immunologic system of the host and decreases the penetration and therefore the effectiveness of antibiotics. Reports of increased resistance to infection of polytetrafluorethylene (PTFE) compared with Dacron may be related to the 100-fold decrease in bacterial adherence to PTFE. This difference between the 2 prosthetic materials has been used to select PTFE over Dacron when other parameters are similar.

Treatment

The classic principles of treatment for graft infection are the complete removal of the prosthetic material, débridement of infected arterial tissues, revascularization through noncontaminated extra-anatomic routes and long-term organism-specific parenteral antibiotics. Occasionally, exceptions to these principles are made, and an increasing number of cases are reported with either partial removal of the prosthetic material or in situ replacement with a new prosthetic. If possible, revascularization should be delayed until adequate local control of the infection is obtained. Unfortunately, this is rarely possible.

Initial antibiotic therapy should be guided by a knowledge of likely pathogens in the given clinical situation. Efforts should be made to obtain fluid for culture and sensitivities as quickly as possible to ensure that adequate coverage is provided for the patient. When the intestine is involved, the patient should be started on broad-spectrum antibiotic coverage with activity against both gram-positive cocci and aerobic and anaerobic bowel flora. When the intestine is not involved, anaerobic coverage is not required but coverage for *S epidermidis* with vancomycin is required.

Patients with gastrointestinal bleeding and aortic grafts should be approached with a sense of urgency even if the bleeding is minor. These patients often have "herald" bleeds, which are minor episodes that stop spontaneously and forewarn of a major hemorrhage. Patients with massive gastrointestinal bleeding and aortic grafts should undergo immediate exploration even when diagnostic studies are normal. Upper tract endoscopy may show blood coming from the fourth portion of the duodenum, but the absence of pathology in the stomach and proximal duodenum is often sufficient to justify exploration.

The operative sequence in the treatment of aortic graft infections depends on whether active bleeding is present. Ideally, if revascularization is required, it should precede removal of the infected prosthesis. When hemorrhage is present, however, the aorta must be controlled immediately and revascularization should follow. Control of hemorrhage is best obtained by controlling the supraceliac aorta after dividing the crus of the diaphragm. After proximal control has been obtained, the aortic graft should be removed, the tissues débrided, the duodenum repaired, and the aortic stump closed. If the proximal anastomosis was initially end to side, a venous patch can be used to close the aorta. In the more common end-to-end anastomosis, the aortic stump must be sutured with a monofilament material. Prevertebral fascia can be used to buttress this closure and the stump covered with omentum.

The retroperitoneum can be irrigated with large sump catheters and dilute (0.1%) povidine-iodine solution. The abdomen is closed and the patient reprepped with a completely rescrubbed team and new instruments. The extra-anatomic repair follows and usually consists of bilateral axillofemoral bypass grafts. Alternative inflow sites are the supraceliac aorta, the descending thoracic aorta, and the ascending aorta. The operative mortality rate for patients with this procedure is about 25%, and the actuarial primary patency rates at 2 and 5 years are 82% and 65%, respectively. The rate of reocclusion in ringed reinforced grafts is lower (9%) than in nonreinforced grafts (22%).

When the patient presents with a graft infection and no bleeding, the extra-anatomic reconstruction is performed initially through uninfected routes. When the wounds are closed, the abdomen is opened and the infected graft removed. Local débridements, arterial and aortic stump closures, and irrigation systems are similar to the prior example. When the graft infection extends into the groin, the revascularization is more complicated. In these cases, the femoral vessels should be approached laterally with the new conduit under the sartorius muscle and rectus femoris fascia for an anastomosis into the mid-profunda femoris artery. The femoral arteries can be repaired with an autogenous venous patch or ligated. The former is preferable when retrograde flow into the pelvis through the external iliac artery is desired. Reconstruction of the artery rather than ligation increases the possibility of hemorrhage, and wound irrigation systems with dilute povidine-iodine solution should be used.

The conditions for leaving prosthetic graft material in place as defined by Calligaro and associates (1991) are (1) the graft must be noncavitary and patent with the anastomoses intact; (2) the patient does not have systemic sepsis; and (3) the wounds can be widely and often repetitively débrided. For instance, if only one groin is infected in a graft that has been well incorporated, a unilateral replacement can be done. The graft is initially detached through a retroperitoneal incision and then removed through the groin. If the graft is surrounded by fluid in the retroperitoneum, it must be considered infected and a local approach should be abandoned. The common femoral artery is either ligated or repaired with a vein patch. Reconstruction may be done with an obturator bypass from the contralateral femoral artery or from the ipsilateral axillary artery via a new uninfected pathway to an uninvolved vessel, namely, the distal profunda femoris or the above-knee popliteal artery.

Some anecdotal evidence suggests that infected aortic grafts can be managed with in situ graft replacement after adequate débridement has been performed. These grafts are covered with an omental flap, and long-term antibiotics are given. This treatment should be considered only for patients with low-grade infection with negative perigraft and blood cultures; it must be considered experimental until safety and efficacy are confirmed by adequate clinical trials.

URETERAL INJURY

Essentials of Diagnosis
- Leakage of urine.
- Ureteral obstruction with hydronephrosis.

The ureters can be injured during dissection at the iliac bifurcation in the transperitoneal approach to the aorta, during mobilization of the aorta from the retroperitoneal approach, during the creation of the tunnels for an aortofemoral bypass, or during the removal of an infected prosthesis. Most injuries arise from direct trauma or ischemia from dissection. Compression of the ureters by the prosthesis may cause obstruction, but this is an unusual event. Obstruction can be avoided by placing the graft limb under the ureter. The results of ureteral trauma are either leakage or obstruction with hydronephrosis or both. Either can result in sepsis and graft infection. The risk of ureteral injury is significantly increased during reoperations.

Several studies have examined the incidence of hydronephrosis after aortic surgery. The incidence ranges from 2% to 20%. Most cases of early postoperative hydronephrosis are transient and require no further therapy. Delayed hydronephrosis is more ominous since many of these patients also present with graft complications. Delayed hydronephrosis should be evaluated to determine its precise nature and cause.

Diagnosis
Dynamic CT scans are useful diagnostic tools in determining the nature and cause of delayed hydronephrosis. Perigraft fluid collections should be aspirated with image guidance to obtain culture and sensitivity information. Extravasated urine provides an ideal culture medium that can infect the prosthetic material. Sinograms through draining fistulas are helpful in identifying perigraft collections.

Treatment

The treatment of ureteral injuries is dependent on the status of the graft. If a ureteral injury is suspected at operation, indigo carmine dye can be injected intravenously and will appear in the retroperitoneum if a leak is present. If a ureteral injury is recognized and the graft is to remain in the retroperitoneum, the dangers of a failed repair with urine extravasation and subsequent graft infection are significant. A difficult choice must be made between repair or primary nephrectomy. This decision is influenced by the site and mechanism of ureteral injury and the status of the contralateral kidney. If the injury is distal and enough length is available, a ureteroneocystostomy is an appropriate choice. The options are not as appealing for more proximal injuries. When a ureteral injury is discovered in the postoperative period and the graft remains in the retroperitoneum, attempted repair is usually too dangerous and a nephrectomy should be performed. When the ureteral injury follows graft removal, repair should be attempted because prosthetic infection is no longer a risk.

Some ureteral injuries may be avoided by placing stents prior to operation and after the induction of anesthesia. The stents make identification of the ureter easier. Situations in which stents might benefit are reoperations, inflammatory aneurysms, complex aneurysms involving the aorta and iliac arteries, and graft removal.

ISCHEMIC COLITIS

Essentials of Diagnosis

- Severe: bloody diarrhea, left lower quadrant pain, signs of peritonitis, blackened mucosa on sigmoidoscopy.
- Mild: abdominal tenderness, leukocytosis, prolonged ileus, or diarrhea, mucosal changes only.

General Considerations

Ischemic colitis following operations on the abdominal aorta is usually due to interruption of prograde flow in the inferior mesenteric artery (IMA) in the setting of compromised collateral flow from the superior mesenteric artery (SMA) system and the hypogastric arteries. The incidence of this complication depends on the criteria used to establish the diagnosis. If patients undergo routine sigmoidoscopy, the incidence of ischemic colitis following aortic grafting ranges from 6% to 10%. Clinically significant colitis occurs in a smaller percentage of patients (1–2%). Less common causes are atheroemboli and inadvertent dissection in the sigmoid mesentery and damage of important collateral arteries.

The preoperative arteriogram is helpful in assessing the status of the inferior mesenteric circulation. Large collateral vessels connecting the inferior and superior mesenteric circulations (**meandering artery**) should raise questions about the safety of IMA ligation. The arteriogram in Figure 17–4 shows a meandering artery

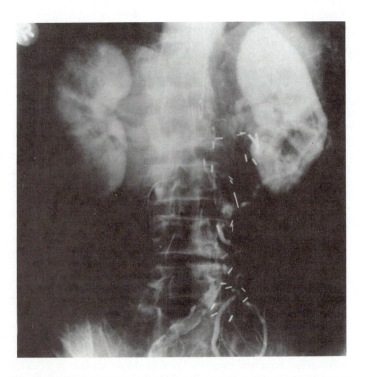

Figure 17–4. Arteriogram showing a large meandering artery in a patient with aortoiliac occlusive disease. Inflow was documented intraoperatively from the superior mesenteric artery so the inferior mesenteric artery was not reimplanted.

in a patient with aortoiliac occlusive disease. At operation, the Doppler analysis showed that inflow was clearly from the SMA so that the IMA could be ligated safely. The IMA only can be ligated in this instance when flow is clearly in the direction of SMA to IMA. A number of methods have been described to determine whether the IMA can be ligated. Ernst (1985) has shown that if the back pressure is 40 mmHg in the IMA the IMA could be safely ligated. Otherwise, reimplantation of the IMA is required. Hobson has determined that if a Doppler signal is present in the distal colonic mesentery at the conclusion of the procedure, IMA ligation is safe. Occlusion of both hypogastric arteries or devascularization of them because of the setup of the bypass also raises the incidence of colonic ischemia. Every effort should be made to perfuse at least one hypogastric artery. If this is impossible, the IMA, if patent, should be reimplanted.

Clinical Findings

A. Severe Form: Colon ischemia can take many forms after operation. In the most extreme variety, the patient has bloody diarrhea within the first few postoperative days. The patient will complain of left lower quadrant pain, and signs of peritonitis will be present. Sigmoidoscopy reveals blackened mucosa. Affected patients must be operated on emergently because of the presence of transmural infarction of the sigmoid colon. Prompt operation may prevent contamination of the graft. The involved intestine should be resected and the proximal end brought out as a colostomy. The mortality rate for this form of ischemic colitis is 50%.

B. Mild Form: The mildest and most common form of ischemic colitis involves the mucosa only. Clinical symptoms may be absent, and the diagnosis is made when routine postoperative sigmoidoscopy is performed. No treatment is required. An intermediate form involves both the mucosa and the muscularis. Patients with the mild form of colonic ischemia have abdominal tenderness, leukocytosis, prolonged ileus, or diarrhea. These patients require treatment with antibiotics, bowel rest, and a diverting colostomy. Many will progress to form a colonic stricture, which requires resection at the time of colostomy closure.

Treatment

Prompt diagnosis and an aggressive operative approach to patients with ischemic colitis are important in increasing survival and reducing the likelihood of graft infection. Patients who develop lower abdominal pain with diarrhea following aortic grafting should have prompt sigmoidoscopy. Patients can be stratified on the basis of the findings. Those with involvement of the mucosa alone can be placed at bowel rest and followed up with repeat studies. Those with deeper involvement should have surgical exploration. Nontransmural ischemia involving the muscularis should be treated by a diverting colostomy. Full-thickness involvement requires resection of the involved intestine with an end colostomy. If the graft limb of an aortoiliac or femoral bypass has been contaminated, it should be covered with omentum. If frank fecal contamination of the graft has occurred, the graft should be removed.

Several technical maneuvers at operation can reduce the incidence of ischemic colitis. Dissection around the diseased areas should be minimized. Large IMAs should be protected from emboli by a bulldog clamp. Dissection around the IMA should be done only at its aortic origin to prevent important collateral branches from being injured. The aortic anastomosis should be end to side in occlusive disease when the IMA is large. Large IMAs should be reimplanted when end-to-end anastomoses are required. The sigmoid colon should be inspected at the conclusion of the procedure. If Doppler signals are identified at the mesenteric border, the colon is almost always viable. If the sigmoid colon is ischemic, an attempt should be made to improve flow. This can be done by reimplanting a patent IMA that had been ligated, by correcting a superior mesenteric artery stenosis (if present), and by ensuring that the hypogastric arteries are perfused.

SPINAL CORD ISCHEMIA

Essentials of Diagnosis

- Paralysis.
- Buttocks and colon ischemia.

General Considerations

Spinal cord ischemia and paraplegia are very rare after operations on the infrarenal abdominal aorta. When they do occur, the complication often involves the cauda equina or the spinal roots and the patient presents with an asymmetric reduction in neurologic function. Although interruption of the greater medullary artery of Adamkiewicz (T9–T10) has been incriminated in cases of paraplegia following operation on the thoracic and upper abdominal aorta, it is not the main cause of paraplegia after operations below the renal arteries. When the greater medullary artery is low-lying and arises below the renal arteries, its interruption is unavoidable, as is the resultant complication.

The typical cause of paraplegia following infrarenal procedures is the interruption of the circulation to the lower spinal cord and cauda because of pelvic devascularization (Fig 17–5). Often, paraplegia occurs with colon and buttock ischemia and increases the mortality from this complication. The devascularization may be unavoidable as well, but there are circumstances in which the pelvic blood supply can be maintained. The critical anatomic fact is that the blood supply to the lower spinal cord comes partly from the hypogastric artery via iliolumbar and lateral sacral arteries. The same precautions that apply to preventing colon is-

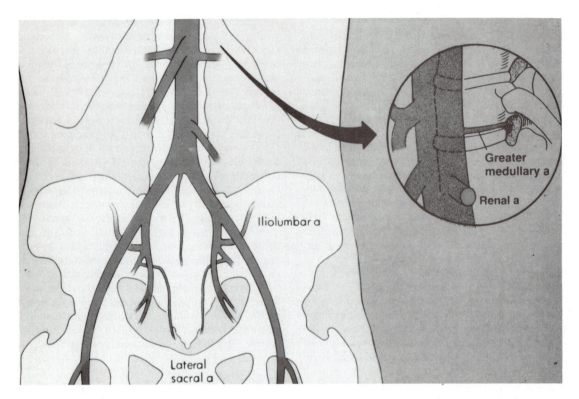

Figure 17–5. The anatomy of the spinal cord circulation. The greater medullary artery arises above the renal arteries and should not be interfered with during operations on the infrarenal aorta. The distal spinal cord is perfused form the iliolumbar and lateral sacral arteries. Interruption by either lack of perfusion of the hypogastric system or embolization can result in spinal cord ischemia.

chemia apply here. At least one hypogastric artery should be perfused if at all possible. This may mean performing an end-to-side aortic anastomosis when the external iliac arteries are occluded and retrograde flow to the hypogastric arteries is not possible.

Prevention

Although spinal cord ischemia is not always preventable, some important considerations can reduce its incidence. The preoperative arteriogram should be examined for external iliac artery disease. Bilateral occlusions mandate an end-to-side proximal anastomosis when operating for occlusive disease or reimplantation of an IMA when operating for aneurysms. A lateral aortogram may identify a large proximal posterior lumbar vessel, which may represent an anomalously low artery of Adamkiewicz that should be preserved. Avoid excessive manipulation of a diseased aorta, and if manipulation is necessary it should be done only when the outflow vessels are protected from atheroembolization. Hypogastric arterial flow should be evaluated prior to completion of any aortic procedure with Doppler signals and palpation. If bilateral hypogastric aneurysms are resected, one hypogastric artery should be revascularized, if possible, with a limb to the outflow vessels.

Prognosis

After paraplegia is recognized in the postoperative period, little can be done. Early reoperation to maximize pelvic blood flow may help to limit the amount of buttock and colon ischemia and may help ischemic, still viable areas of the spinal cord. However, no direct evidence exists to support this consideration.

FALSE ANEURYSMS (Pseudoaneurysms)

Essentials of Diagnosis

- Pulsatile femoral mass.
- Back pain (in case of retroperitoneal false aneurysm).

False aneurysms or pseudoaneurysms are aneurysms that form without a complete arterial wall. They are really localized hematomas contained by surrounding tissues. The wall is composed of fibrous tissue. False aneurysms may rupture, cause thrombosis, or embolization of mural thrombus, and therefore should be repaired when recognized. Their incidence ranges from 3% to 5% after aortofemoral bypass, and they occur most often at the femoral anastomosis.

Numerous factors are responsible for the development of a false aneurysm. Prior to the use of non-absorbable monofilament suture material, false aneurysms were due mainly to the absorption and fragmentation of the silk used for making the anastomosis. Suture failure is no longer a factor. The most common cause of false aneurysms is the degeneration of the arterial wall with the partial dehiscence of an intact suture line. Infection may also be a factor and should always be considered, particularly when *S epidermidis* is involved because an inflammatory response with purulent material will not be present. Send samples of the graft for culture and instruct the lab to use sonication techniques to increase the yield of positive results. Faulty operative technique with inadequate bites, tension on the anastomosis due to a short graft, or endarterectomy of the host vessel may also lead to the development of a pseudoaneurysm.

Clinical Findings

The diagnosis of a femoral pseudoaneurysm is by palpation of a pulsatile mass, which may be confirmed by ultrasonography. When a femoral pseudoaneurysm is diagnosed, a search for others should be undertaken. Most femoral artery aneurysms are bilateral, and around 15% to 20% will have associated aortic false aneurysms. Arteriography is not necessary unless the outflow is in question. The arteriogram in Figure 17–6 shows bilateral false aneurysms after an aortofemoral bypass. The diagnosis of a retroperitoneal false aneurysm is more difficult; therefore, patients are more likely to present with symptoms of back pain as the retroperitoneal false aneurysm enlarges or ruptures.

Treatment

Most false aneurysms should be repaired. They are treated by excision with graft extension. The most important element of the operation is control of the vessels in a reoperative area. The best place to obtain control for an aortic pseudoaneurysm is at the supraceliac aorta after division of the crus of the diaphragm. The aorta can be safely controlled here, and the old graft and anastomosis can be isolated. The diagram in Figure 17–7 depicts the difficulty in trying to control an aortic pseudoaneurysm directly. Dissection risks severe hemorrhage due to inadvertent entry into the sac and damage to the left renal vein, renal arteries, or duodenum. Repair requires the insertion of a new graft from the débrided aorta to the old graft. This graft can be short, but do not attempt to repair the defect primarily. The distal graft can be either dissected out and clamped or controlled with a balloon catheter.

Proximal control of a femoral pseudoaneurysm requires a clamp on the graft limb. This is best done by reflecting the inguinal ligament and clamping the prosthesis in the retroperitoneum. Again, the false aneurysm sac should not be entered until proximal control has been obtained. The outflow vessels and the

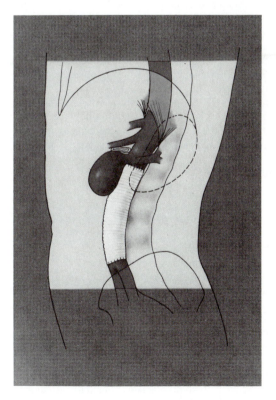

Figure 17–7. Diagram showing the difficulty in controlling a false aneurysm at the proximal anastomosis of an aortic graft. Not only can serious hemorrhage occur from inadvertent entry into the sac, but the dudodenum left renal vein and renal arteries can be damaged.

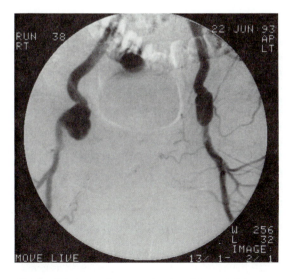

Figure 17–6. Arteriogram showing bilateral false aneurysms after aortofemoral graft. Arteriography is not necessary to make this diagnosis but is helpful in defining outflow vessels.

common femoral artery also require control. If the superficial femoral artery is chronically occluded, the easiest way to obtain distal control is to divide it and lift it upward. This allows access to the posterior surface of the common femoral artery and the deep femoral artery. Continuing this dissection allows for control of the proximal common femoral artery. The graft limb is detached from the anastomosis and the artery débrided. A short interposition graft is then sewn to the limb of the graft and to the new outflow.

If the superficial femoral is patent, the dissection is more difficult and the deep femoral artery can be safely controlled by inserting a balloon-tipped catheter to prevent backbleeding.

MATERIAL FAILURE

Essential of Diagnosis
• Significant dilatation of prosthesis.

Structural failure of a polyester prosthesis is an exceedingly rare event. This type of failure may be due to degeneration of the fabric or failure in fabrication. A modest dilatation occurs in most prostheses over time. In one study performed at 33 months after implantation, Dacron grafts dilated 15% in normotensive patients and 21% in hypertensive patients. This amount of dilatation is consistent with manufacturers' specifications and should not be considered as a major complication. Sporadic reports have appeared regarding localized saccular dilatations in the body of the grafts (Fig 17–8), which have been successfully repaired with segments of new prosthetic material. Dilatation is not associated with the development of anastomotic false aneurysms. Graft segments analyzed after repair of false aneurysms show no evidence of fabric failure.

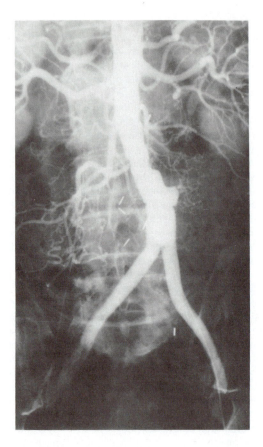

Figure 17–8. Occasionally, a false aneurysm forms as a saccular outpouching from the body of a prosthetic graft. This is a defect in fabric manufacturing and fortunately is rare. Treatment is excision and replacement with a new prosthesis.

SEXUAL DYSFUNCTION

Essentials of Diagnosis
• Erectile dysfunction.
• Retrograde ejaculation.

The association of male sexual dysfunction and aortoiliac occlusive disease was recognized by Réné Leriche in 1923. It became apparent that with operative correction, sexual dysfunction improved in some and deteriorated in others. A complete sexual history must be taken for any man considering an aortic reconstruction. Two mechanisms potentially affect sexual function in men after surgery on the abdominal aorta: (1) operative division of the genital autonomic nerves causing retrograde ejaculation and (2) interruption of the pelvic blood supply causing erectile dysfunction. Operations on the abdominal aorta should

therefore be aimed at preserving both the autonomic nerves and the pelvic blood supply. The risk of retrograde ejaculation in a man who desires to have children should preclude a dissection in the region of the autonomic nerves.

Two preventive measures for reducing sexual dysfunction consist in using a nerve-sparing technique for the aortic dissection and ensuring that the hypogastric arteries are perfused. The nerve-sparing technique makes use of the knowledge that the autonomic nerves course on the left anterior surface of the aorta surrounding the IMA and traveling to the aortic bifurcation in the midline. The aortotomy should then be made to the right of midline, the nerves retracted, and the IMA sutured from within. It is also important to know the status of the hypogastric arteries and to create the bypass so that flow is at least as good as it was preoperatively. This may mean creating a third limb from an aortobifemoral graft to the hypogastric artery. These maneuvers can reduce but not eliminate the incidence of sexual dysfunction.

REFERENCES

Bergen JJ et al: Ureteral changes after aortic surgery: Significance in diagnosis and treatment. In: *Current Critical Problems in Vascular Surgery,* vol 4. Veith F (editor). Quality Medical Publishing, 1992:267.

Brewster DC et al: Reoperation for aortofemoral graft limb occlusion: Optimal methods and long-term results. J Vasc Surg 1987;5:363.

Calligaro KD et al: New method for managing infected prosthetic grafts in the groin. In: *Current Critical Problems in Vascular Surgery,* vol 3. Veith FV (editor). Quality Medical Publishing, 1991:374.

Ernst CB: Intestinal ischemia following abdominal aortic reconstruction. In: *Complications in Vascular Surgery.* Bernard VM, Towne JB (editors). Grune & Stratton, 1985:325.

Hobson RW II et al: Assessment of colonic ischemia during aortic surgery by Doppler ultrasound. J Surg Res 1976; 20:231.

May AG, DeWeese JA, Rob CG: Changes in sexual function following operation on the abdominal aorta. Surgery 1969;65:41.

Picone AL et al: Spinal cord ischemia following operations on the abdominal aorta. J Vasc Surg 1986;3:94.

Reilly LM et al: Improved management of aortic graft infection: The influence of operation sequence and staging. J Vasc Surg 1987;5:421.

18 Aneurysms of the Abdominal Aorta & Iliac Arteries

Jack L. Cronenwett, MD, & Lawrence N. Sampson, MD

Aneurysms are defined as localized dilatations at least 1.5 times the diameter of the normal artery. They may be saccular or fusiform and are adjacent to a normal-sized arterial segment. Diffuse arterial dilation is termed **ectasia,** whereas **arteriomegaly** refers to ectasia of several arterial segments, usually associated with multiple aneurysms. Because arteriomegaly is rare, most patients with multiple aneurysms have intervening segments of normal-sized artery.

Abdominal aortic aneurysms (AAAs) are the 13th leading cause of death, accounting for more than 15,000 deaths per year. Based on autopsy series, the incidence of AAAs in 60–70-year-old patients is 4% in men and 1% in women. Death rates from ruptured AAA follow a similar age distribution (Fig 18–1).

Essentials of Diagnosis
- Abdominal/back pain of sudden onset.
- Hypotension.
- A pulsatile abdominal mass.

General Considerations
The normal aortic diameter gradually decreases from the thorax to the aortic bifurcation, is larger in men than women, and increases with age. Thus, the precise definition of AAA varies among individuals. For practical purposes, a diameter of 3 cm is a useful minimum size criterion. AAAs are 4–6 times more common in men than in women, and their incidence increases with age in both sexes. During a recent 30-year interval, the incidence of AAAs increased 4-fold. This was due to both increased detection with better imaging techniques and a real increase in age-adjusted AAA incidence.

The infrarenal aorta is the most common location for clinically significant aneurysms. Among AAAs undergoing surgical repair, about 95% are infrarenal; only 5% involve the suprarenal aorta. Although 50% of AAAs extend to involve the iliac arteries, isolated iliac artery aneurysms are rare. Isolated aneurysms of the suprarenal aorta are extremely rare unless they have an associated thoracic or infrarenal component. Concomitant thoracic aneurysms are more common and may occur in up to 12% of patients with AAAs. Peripheral aneurysms (femoral or popliteal) are present in about 15% of patients with AAAs. As dilatation of the aorta occurs, elongation also results, leading to a tortuous configuration of the aneurysmal aorta and iliac arteries.

A. Pathophysiology: AAAs represent a degenerative process that has often been attributed to atherosclerosis because of the elderly age of the patients affected and the universal atherosclerotic changes in their arteries (Fig 18–2). This theory fails to account for the alternative development of occlusive disease in many atherosclerotic aortas, which implies a more complex cause of AAAs. The normal aortic tunica media consists of elastin and collagen fibers with smooth muscle cells and matrix. Elastin is known to provide compliance, whereas collagen provides strength in the normal aorta. Moreover, digestion of elastin leads to aortic dilatation, whereas digestion of collagen leads to aortic rupture in experimental models.

Histologically, AAAs demonstrate fragmentation of elastin layers and decreased elastin content. Ultimately, the aneurysmal aorta has a thin and fibrotic tunica media with only a few elastin layers remaining. Intimal atherosclerosis is typical, but the medial degenerative process distinguishes aneurysms from the intimal-medial thickening that occurs in occlusive atherosclerosis. As AAAs enlarge, thrombus is laminated on the intimal surface in progressively greater quantity.

Elastin and collagen are continually synthesized by aortic smooth muscle cells and degraded by proteinases in the normal remodeling of arterial wall matrix. An imbalance of these processes could lead to AAA formation. Increased elastase levels and decreased elastin have been found in aneurysmal aortas compared with normal aortas or in patients with occlusive disease. Increased collagenase and decreased collagen have been found in larger aneurysms, particularly in those that ruptured. Increased proteinase activity could be related to increased production or to a decreased inhibitor level. Reduced levels of proteinase inhibitors (tissue inhibitor of metalloproteinase-1 and α_1-antitrypsin) have been shown in some AAA patients.

The infrarenal location of most aortic aneurysms has been attributed to both hemodynamic and structural influences. Reflected waves from the aortic bi-

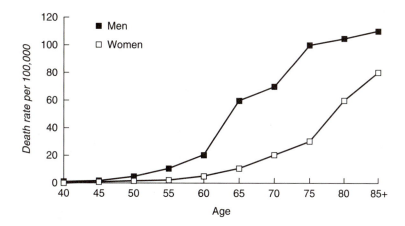

Figure 18–1. Death rate by age from ruptured AAA for men and women.

furcation increase pulsatility and wall tension in a non-compliant, atherosclerotic aorta. Increased aortic pulsatility due to other increases in peripheral resistance, such as lower extremity amputation, has also increased the incidence of AAAs. Structural differences in the infrarenal aorta may also influence the propensity for aneurysm formation in this location.

Immune mechanisms may contribute to the formation of AAAs. An increased presence of inflammatory cells, immunoglobulins, and cytokines has been found within AAAs compared with normal aortas.

Inflammatory cells are an important potential source of collagenase or elastase, which could lead to structural damage; however, an association between the location of these cells and the specific site of elastin/collagen loss is not clear.

The correlation between genetic inheritance and AAA is being investigated.

B. Gender and Family History: Because of their high incidence and propensity for rupture, AAAs are the 10th leading cause of death in men over 55 years of age in the USA. In men, AAAs begin to occur at age 50 and reach peak incidence at age 80. In women, their onset appears delayed, beginning at age 70 and peaking in incidence at age 90.

Studies of patients undergoing AAA repair indicate that family history is an important predictor of aneurysm development. Fifteen to 25% of patients with AAAs have a first-degree relative with an AAA, compared with only 2–3% of control patients without AAAs. Conversely, 8% of first-degree relatives of patients with AAAs have a clinically apparent AAA. The familial incidence of AAAs increases in relatives of women. In a surgical series of patients undergoing repair, women accounted for 35% of patients with a family history of AAA, but for only 14% of patients without familial AAAs. Furthermore, the incidence of AAA rupture in women with familial AAAs was 30% compared with 17% in male patients with familial AAAs.

Clinical Findings

A. Physical Examination: Although AAAs can be detected by physical examination, the sensitivity of physical examination depends on the aneurysm size,

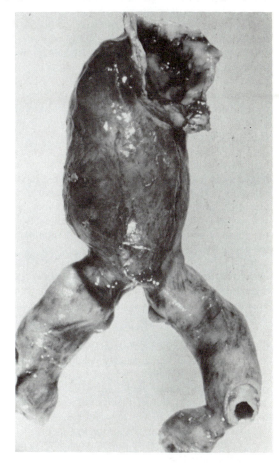

Figure 18–2. Autopsy specimen of an infrarenal AAA not involving the iliac arteries. Proximal aorta has been transected at the neck just below the renal arteries.

the obesity of the patient, the skill of the examiner, and the focus of the examination. In a population-based study, the positive predictive value of physical examination for detecting AAAs larger than 3.5 cm was only 15%. Conversely, AAAs may be suspected in thin patients with a prominent, but normal-sized aorta or in patients with a mass overlying the aorta that transmits a prominent pulse. The accuracy of physical examination for AAA size measurement is poor, resulting in an overestimation of size based on intervening abdominal structures. Therefore, patients (especially men over age 60) who present with new abdominal or back pain should have the diagnosis of AAA excluded by an imaging study.

B. Signs and Symptoms: Most AAAs (about 75%) cause no symptoms unless they rupture. Some patients with AAAs experience abrupt abdominal or back pain and undergo emergency laparotomy for presumed rupture, at which time no hemorrhage is found. These AAAs, which are usually tender and may have surrounding localized edema, are termed **acutely expanding aneurysms** and are considered an immediate precursor of rupture. These account for 8–26% of AAAs explored for presumed AAA rupture.

Aneurysm rupture means disruption of the aortic wall with extravasation of blood. The severity of accompanying hypotension and shock depends on both the extent of blood loss and the cardiovascular compensation by patients with ruptured AAAs. Although the classic presentation of ruptured AAA includes abdominal/back pain, hypotension, and a pulsatile abdominal mass, all 3 findings are found in only 20% of patients with proven AAA rupture.

Most patients with ruptured AAAs present with at least transient hypotension, which develops into frank hypotension and shock over a period of hours. Rarely, rupture is effectively contained within the retroperitoneum, and symptoms can persist for a period of days or even weeks. Such patients appear to manifest acute or chronic inflammatory conditions, thus confusing the diagnosis.

Most ruptured AAAs in patients who survive long enough to receive medical attention have ruptured into the retroperitoneal space with some containment of blood loss, resulting in a retroperitoneal hematoma. Autopsies indicate that 18% of AAAs rupture anteriorly into the peritoneal cavity and 82% posteriorly into the retroperitoneal space (Fig 18–3). Acute pain in the back, flank, and abdomen usually results, sometimes with radiation to the thigh, groin, or testicles. Ecchymoses can result in the flank (Grey Turner's sign), scrotum, or thighs as blood dissects in these retroperitoneal planes.

Occasionally, large AAAs cause symptoms from local compression (eg, early satiety, nausea or vomiting from duodenal compression, hydronephrosis from ureteral compression, or venous thrombosis from iliocaval venous compression). Posterior erosion of AAAs into adjacent vertebrae can lead to back pain.

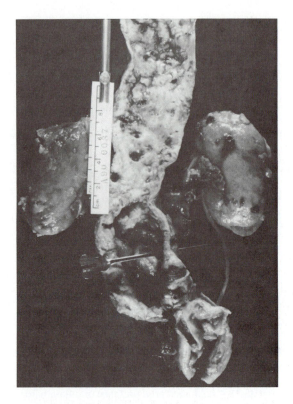

Figure 18–3. Autopsy specimen of the abdominal aorta demonstrating posterolateral rupture of infrarenal AAA (probe through site of rupture). Note associated atherosclerotic plaque in the suprarenal aorta.

Even without bony involvement, AAAs may cause chronic back or abdominal pain that is vague and ill defined. Acute ischemic symptoms can also occur from distal embolization of thrombotic debris contained within the AAA or from acute aneurysmal occlusion, presumably due to local dissection within the bulky intraluminal thrombus. Embolism is much more common than acute thrombosis, but both combined occur in less than 2–5% of patients with AAA. In patients with distal emboli, a proximal aneurysm source must always be considered, especially in those without apparent occlusive disease (ie, with normal peripheral pulses; Fig 18–4).

C. Imaging Studies: Since most patients with AAAs are asymptomatic, it is not surprising that AAAs are often discovered incidentally by imaging studies performed for the evaluation of unrelated symptoms. Increasing use of ultrasonography, computed tomography (CT), and magnetic resonance imaging (MRI) providing accurate diagnostic and measurement techniques has led to more frequent detection of very small AAAs.

1. Ultrasonography–Ultrasound scanning is the least expensive and most frequently used examination, particularly for initial confirmation of a suspicion of

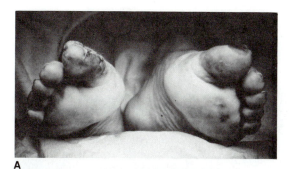

A

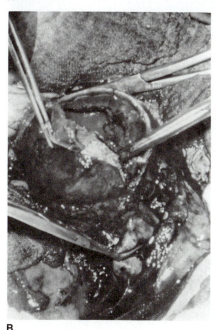

B

Figure 18–4. *A:* This patient experienced multiple emboli to the foot from a proximal AAA. ***B:*** The AAA contained degenerating thrombus that was loose and easily accounted for the embolic source.

AAA during physical examination and long-term follow-up of small AAAs. Size measurements are more accurate in the anteroposterior than the lateral dimension (accuracy about 3 mm). Bowel gas can cause images of the suprarenal aorta and iliac arteries to be more difficult to obtain. Ultrasonography cannot accurately determine the presence of retroperitoneal hemorrhage and often cannot accurately determine the upper extent of an AAA (Fig 18–5).

2. **CT**–CT scanning is more expensive than ultrasonography and involves radiation exposure, but is more accurate and provides a more precise definition of the extent of the AAA. The technique of spiral-CT scanning provides rapid imaging with better resolution of the visceral aortic branches when thin slices are obtained. CT scanning is particularly useful for excluding a potentially contained rupture in a minimally symptomatic patient, for defining the superior extent of an AAA, and for detecting other unsuspected pathology such as an inflammatory aneurysm.

3. **MRI and MRA**–Although less commonly available, MRI appears comparable to CT scanning, while avoiding radiation exposure. Magnetic resonance angiography (MRA) may also be obtained with special equipment to provide noninvasive arterial flow visualization combined with spatial resolution of the AAA and adjacent arteries. This modality, still under active evaluation, may supplant the need for both arteriography and CT scanning for the preoperative evaluation of AAAs if the resolution of MRA can be improved for the visceral arteries.

4. **Arteriography**–Arteriography is not an accurate technique to determine the presence or size of AAAs due to thrombus usually contained within the aneurysm, which diminishes the size of the contrast-filled lumen. However, it is useful for preoperative evaluation before AAA repair, especially in patients with known or suspected renal, mesenteric, or iliac artery occlusive disease, which might modify the surgical approach. With the advent of high-resolution CT and MRI, many surgeons believe that routine arteriography is not cost-effective unless specific clinical factors indicate potentially complicated AAA surgery. These factors include hypertension or renal insufficiency, symptoms of mesenteric ischemia, decreased femoral pulses, suprarenal aneurysm involvement, and other known anomalies such as horseshoe kidney and pelvic kidney. Arteriography is not able to detect unsuspected pathology such as cholelithiasis, intra-abdominal malignancy, venous anomalies, and large iliac aneurysm, but it has the ability to detect multiple renal arteries and to define the patency of the inferior mesenteric artery (IMA) and the pelvic circulation, which may have an important impact on the adequacy of pelvic circulation after AAA repair.

Risk Factors

Factors that significantly increase the incidence of AAAs in screening studies are coronary artery disease (CAD), hypertension, peripheral artery occlusive disease, smoking, and chronic obstructive pulmonary disease (COPD). Depending on the distribution of these risk factors, ultrasound screening studies yield a different prevalence of asymptomatic AAA detection (Table 18–1). In selected patients with several risk factors, occurrence of AAAs may be as high as 35%. The presence of other peripheral aneurysms is also an important marker for an increased probability of AAA. Of patients with popliteal aneurysms, 41% have a concomitant AAA, whereas 66% of patients with femoral aneurysms have an AAA.

The decision to electively repair a specific AAA depends on a careful comparison of AAA rupture risk with elective operative risk, taken in the context of a patient's overall life expectancy.

A. AAA Rupture Risk: Independent studies have confirmed that AAA rupture risk increases with

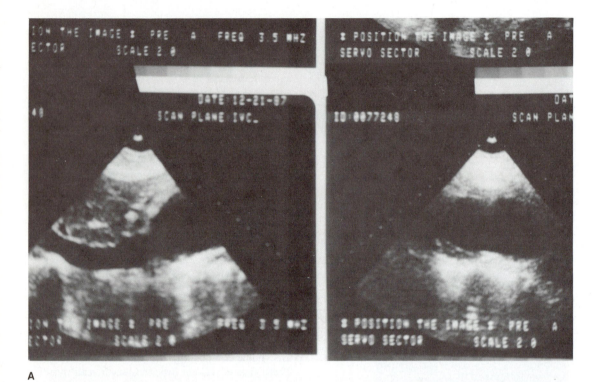

A

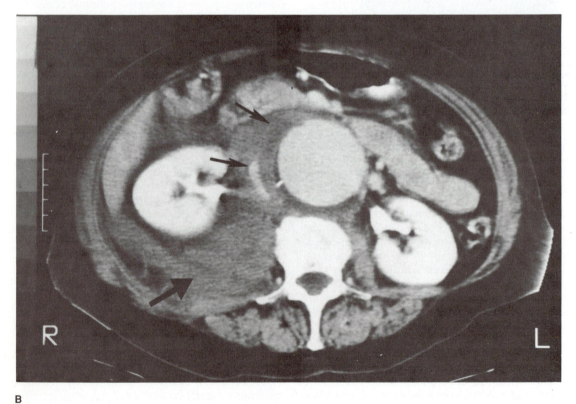

B

Figure 18–5. ***A:*** Longitudinal views of ultrasound scan of an AAA, clearly showing the aneurysm neck with no evidence of rupture. ***B:*** Computed tomography of the same patient as in ***A*** demonstrating right lateral rupture (*small arrows*) and a retroperitoneal hematoma not visible by ultrasonography (*large arrow*).

Table 18–1. Prevalence of AAA larger than 3 cm in men.

Risk Factor	Men	
	Present	Absent
Overall	8%	
CAD	11%	7%
Smokers	13%	6%
PVD	13%	6%
COPD	12%	8%
Hypertension	12%	6%
COPD + hypertension	35%	4%

From ultrasound screening methods.
CAD, Coronary artery disease; PVD, peripheral vascular disease; COPD, chronic obstructive pulmonary disease.

aneurysm size, hypertension, and chronic obstructive pulmonary disease (COPD). Size is the most widely accepted predictor of AAA rupture and the usual criterion for elective repair (Fig 18–6). Hypertension is an intuitive risk factor based on Laplace's law, in which tension responsible for rupture in the aneurysm wall equals blood pressure multiplied by the AAA radius ($t = p \times r$). COPD and bronchiectasis are also considered to be important independent predictors of AAA rupture, which together with hypertension, appear to explain why some small AAAs rupture. The mechanism of the relation between AAA rupture and COPD is uncertain, but it may be related to increased proteinase destruction of connective tissue in both aortic wall and pulmonary parenchyma. Other less certain factors such as smoking, rapid AAA expansion rate, and a positive family history have also been suggested to increase AAA rupture risk.

AAAs generally increase nonlinearly as a function of size at the rate of 10% diameter increase per year. Thus, larger aneurysms expand more rapidly. Greater pulse pressure (systolic minus diastolic pressure) is also well correlated with increased expansion. Whether an increased AAA expansion rate translates into increased rupture rate (independent of absolute size) has not been proved.

B. Small AAAs: Considerable disagreement exists about the rupture risk of small AAAs (<4–5 cm diameter) and thus the appropriateness of elective repair. Based on autopsy results, 24% of AAAs 4–5 cm in diameter had ruptured at the time of death, as had 10% of AAAs less than 4 cm. However, these studies probably overestimate the risk of AAA rupture, since autopsies are more frequently performed after sudden deaths from unknown cause. Follow-up studies of patients with small AAAs variously estimate the rupture risk to be 0.4–5.4% per year. Differences are probably due to variation in other risk factors that influence rupture (eg, hypertension, COPD), differing case mix in referral-based studies, and patients undergoing elective repair during follow-up who artificially decrease the apparent rupture risk.

Most surgeons agree that 5-cm AAAs warrant elective repair in good-risk patients. However, some have recommended "selective management" in which small AAAs are followed up with ultrasound size measurements at 6-month intervals, reserving operation for patients who experience rapid AAA expansion (≥ 1 cm/yr) or symptoms suggesting acute expansion, or whose AAA reaches a given threshold diameter (eg, 6 cm). The 3-year outcome of this approach was that 27% of patients were still alive without AAA repair; 29% had died of other causes; 39% had required elective or urgent AAA repair; and 4% had experienced AAA rupture. Thus, the frequent need for elective AAA repair during follow-up has raised the question of whether early elective repair at the time of AAA diagnosis would be cost-effective, since rupture would be avoided, patients would be operated on when younger (and presumably healthier), and surgery might be less complicated when dealing with smaller AAAs.

Computed decision analysis models have indicated that early surgery, even for 4-cm AAAs in younger patients yields a survival benefit compared with watchful waiting until a 5-cm threshold size is reached. Cost-effectiveness analysis indicates that early repair of such 4-cm AAAs is cost-effective if the AAA rupture rate is 3% or more per year, the elective operative mortality rate of 5% or less, and the patient age is 70 years or less.

C. Cardiac Risk: Clinical criteria are useful for stratifying cardiac risk preoperatively. Angina, history of myocardial infarction (MI), Q wave on ECG, ventricular arrhythmia, congestive heart failure (CHF), diabetes, and age over 75 years have been found to increase the risk of postoperative cardiac events (unstable angina, MI, ischemic CHF, or cardiac death). Various combinations of these risk factors have been used to generate prediction criteria (Goldman, Detsky, Eagle) for perioperative cardiac morbidity. When few risk factors are present, the sensitivity for excluding a postoperative cardiac event varies from 54% to 92%, whereas the specificity for predicting such an event increases from 26% to 94% as the number of risk factors increase. It is well established that patients with AAAs have a high incidence of CAD. In consecutive series of patients with AAAs undergoing routine preoperative coronary arteriography, 6% had normal arteries, 29% had mild to moderate CAD, 29% had advanced compensated CAD, 31% had severe correctable CAD, and 5% had severe uncorrectable CAD. In patients without clinical evidence of CAD, 18% had severe correctable CAD, whereas in patients with clinically suspected CAD, 44% had severe correctable lesions. The inability to precisely assess preoperative cardiac risk with standard clinical evaluation has led to the application of a variety of more sensitive and sophisticated techniques.

1. Radionuclide thallium scanning–This diagnostic method effectively demonstrates areas of previous MI (no isotope uptake). When combined with exercise stress, this scan also demonstrates areas of

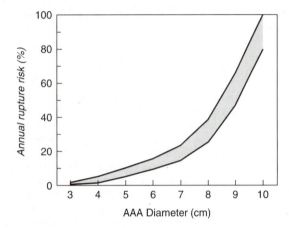

Figure 18–6. Estimated annual rupture risk as a function of AAA size. The range shown reflects differences in published estimates and probably reflects the influence of other important influences on rupture (hypertension and COPD).

marginal perfusion (late thallium uptake or redistribution) that are susceptible to infarction. Since many patients with AAAs are unable to undergo conventional stress testing due to exercise limitation, dipyridamole (Persantine) thallium scanning (DTS), which mimics stress by coronary vasodilatation, is an effective substitute. The sensitivity of this test is high (a patient without ischemic redistribution has a 0–10% risk of postoperative MI). However, the specificity is low, since only 25–50% of patients who have a positive test (redistribution) will have a postoperative MI. The specificity of DTS can be improved by quantitating the extent of ischemia. Patients with thallium redistribution in 2 or 3 different views (anterior, lateral, oblique) had a 36% likelihood of postoperative ischemic events, whereas none of the patients with single view redistribution had an event.

2. Echocardiography–Also useful for preoperative cardiac evaluation, echocardiography assesses valvular function and overall ventricular function by estimating ejection fraction (EF). Patients with markedly reduced EF (<35%) have been shown to have an operative mortality rate comparable to patients with more normal cardiac function. However, EF is a useful predictor of late survival after AAA repair. Patients with an EF of less than 35% had a 1-year survival rate of 57%, substantially lower than the 90% of those with an EF of 35% or more. Inability of echocardiography to stratify early postoperative risk is probably due to its failure to identify patients with good cardiac performance but substantial CAD and who might experience MI due to perioperative stress. If dobutamine (a predominately β_1-agonist) is infused during echocardiography, enhanced contractility results in normal segments, whereas areas with marginal perfusion demonstrate wall motion abnormality. As with

DTS, sensitivity of dobutamine stress echocardiography is high (95%), whereas the specificity is low (29%).

3. Continuous ECG (Holter) monitoring–Holter monitoring of patients after AAA surgery has demonstrated a high incidence of ST-segment depression, which has been positively correlated with development of MI occurring an average of 2 days postoperatively. Extension of such monitoring to the preoperative interval has also demonstrated a correlation with postoperative MI.

4. Angiography–Angiography is the gold standard for evaluating the details of coronary anatomy and for determining whether disease can be treated either by coronary artery bypass grafting (CABG) or by balloon angioplasty. Patients with minimal or no CAD demonstrated by angiography have a near 0% risk of postoperative MI. The specificity of arteriography is more difficult to evaluate, since not all patients with coronary lesions will experience postoperative MI, especially given the current techniques of perioperative management. Patients with severe, uncorrectable CAD who underwent AAA surgery have a higher mortality rate, but most deaths do not occur until several years postoperatively.

D. Operative Risk: Elective operative mortality rate after AAA repair is less than 5% in contemporary series and is strongly influenced by CAD, renal failure, and pulmonary disease. Without these risk factors, elective operative mortality rate is less than 2%, but may be as high as 50% if all 3 risk factors are severe. Age does not appear to be an important risk factor for increased mortality after elective AAA repair, indicating that physiologic rather than chronologic age is the important determinant of outcome. However, age alone is an important predictor of death after ruptured AAA repair, presumably because of the increased stress of the operation and the diminished reserve of older patients.

In addition to patient-specific risk factors, surgeons or hospitals who perform few AAA repairs (<5/year) experience an operative mortality rate 2–3 times higher than normal. Of patients with ruptured AAAs who arrive at hospitals, mortality rates range from 15% to 87%, with an average of 54%. A number of specific factors have been shown to predict increased risk of death from ruptured AAA, including age over 75–80 years, female gender, persistent preoperative hypotension despite volume replacement, preoperative hematocrit less than 25–30%, acute preoperative ECG abnormality or cardiac arrest, and preoperative renal or pulmonary dysfunction. The best predictor appears to be the extent of hemorrhage and shock prior to AAA repair. Following free intraperitoneal rupture with hemorrhage and shock, less than 10% of patients survive AAA repair. In contrast, survival is high (>80%) if AAA rupture is associated with only a small, well-contained retroperitoneal hematoma in a stable patient.

Intraoperative factors shown to correlate with high mortality during ruptured AAA repair include massive transfusion requirement, suprarenal AAA, free intraperitoneal rupture, technical difficulties such as venous injury, and prolonged aortic cross-clamp time. Unfortunately, no combination of these risk factors predicts outcome with certainty in individual patients. Thus, in the emergency setting, most patients should undergo attempted AAA repair if rupture is suspected, since there is usually not time for the extensive discussions on whether it is appropriate to withhold treatment.

An analysis of patients who died from ruptured AAAs indicates that 4 factors were primarily responsible: (1) failure to electively treat known AAAs; (2) errors in diagnosing AAA rupture leading to delayed treatment; (3) technical error during AAA repair, usually involving venous injury; and (4) undue delay in operative treatment after recognizing AAA rupture. Not only is AAA rupture associated with a high mortality rate, but it is extremely expensive because of the high rate of complications following surgery. Many patients ultimately die, but not without experiencing days to weeks of intensive care for multisystem organ failure.

Differential Diagnosis

Unstable patients with a distended abdomen, a known history of AAA, or a pulsatile mass should be expeditiously explored. Occasionally, a cause other ruptured AAA is found, but nearly always requires surgical treatment anyway. An ECG can be obtained rapidly to exclude an acute transmural MI, which might be aggravated by a negative laparotomy. Most common misdiagnoses are renal colic, diverticulitis, gastrointestinal (GI) hemorrhage, acute MI, and nonspecific low back pain. In the absence of hypotension, unless a pulsatile abdominal mass is noted, patients with AAA rupture who present with abdominal pain or back pain are especially likely to be misdiagnosed initially. For the patient in whom there is much diagnostic uncertainty, an ultrasound examination performed in the emergency room may reveal an AAA and thus expedite treatment. CT can exclude hemorrhage and thus allow delayed, elective repair after careful in-hospital evaluation, an approach that has been shown to reduce operative mortality compared with urgent repair of expanding, nonruptured AAAs. However, the evaluation of a potentially ruptured AAA with CT scanning must be performed expeditiously and in a hospital where emergency AAA repair can be performed if the patient becomes unstable.

Management

A. Perioperative: Improvements in perioperative care have led to significant reductions in morbidity and mortality following AAA surgery. Individualized care includes preoperative antibiotics (usually a cephalosporin) to reduce the risk of prosthetic graft infection. Ample intravenous access, intra-arterial pressure recording, and Foley catheter monitoring of urine output are routine. Because of the frequent association of cardiac abnormalities, pulmonary artery catheters are often useful to guide volume replacement therapy. Mixed venous oxygen tension measuring, available with these catheters, provides an additional estimate of global circulatory function. Transesophageal echocardiography has been recommended to monitor ventricular volume and wall motion abnormalities, especially during aortic clamping and declamping, to guide fluid administration and the use of vasoactive drugs.

When clinical evidence of pulmonary dysfunction exists, preoperative baseline arterial blood gases and pulmonary function testing is appropriate. Preoperative renal function is easily evaluated with blood urea nitrogen (BUN) and creatinine measurements. Preoperative arteriography must be cautiously used in a patient with renal failure because of the potential aggravating effects of intravenous contrast material.

B. Anesthesia: Nearly all patients undergo general anesthesia for AAA repair. The supplemental use of continuous epidural anesthesia, begun preoperatively and continued for postoperative pain control, is being carried out more frequently. This technique allows a lighter plane of general anesthesia to be maintained. Additional benefits are reduction in the sympathetic-catecholamine stress response and thus possible reduction of cardiac complications. One randomized trial found that general-epidural anesthesia demonstrated decreased deaths, cardiac events, infection, and overall complications. Although concern has been raised about possible complications of epidural hematoma in patients who are anticoagulated, this has proved to be rare if the epidural catheter is inserted before and removed after anticoagulation.

Surgical Treatment

Both "AAA repair" and "AAA resection" are terms used to describe contemporary operative treatment of AAAs, which actually consists of endoaneurysmal graft placement to exclude the aneurysm (Fig 18–7).

A. Emergent Repair: Prior to laparotomy overresuscitation of these unstable patients with blood or saline should be avoided, since high blood pressure increases aneurysm bleeding and disruption. Thus, systolic blood pressures of 80–100 mmHg can be tolerated if patients are not experiencing neurologic or cardiac compromise. For patients with frank shock, MAST trousers may be beneficial during transport to a surgical center, but the eventual outcome of these patients is poor.

Patients with known ruptured AAAs should be brought immediately to the operating room even when hemodynamically stable, where venous access, arterial catheterization, and other preanesthetic preparation can be accomplished urgently.

The abdomen should be prepped and draped prior to anesthesia, since anesthetic-induced loss of abdominal

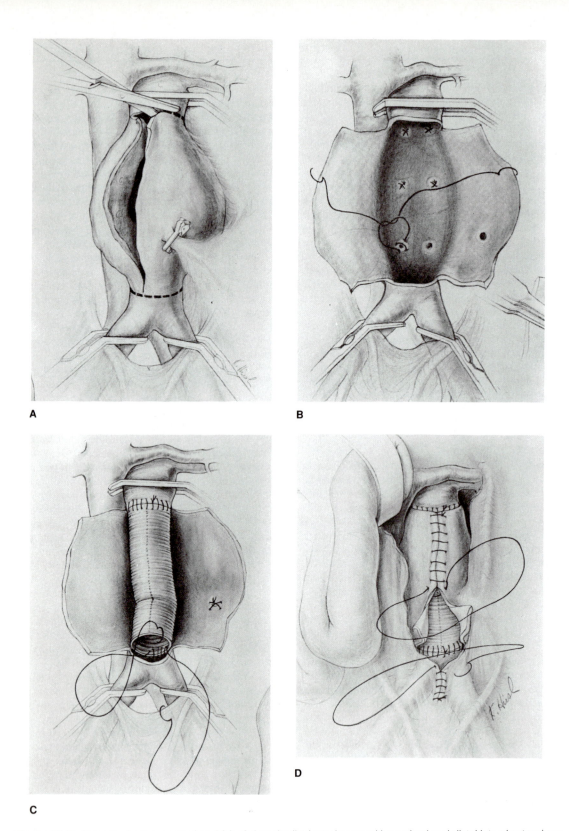

Figure 18–7. Steps in elective repair of an AAA. **A:** Longitudinal arteriotomy with proximal and distal lateral extensions, leaving posterior wall intact. Note infrarenal location of the clamp and the miniclamp on the inferior mesenteric artery. **B:** Open AAA with laminated thrombus removed and suture ligation of patent lumbar arteries. **C:** Endoaneurysmal placement of a tube graft with proximal anastomosis completed. **D:** Closing aneurysm over graft to prevent aortoenteric fistula. (Reproduced, with permission, from Cronenwett JL, Sampson LN: Aortoiliac aneurysms. In: *Atlas of Vascular Surgery.* Zarins CK, Gewertz BL [editors]. Churchill Livingstone, 1989.)

wall and peripheral vascular tone may precipitate sudden hypotension. The surgical approach for a ruptured AAA must emphasize rapid proximal aortic control, avoidance of venous injury, endoaneurysmal graft placement, adequate blood product replacement, and avoidance of hypothermia by various warming methods.

A midline incision should be rapidly performed and the extent of hemorrhage ascertained. Proximal aortic control is best obtained by compression through the lesser space or by actual dissection and clamping of the supraceliac aorta at this level. The retroperitoneal hematoma and aneurysm can then be directly entered and the neck of the aneurysm identified internally without the need for dissection of the renal or iliac veins. Distal aortic backbleeding can be controlled with iliac balloon occlusion catheters placed from within the AAA. The aortic graft is then anastomosed with minimal division of the proximal aorta to avoid any danger of venous injury. After completing the proximal aortic suture line, the supraceliac clamp is moved onto the graft below the renal arteries to minimize mesenteric and renal ischemic time.

If the retroperitoneal hematoma is minimal, AAA repair can proceed similarly to the elective technique with infrarenal aortic clamping. Because of the large volume of hemorrhage usually encountered with ruptured AAAs, a massive transfusion protocol coordinated with the blood bank is appropriate in addition to rapid autotransfusion devices. Heparin is usually not administered in this case because extensive hemorrhage and loss of coagulation products usually eliminate the risk of distal arterial thrombosis.

B. Elective Repair:

1. Transperitoneal vs. retroperitoneal–The aorta can be approached through a transperitoneal incision (midline or transverse) or through a retroperitoneal approach. In recent years, the left retroperitoneal approach has enjoyed a resurgence in popularity due to suggestions that pulmonary morbidity, ileus, and intravenous fluid requirements are decreased postoperatively. Relative indications for retroperitoneal exposure include a "hostile" abdomen caused by multiple previous transperitoneal operations, an abdominal wall stoma, a horseshoe kidney, an inflammatory aneurysm, or anticipated need for suprarenal endarterectomy or anastomosis. Relative indications for a transperitoneal approach include a ruptured AAA, coexistent intra-abdominal pathology, uncertain diagnosis, left-sided vena cava, large bilateral iliac aneurysms, or need for access to both renal arteries.

2. Operative conduct–Exposure of sufficient normal aorta proximal to an AAA may be difficult with a transperitoneal incision if the AAA originates just below the renal arteries. Ligation and division of the left renal vein is an alternative, but occasionally leads to renal dysfunction. If the left renal vein must be ligated, it should be done at its junction with the vena cava to maintain patency of collateral drainage through the gonadal vein. Left retroperitoneal exposure, with displacement of the left kidney anteriorly, avoids this problem and facilitates suprarenal exposure.

After obtaining exposure of the AAA and adjacent aorta and iliac arteries, a region of normal proximal aorta is identified to avoid embolization of intra-aortic plaque or thrombus during aortic clamping. If the iliac arteries are not diseased, the distal clamps should be applied first to further reduce risk of embolization. When the AAA approaches or involves the renal arteries, it is usually safer to apply the proximal cross-clamp above the celiac artery rather than risk injury to the intervening visceral arteries by clamping between the renal arteries and the superior mesenteric artery (SMA).

Regardless of the extent of an infrarenal AAA, it is desirable to construct the proximal aortic anastomosis near the renal arteries to avoid subsequent aneurysmal degeneration of residual infrarenal aorta. After the aneurysm is excluded, it is incised. Backbleeding lumbar arteries are controlled with sutures. If patent, the inferior mesenteric artery (IMA) is temporarily clamped to allow later assessment of backbleeding to discern the need for reimplantation.

Graft replacement can be accomplished with a straight tube graft of the infrarenal aorta in 40–50% of patients in whom the iliac arteries are uninvolved. Extension to the iliac arteries with an inverted Y-shaped graft is necessary in 50–60% of patients, because of aneurysmal involvement of the iliac arteries or severe calcification of the aortic bifurcation. Extension of this graft to the femoral level is indicated for severe concomitant iliac occlusive disease or rarely because of technical difficulties anticipated with a deep pelvic anastomosis. Iliac anastomoses are preferred because of increased infection and pseudoaneurysm complications associated with femoral anastomoses.

Graft material consists of either woven or knitted Dacron, or polytetrafluoroethylene. Anastomoses are constructed with permanent, usually polypropylene, monofilament sutures, in a continuous running fashion. For a thin or friable aortic wall, interrupted sutures or sutures reenforced with Teflon pledgets may be useful. Autotransfusion devices have been shown to be cost-effective during AAA surgery because of obligatory blood loss from lumbar branches, backbleeding, flushing, and so on. Systemic anticoagulation with heparin is used by most surgeons, with protamine reversal of this anticoagulant effect after flow restoration. Intraoperative measurement of activated clotting time allows accurate titration of anticoagulant effect and its reversal.

After graft placement, the aneurysm wall is used to wrap the prosthesis, effectively isolating it from the small intestine to prevent an aortoenteric fistula. IMA reimplantation, although not usually required, must be carefully considered when the pelvic circulation is compromised by internal iliac disease or when SMA collateral flow is inadequate as from SMA occlusive disease or previous intestinal surgery.

3. Concomitant revascularization–Indications for concomitant mesenteric/renal artery revascularization during elective AAA surgery are comparable to those used for disease isolated to these arteries. Occasionally, asymptomatic, high-grade stenoses of these visceral arteries warrant prophylactic reconstruction if the patient is at low operative risk and the AAA repair proceeds uneventfully. Since the natural history of asymptomatic renal and mesenteric stenoses is not precisely known, prophylactic repair appears justified only for high-grade stenoses.

C. Endovascular Repair: The **endovascular approach** is a promising approach with endovascular exclusion of AAAs using a stented graft (Fig 18–8). This technique, which has been developed in animals and is now in human trials, consists of the transfemoral placement of a thin-walled prosthetic graft that is attached to the proximal aorta with an internal wire stent with barbs that fix its location in the aorta. The proportion of patients ineligible for this approach due to anatomic factors such as the absence of a normal proximal aortic neck is not clear. This technique may further reduce the risk of elective AAA repair and may be especially appropriate for high-risk patients.

Complications

A. General Complications: Aortic surgery is technically demanding and, despite a low incidence, operative complications can be severe and fatal. Sig-

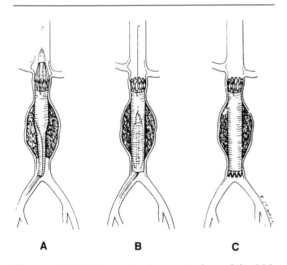

Figure 18–8. Endovascular placement of a graft for AAA repair. **A:** Inflating balloon, expanding stent to form proximal anastomosis. **B:** Balloon expansion of graft. **C:** Graft in place after distal stent expanded. (Reproduced, with permission, from Parodi JC: Endovascular repair of abdominal aortic aneurysms. In: *Advances in Vascular Surgery.* Whittemore AD, Bandyck DF, Cronenwett JL, Hertzer NR, White RA [editors]. Mosby-Yearbook, 1993.)

nificant hemorrhage usually results from difficulties with the proximal anastomosis or from venous injury. Juxtarenal aneurysms may compromise the length and quality of the proximal aortic neck if an infrarenal clamp is used. In these situations, proximal suture line bleeding, particularly when posterior, may be difficult to control. Occasionally, a friable aortic wall can lead to suture line disruption. Here, temporary aortic control at the supraceliac level facilitates anastomotic repair without excessive additional blood loss.

1. Injury–Venous bleeding usually results from injury to the iliac or left renal veins during initial exposure. Often, the distal AAA or common iliac aneurysm is densely adherent to the associated iliac vein, making circumferential arterial isolation hazardous. Occasionally, a posterior left renal vein or a large lumbar vein may pose similar hazards for proximal dissection. Careful suture repair of these venous injuries is required, occasionally facilitated by temporary division of the overlying artery.

Aortic cross-clamping results in a sudden increase in cardiac afterload, evidenced by hypertension, which can precipitate myocardial ischemia. Gradual clamp application carefully coordinated with anesthetic and vasoactive drug administration are required to avoid this problem. In contrast, aortic declamping with suddenly reduced afterload may cause significant hypotension. Adequate fluid and blood replacement is critical to avoid this complication.

Rarely, injury to an adjacent organ occurs during AAA repair. Ureteral injury should be repaired with a primary, spatulated anastomosis using fine, interrupted absorbable sutures over a removable stent. Splenic injury due to excessive retraction may result in hemorrhage that should be controlled by splenectomy, since late hemorrhage is poorly tolerated if attempted splenic repair fails. Inadvertent enterotomy usually prompts termination of the procedure with subsequent AAA repair.

2. Ischemia–Sigmoid colon ischemia following AAA repair is a rare but devastating complication, more likely to occur following ruptured AAA repair. It may result from embolization into or ligation of the IMA and internal iliac arteries. Fortunately, the abundance of collateral flow to the sigmoid colon usually prevents this problem. Careful inspection of the sigmoid colon following graft placement is important and may be facilitated by Doppler insonation of the bowel wall and mesentery.

Preoperative arteriographic indicators of risk for sigmoid ischemia include a stenotic or occluded SMA, a large patent IMA with ascending collateral flow, and occlusion of both internal iliac arteries. Postoperatively, colon ischemia should be suspected in the presence of cramping abdominal pain or early diarrhea, usually containing blood. This should prompt immediate flexible sigmoidoscopy or colonoscopy. In most cases, patchy, partial-thickness mucosal necrosis and sloughing can be detected. In more severe cases of transmural infarction, early reexploration is indicated to avoid the 90% or more fatality rate reported with delayed recognition of sigmoid ischemia. Treatment requires sigmoid resection and colostomy, often combined with aortic graft excision followed by extra-anatomic bypass if substantial contamination has occurred.

Lower extremity ischemia may occur after AAA surgery, usually from embolization of aneurysmal debris that occurs during AAA mobilization or aortoiliac clamping. Usually, such emboli are small, resulting in transient, patchy areas of skin erythema or dusky blue toes not amenable to surgical treatment. Occasionally, larger emboli or distal intimal flaps, particularly in diseased iliac arteries, may require operative intervention. For this reason, the lower extremities should be carefully inspected and monitored intraoperatively following AAA repair.

Impotence or retrograde ejaculation may result after AAA repair due to injury of autonomic nerves in the para-aortic dissection. The incidence of this complication is difficult to determine because of the many causes of impotence in this older age group and the frequent underreporting. Careful preservation of nerve trunks, particularly in the distal left para-aortic region is important to limit this complication, which otherwise may occur in 25% of cases.

Paraplegia, due to spinal cord ischemia, is rare following infrarenal AAA repair (occurring in less than 0.2%). This appears to result when important spinal artery collateral flow via the internal iliac arteries or an abnormally low origin of the main spinal artery (arterial magna radicularis) is obliterated or embolized during AAA repair. Recovery from this complication is unusual and mortality rate is high.

B. Cardiac Complications: Despite careful preoperative screening and intraoperative management, cardiac complications, particularly MI, constitute the most serious threat to patients following AAA repair. This type of complication remains the leading cause of death after elective AAA surgery (Table 18–2). Most of these events occur within the first 2 days after surgery during which time intensive care monitoring is appropriate for high-risk patients. Maximizing myocardial function with adequate preload, controlling oxygen consumption by reduced heart rate and blood pressure product, ensuring adequate oxygenation, and establishing effective analgesia are important techniques for preventing myocardial ischemia postoperatively. Patients with cardiac dysfunction have a greater risk of MI when the postoperative hematocrit is less than 28%, even though this is well tolerated by normal persons. In addition to providing excellent pain control, postoperative epidural analgesia may reduce myocardial complications by decreasing the catecholamine stress response.

C. Pulmonary Complications: Pneumonia and atelectasis are common but seldom fatal following AAA repair. Pulmonary embolism is rare, and deep venous thrombosis (DVT) is seldom of clinical signif

Table 18–2. Prevalence of early (30-day) postoperative complications after elective AAA repair.

Complication	Prevalence
All Cardiac	15%
Myocardial infarction	2–8%
All Pulmonary	8–12%
Pneumonia	5%
Worsening renal function	5–12%
Dialysis	1–6%
Deep venous thrombosis	8%
Bleeding	2–5%
Ureteral injury	<1%
Stroke	1%
Leg ischemia	1–4%
Colon ischemia	1%
Wound infection	<5%
Spinal cord ischemia	<1%

icance after AAA repair, perhaps because of intraoperative anticoagulation. Unrecognized DVT may occur in 18% of untreated patients; therefore, perioperative prophylaxis with intermittent pneumatic compression stockings is appropriate, with the addition of subcutaneous heparin in high-risk patients.

D. Renal Complications: Renal failure, once a frequent complication of AAA repair, is now unusual, and dialysis requirement is rare except after complicated, ruptured AAA repair. Possible causes are intraoperative hypotension, embolization associated with pararenal clamping, and a poorly understood renal response to infrarenal aortic clamping and declamping per se. Careful monitoring of intravascular volume with adequate pre- and intraoperative replacement are important factors for reducing postoperative renal failure. Adjuvant use of mannitol, loop diuretics, or low-dose dopamine, although frequently used, are of less proven benefit.

E. Late Complications: Late complications after successful AAA or iliac aneurysm repair are infrequent.

1. Pseudoaneurysm–Anastomotic disruption, usually due to arterial degeneration or graft infection, can result in a pseudoaneurysm, which is an expanding hematoma, locally contained by surrounding connective tissue. After a 3-year follow-up, the incidence of anastomotic pseudoaneurysm is 0.2% for aortic anastomoses, 1.2% for iliac anastomoses, and 3% for femoral anastomoses. Aortic pseudoaneurysms appear to increase progressively with time. A recent study reported an incidence of aortic pseudoaneurysms of only 1% after 8 years, but 20% after 15 years, suggesting the appropriateness of CT scans about 10 years postoperatively. When identified, aortic and iliac pseudoaneurysms warrant repair because of the high risk of mortality if rupture occurs.

2. Graft infection–After AAA repair, graft infection is unusual unless a femoral anastomosis is required. Patients with aortoiliac grafts have an incidence of infection of 0.5%, usually manifesting 3–4 years after implantation. The development of a secondary aortoenteric fistula after AAA repair is also unusual (0.9%), but much more common than a primary aortoenteric fistula associated with an AAA. These fistulas develop about 5 years after AAA repair, nearly always involving the duodenum at the proximal suture line and manifesting GI hemorrhage. Less frequently, aortoenteric fistulas may involve the central portion of the graft and lead to infection rather than hemorrhage. Both aortic graft infection and aortoenteric fistula usually require graft resection and extra-anatomic replacement. Unfortunately, both these complications have a high associated mortality rate, usually greater than 50%.

3. Thrombosis—Thrombosis of an aortoiliac graft following AAA repair is unusual, unless extensive iliac occlusive disease coexists, which may lead to early graft thrombosis if unrecognized.

4. Other aneurysms—After AAA repair, about 5% of patients develop complications due to other aneurysms, at a mean interval of 5 years postoperatively. Usually, these are true aneurysms of the thoracic or more proximal abdominal aorta or occasionally of the iliac arteries. If these secondary aneurysms rupture, less than 5% of patients survive. Thus, it is important to detect these aneurysms before rupture occurs. Hypertension significantly increases the risk of secondary aneurysm complications. It suggests that initial screening should be performed for other aneurysms when a patient with an AAA is hypertensive or if a tortuous, possibly dilated thoracic aorta is seen on chest radiographs.

In total, only 3–5% of patients experience late complications of AAA/iliac aneurysm repair, but most are severe and often fatal. Complications have been prevented by the use of prophylactic perioperative antibiotics, careful closure of viable tissue between the aortic graft and duodenum, and detection and treatment of other associated aneurysms.

Prognosis

After elective AAA repair, cardiac complications are the predominant cause of death, while after ruptured AAA repair, multisystem organ failure and hemorrhage are the principal causes (Table 18–3).

Five-year survival rate after successful AAA repair in modern series is 70%, with a 10-year survival rate of 40%. Survival is comparable after successful elective and ruptured AAA surgery, if the patient survives the initial 30 days. Systemic complications of atherosclerosis cause most late deaths after AAA repair in this predominantly elderly male population. The cause of late deaths after AAA repair are cardiac problems (44%), cancer (15%), rupture of another aneurysm (11%), stroke (9%), and pulmonary conditions (6%). The existence of cardiac causes, aneurysmal disease, and stroke indicates that vascular complications account for two-thirds of the late deaths following AAA repair. When outcome is stratified according to these risk factors, the 5-year survival rate improves to 84%

Table 18–3. Causes of early (30-day) mortality after elective and ruptured AAA repair.

Cause	Elective	Ruptured
Cardiac	58%	20%
Pulmonary	6%	3%
Renal	4%	9%
Colon infarction	1%	9%
Hemorrhage	0%	18%
MSOF	1%	35%
Other	24%	6%

MSOF, multisystem organ failure.

in patients without heart disease (identical with that of normal age-matched controls), which is substantially better than the 54% survival rate observed in patients with known heart disease.

An analysis of CABG performed in preparation for AAA repair indicates that improved long-term survival is likely in patients under age 70 years with severe CAD, but that older patients do not benefit from this aggressive approach.

SPECIAL PRESENTATIONS

Inflammatory AAAs

Inflammatory AAAs are a distinct entity characterized by marked thickening of the aneurysmal wall, especially in the anterior and lateral aspects. This surrounding "peel" consists of an intense fibrotic inflammatory response in the adventitial and periadventitial layers with a lymphocyte (primarily T cells) and plasma cell infiltrate. Although these changes suggest an immune mechanism, the exact cause is not clear. This process may be related to more diffuse retroperitoneal fibrosis, but it is unique because of its predominance in the aneurysmal wall.

Patients with inflammatory AAAs nearly always complain of pain, which frequently (>85%) leads to urgent exploration for suspected ruptured AAA. They may present with a febrile illness, elevated sedimentation rate, and systemic symptoms, which confuse the diagnosis. Treatment with corticosteroids has been used to reduce acute inflammatory symptoms and even reduce the fibrotic reaction. The benefit of reducing aneurysmal wall thickness is not clear, since reduced strength and potential rupture may result.

The diagnosis of inflammatory aneurysm can be made preoperatively by CT scanning, which reveals a "halo" of soft tissue around the anterior AAA enhanced by intravenous contrast. Preoperative recognition of an inflammatory aneurysm may facilitate management with a retroperitoneal approach to avoid the most thickened and inflamed portion of the anterior wall. Although the dense fibrotic reaction around inflammatory AAAs might suggest a protection from rupture, this is not the case, probably because of rupture through the less thickened posterior wall.

Thus, current indications for repair of inflammatory AAAs are identical with those for noninflammatory aneurysms.

When approached transabdominally, an inflammatory aneurysm has a characteristic shiny, pearly-gray appearance, which resembles the head of a newborn baby. Fibrosis of the AAA wall often extends to involve the duodenum, ureters, and adjacent structures. To avoid injuring these during operative repair, supraceliac control, direct AAA incision without infrarenal dissection, and endoaneurysmal repair (analogous to a ruptured AAA) are recommended if the transperitoneal approach is used. By avoiding the anterior fibrosis, the left retroperitoneal approach reduces the risk to adjacent structures and is recommended when inflammatory AAAs are recognized preoperatively.

Complications associated with injury to adjacent structures should be minimal if appropriate techniques are used. Preoperative ureteral stenting facilitates identification of ureters and treats hydronephrosis, if present. Ureterolysis is not recommended, since injury is common, ureteral obstruction can be treated with a stent, and hydronephrosis usually resolves after inflammatory AAA repair. In more than 50% of patients, associated retroperitoneal fibrosis regresses after AAA treatment, suggesting that a hemodynamic influence or an interaction of blood with the aneurysm wall sustains this diffuse inflammatory reaction.

Infected AAAs

An infected aneurysm can result from degenerative changes caused by primary infection of a previously normal artery (<1%) or a secondary infection of an already established aneurysm. If sufficiently severe, primary aortic infection can lead to aortic degeneration, localized wall disruption, and pseudoaneurysm formation, usually in a localized, asymmetric fashion. The term **mycotic** describes these primary infected aneurysms, not because of a fungal origin, but because of the saccular, asymmetric pseudoaneurysm reminiscent of a mushroom. The source of aneurysm infection may be septic embolization from a distant site or contiguous spread from a local infection. Although any bacterial or fungal infection can lead to an infected aneurysm, the most common pathogens are *Salmonella* sp and *Staphylococcus aureus.*

Clinically significant secondary infection of an already established AAA is also rare. However, unapparent infection, more appropriately described as bacterial colonization is common, since up to 37% of AAAs demonstrate positive intraoperative cultures. The significance of this bacterial colonization appears minimal, since the finding of a positive intraoperative culture has not increased the rate of subsequent prosthetic graft infection.

Since infected AAAs are rare and the symptoms are nonspecific, diagnosis can be delayed or unsuspected until surgery. Abdominal pain, fever, bacteremia, and a pulsatile abdominal mass should suggest an infected AAA, but all these findings may not be present and the AAA may be small enough to escape detection. For this reason, an infected AAA should be considered in the differential diagnosis of fever of unknown origin, particularly if *Salmonella* is cultured from the blood of a patient older than 50 years. In the absence of systemic signs of infection, a localized, noncalcified, asymmetric AAA in an otherwise normal-appearing aorta should suggest a primary infected AAA.

Traditionally, the treatment for an infected infrarenal AAA has been aortic excision with proximal and distal closure, débridement of surrounding infected tissue, and extra-anatomic (axillobifemoral) bypass. Complications of proximal aortic stump ("blowout") after this procedure have led some to recommend in situ graft replacement after débridement of all infected tissue.

Experience suggests that aortic excision with extra-anatomic bypass is optimal for patients with overtly purulent infection, especially those caused by *Salmonella, Pseudomonas,* or other gram-negative organisms. In situ replacement is more applicable to less purulent infections, especially from gram-positive organisms or infections involving the suprarenal aorta in which visceral reconstruction requires in situ replacement.

Primary Aortocaval Fistulas

Rarely, large expanding AAAs may erode into the adjacent vena cava or proximal left iliac vein leading to a direct aortovenous fistula. Most often, affected patients experience symptoms of pain associated with AAA rupture, and rarely a chronic, stable AV fistula may result. Sudden AAA rupture into the vena cava may also be associated with more typical retroperitoneal rupture, in which case the aortocaval fistula may not be recognized until emergency surgery is performed.

The extent of hemodynamic compromise due to the aortocaval fistula, depends on its size. A typical machinery bruit is present in over 50% of cases, whereas venous hypertension leads to leg swelling in one-third. Renal vein hypertension may lead to microscopic or gross hematuria. Acute congestive heart failure (CHF) results in 25% of patients when the fistula is large or when baseline cardiac function is poor. In the rare case of a stable, chronic aortocaval fistula, sustained increased venous pressure can result in lower extremity swelling, venous thrombosis, perineal and hemorrhoidal varices, scrotal edema, and hematuria. In these cases, an abdominal bruit and high-output CHF may aid an otherwise confusing diagnosis, which is best confirmed by arteriography.

Surgical treatment of an aortocaval fistula consists of conventional repair of the AAA with closure of the fistula from within the aneurysm. Dissection of the vena cava or iliac vein away from the aneurysm is extremely hazardous. Control of the vena cava adjacent to the fistula with direct pressure from within the aneurysm allows the fistula to be closed without excessive bleeding or air embolization. Mortality rate from an aortocaval fistula remains high (35%):

Primary Aortoenteric Fistulas

Expanding AAAs may possibly erode into adjacent intestine, usually the 3rd or 4th portion of the duodenum because of its adjacency to the AAA. This rare but dramatic complication is usually associated with large AAAs. Much more common is the secondary aortoenteric fistula, which arises as a late anastomotic complication of a prosthetic aortic graft. Initially, GI bleeding may be limited, leading to melena or anemia. Eventually, and often abruptly, severe hemorrhage leads to hematemesis and shock. Classically, patients with aortoenteric fistulas present with a small herald hemorrhage due to bowel mucosal bleeding, prior to sudden brisk hemorrhage and collapse.

A primary aortoduodenal fistula should be suspected in a patient with GI hemorrhage, abdominal pain, and a pulsatile abdominal mass. Because of the rarity of this complication, however, it is much more common for patients with AAAs to develop upper GI hemorrhage from the more common causes of peptic ulcer disease, gastritis, or even esophageal varices. Therefore, the first diagnostic step in these patients should be upper GI endoscopy, which often locates the source of the bleeding. An aortoenteric fistula should be suspected when no obvious source of bleeding is found.

Rarely, a mucosal defect may be seen in the 3rd or 4th portion of the duodenum. Since severe hemorrhage can occur suddenly, evaluation must proceed rapidly in a patient with a known or suspected AAA and GI hemorrhage. A CT scan can confirm the diagnosis of AAA, but usually cannot demonstrate local inflammatory changes diagnostic of an aortoduodenal fistula. Similarly, arteriography usually is not beneficial unless it identifies an alternative source of GI hemorrhage. Often, the diagnosis of primary aortoduodenal fistula cannot be definitively established. Thus, when other more common sources of GI bleeding have been excluded, exploratory laparotomy is indicated because of the universal mortality of an untreated aortoduodenal fistula. Similar to that of infected AAAs, treatment may consist of in situ AAA repair, duodenal closure, and interposition of aneurysm wall, retroperitoneal tissue, or omentum between the aortic graft and duodenum. If substantial contamination of the operative field has occurred, aortic ligation with extra-anatomic bypass may be required.

Suprarenal Aneurysms

AAAs that extend above the renal arteries, but end below the diaphragm are termed **suprarenal** and constitute about 5% of AAAs. The term **pararenal** is used to describe AAAs that involve the renal but not the mesenteric arteries, when at least one renal artery

needs reimplantation for AAA repair. **Juxtarenal** refers to AAAs that do not involve the renal arteries, but whose proximity often requires clamping above the renal arteries. (If an AAA extends above the diaphragm, it is referred to as a thoracoabdominal aneurysm, discussed in Chapter 11.)

The natural history of suprarenal AAAs is even less well defined than infrarenal AAAs, because these AAAs are less frequently encountered. Lacking other data, rupture risk should be considered comparable to infrarenal AAAs.

CT or MRI is required to define the exact size and extension of a suprarenal AAA. Arteriography can usually demonstrate suprarenal extension and is useful to define potentially associated renal/mesenteric occlusive disease, but may underestimate overall aneurysm size. An AAA is rarely isolated to the suprarenal component unless an infrarenal AAA has been previously repaired.

Surgical risk is higher in suprarenal than in infrarenal AAAs because of the necessity for renal/mesenteric artery revascularization and the possibility of ischemic injury during supraceliac cross-clamping. Thus, most surgeons use a threshold size for elective repair of a suprarenal AAA that is about 1 cm larger than an infrarenal AAA in the same patient. Surgical treatment of ruptured suprarenal AAAs is even more complicated and is associated with nearly a 100% mortality rate.

Suprarenal AAAs are best approached surgically by a left retroperitoneal incision, which can be extended into the chest as a thoracoabdominal incision as required for proximal exposure. If an unsuspected suprarenal aneurysm is discovered during transperitoneal exposure, medial visceral rotation (reflecting the left colon, spleen, pancreas, and stomach medially to gain proximal retroperitoneal exposure) can be used. The inclusion technique popularized by Crawford is used for these AAAs, so that the mesenteric and renal arteries are incorporated onto the bypass graft as an onlay patch.

The celiac, SMA, and right renal artery usually can be incorporated as one large patch, whereas the left renal artery generally has to be reimplanted separately. Often, the upper aortic anastomosis for a suprarenal aneurysm can incorporate the visceral artery origins using a beveled technique that excludes the entire aneurysm except for the small portion of the wall where these visceral arteries originate. Ischemic injury to the liver, intestines, and kidneys is unlikely if proximal aortic clamp time can be kept below 30 minutes.

After the visceral arteries are revascularized, the aortic clamp is moved onto the graft, distal to these vessels before completing the distal aortic or iliac anastomosis. Intraoperative cooling by iced saline perfusion of the renal or mesenteric arteries can be used if a prolonged aortic clamp time is anticipated, especially for the left renal artery when this must be reimplanted separately. Significantly greater changes in resistance occur with aortic clamping and declamping above the celiac artery, necessitating careful coordination of anesthesia, fluid administration, and vasoactive drug use.

Long-term prognosis for patients with successful repair of suprarenal AAAs is comparable to that of those with infrarenal AAAs, although operative mortality rate for suprarenal AAA patients is higher on average (4–10%).

Associated Anatomic Anomalies

Renal developmental anomalies may complicate AAA repair. Multiple renal arteries are relatively common (15–30%), whereas pelvic kidney, horseshoe kidney, and multiple ureters are rare. If detected by preoperative arteriography, accessory renal arteries that supply distinct areas of renal parenchyma can be reimplanted onto the aortic graft if they arise from the AAA. If arteriography is not performed, these accessory renal arteries can be found during careful dissection of the aorta, usually arising more anteriorly than the normal lateral renal artery orifices.

Reimplantation of these arteries is facilitated by excising a "button" of associated aortic wall along with the orifice, Carrel's patch technique. **Pelvic kidneys** usually have a single renal artery, but their origin may be displaced to the distal aorta or even iliac arteries and thus require reimplantation. Distal origins of a renal artery require special consideration to avoid prolonged ischemic injury when clamping the more proximal aorta.

Horseshoe kidneys pose more technical difficulty, both because they limit access to the distal aorta and because they usually are supplied by multiple renal arteries. The isthmus of the horseshoe kidney should not be divided unless it is extremely thin and atrophic. Rather, the graft can be tunneled beneath the kidney if the aorta is approached anteriorly. Care must be taken to revascularize the major multiple arteries with reimplantation. Preoperative arteriography facilitates identification of these branches, but careful intraoperative dissection and inspection are required to avoid injury. A retroperitoneal approach to the AAA offers significant advantages because the graft can be easily placed behind the horseshoe kidney and the renal arteries reimplanted similar to the inclusion technique used for suprarenal aneurysms.

Major venous anomalies, although rare, can also pose technical difficulties during AAA repair. Failure to recognize these anomalies can lead to venous injury and significant hemorrhage. A **retroaortic left renal vein** (incidence 2–3%) or a **circumaortic anterior** and **posterior left renal vein** (incidence ≤ 7%) are the most common anomalies. These should be suspected if the left renal vein is not encountered anteriorly during the proximal aortic dissection or if it appears small. Preoperative CT scanning discloses these anomalies, as well as less common **left-sided** or **duplicated inferior vena cava.** Except in cases of situs inversus, a left-sided vena cava usually crosses anteriorly to the right side of the aorta at the level of the renal veins.

Venous anomalies complicate aortic exposure and must be approached with care. Duplicated veins may often be ligated to facilitate exposure, but the details of venous anatomy must be fully appreciated to avoid inadvertent ligation of a nonduplicated system.

Associated Abdominal Disease

Not infrequently, an AAA is detected during the evaluation of another disease process such as prostate cancer, lumbar disk disease, cholelithiasis, or even colon cancer. If such an AAA warrants surgical repair, a decision must be made concerning the prioritization of treatment for these 2 disease processes. The general guideline is to treat the most life-threatening process first and to avoid simultaneous operations unless a high complication rate would otherwise be anticipated. Usually, the AAA takes priority, such as in patients with lumbar disk disease or prostate cancer, when the other procedure can be secondarily staged without increased risk. More difficult decisions arise with cholelithiasis or colon cancer, in which simultaneous surgical treatment is attractive, but increases the risk of prosthetic graft contamination. This is especially true of colon operations, so that AAA repair and colon resection should be staged except in extraordinary circumstances.

The larger the AAA, the more important it is to treat it first. Alternatively, colon cancers that are obstructing—and potentially liable to perforate or cause total obstruction (particularly those on the left side)—should usually be treated prior to AAA repair. Patients who require surgical treatment of another urgent problem but who have an AAA of 6 cm or more should usually be observed postoperatively in hospital until the AAA can be repaired because of the possibility of postoperative rupture. There is controversy concerning the advisability of cholecystectomy associated with AAA repair. Because of a 15% incidence of positive bile cultures during routine cholecystectomy, many surgeons have avoided concomitant cholecystectomy for asymptomatic cholelithiasis. Concomitant cholecystectomy has been successfully performed in many patients, however, without an apparent increase in graft infection. The incidence of graft infection is low and the onset delayed, so that results must be viewed cautiously when an unsuspected intra-abdominal problem is discovered during AAA repair. Usually, the AAA reconstruction should proceed and the other (probably asymptomatic) condition dealt with secondarily, if concomitant treatment would lead to an increased risk of prosthetic graft infection.

Isolated Iliac Artery Aneurysms

Isolated iliac aneurysms, without an associated AAA, are rare. Their deep location in the pelvis makes detection by physical examination nearly impossible, although large internal iliac aneurysms are occasionally discovered by rectal examination. The common iliac artery is most frequently involved, followed by the internal iliac artery, with the external iliac usually spared, for reasons not understood. There is a clear male predominance (male/female ratios 5–16:1), and most affected patients are 65–75 years old. Although iliac artery aneurysms are usually asymptomatic until rupture, patients may present with unique signs caused by local compression of adjacent pelvic structures. Ureteral obstruction, hematuria, iliac vein thrombosis, large bowel obstruction, and lower extremity neurologic deficit may be present, but are more frequently caused by other entities, thereby confusing the initial diagnosis of an iliac aneurysm.

The natural history of small iliac aneurysms is not well defined, because these aneurysms are rare and usually have not been followed up with sequential imaging. In most surgical series, the average size of small iliac aneurysms is 4–5 cm, whereas the average size of ruptured iliac aneurysms has been estimated to be 6 cm. During follow-up of iliac aneurysms, varying rates of rupture have been reported ranging from 10% to 70% after 5 years.

Mortality rate from rupture is 25–57%, whereas mortality rate from elective repair is less than 5%. Despite the vagaries concerning natural history, most surgeons recommend elective repair of isolated iliac aneurysms at a threshold diameter of about 3 cm in good-risk patients.

Repair consists of replacement of the common iliac artery, extending this replacement to include the infrarenal aorta as necessary, depending on its quality. Iliac aneurysms may be approached through a lower abdominal retroperitoneal incision, but when bilateral or potentially requiring aortic repair, a transabdominal approach is more versatile. Proximal ligation of an internal iliac aneurysm without distal ligation or endoaneurysmorrhaphy may lead to persistent aneurysm expansion and rupture. Therefore, internal iliac artery aneurysms should be excluded by distal ligation with endoaneurysmal ligation of branches.

When internal iliac aneurysms are bilateral or the contralateral artery is occluded, pelvic blood flow must be carefully assessed. In these circumstances, one internal iliac artery may require direct graft revascularization. Although back pressure recording from the distal internal iliac artery is possible, the adequacy of pelvic circulation is usually assessed by clinical grading of backbleeding, as well as visual and Doppler assessment of the sigmoid colon blood flow following temporary iliac clamping.

REFERENCES

Akkersdijk GJ, Puylaert JB, de Vries AC: Abdominal aortic aneurysm as an incidental finding in abdominal ultrasonography. Br J Surg 1991;78:1261.

Bengtsson H, Bergqvist D: Ruptured abdominal aortic aneurysm: A population-based study. J Vasc Surg 1993; 18:74.

Bengtsson H, Bergqvist D, Sternby NH: Increasing prevalence of abdominal aortic aneurysms: A necropsy study. Eur J Surg 1992;158:19.

Bernstein EF, Chan EL: Abdominal aortic aneurysm in high-risk patients. Ann Surg 1984;200:255.

Breckwoldt WL et al: The effect of suprarenal cross-clamping on abdominal aortic aneurysm repair. Arch Surg 1992;127:520.

Brewster DC et al: Aortocaval and iliac arteriovenous fistulas: Recognition and treatment. J Vasc Surg 1991;13:253.

Brewster DC et al: Intestinal ischemia complicating abdominal aortic surgery. Surgery 1991;109:447.

Brin BJ, Busuttil RW: Isolated hypogastric artery aneurysms. Arch Surg 1982;117:1329.

Brunkwall J et al: Solitary aneurysms of the iliac arterial system: An estimate of their frequency of occurrence. J Vasc Surg 1989;10:381.

Bunt TJ: Synthetic vascular graft infection. II. Graft-enteric erosions and graft-enteric fistulas. Surgery 1983;94:1.

Calcagno D et al: Late iliac artery aneurysms and occlusive disease after aortic tube grafts for abdominal aortic aneurysm repair. Ann Surg 1991;214:733.

Calligaro KD et al: Pulmonary risk factors of elective abdominal aortic surgery. J Vasc Surg 1993;18:914.

Cambria RP et al: The impact of selective use of dipyridamole-thallium scans and surgical factors on the current morbidity of aortic surgery. J Vasc Surg 1992;15:43.

Cambria RP et al: Transperitoneal versus retroperitoneal approach for aortic reconstruction: A randomized prospective study. J Vasc Surg 1990;11:314.

Chuter TA et al: Transfemoral endovascular aortic graft placement. J Vasc Surg 1993;18:185.

Cohen JR et al: Abdominal aortic aneurysm repair in patients with preoperative renal failure. J Vasc Surg 1986;3:867.

Cohen JR et al: Role of the neutrophil in abdominal aortic aneurysm development. Cardiovasc Surg 1993;1:373.

Crawford ES, Beckett WC, Greer MS: Juxtarenal infrarenal abdominal aortic aneurysm: Special diagnostic and therapeutic considerations. Ann Surg 1986;203:661.

Crawford ES et al: Infrarenal abdominal aortic aneurysms: Factors influencing survival after operation performed over a 25-year period. Ann Surg 1981;193:699.

Crawford ES et al: The impact of renal fusion and ectopia on aortic surgery. J Vasc Surg 1988;8:365.

Crawford ES et al: Celiac axis, superior mesenteric artery, and inferior mesenteric artery occlusion: Surgical considerations. Surgery 1977;82:856.

Cronenwett JL: Factors influencing the long-term results of aortic aneurysm surgery. In: Vascular Surgery: Long-Term Results. Yao JST, Pearce WH (editors). Appleton & Lange, 1993.

Cronenwett JL et al: Actuarial analysis of variables associated with rupture of small abdominal aortic aneurysms. Surgery 1985;98:472.

Cronenwett JL et al: Variables that affect the expansion rate and outcome of small abdominal aortic aneurysms. J Vasc Surg 1990;11:260.

Darling RC III et al: Are familial abdominal aortic aneurysms different? J Vasc Surg 1989;10:39.

Darling RC et al: Autopsy study of unoperated abdominal aortic aneurysms: The case for early resection. Circulation 1977;56(Suppl 2):II-161.

Detsky AS et al: Cardiac assessment for patients undergoing noncardiac surgery: A multifactorial clinical risk index. Arch Intern Med 1986;146:2131.

Dobrin PB: Pathophysiology and pathogenesis of aortic aneurysms: Current concepts. Surg Clin North Am 1989; 69:687.

Durham SJ et al: Probability of rupture of an abdominal aortic aneurysm after an unrelated operative procedure: A prospective study. J Vasc Surg 1991;13:248.

Eagle KA et al: Combining clinical and thallium data optimizes preoperative assessment of cardiac risk before major vascular surgery. Ann Intern Med 1989;110:859.

Farkas JC et al: Long-term follow-up of positive cultures in 500 abdominal aortic aneurysms. Arch Surg 1993; 128:284.

Frame PS, Fryback DG, Patterson C: Screening for abdominal aortic aneurysm in men ages 60 to 80 years: A cost-effectiveness analysis. Ann Intern Med 1993;119:411.

Giordano JM, Trout HH III: Anomalies of the inferior vena cava. J Vasc Surg 1986;3:924.

Gloviczki P et al: Ruptured abdominal aortic aneurysm: Repair should not be denied. J Vasc Surg 1992;15:851.

Goldman L et al: Multifactorial index of cardiac risk in noncardiac surgical procedures. N Engl J Med 1977;297:845.

Hermreck AS: Prevention and management of surgical complications during repair of abdominal aortic aneurysms. Surg Clin North Am 1989;69:869.

Hertzer NR et al: Coronary artery disease in peripheral vascular patients: A classification of 1000 coronary angiograms and results of surgical management. Ann Surg 1984;199:223.

Hessel EA III: Intraoperative management of abdominal aortic aneurysms: The anesthesiologist's viewpoint. Surg Clin North Am 1989;69:775.

Hollier LH et al: Conventional repair of abdominal aortic aneurysm in the high-risk patient: A plea for abandonment of nonresective treatment. J Vasc Surg 1986;3:712.

Hollier LH et al: Late survival after abdominal aortic aneurysm repair: Influence of coronary artery disease. J Vasc Surg 1984;1:290.

Johnston KW: Multicenter prospective study of nonruptured abdominal aortic aneurysm. Part II. Variables predicting morbidity and mortality. J Vasc Surg 1989;9:437.

Johnston KW, Scobie TK: Multicenter prospective study of nonruptured abdominal aortic aneurysms. I. Population and operative management. J Vasc Surg 1988;7:69.

Katz DA, Littenberg B, Cronenwett JL: Management of small abdominal aortic aneurysms: Early surgery vs watchful waiting. JAMA 1992;268:2678.

Kazmers A, Cerqueira MD, Zierler RE: Perioperative and late outcome in patients with left ventricular ejection fraction of 35% or less who require major vascular surgery. J Vasc Surg 1988;8:307.

Komori K et al: Management of concomitant abdominal aortic aneurysm and gastrointestinal malignancy. Am J Surg 1993;166:108.

Kvilekval KHV et al: The value of computed tomography in the management of symptomatic abdominal aortic aneurysms. J Vasc Surg 1990;12:28.

Lalka SG et al: Dobutamine stress echocardiography as a predictor of cardiac events associated with aortic surgery. J Vasc Surg 1992;15:831.

Lette J et al: Multivariate clinical models and quantitative dipyridamole-thallium imaging to predict cardiac morbidity and death after vascular reconstruction. J Vasc Surg 1991;14:160.

Levinson JR et al: Usefulness of semiquantitative analysis of dipyridamole-thallium-201 redistribution for improving risk stratification before vascular surgery. Am J Cardiol 1990;66:406.

Lilienfeld DE et al: Epidemiology of aortic aneurysms: I. mortality trends in the United States, 1951 to 1981. Arteriosclerosis 1987;1:637.

MacSweeney ST et al: High prevalence of unsuspected abdominal aortic aneurysm in patients with confirmed symptomatic peripheral or cerebral arterial disease. Br J Surg 1993;80:582.

Majumder PP et al: On the inheritance of abdominal aortic aneurysm. Am J Hum Genet 1991;48:164.

Marston WA et al: Misdiagnosis of ruptured abdominal aortic aneurysms. J Vasc Surg 1992;16:17.

Michaels JA: The management of small abdominal aortic aneurysms: A computer simulation using Monte Carlo methods. Eur J Vasc Surg 1992;6:551.

Nachbur BH, Inderbitzi RG, Bar W: Isolated iliac aneurysms. Eur J Vasc Surg 1991;5:375.

Nelson AH, Fleisher LA, Rosenbaum SH: Relationship between postoperative anemia and cardiac morbidity in high-risk vascular patients in the intensive care unit. Crit Care Med 1993;21:860.

Nypaver TJ et al: Repair of pararenal abdominal aortic aneurysms: An analysis of operative management. Arch Surg 1993;128:803.

Olin JW et al: The incidence of deep venous thrombosis in patients undergoing abdominal aortic aneurysm resection. J Vasc Surg 1993;18:1037.

Olsen PS et al: Surgery for abdominal aortic aneurysms: A survey of 656 patients. J Cardiovasc Surg 1991;32:636.

Parodi JC: Endovascular repair of abdominal aortic aneurysms. In: *Advances in Vascular Surgery*. Whittemore AD et al (editors). Mosby-Yearbook, 1993.

Pasternack PF et al: The value of silent myocardial ischemia monitoring in the prediction of perioperative myocardial infarction in patients undergoing peripheral vascular surgery. J Vasc Surg 1989;10:617.

Paty PSK et al: Aortic replacement for abdominal aortic aneurysm in elderly patients. Am J Surg 1993;166:191.

Pavone P et al: Abdominal aortic aneurysm evaluation: Comparison of US, CT, MRI, and angiography. Magn Reson Imaging 1990;8:1990.

Plate G et al: Recurrent aneurysms and late vascular complications following repair of abdominal aortic aneurysms. Arch Surg 1985;120:590.

Reddy DJ et al: Management of infected aortoiliac aneurysms. Arch Surg 1991;126:873.

Robison JG et al: Aortic reconstruction in high-risk pulmonary patients. Ann Surg 1989;210:112.

Roger VL et al: Influence of coronary artery disease on morbidity and mortality after abdominal aortic aneurysmectomy: A population-based study, 1971–1987. J Am Coll Cardiol 1989;14:1245.

Stella A et al: Postoperative course of inflammatory abdominal aortic aneurysms. Ann Vasc Surg 1993;7:229.

Sterpetti AV et al: Factors influencing the rupture of abdominal aortic aneurysms. Surg Gynecol Obstet 1991;173:175.

Sterpetti AV et al: Sealed rupture of abdominal aortic aneurysms. J Vasc Surg 1990;11:430.

Strachan DP: Predictors of death from aortic aneurysm among middle-aged men: The Whitehall study. Br J Surg 1991;78:401.

Svensson LG et al: A prospective study of respiratory failure after high-risk surgery on the thoracoabdominal aorta. J Vasc Surg 1991;14:271.

Tayor LM et al: The incidence of perioperative myocardial infarction in general vascular surgery. J Vasc Surg 1991;15:52.

Thomas B, Lund K, Skau T: Isolated aneurysms of the iliac artery: What are the chances of rupture? Eur J Vasc Surg 1988;2:213.

Thompson JE et al: Surgical management of abdominal aortic aneurysm: Factors influencing mortality and morbidity-a 20-year experience. Ann Surg 1975;181:654.

Tilson MD: Rationale for molecular approaches to the etiology of abdominal aortic aneurysm disease. J Vasc Surg 1992;15:924.

Todd GJ et al: The accuracy of CT scanning in the diagnosis of abdominal and thoracoabdominal aortic aneurysms. J Vasc Surg 1991;13:302.

Tromp G et al: Sequencing of cDNA from 50 unrelated patients reveals that mutations in the triple-helical domain of type III procollagen are an infrequent cause of aortic aneurysms. J Clin Invest 1993;91:2539.

Valentine RJ et al: Nonvascular emergencies presenting as ruptured abdominal aortic aneurysms. Surgery 1993;113:286.

van Laarhoven CJ et al: Chronic obstructive pulmonary disease and abdominal aortic aneurysms. Eur J Vasc Surg 1993;7:386.

Veith FJ et al: The need for quality assurance in vascular surgery. J Vasc Surg 1991;13:523.

Webster MW et al: Ultrasound screening of first-degree relatives of patients with an abdominal aortic aneurysm. J Vasc Surg 1991;13:9.

Wheeler WE, Hanks J, Raman VK: Primary aortoenteric fistulas. Am Surg 1992;58:53.

Wong T, Detsky AS: Preoperative cardiac risk assessment for patients having peripheral vascular surgery. Ann Intern Med 1992;116:743.

Yeager MP et al: Epidural anesthesia and analgesia in high-risk surgical patients. Anesthesiology 1987;66:729.

Peripheral Arterial Aneurysms

19

Richard H. Dean, MD

Aneurysms located in peripheral arteries collectively are much less common than aortic aneurysms. Although there are many causes of peripheral aneurysms, atherosclerosis remains the most common cause. In ascending order of frequency, these aneurysms affect the carotid, subclavian/axillary, femoral, and popliteal arteries. Small series and case reports of aneurysms located at other sites of the arterial tree underscore the potential for development at any site. However, these aneurysms are so rare that they do not merit further individual discussion. Aneurysms at the above-mentioned locations are reviewed individually, since the natural history and methods of management are relatively specific to each site.

CAROTID ARTERY ANEURYSMS

General Considerations

Extracranial aneurysms of the carotid artery are rare. Carotid artery aneurysms are most frequently found in the common carotid artery, particularly at its bifurcation. The middle and distal portions of the internal carotid artery are the next most common sites. Aneurysms at the bifurcation are usually fusiform, whereas those located in the internal carotid artery are most often saccular. Atherosclerosis is responsible for over 50% of all carotid artery aneurysms. Trauma and previous carotid artery surgery are less common causes. Although syphilis was the most common cause 50 years ago, it is a rare cause of carotid artery aneurysm today.

The most common serious risks associated with carotid artery aneurysms are transient ischemic attacks and stroke. Most such central nervous system defects are caused by embolization of laminated thrombus lining the wall of the aneurysm. Less frequently, cerebral symptoms are caused by diminished flow through the carotid artery secondary to its compression by the mass of an adjacent saccular aneurysm. Although common in reports during the late 19th and early 20th centuries, rupture of carotid artery aneurysms is rare today. When rupture does occur, it is manifested by hemorrhage from the pharynx, ear, or nose and may lead to death by suffocation.

Clinical Findings

A. Signs and Symptoms: Since most carotid artery aneurysms are identified because of clear symptoms, the true risk associated with the presence of an aneurysm is poorly defined. Nevertheless, their natural history is generally unfavorable. The clinical presentation of carotid artery aneurysms varies according to their location and size.

Distal internal carotid artery aneurysms may be completely hidden. By contrast, almost every common carotid artery and bifurcation aneurysm are first discovered as a pulsatile mass just below the angle of the mandible. Occasionally, an aneurysm patient may present with a pulsatile mass in the tonsillar fossa or oropharynx without external manifestation. With either presentation, the aneurysms may cause symptoms of pain and tenderness, or they may cause no symptoms. Distal internal carotid artery aneurysms may produce recurrent facial pain, 5th or 6th cranial nerve palsy, deafness, or even Horner's syndrome when they compress adjacent structures at the base of the skull. Even **Raeder's paratrigeminal syndrome,** the combination of intermittent facial pain and oculosympathetic paresis, has been caused by aneurysms situated at the base of the skull.

B. Imaging Studies: Duplex sonography with B-mode imaging usually confirms or excludes the presence of an aneurysm of the extracranial carotid artery. Nevertheless, high internal carotid artery aneurysms cannot be diagnosed accurately by this method because of the limitations in visualizing that region. Computed tomography and magnetic resonance imaging are useful substitutes for B-mode imaging for the diagnosis of such lesions located high in the neck.

Angiography remains the definitive diagnostic test on which to base therapy, even when the diagnosis has been established by one of the noninvasive methods (Fig 19–1). Visualization of the entire length of both extracranial and intracranial components of the carotid artery and the vertebrobasilar system is required for any treatment strategies to be adequate.

Differential Diagnosis

Elongation with kinking of the carotid artery is the most frequently found lesion masking as a carotid artery aneurysm. Usually, this lesion presents as a pul-

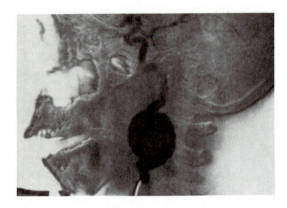

Figure 19–1. Arteriogram of fusiform carotid artery aneurysm.

satile mass at the base of the right side of the neck, typically in older hypertensive women. Careful palpation may suggest that the pulsatile mass is an elongated tortuous vessel. This mass is easily distinguished from an aneurysm by the fact that the pulsation is along the long axis of the vessel. A prominent carotid artery bifurcation in a patient with a thin neck, carotid body tumor, enlarged lymph nodes, branchial cleft cyst, or other masses that overlie and transmit the carotid pulse can be mistaken for an aneurysm. Usually, careful palpation differentiates these entities from a true aneurysm of the carotid bifurcation.

Treatment

Since most carotid artery aneurysms are associated with an elongated, tortuous vessel, aneurysm resection and simple reanastomosis of the 2 ends can be used in about 50% of patients. Most other aneurysms are treated by resection and interpositional placement of either a saphenous vein graft or a polytetrafluoroethylene graft. Occasionally, saccular aneurysms can be treated by resection and lateral arteriorrhaphy or patch angioplasty.

Through the use of electroencephalography, stump pressure measurements, or test clamping of the carotid artery while using regional anesthesia, the need for temporary shunting can be identified. When a neurologic deficit is produced by test cross-clamping or identified by electroencephalographic monitoring or when the distal stump pressure is lower than 50 mmHg, one of the following procedures may be carried out: resection, reanastomosis, or graft interposition is performed over a temporary shunt.

Prognosis

Using the techniques of cerebral protection as well as intraoperative heparin anticoagulation and modern anesthetic techniques, the operative mortality rate should be no higher than 1% and permanent neurologic deficits should be less than 5%.

Goldstone J: Aneurysms of the extracranial carotid artery. In: *Vascular Surgery,* 3rd ed. Rutherford, RB (editor). WB Saunders, 1989:1418.

Hardin CA: Surgical treatment of extracranial carotid aneurysms with excision and arterial restoration. Vasc Surg 1973;7:247.

Zwolak RM et al: Atherosclerotic extracranial carotid artery aneurysms. J Vasc Surg 1984;1:415.

SUBCLAVIAN/AXILLARY ARTERY ANEURYSMS

General Considerations

Subclavian and axillary artery aneurysms account for about 1% of all peripheral artery aneurysms. Thoracic outlet syndrome is the dominant cause of subclavian artery aneurysms accounting for almost 75% of such lesions. Through impingement of the subclavian artery by the first rib, turbulent flow and subsequent vessel wall failure lead to poststenotic dilatation and ultimately aneurysmal degeneration. In contrast, most distal axillary artery aneurysms are caused by crutch trauma to the vessel and subsequent degeneration with aneurysmal formation.

Clinical Findings

Most subclavian and axillary artery aneurysms are manifested as a consequence of distal embolization of laminated clot from within the aneurysm. Digital ischemia secondary embolization of intramural laminated clot leading to digital artery occlusion is the most common presenting symptom. Such aneurysms infrequently may produce neurologic sequelae by stretching fibers of the surrounding brachial plexus. Similarly, right subclavian artery aneurysms may stretch the recurrent laryngeal nerve and cause hoarseness by producing vocal cord paralysis. Thrombosis of these aneurysms is unusual but when present may cause variable degrees of arm ischemia, depending on the magnitude of collateral circulation. Although rupture can occur, it is a rare presentation in patients with aneurysms in the subclavian or axillary artery sites.

Diagnosis

Proximal subclavian artery aneurysms may be identified by plain chest radiographs. Such films may reveal an upper mediastinal or apical mass. More distal subclavian and axillary artery aneurysms may be identified on physical examination as a pulsatile mass in the supraclavicular region or axilla. In both instances, arch and selective upper extremity arteriography is the definitive diagnostic study. Complete arteriographic studies should be performed not only to evaluate the aneurysm location but also to assess distal sites for thromboembolism and vessel occlusions (Fig 19–2). Similarly, the site of vertebral artery origin in relation to the aneurysm also is of importance for planning aneurysm replacement.

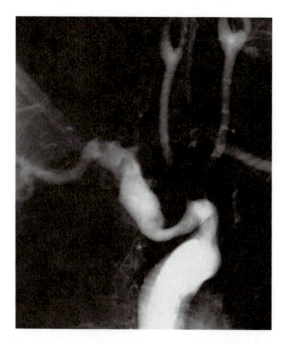

Figure 19–2. Arteriogram of subclavian artery aneurysm.

Hobson RW II, Israel MR, Lynch TG: Axillosubclavian arterial aneurysms. In: *Aneurysms.* Bergan JJ, Yao JST (editors). Grune & Stratton, 1982:435.

Hobson RW, Sarkaria J, O'Donnell J, Neville W: Atherosclerotic aneurysms of the subclavian artery. Surgery 1979;85:358.

Pairolero PC et al: Subclavian-axillary artery aneurysms. Surgery 1981;90:757.

FEMORAL ARTERY ANEURYSMS

General Considerations

Femoral artery aneurysms are the second most common site of peripheral artery aneurysms. Most are caused by atherosclerosis. Other causes include false aneurysm at sites of vascular reconstructive grafting, penetrating trauma, and infected or mycotic aneurysms. Most atherosclerotic femoral artery aneurysms are benign. Those that become symptomatic do so by either distal embolization of intramural thrombus or acute thrombosis causing limb-threatening ischemia. Rarely do these aneurysms rupture. Since the muscular fascial compartment surrounding the femoral artery confines expansion, rapid exsanguination following rupture is rare. In contrast, the tamponading effect of the pressure in the confined rupture may cause pressure occlusion of the femoral artery and severe distal ischemia.

Diagnosis

Femoral artery aneurysms are usually diagnosed by a careful physical examination. Palpation of a smooth fusiform dilatation of the femoral artery with expansile pulsations is usually sufficient to definitively establish the diagnosis of a femoral artery aneurysm.

Definitive diagnostic evaluation is obtained by arteriography whenever an aneurysm is suspected or diagnosed by physical examination (Fig 19–3). Since 85% of patients with atherosclerotic femoral artery aneurysms have associated aortic, iliac, or popliteal artery aneurysms, a complete arteriographic assessment of the abdominal aorta and its run-off through the pedal level is appropriate. In over 70% of patients, arteriographic study will reveal the presence of a contralateral femoral artery aneurysm as well.

Treatment

Isolated femoral artery aneurysms are replaced with an interpositional synthetic 8-mm Dacron or polytetrafluoroethylene graft. Frequently, simultaneous correction of coexistent aortic or iliac aneurysms may require aortofemoral grafting. Similarly, coexistent popliteal aneurysms may require femoropopliteal saphenous vein bypass grafting in conjunction with femoral aneurysm replacement.

Prognosis

Long-term results of femoral artery aneurysm replacement are excellent with the operative mortality

Since distal subclavian and proximal axillary artery aneurysms are almost always associated with thoracic outlet syndrome, diagnostic evaluation should include assessment for cervical ribs and anomalous first rib anatomy by use of neck and upper rib plain x-rays. Further consideration of both the vascular and neurogenic sequelae of thoracic outlet syndrome are provided in Chapter 12.

Treatment

Symptomatic subclavian and axillary artery aneurysms and asymptomatic aneurysms of at least 2.5 times the normal vessel diameter generally should be replaced. In all instances, the preferred procedure is to replace subclavian artery aneurysms with an interpositional synthetic graft and axillary artery aneurysms with a saphenous vein graft. Proximal right subclavian artery aneurysms are exposed by median sternotomy with extension of the cervical end of the incision into the right supraclavicular area. Proximal left subclavian artery aneurysms are approached through a left lateral thoracotomy. More distal subclavian and proximal axillary artery aneurysms are exposed through a supraclavicular incision. Occasionally, this exposure can be combined with an infraclavicular incision to expose the axillary artery beyond the aneurysm for the distal anastomosis. Exposure of these areas of the thoracic outlet and associated points regarding surrounding anatomy are described in Chapter 12.

Abbott WM, Darling RC: Axillary artery aneurysms secondary to crutch trauma. Am J 1973;125:515.

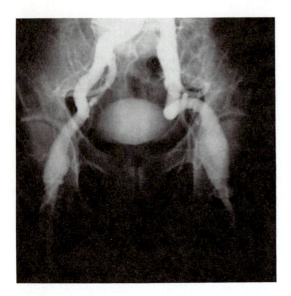

Figure 19–3. Arteriogram of femoral artery aneurysm.

rate approaching zero and patency rate greater than 95%. All patients should be followed up at regular intervals with repetitive ultrasound scans of the unreplaced segments of the abdominal aorta, iliac, femoral, and popliteal arteries to identify developing aneurysms at any of these sites.

Cutler BS, Darling RC: Surgical management of arteriosclerotic femoral aneurysms. Surgery 1973;74:764.

Pappas G et al: Femoral aneurysms: Review of surgical management. JAMA 1963;190:489.

Queral LA, Flinn W, Yao JST, Bergan JJ: Management of peripheral artery aneurysms. Surg Clin North Am 1979;59:693.

Tolstedt GE, Radke HM, Bell JW: Late sequelae of arteriosclerotic femoral aneurysms. Angiology 1979;12:601.

POPLITEAL ARTERY ANEURYSMS

General Considerations

Popliteal artery aneurysms remain a challenge for the most skilled surgeon. Atherosclerosis is the underlying cause of most such aneurysms, and 50% of patients present with bilateral aneurysms. Over 75% of popliteal artery aneurysms are associated with aneurysms at other sites in the aorta-iliac-femoral-popliteal arterial segment.

Clinical Findings

A. Signs and Symptoms: The most common clinical presentation of a popliteal artery aneurysm is thrombosis and extreme distal ischemia. Frequently, examination of the distal extremity reveals petechial hemorrhages due to small emboli. As the popliteal artery aneurysm increases in size, progressive deposi-

tion of laminated thrombus occurs within its wall. Dissection of this mural thrombus acutely occludes the previously nonstenotic vessel. Since little collateral flow is present at the time of thrombosis, distal propagation of the clot frequently leads to irretrievable limb-threatening ischemia. Occasionally, the presenting symptoms are secondary to pressure on the popliteal nerve by a large aneurysm. Such pressure can cause neuropraxia, numbness, and calf muscle dysfunction. Popliteal vein compression may cause symptoms of calf swelling and superficial venous varicosities. Rarely do popliteal aneurysms rupture. When rupture occurs, exsanguination is uncommon. More likely, the tamponaded hematoma compresses the artery and causes severe ischemia of the distal leg.

B. Imaging Studies: A careful physical examination is usually sufficient to make the diagnosis of popliteal artery aneurysm. Nevertheless, smaller aneurysms and those located high in a muscular leg may be difficult to identify. This is especially true for the inexperienced examiner. Popliteal artery aneurysms are rarely located in the distal popliteal space; they are usually found just behind or above the knee joint.

Ultrasound scanning can readily confirm the diagnosis when physical examination is not definitive. Scanning of the contralateral popliteal artery should always be performed to identify the presence or absence of bilateral aneurysms. As with femoral artery aneurysms, the abdominal aorta and iliac and femoral arteries also should be measured by ultrasonography to exclude the simultaneous presence of aneurysms at these sites.

The role of arteriography is to plan operative correction by identifying the extent of the aneurysm and the status of inflow and run-off vessels available for bypass graft attachment (Fig 19–4). Nevertheless, previously unrecognized small popliteal aneurysms may be uncovered during angiography for distal ischemia caused by emboli originating from the popliteal artery aneurysm's laminated clot. Arteriography may be misleading and not capture the presence of popliteal artery aneurysms when patients present with acute thrombosis. Clues to their presence in such circumstances can be obtained by finding an enlarged, patent contralateral popliteal artery.

Treatment

Because of the risk of limb loss after acute popliteal artery thrombosis, replacement of popliteal artery aneurysms is usually indicated based solely on their presence. Since associated atherosclerotic stenoses or aneurysmal disease of the superficial femoral artery is usually also present, replacement of popliteal artery aneurysms usually requires a common femoral to distal popliteal or tibial vessel bypass with exclusion of the aneurysm by proximal and distal ligation. The presence of tibial vessel occlusions secondary to embolism of laminated clot from the aneurysm frequently

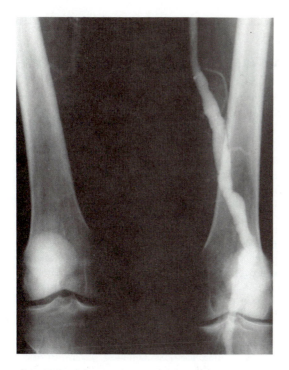

Figure 19–4. Arteriogram of popliteal artery aneurysm.

can be performed through a posterior popliteal approach, the medial approach is more versatile. All levels of the limb arterial tree can be approached by this route with the patient supine. Furthermore, it allows harvest of the entire length of saphenous vein if a long bypass is required. In all instances, autogenous saphenous vein is the conduit of choice.

Prognosis

Results of popliteal artery aneurysm replacement primarily depend on the clinical presentation at the time of operation, the status of the tibial outflow tract, and the availability of a satisfactory autogenous saphenous vein. Early amputation with or without failed attempts at salvage occurs in almost 40% of patients presenting with limbs with acute aneurysm thrombosis. In contrast, limb loss is rare after elective replacement prior to any clinical manifestations.

Dent TL et al: Multiple arteriosclerotic arterial aneurysms. Arch Surg 1972;105:338.

Evans WE, Vermilion BD: Popliteal and femoral aneurysms. In: *Vascular Surgery.* Rutherford RB (editor). WB Saunders, 1984:814.

Shortell CK, DeWeese JA, Ouriel K, Green RM: Popliteal artery aneurysms: A 25 year experience. J Vasc Surg 1991;14:771.

Szilagyi DE, Schwartz RL, Reddy DJ: Popliteal arterial aneurysms: Their natural history and management. Arch Surg 1981;116:724.

Vermilion BD et al: A review of one hundred forty seven popliteal aneurysms wit long-term follow-up. Surgery 1981;90:1009.

demands that the distal attachment of the replacement graft be at the distal tibial level.

Although exposure for replacement of an isolated popliteal artery aneurysm without associated disease

20 Visceral Artery Aneurysms

James C. Stanley, MD

Aneurysms of the visceral branches of the abdominal aorta represent an unusual but important group of vascular diseases. More than 3300 splanchnic and renal artery aneurysms have been reported in the English literature. Splanchnic aneurysms are twice as common as renal aneurysms. Because of the variability in their biologic character and their clinical relevance, visceral artery aneurysms are presented separately.

SPLANCHNIC ARTERY ANEURYSMS

The major splanchnic artery aneurysms, in decreasing order of incidence, affect the splenic, hepatic, superior mesenteric, celiac, gastric-gastroepiploic, jejunal-ileal-colic, pancreaticoduodenal-pancreatic, and gastroduodenal arteries (Table 20–1). The natural history of splanchnic artery aneurysms has become better defined in recent times (Table 20–2). Nearly 22% of splanchnic aneurysms are seen as surgical emergencies, of which 8.5% result in the patient's death.

Splenic Artery Aneurysm

Splenic artery aneurysms account for 60% of splanchnic artery aneurysms. The prevalence of splenic artery aneurysms in the general population is nearly 0.8%. Women are affected with splenic artery aneurysms 4 times more often than men.

A. Preexisting Conditions and Causes: Three distinct conditions predispose to the development of splenic artery aneurysms. The first is arterial fibrodysplasia, usually with hypertension secondary to renal artery medial fibrodysplasia. This association has been identified only in women. About 2% of patients known to have renal artery fibrodysplasia have splenic artery aneurysms. The second is pregnancy. Increases in splenic blood flow and alterations in vessel wall elastin during gestation appear to contribute to these aneurysms. This is particularly evident with repeated pregnancies, since 40% of women reported to have splenic artery aneurysms have been grand multiparas. The third is portal hypertension and splenomegaly. Splenic artery aneurysms have been observed in 10% of patients with these disorders. Loss of vessel wall integrity may accompany the marked increases in splenic blood flow as well as the increased estrogen activity associated with cirrhosis in these

cases. Aneurysms in the latter category have been recognized more frequently after orthotopic liver transplantation.

Splenic artery aneurysms often exhibit typical calcific arteriosclerotic changes, but this is more likely to represent a secondary event than a primary etiologic process. Most splenic artery aneurysms are saccular and occur at vessel branchings (Fig 20–1). Discontinuities in the internal elastic lamina exist in normal vessels at these sites, precisely where aneurysmal changes are most likely to evolve. Splenic artery aneurysms are multiple in 20% of patients. Periarterial inflammation with chronic pancreatitis and penetrating trauma are less common causes of these aneurysms. Inflammatory aneurysms associated with pancreatitis usually represent false aneurysms due to pseudocyst erosion into the main splenic artery (Fig 20–2).

B. Signs and Symptoms: Vascular calcifications that have a signet-ring appearance on plain abdominal radiographs were often the first evidence of a splenic artery aneurysm in past years. Currently, arteriographic diagnosis of these aneurysms is more likely during studies undertaken for other diseases. Ultrasonography, computed tomography (CT), and magnetic resonance imaging (MRI) are also useful in establishing the presence of these lesions.

Symptoms of left upper quadrant or epigastric pain accompany a minority of splenic artery aneurysms. Most of these aneurysms are asymptomatic, being referred to as **bland aneurysms.** The most serious man-

Table 20–1. Incidence of gender ratio of splanchnic artery aneurysms.

Location	Incidence Within Splanchnic Circulation	Male:Female Ratio
Splenic artery	60%	1:4
Hepatic artery	20%	2:1
Superior mesenteric artery	5.5%	1:1
Celiac artery	4%	1:1
Gastric and gastroepiploic arteries	4%	3:1
Jejunal, ileal, and colic arteries	3%	1:1
Pancreaticoduodenal and pancreatic arteries	2%	4:1
Gastroduodenal arteries	1%	4:1

Table 20–2. Rupture & mortality associated with splanchnic artery aneurysms.

Location	Incidence of Reported Rupture	Mortality with Rupture
Splenic artery	2% (bland aneurysms)	25% (bland aneurysms); during pregnancy: 70% maternal; 75% fetal
Hepatic artery	20%	35%
Superior mesenteric artery	Uncommon, thrombosis more common	50%
Celiac artery	13%	50%
Gastric and gastroepiploic arteries	90%	70%
Jejunal, ileal, and colic arteries	30%	20%
Pancreaticoduodenal and pancreatic arteries	50%	50%
Gastroduodenal artery	50%	50%

ifestation of these lesions is bleeding following rupture. This often occurs as a double rupture, with initial bleeding usually contained within the lesser sac. Free hemorrhage into the peritoneal cavity eventually occurs when this containment is lost. Pancreatitis-related aneurysms are more likely to cause intestinal hemorrhage following their erosion into the stomach or pancreatic ductal system. Finally, development of an arteriovenous fistula following splenic artery aneurysm rupture into the splenic vein may occur. This is a rare, but recognized cause of gastrointestinal hemorrhage from esophageal varices due to left-sided portal hypertension.

Rupture of bland splenic artery aneurysms occurs in less than 2% of cases. Rupture is just as likely to occur when an aneurysm is calcified, exists in a normotensive patient, or affects the very elderly. Splenic artery aneurysms in liver transplant recipients may be at greater risk for rupture than those in other patients.

Nearly 95% of aneurysms first recognized during pregnancy have ruptured, with a maternal mortality rate close to 70% and fetal mortality exceeding 75%. However, these data are misleading because many aneurysms undoubtedly evolve during repeated pregnancies, and most of these do not rupture during pregnancy. Nevertheless, splenic artery aneurysms encountered during pregnancy must be considered to represent a serious health hazard.

C. Treatment: The reported operative mortality rate in treating splenic artery aneurysm rupture is 25%. Given the fact that most patients experiencing aneurysmal rupture undergo surgical therapy, it would be advisable to undertake elective operation for the small asymptomatic splenic artery aneurysm only when the operative mortality rate is less than 0.5% (this represents the product of the known 25% surgical mortality rate and the 2% rupture rate of bland aneurysms). Treatment in higher-risk patients might better involve percutaneous transcatheter embolization of the aneurysm.

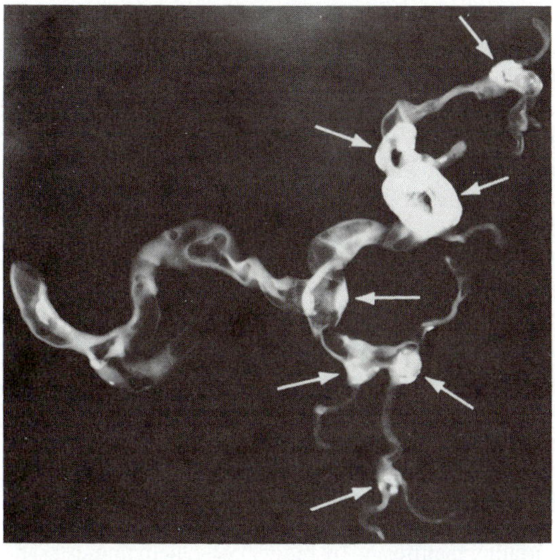

Figure 20–1. Multiple splenic artery aneurysms (*arrows*) occurring at each bifurcation of the distal artery in a grand multiparous female patient. (Reproduced, with permission, from Stanley JC, Thompson NW, Fry WJ: Splanchnic artery aneurysms. Arch Surg 1970;101:689.)

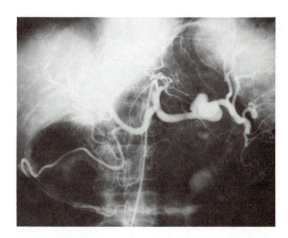

Figure 20–2. Solitary splenic artery aneurysm affecting the midportion of the vessel, caused by arterial erosion from a pancreatic pseudocyst due to alcoholic pancreatitis. (Reproduced, with permission, from Stanley JC, Frey CF, Miller TA, Lindenauer SM, Child CG: Major arterial hemorrhage: A complication of pancreatic pseudocysts and chronic pancreatitis. Arch Surg 1976;111:435.)

Splenectomy was the most common form of surgical therapy for splenic artery aneurysms in the past. However, the immunologic importance of splenic preservation, even in the elderly, has caused splenectomy to lose favor. Simple ligature obliteration or excision of these aneurysms appears to be preferable therapy. A laparoscopic approach to these lesions has appeal in selected cases. Inflammatory splenic artery aneurysms embedded in the tail of the pancreas are best treated by distal pancreatectomy. Others, especially false aneurysms associated with pseudocysts, are most easily treated by incising the aneurysmal sac and ligating entering and exiting vessels from within. Pancreatic resection or cyst drainage in the latter cases depends on the degree of associated inflammation and general condition of the patient.

Bronsther O, Merhav H, Van Thiel D, Starzl TE: Splenic artery aneurysms occurring in liver transplant recipients. Transplantation 1991;52:723.

Busuttil RW, Brin BJ: The diagnosis and management of visceral artery aneurysms. Surgery 1980;88:619.

Hashizame M et al: Laparoscopic ligation of splenic artery aneurysm. Surgery 1993;113:352.

Jorgensen BA: Visceral artery aneurysms: A review. Dan Med Bull 1985;32:237.

Lowry SM, O'Dea TP, Gallagher DI, Mozenter R: Splenic artery aneurysm rupture: The seventh instance of maternal and fetal survival. Obstet Gynecol 1986;67:291.

Stanley JC, Fry WJ: Pathogenesis and clinical significance of splenic artery aneurysms. Surgery 1974;76:889.

Stanley JC, Thompson NW, Fry WJ: Splanchnic artery aneurysms. Arch Surg 1970;101:689.

Trastek VF et al: Splenic artery aneurysms. Surgery 1982; 91:694.

Waltman AC, Luers PR, Athanasoulis CA, Warshaw AL: Massive arterial hemorrhage in patients with pancreatitis: Complementary roles of surgery and transcatheter occlusive techniques. Arch Surg 1986;121:439.

Hepatic Artery Aneurysm

Hepatic artery aneurysms account for 20% of splanchnic artery aneurysms. Men are twice as likely to be affected as women. Nontraumatic and nonmycotic aneurysms are discovered most often during the 6th decade of life. Hepatic artery aneurysms attributed to trauma and infection associated with intravenous drug abuse-related sepsis and endocarditis are more likely to occur in patients during the 3rd and 4th decades of life. With increasing societal violence, a marked increase in the number of reported traumatic aneurysms has been seen (Fig 20–3). The cause of many other aneurysms is unknown, but it has been considered to be due to medial degeneration in nearly 25% of patients. Arteriosclerosis, although often present, is considered a secondary process, not an initiating event in these aneurysms. Connective tissue arteriopathies such as periarteritis nodosa are a cause of microaneurysms involving the hepatic vessels. Hepatic artery aneurysms are usually solitary, affecting

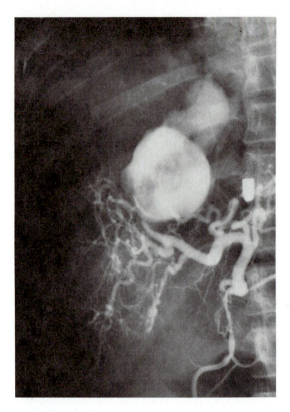

Figure 20–3. Traumatic hepatic artery aneurysm due to a gunshot wound. (Reproduced, with permission, from Whitehouse WM Jr, Graham LM, Stanley JC: Aneurysms of the celiac, hepatic, and splenic arteries. In: *Aneurysms, Diagnosis and Treatment.* Bergan JJ, Yao JST [editors]. Grune & Stratton, 1981.)

extrahepatic vessels in nearly 80% of cases and intrahepatic vessels in 20%.

Most hepatic artery aneurysms are initially recognized as incidental findings during arteriography, CT, or ultrasonography for other illnesses. Most are asymptomatic. When these are aneurysms are symptomatic, they most often cause right upper quadrant or epigastric pain. Large aneurysms have been reported to cause obstructive jaundice, although most are too small to compress the biliary ducts. Hepatic artery aneurysms rarely are seen as pulsatile abdominal masses.

Hepatic artery aneurysm rupture has occurred in 20% of recently reported cases, but the true incidence may be less. The mortality rate from aneurysm rupture is about 35%. Bleeding following rupture occurs equally into the biliary tract and peritoneal cavity. Hemobilia, manifested by biliary colic, hematemesis, and jaundice, is often evident after rupture into the biliary tract. Chronic insidious gastrointestinal hemorrhage is uncommon in these circumstances.

Common hepatic artery aneurysms are often treated by aneurysmectomy or simple ligation with arterial reconstruction. The liver's collateral arterial circulation and portal vein flow usually provide an adequate blood supply to the liver despite interruption of the proximal hepatic artery. Temporary operative occlusion of the aneurysmal artery usually reveals compromised liver blood flow. If such is the case, direct vascular reconstruction must be undertaken with either prosthetic or autologous grafts. In the presence of coexisting liver parenchymal disease, arterial reconstructions should always be undertaken. Casual ligation of extrahepatic branches to control bleeding from intrahepatic aneurysms may cause liver necrosis. Hepatic territory resection in certain of these patients may be the more appropriate therapy. Percutaneous transcatheter obliteration of an aneurysm with balloons, coils, or thrombogenic particulate matter may be a reasonable alternative to surgical therapy in high-risk patients.

Guida PM, Moore SW: Aneurysm of the hepatic artery: Report of five cases with a brief review of the previously reported cases. Surgery 1966;60:299.

Jeans PL: Hepatic artery aneurysms and biliary surgery: Two cases and a literature review. Aust N Z J Surg 1988; 58:889.

Lal RB et al: Hepatic artery aneurysm. J Cardiovasc Surg 1989;30:509.

Stauffer JT, Weinman MD, Bynum TE: Hemobilia in a patient with multiple hepatic artery aneurysms: A case report and review of the literature. Am J Gastroenterol 1989;84:59.

Superior Mesenteric Artery Aneurysms

Aneurysms of the proximal superior mesenteric artery account for 5.5% of splanchnic aneurysms. Men and women are affected equally. Mycotic aneurysms secondary to infection from bacterial endocarditis continue to be a dominant cause of these lesions. Nonhemolytic streptococci and a variety of pathogens associated with parental substance abuse are encountered most often. Medial degeneration, periarterial inflammation, and trauma have also been associated with these aneurysms. Arteriosclerosis is considered a secondary event rather than a cause. Superior mesenteric artery aneurysms are recognized most often during CT and arteriographic studies for nonvascular disease. Most reported superior mesenteric artery aneurysms have been symptomatic, causing mild to severe abdominal discomfort, which is often suggestive of intestinal angina.

Rupture of a superior mesenteric artery aneurysms is unusual, and aneurysmal dissection is uncommon. Gastrointestinal hemorrhage usually reflects acute aneurysmal occlusion with bleeding from areas of mucosal infarction and sloughing. Cessation of flow from sudden aneurysm occlusion proximal to the inferior pancreaticoduodenal and middle colic arteries effectively excludes blood flow into the distal intestinal circulation. Severe intestinal ischemia evolves because the usual collateral networks from the adjacent celiac and inferior mesenteric arterial circulations become ineffective.

Simple ligation of superior mesenteric artery aneurysms without arterial reconstruction is possible in certain patients, especially those who have an adequate collateral circulation to the midgut. It is surprising that ligation and aneurysmorrhaphy have been the most frequently reported means of managing superior mesenteric artery aneurysms. Temporary occlusion of the superior mesenteric artery and Doppler assessment of intestinal blood flow assist in determining the adequacy of collateral vessels in these circumstances. If gut ischemia is apparent, intestinal revascularization by means of an aortomesenteric graft or some other bypass is necessary. Because of the potential for synthetic graft infection if bowel ischemia is present, autologous vein is favored for these reconstructions.

Cormier F et al: Dissecting aneurysms of the main trunk of the superior mesenteric artery. J Vasc Surg 1992;15:424.

DeBakey ME, Cooley DA: Successful resection of mycotic aneurysm of superior mesenteric artery: Case report and review of the literature. Am Surg 1953;19:202.

Friedman SG, Pogo GJ, Moccio CG: Mycotic aneurysm of the superior mesenteric artery. J Vasc Surg 1987;6:87.

Celiac Artery Aneurysm

Celiac artery aneurysms account for 4% of splanchnic artery aneurysms, with men and women affected equally. Most aneurysms are associated with medial defects, although in the distant past most of these aneurysms were mycotic. Arteriosclerosis, a common histologic finding, is considered a secondary process. Celiac artery aneurysms are invariably saccular, affecting the distal vessel at its branching (Fig 20–4).

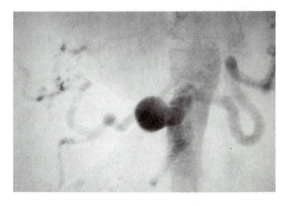

Figure 20–4. Celiac artery aneurysm affecting the distal trunk of the vessel. (Reproduced, with permission, from Stanley JC, Whitehouse WM Jr: Aneurysms of splanchnic and renal arteries. In: *Surgery of the Aorta and its Body Branches.* Bergan JJ, Yao JST [editors]. Grune & Stratton, 1979.)

Celiac artery aneurysms are usually asymptomatic. Diagnosis is most often established as a result of ultrasonography, angiography, or other imaging studies undertaken for nonvascular disease. Rupture has been reported to affect 13% of these aneurysms and carries a mortality rate of 50%. Rupture usually causes exsanguinating hemorrhage into the lesser space first and then into the general peritoneal cavity. Although rare, gastrointestinal bleeding may follow aneurysm erosion into the stomach or pancreatic ductal system.

Operation is recommended for all celiac artery aneurysms unless prohibitive surgical risks exist. Aneurysmectomy with arterial reconstruction of the celiac trunk is the preferred treatment for most celiac artery aneurysms. Simple aneurysm exclusion by ligation of entering and exiting branches may be performed in selected patients whose foregut collateral blood flow to the liver is sufficient to prevent hepatic necrosis. If this is not the case, an aortoceliac artery bypass should be performed with an autologous vein or prosthetic graft. Surgical therapy is successful in greater than 90% of celiac artery aneurysms treated operatively.

Graham LM et al: Celiac artery aneurysms: Historical (1745–1949) versus contemporary (1950–1984) differences in etiology and clinical importance. J Vasc Surg 1985;2:757.

Hertzer NR, Mullally PH: Celiac artery aneurysmectomy with hepatic artery ligation. Arch Surg 1972;104:337.

Shumacker HB Jr, Siderys H: Excisional treatment of aneurysm of celiac artery. Ann Surg 1958;148:885.

Gastric & Gastroepiploic Artery Aneurysms

Gastric and gastroepiploic artery aneurysms represent 4% of splanchnic artery aneurysms. Gastric artery aneurysms are 10 times more common than gastroepiploic artery aneurysms. Men are affected 3 times more often than women. Most of these perigastric aneurysms are discovered in patients over 50 years of age. These aneurysms are usually solitary. They develop as a result of periarterial inflammation or medial degeneration. When arteriosclerosis is present, it is considered a secondary process.

Most gastric and gastroepiploic artery aneurysms have been symptomatic when initially recognized. They usually are seen as emergencies without preceding symptom, with rupture having occurred in greater than 90% of reported cases. Gastrointestinal bleeding is twice as common as intraperitoneal hemorrhage. Rupture of these aneurysms may be catastrophic, as evidenced by the reported 70% mortality rate of such an event.

Surgical treatment of intramural gastric and gastroepiploic artery aneurysms involves aneurysmectomy with excision of the involved portion of the stomach. Extramural aneurysms may be treated by arterial ligation alone, with or without aneurysm excision. A laparoscopic approach to selected extramural aneurysms may be feasible. Many of these perigastric

aneurysms are minute, and a search for them is often tedious if preoperative localization has not been established by CT or arteriographic studies.

Thomford NR, Yurko JE, Smith EJ: Aneurysm of gastric arteries as a cause of intraperitoneal hemorrhage: Review of literature. Ann Surg 1968;168:294.

Uchikoshi F et al: Aneurysm of the right gastroepiploic artery: A case report of laparoscopic resection. Cardiovasc Surg 1993;1:550.

Varekamp AP, Minder WH, VanNoort G, Wassenaar HA: Rupture of a submucosal gastric aneurysm, a rare cause of gastric hemorrhage. Neth J Surg 1983;35:100.

Jejunal, Ileal, & Colic Artery Aneurysms

Aneurysms of the jejunal, ileal, and colic arteries represent 3% of splanchnic artery aneurysms. They generally occur in patients over 60 years of age, with men and women equally affected. Solitary aneurysms occur in 90% of cases. Acquired medial defects are considered the cause of most of these aneurysms. Infected emboli associated with subacute bacterial endocarditis and connective tissue diseases such as periarteritis nodosa may underlie some multiple aneurysms affecting these intestinal branch arteries. Arteriosclerosis, evident in 20% of these aneurysms, is considered a secondary finding not an etiologic process.

Many intestinal branch aneurysms are asymptomatic, being incidental findings during arteriography for other diseases. However, most of the aneurysms described in the literature have ruptured. Actual rupture rate is probably less than 30%. Rupture has been associated with a mortality rate of 20%. Rupture usually occurs into the gastrointestinal tract, with rupture into the mesentery or free peritoneal cavity being uncommon. Nevertheless, mesenteric branch aneurysm rupture is responsible for abdominal apoplexy more frequently than any other splanchnic artery aneurysm.

Operation for extraintestinal branch aneurysms usually entails arterial ligation, with or without aneurysmectomy. Intramural aneurysms or those associated with intestinal infarction require resection of the affected segment of bowel. Inferior mesenteric artery aneurysms are rare, and definition of their clinical importance is anecdotal at best.

Geelkerken RH, van Bockel JH, deRoos WK, Hermans J: Surgical treatment of intestinal artery aneurysms. Eur J Vasc Surg 1990;4:563.

Graham LM, Hay MR, Cho, KJ, Stanley JC: Inferior mesenteric artery aneurysms. Surgery 1985;97:158.

Trevisani MF, Ricci MA, Michaels RM, Meyer KK: Multiple mesenteric aneurysms complicating subacute bacterial endocarditis. Arch Surg 1987;122:823.

Pancreaticoduodenal, Pancreatic, & Gastroduodenal Artery Aneurysms

Pancreatic and pancreaticoduodenal artery aneurysms represent 2% and gastroduodenal artery aneurysms represent an additional 1.5% of splanchnic artery aneurysms. Men are 4 times more likely than women to be affected. Aneurysms of these vessels are usually encountered in patients older than 50 years of age. In general, these aneurysms are the most difficult of all splanchnic artery aneurysms to treat. About 60% of gastroduodenal and 30% of pancreaticoduodenal artery aneurysms are associated with pancreatitis-related vascular necrosis or vessel erosion by an adjacent pancreatic pseudocyst (Fig 20–5). Medial degeneration and trauma are less common causes. Arteriosclerosis is invariably a secondary, not a causal process, when present in these lesions.

Most of these aneurysms are associated with epigastric pain and discomfort. This is often due to underlying pancreatic inflammatory disease. Gastroduodenal and pancreaticoduodenal aneurysm rupture has occurred in 50% of reported cases. Bleeding in these circumstances may be into the stomach, biliary tract, or pancreatic ductal system. Hemorrhage into the peritoneal cavity is less common, occurring about 15% of the time. Mortality rates with rupture are nearly 50%. Arteriography is an important means of confirming the presence of these lesions. CT and MRI are of increasing importance in diagnosis and are helpful in detecting the presence of rupture or extent of associated pancreatic pathology.

Surgical therapy is indicated in all but the highest-risk patient with gastroduodenal, pancreaticoduodenal, or pancreatic arterial aneurysms. Treatment of large pancreatitis-related false aneurysms is best accomplished by arterial ligation from within the aneurysmal sac, rather than by extra-aneurysmal arterial ligation within an inflamed pancreas. If a pancreatic pseudocyst or abscess has caused a false aneurysm, some form of drainage procedure should accompany ligature control of the involved vessel. Pancreatic resections, including distal pancreatectomy

or pancreaticoduodenectomy, are appropriate in selected patients. Although transcatheter embolization and electrocoagulation have been recommended as an alternative treatment, rebleeding and late aneurysmal rupture with such therapy occur, thus limiting its routine use.

Eckhauser FE et al: Gastroduodenal and pancreaticoduodenal artery aneurysms: A complication of pancreatitis causing spontaneous gastrointestinal hemorrhage. Surgery 1980;88:335.

Gangahar DM et al: True aneurysm of the pancreaticoduodenal artery: A case report and review of the literature. J Vasc Surg 1985;2:741.

Mandel SR, Jaques PF, Mauro MA, Sanofsky S: Nonoperative management of peripancreatic arterial aneurysms: A 10-year experience. Ann Surg 1987;205:126.

RENAL ARTERY ANEURYSMS

Renal artery aneurysms are a relatively rare vascular disease. The clinical importance of these aneurysms has been better defined in recent years. Clear differences exist between true and dissecting renal artery aneurysms (Table 20–3).

True Renal Artery Aneurysms

The incidence of true renal artery aneurysms is nearly 0.1% in the general population. Although women are more likely than men to have these aneurysms, when patients with renal arterial dysplasia are excluded, there is no gender predilection. The right renal artery is more likely than the left to exhibit these aneurysms. This may reflect the fact that dysplastic disease is more common and more severe on the right.

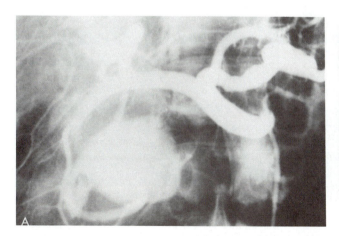
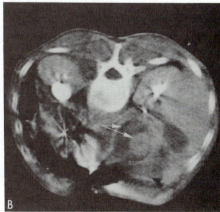

Figure 20–5. Gastroduodenal artery aneurysm. Selective celiac arteriogram. (**A**) and computed tomography (**B**). (Reproduced, with permission, from Eckhauser FE et al: Gastroduodenal and pancreaticoduodenal artery aneurysms: A complication of pancreatitis causing spontaneous gastrointestinal hemorrhage. Surgery 1980;88:335.)

Table 20–3. Renal artery aneurysms.

Lesion	Incidence of Reported Rupture	Male:Female Ratio	Mortality with Rupture
True renal artery aneurysm	3%	1:1.2	10% (bland aneurysms); during pregnancy: 55% maternal, 85% fetal
Dissecting renal artery aneurysm	Uncommon, thrombosis more common	10:1	Undefined

Most true renal artery aneurysms are saccular, occurring at extraparenchymal primary or secondary renal artery bifurcations (Fig 20–6). The average diameter of these lesions is 1.4 cm. Intraparenchymal aneurysms occur in less than 10% of patients. Renal artery aneurysms usually evolve as a consequence of medial degeneration, with internal elastic lamina fragmentation invariably being present. In many instances, renal artery aneurysms appear directly related to medial fibroplasia (Fig 20–7). Arteriosclerosis is thought to represent a secondary event rather than a primary process. Multiple microaneurysms secondary to necrotizing arteridites such as polyarteritis nodosa are a rare but important cause of certain aneurysms.

Very few renal artery aneurysms are symptomatic. Nevertheless, aneurysmal expansion, rupture, or renal infarction from dislodged aneurysmal thrombus may accompany these lesions. Rupture of a renal artery aneurysm affects less than 3% of cases, although rupture may be more common with intrarenal lesions. The mortality rate accompanying rupture is about 10%. Loss of the kidney is almost inevitable with aneurysm rupture. Renal artery aneurysm rupture during pregnancy is life-threatening. Rupture in pregnancy has been associated with an 85% fetal mortality rate and a 45% maternal mortality rate. It is surprising that the affected kidney has been salvaged in nearly 20% of surviving women.

A cause-effect association of renal artery aneurysms to systemic hypertension is controversial. Aneurysmal thrombus may undergo embolization or propagate and occlude a distal artery, thereby producing renal ischemia and renovascular hypertension in some cases. Aneurysmal compression of an adjacent artery may be an additional cause of renovascular hypertension, but such is very uncommon. Intrinsic stenotic disease adjacent to an aneurysm may be a more likely cause of secondary hypertension in most cases.

Symptomatic patients with suspected expansion of a true renal artery aneurysm should undergo surgical

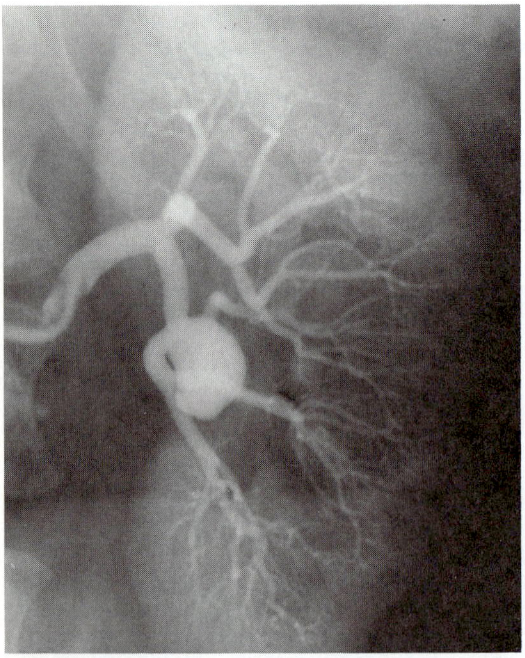

Figure 20–6. Saccular renal artery aneurysm occurring at segmental branching. (Reproduced, with permission, from Stanley JC, Whitehouse WM Jr: Renal artery macroaneurysms. In: *Aneurysms, Diagnosis and Treatment.* Bergan JJ, Yao JST [editors]. Grune & Stratton, 1981.)

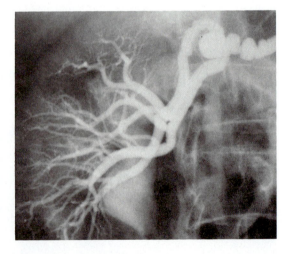

Figure 20–7. Renal artery macroaneurysm affecting the primary bifurcation of a vessel exhibiting medial fibrodysplasia. (Reproduced, with permission, from Stanley JC, Whitehouse WM Jr: Renal artery macroaneurysms. In: *Aneurysms, Diagnosis and Treatment.* Bergan JJ, Yao JST [editors]. Grune & Stratton, 1981.)

repair. Similarly, aneurysms with coexisting renal artery stenoses are best treated operatively. Surgical therapy is also warranted for aneurysms that contain thrombus, if distal embolization is evident. Large asymptomatic aneurysms, exceeding 2 cm in diameter, may be appropriately treated operatively by experienced surgeons. Finally, surgical therapy is recommended for aneurysms in women of childbearing age, who might possible conceive in the future.

Surgical therapy is aneurysmectomy without loss of the kidney substance or compromise of normal renal blood flow. An exception exists in the management of ruptured aneurysms, where nephrectomy is usually required. Large aneurysms may often be excised with direct repair of the artery. Removal of smaller aneurysms usually necessitates an angioplastic vein patch closure or implantation of the involved artery into an adjacent renal artery. Renal artery reconstruction in situ with an aortorenal bypass using autogenous saphenous vein or internal iliac artery is perhaps the most common means of treating patients with these lesions. Occasionally, in patients with complex disease, ex vivo repairs are appropriate. Partial nephrectomy may be necessary for intraparenchymal aneurysms.

Cohen JR, Shamash FS: Ruptured renal artery aneurysms during pregnancy. J Vasc Surg 1987;6:51.

Henriksson C, Bjorkerud S, Nilson AE, Pettersson S: Natural history of renal artery aneurysms elucidated by repeated angiography and pathoanatomical studies. Eur Urol 1985;11:244.

Stanley JC et al: Renal artery aneurysms: Significance of macroaneurysms exclusive of dissections and fibrodysplastic mural dilations. Arch Surg 1975;110:1327.

Tham G et al: Renal artery aneurysms: Natural history and prognosis. Ann Surg 1983;197:348.

Dissecting Renal Artery Aneurysms

Isolated dissections of the renal arteries occur most often after blunt abdominal trauma or intraluminal catheter-induced injury. Others occur spontaneously. Dissections may be associated with false aneurysm formation (Fig 20–8). Men are 10 times more likely than women to be affected with these lesions. The right renal artery is involved more frequently than the left, perhaps because of increased physical stresses on this artery with the known greater ptosis of the right kidney compared with the left. One third of renal artery dissections are bilateral.

Renal artery dissections due to blunt abdominal trauma usually develop after displacement of the kidney during deceleration, causing marked stretching of the vascular pedicle and fracture of the intima, which is the least elastic arterial wall component. These dissections usually occur in the inner media. Direct trauma of the renal artery over unyielding vertebral bodies may cause medial hemorrhage and subsequent

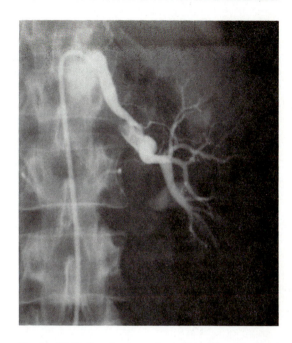

Figure 20–8. Renal artery dissection with associated false aneurysm. (Reproduced, with permission, from Gewertz BL, Stanley JC, Fry WJ: Renal artery dissections. Arch Surg 1977;112:409.)

false aneurysm formation. Renal artery injury during diagnostic arteriography occurs frequently, but limited dissections associated with percutaneous balloon angioplasty are commonplace.

Spontaneous dissections affect the renal arteries more than any other peripheral artery, usually in association with coexisting renovascular disease. These dissections are most likely to extend within the outer media. Spontaneous renal artery dissections usually begin in the proximal renal artery and terminate at the first branching of this vessel.

Pain, hematuria, and systemic hypertension are common manifestations of acute renal artery dissections. Chronic manifestations are often associated with compromised renal function and renovascular hypertension. Delayed rupture is rare. The initial clinical diagnosis in these patients is usually incorrect. Urography, often with CT, may establish the presence of renal ischemia is these cases, but the accuracy of this study is limited and prompt arteriography is favored. Arteriographic criteria of renal artery dissections include the following: (1) luminal irregularities with aneurysmal dilatations or saccular dissections associated with segmental stenoses, (2) extension of the dissection distally to the first renal artery branch, and (3) cuffing at branchings causing a "rolled-down sock" appearance.

Dissections secondary to severe blunt trauma usually necessitate emergency renal artery reconstruction. Reconstructions using autogenous saphenous vein or hypogastric artery may be complex, and ex vivo repairs are appropriate in selected cases. If hypertension persists or renal function deteriorates in instances of seemingly minor injury, then late repair is appropriate. Treatment using endovascular stents has appeal, but as yet remains an unproven therapy. Spontaneous dissecting aneurysms should be subjected to early surgical therapy once hemodynamically significant stenoses or occlusions are recognized as causing systemic hypertension or deterioration in renal function.

Edwards BS, Stanson AW, Holley KE, Sheps SG: Isolated renal artery dissection: Presentation, evaluation, management and pathology. Mayo Clin Proc 1982;57:564.

Gewertz BL, Stanley JC, Fry WJ: Renal artery dissections. Arch Surg 1977;112:409.

Reilly LM et al: The role of arterial reconstruction in spontaneous renal artery dissection. J Vasc Surg 1991;14:468.

Mycotic Aneurysms

21

Richard L. McCann, MD, & Mark C. Sebastian, MD

During his 1885 Golstonian lecture, Sir William Osler coined the term **mycotic aneurysm.** In this lecture, Osler disclosed the relation between abnormal cardiac valves and infection with micrococci, not with fungi. He presented a case of bacterial endocarditis which on postmortem examination was found to have infection extending into the aorta that had the appearance of fresh "fungus vegetations." Osler's description of "mycotic endarteritis," resulted in a new term, which endures today. The term, "mycotic aneurysm," is now understood to refer to aneurysms associated with infection from any type of microorganism, and is not limited to fungal infections. These lesions are uncommon but not rare. The epidemiology of mycotic aneurysms has been affected by advances in vascular surgery and medicine in general. The nature of these lesions has also been influenced by cultural changes; for example, most surgeons have never seen a syphilitic aneurysm, whereas the arterial infection due to bizarre organisms related to intravascular injection of illicit drugs is increasing in incidence. Bacterial endocarditis was the most prominent cause of arterial infection during the preantibiotic era. However, the introduction of effective antibiotic therapy, infection of a preexisting atherosclerotic or aneurysmal arterial lesion has become a more prominent cause of mycotic aneurysms.

Essentials of Diagnosis
- Infection in the wall of a large or small artery.
- Often loss tensile strength of arterial wall, which becomes aneurysmal.
- Culture of a microorganism from the wall of the vessel.
- Arterial rupture, if untreated.

General Considerations
Several classifications of vascular infection have been proposed but because of the heterogenous nature of mycotic aneurysms, none has been universally accepted. The important considerations include the source of infection, the nature of the affected vessel, and the specific organism involved (Table 21–1). The source of the infection may be intrinsic to the vascular tree, such as in the classic mycotic organism of Osler, in which heavily colonized cardiac valve vegetations are the source of micro- or macroemboli to distant sites. In these sites, the emboli lodge in vessel branch points or in vasa vasorum, accounting for infection of large vessels. The infection may also spread contiguously and involve the adjacent ascending aorta. A second source of infection is extravascular, resulting from osteomyelitis, pneumonia, abscesses, or other extravascular infections. These processes may cause vascular infection by means of bacteremia or by local spread. A perivascular infection, such as spinal osteomyelitis adjacent to the aorta, may weaken the wall of a blood vessel and result in local aneurysm formation. A third source of infection is direct inoculation. This mechanism occurs from injection of illicit drugs, occasionally from invasive vascular procedures in the medical setting, or from civilian or military trauma. The nature of the affected vessel must also be considered. The normal arterial wall is highly resistant to infection, except in unusual circumstances. A heavy inoculum of a very virulent organism is required to establish infection in a normal vessel wall. Infection can be promoted by local trauma, which may be a result of some underlying disease or which may be iatrogenic or accidental. The atherosclerotic intima, containing ulcerated plaques consisting of necrotic cellular debris and thrombus, may provide a fertile ground for microorganisms to establish local infection. Finally, the mural thrombus associated with aneurysm, particularly abdominal aortic aneurysms, is known to be frequently contaminated with microorganisms. Occasionally, this becomes a significant clinical event, and infection of a preexisting abdominal aortic aneurysm is a distinct clinical entity, which will be described later in the chapter. The particular microorganism involved also plays a role in clinical management and outcome of patients with vascular infections.

The adjective "mycotic," when originally used in the late 19th century, referred to the entire spectrum of microorganisms. Recently, the term is known to refer to fungi. These fungal organisms very rarely cause vascular infection today. Only the rare case of *Candida* involvement or *Aspergillus* in the very unusual clinical circumstance has been reported.

Certain microorganisms have long been known to have a predilection for vascular infection. Among these are *Salmonella, Staphylococcus,* and *Streptococcus.* Although the relative incidence of these organisms has changed moderately in the decades since the introduction of effective antibiotic chemotherapy, they remain the most frequently observed organisms in vascular in-

Table 21–1. Classification of vascular infections.

Source of Infection
  Intrinsic—endocarditis or other intravascular infection
  Extrinsic—osteomyelitis, pneumonia, other infection
    by local spread or bacteremia
  Inoculation—inadvertent during medical procedures,
    unhygienic injections, eg, infecting drug use
Affected Vessel
  Normal—resistant except in high virulence or large inocula
  Atherosclerotic—susceptible, especially to *Salmonella*
    and *Staphylococcus*
  Aneurysmal—many more culture-positive than infections
Causative Microorganism
  Salmonella—most common; 65% involve aorta
  Staphylococcus—next most common
  Streptococcus—seen especially with endocarditis
  Other unusual organisms—as seen in unhygienic
    injections, eg, IV drug abuse, and in immune deficiency

fections. More recently, a number of bizarre organisms, such as *Aspergillus, S Arizona, Campylobacter, Histoplasma, Yersinia, Clostridium, Candida,* and *tuberculosis,* have been observed occasionally with vascular infection. Most patients diagnosed with mycotic aneurysms have impaired immune function caused by corticosteroid therapy, diabetes, or malnutrition.

Clinical Findings

A. Signs and Symptoms: Most patients with mycotic aneurysm present with signs and symptoms of infection such as fever, leukocytosis, and local tenderness or inflammation from erythema. If the infectious component is not recognized or not adequately treated, disruption of the tensile strength of the arterial wall may lead to rupture. In a large vessel, this may result in exsanguinating hemorrhage. Some patients, such as those with bacterial endocarditis, vertebral osteomyelitis, or other periarterial abscesses, tend to develop infection in their arterial system. Others may be predisposed to infection because of pathologic changes in the affected vessel itself. These patients are distinguished from others with uninfected vascular disease by the presence of systemic signs of infection. Only rarely is pus or exudate observed in these patients. By the time that suppuration occurs, the vessel wall has become so weak that it ruptures and results in hemorrhage.

B. Imaging Studies: The importance of early diagnosis cannot be overemphasized. This requires a high index of suspicion and sophisticated radiologic evaluation. The survival of patients once rupture has occurred is very low and thus the importance of prompt and efficient investigation. The arteriographic characteristics that suggest a mycotic nature for aneurysmal disease include a saccular aneurysm with a narrow neck giving a lobular appearance (Fig 21–1). In cases of bacterial endocarditis, many lesions may be present. Osler's original description included a budding fungus-like appearance of the thoracic aorta; this is frequently observed angiographically. The arteriogram outlines only the lumen, and, especially in cases

of rupture with retroperitoneal hematoma, it may underestimate the size of the lesion. Leukocyte may yield a diagnostic study. This test is performed by labeling leukocytes with indium-III-oxine (^{III}Im) and viewing with a gamma camera that produces scintigraphic image. However, false-negative and false-positive studies occur, and clinical correlation is required. In the setting of suspected arterial infection and a positive study, the diagnosis should be considered established. Suspected intra-abdominal infection is often evaluated with abdominal computed tomography. (CT) The characteristics suggestive of infected aneurysm are periaortic soft tissue rim enhancement, and nondisplaced intimal calcifications or an aneurysm without any calcification in the wall. Another interesting observation is the rapid expansion of an aortic aneurysm that strongly suggests a contribution of infection (Fig 21–2). Extraluminal gas has occasionally been observed, and CT-guided needle aspiration cultures may be helpful in establishing the diagnosis. Adjacent vertebral osteomyelitis is also a suggestive finding. Magnetic resonance imaging (MRI), although an excellent technique for evaluation of bland aneurysms probably does not contribute as much information as conventional CT scanning in patients suspected of mycotic infection.

C. Laboratory Findings: The laboratory findings specific to a diagnosis of mycotic aneurysm are indicative of infection, such as leukocytosis, fever, elevated sedimentation rate, and positive cultures. Positive cultures should be obtained from the actual

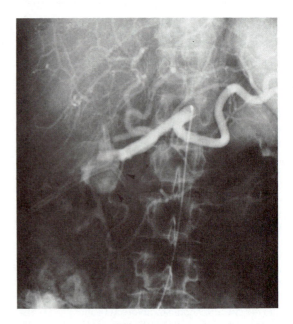

Figure 21–1. Lateral aortogram of a patient who presented with back pain after being treated for bacterial endocarditis with antibiotics and valve replacement. A peculiar posterior pseudoaneurysm of the aorta is found at the level of the celiac axis.

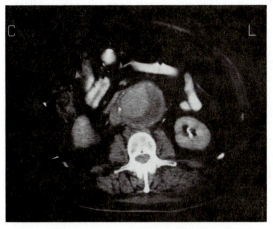
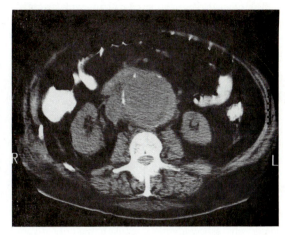

A   B

Figure 21–2. **A:** Abdominal CT scan showing a infrarenal abdominal aortic aneurysm in a patient with *Escherichia coli* sepsis related to urinary tract infection. Because of back pain, the CT scan was repeated 1 week later. **B:** Acute expansion of the aneurysm is noted, which is now more than 9 cm in diameter. *E coli* were cultured from the aneurysm wall at time of surgery.

arterial wall to establish the diagnosis. It is interesting that as much as 15% of bland-appearing abdominal aortic aneurysms have positive culture of the mural thrombus even when infection is not suspected. It is not clear why only 1% or less of these subsequently have any evidence of infection.

D. Principles of Diagnosis: The diagnosis can be made definitely only when organisms are cultured from the vascular wall. Cultures should be sent whenever a chance exists that the arterial lesion may be due to or exacerbated by infection. Certain clinical situations are highly suggestive of mycotic aneurysm. Mycotic aneurysm should be strongly suspected in the setting of bacterial endocarditis if pseudoaneurysm of the mesenteric or other arterial bed is encountered. The presence of fever and toxicity in the setting of rapid expansion of an abdominal aortic aneurysm also strongly suggests mycotic aneurysm.

Treatment

The treatment of patients with a mycotic aneurysm is site specific. Aneurysms in nonessential arteries can be simply ligated proximal and distal to the infectious process and the infected segment excised. The surgical challenge occurs in situations in which an infected artery must be replaced or bypassed to provide adequate circulation for essential organs and limbs. Avoidance of infection of the autogenous or synthetic reconstruction is often difficult and may require ingenuity.

CLASSIC MYCOTIC ANEURYSM

"Classic mycotic aneurysm" is a designation that now refers to the narrow clinical spectrum of infection

of the arterial wall found in association with endocarditis. Before the introduction of effective antimicrobial agents and the ability to treat endocarditis both medically and surgically, this was the most common form of arterial infection and accounted for 80% of cases. Recently, less than 10% of cases of infected aneurysms were related to bacterial endocarditis. There are 3 potential mechanisms by which arterial infection can occur in this clinical situation: (1) local extension of the infection to the adjacent regions of the sinuses of Valsalva and the ascending aorta, (2) embolization of small or large microorganism-rich vegetation particles with lodgment of these embolic particles in vasa vasorum, and (3) impaction of larger particles within smaller vessels in the peripheral arterial tree. In early series, the ascending aorta was most frequently affected, followed by the visceral vessels, the intracranial circulation, and the extremities. Before the introduction of effective antibiotics, 4.5% of patients with bacterial endocarditis died of rupture of a mycotic aneurysm, and emboli were thought to occur in up to 35% of patients with bacterial endocarditis. Treatment at that time was supportive only, and without effective treatment of the underlying endocarditis, the prognosis was hopeless. Although the incidence of this problem has dramatically decreased, coincident with the medical and surgical control of rheumatic heart disease and bacterial endocarditis, it still remains a clinical problem not infrequently seen. With the epidemic of injection drug use in this country, bacterial endocarditis related to this activity is increasing and a larger number of peripheral vascular complications associated with injection drug use will probably be encountered.

The clinical presentation of patients with mycotic aneurysm is that of infection. Systemic signs of myalgias, arthralgias, and fever may be seen. Pain is a frequent accompaniment of embolization, particularly to the lower extremity. These lesions tend to be small and not apparent on physical or radiographic examination except arteriography. Infection clearly plays a role in the development of arterial aneurysm and rupture. This is emphasized by the fact that aneurysm and vessel rupture is not seen in the presence of bland embolization, but is seen only when embolization occurs with emboli containing viable microorganisms. Frequently, the affected vessels are multiple and sometimes numerous.

Although spontaneous healing of mycotic aneurysms has been reported, it is probably rare. Large aneurysms, especially those jeopardizing critical vascular flow and those with active infection, must be managed surgically. The surgical therapy applied may be proximal and distal ligation with débridement and resection of all infected tissue for a noncritical artery or anatomic or extra-anatomic bypass for more critical vessels. Occasionally, the femoral artery can be sacrificed but more frequently it requires bypass. Management of visceral artery disease may be individualized. In most cases, however, bypass, in-line grafting, or endoaneurysmorraphy has been applied with varying success. All treatment depends on adequate control of systemic infection related to the underlying bacterial endocarditis.

The arteriographic appearance of classic mycotic aneurysm is often striking. The vessel involved is usually normal except for the site of involvement. The infections tend to produce well-lobulated saccular aneurysms and pseudoaneurysms. These aneurysms have a tendency for early rupture; thus, treatment must be prompt and efficacious to avoid unfavorable results.

INFECTED ABDOMINAL AORTIC ANEURYSMS

Infection of an atherosclerotic aorta results in a localized weakening or the aortic wall. These aneurysms are most commonly saccular and may involve any section of the aorta. Common risk factors are prior catheterization, intravascular drug use, depressed immune competence, diabetes, and neoplastic disease. *Salmonella* and *Staphylococcus* infections predominate. Most patients have evidence of sepsis, and blood cultures are often positive. Morphologically, the lesions tend to be saccular, localized, and sometimes multiple. The aneurysms may be true aneurysms containing all layers of the vessel wall, or they may be false aneurysms, which result from localized contained rupture because of weakening of the aortic wall by the infectious process. An abdominal aortic aneurysm has a tendency toward early rupture, especially those with infections due to *Salmonella*.

The second type of aortic aneurysm infection results from secondary contamination of an existing atherosclerotic aneurysm, presumably by hematogenous inoculation. These aneurysms may be difficult to distinguish from bland, uninfected aneurysms. It is interesting that studies have repeatedly shown that routine cultures of aortic thrombus material removed from aneurysms at the time of routine aneurysm repair show a high incidence of positive bacterial culture findings. The incidence of positive cultures has varied from 8% to 15%, and the incidence of positive cultures in ruptured aneurysms is twice the rate of positive culture in unruptured aneurysms, suggesting that infection may play a role in aneurysm rupture. The paradoxical observation is that many patients with positive cultures fail to demonstrate any subsequent evidence of infection despite in-line replacement with synthetic arterial prostheses. The dilemma remains about what to do when a culture of apparently bland abdominal aortic aneurysm contents unexpectedly yields bacterial growth. Most favor long-term if not indefinite organism-specific antibiotic therapy.

A particular clinical syndrome is recognized when *Salmonella* causes aortic infection. Vascular infections are due to 3 species of *Salmonella*: *S choleraesuis, S typhirmurium,* and *S enteritidis.* Seventy-five percent of aneurysms caused by *Salmonella* are of the aorta. Fifty percent of these involve the abdominal aorta. Rupture of the vessel and pseudoaneurysm formation are very common. When rupture occurs, mortality rate exceeds 80%. Even when treatment precedes rupture, nearly 50% of patients do not survive. Opinions differ regarding management of aortic infection. When the infection involves the suprarenal aorta or the great vessels, in-line grafting is almost always necessary and has been successful. However, recurrent infection of the graft remains a significant risk. With the infrarenal aorta an alternate strategy is possible.

Some clinicians continue to advocate débridement of the aorta with removal of as much infected vascular and retroperitoneal tissue as practical and then placement of an in-line prosthetic graft by traditional techniques. The contrary opinion holds that placement of a bypass graft through uninfected planes—through either a thoracic retroperitoneal route or more commonly an axillofemoral or axilloiliac graft—is a preferable strategy. Proponents of the in situ graft replacement emphasize its simplicity, optimal long-term patency rates, and empirical success. Proponents of the alternative extra-anatomic bypass point out that overall morality rate with in situ grafting remains 32%, with 50% of these deaths being due to recurrent sepsis. This is particularly true in cases of *Salmonella* aortitis.

Long-term results with axillofemoral reconstructions have been continuously improved. Long-term patency rates now approach 85% with limb salvage in a similar range. Also, if infection has been controlled and a delayed thrombosis of the axillofemoral reconstruction occurs, conversion to intracavitary bypass can be used with the new graft taking origin from uninvolved thoracic or upper abdominal aorta (Fig 21–3).

The most serious complication of aneurysm excision and extra-anatomic bypass is rupture of the aortic stump as long as 13 months following aortic closure. When aortoenteric fistula is present, the risk of aortic stump rupture is even greater. Several methods have been recommended for closing the aortic stump. It is not known whether any of these is truly protective. The use of omentoplasty to cover the stump does not appear to be helpful since 6 ruptures occurred in a series of 8 patients. It is surprisingly that 2 patients with stump rupture were salvaged, but most instances are fatal (Fig 21–4).

No consensus exists regarding the duration of antibiotic therapy after surgical treatment. Many continue to advocate indefinite use of antibiotics, which seems a reasonable approach considering the potential for life-threatening aortic stump rupture.

SUPRARENAL AORTIC MYCOTIC ANEURYSMS

A particularly challenging clinical situation is mycotic aneurysm of the thoracic or suprarenal aorta. Although this occurs less commonly than infrarenal aortic infection, when it does occur it presents a difficult challenge. Restoration of arterial continuity through uncontaminated tissues is technically difficult because of the requirement to maintain visceral and lower extremity perfusion. Lifelong, organism-specific antibiotics are usually recommended in this setting, especially if in-line grafting has been performed.

VISCERAL ARTERY MYCOTIC ANEURYSMS

A large percentage of visceral artery aneurysms are found to be mycotic in origin. The superior mesenteric artery is the most commonly involved visceral vessel. Infection is thought to be the cause of as much as 60% of superior mesenteric artery aneurysms. Because of

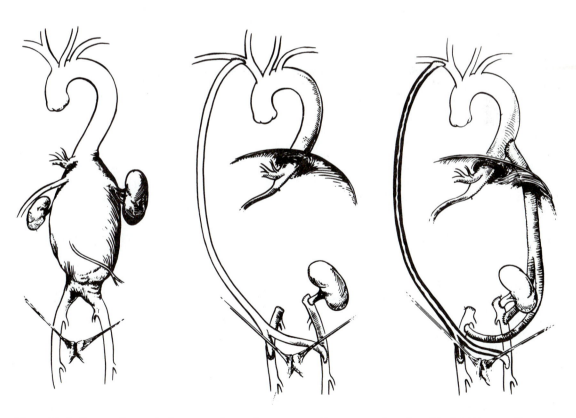

Figure 21–3. Strategy for repair of suprarenal mycotic aneurysm with autotransplantation of the left kidney and lower extremity revascularization via axillobifemoral grafting with aortoplasty. After eradiction of all infection, lower extremity circulation can be improved by thoracoaortic to iliac bypass (Reproduced, with permission, from Reddy DJ, Ernst CB: Infected aortic aneurysms: Recognition and management. Semin Vasc Surg 1988;1:174.)

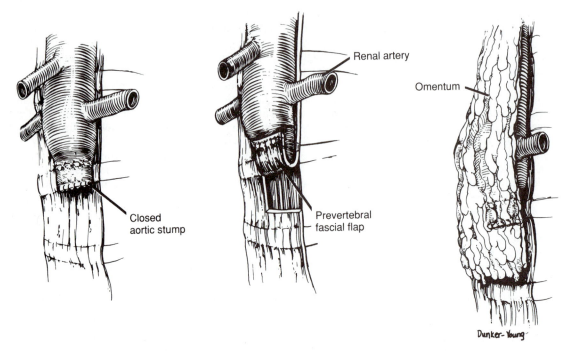

Figure 21–4. Method for closure of the aortic stump using a prevertebral flap to aortic closure and coverage with a pedicle graft of omentum. (Reproduced, with permission, from Ernest, CB: Aortoenteric fistulas. In: *Vascular Emergencies.* Haemovichi H (editor). Appleton-Century-Crofts, 1982.)

their small size, these aneurysms are often not apparent on physical or radiographic evaluation except for angiography. Despite their small size, the incidence of preoperative rupture is high. Free peritoneal rupture is usually fatal. Aneurysms may rupture into the lessor sac and be contained there; occasionally, celiac artery aneurysms may rupture into the thorax. Simple ligation with excision or endoaneurysmorrhaphy has been performed for visceral artery lesions. This frequently leads to mesenteric vascular insufficiency and the need for bowel resection. Mesenteric revascularization by use of saphenous vein graft from the aorta has been reported and is a good strategy if the bowel is threatened after ligation. Most visceral artery mycotic lesions are found in the setting of bacterial endocarditis, and if the diagnosis is not obvious preoperatively, it should be suspected and echocardiography should considered.

MYCOTIC CAROTID ARTERY ANEURYSM

The cerebral circulation is a common site for lodgment of embolic vegetations in patients with bacterial endocarditis. The controversy regarding the strategy of arterial reconstruction versus ligation for mycotic carotid artery aneurysm remains unresolved. Most authors in the past have favored ligation. Recently, the safety of carotid ligation has been determined by measuring carotid stump back pressure at surgery. Temporary balloon occlusion has been used in the angiography suite together with monitoring of the neurologic status of the awake patient to determine the safety of carotid occlusion in cases with carotid artery aneurysm. Gradual occlusion of the carotid artery with a screw clamp has been used since the days of syphilitic aneurysms. Reconstruction has been performed both by resection and direct anastomosis and also by saphenous vein graft interposition.

SPECIAL CLINICAL SITUATIONS

With the decline in bacterial endocarditis and control of infectious diseases in general, mycotic aneurysm is now seen most frequently in special clinical situations. Intravenous drug abuse continues to increase despite all efforts to the contrary. Mycotic aneurysm associated with unhygienic self-injection is seen frequently, particularly at major urban medical centers. Parallel with this increase is the epidemic of HIV infection, which is associated with infection diminished resistance. Finally, explosive growth has been seen in the use of solid organ transplants with attendant deliberate immunosuppression. The vascular connection of these organ transplants place a patient are at particular risk of infective aneurysm formation.

Drug Abuse

Perhaps the most common clinical setting for mycotic aneurysm involves illicit injection of drugs. Large series have been reported from major metropolitan centers. It is interesting that despite the use of unhygienic techniques for vascular self-injection of illicit drugs, the most common organism isolated from vascular infection under these circumstances is still *Staphylococcus aureus*. These lesions are frequently misdiagnosed as cellulitis or abscess formation, and a high index of suspicion must be maintained. Only a minority of lesions involve the upper extremity. Usually no vascular morbidity results from resection of radial or brachial artery lesions, and reconstruction generally is not necessary when these vessels are involved.

Treatment for femoral artery lesions is more controversial. Ligation and excision of iliac and deep femoral artery lesions may not result in limb-threatening ischemia. However, resection of femoral artery lesions without reconstruction often results in severe limb ischemia, and one-third of patients treated in this fashion experience limb loss. Despite this, some clinicians continue to recommend deferring revascularization in cases in which an audible Doppler signal persists after resection of infected femoral artery aneurysm. The alternative strategy suggests the use of extra-anatomic revascularization, often placed prior to aneurysm ligation and resection.

The route for the bypass should completely avoid the septic area by using the obturator foramen approach or a lateral subcutaneous route with an axillopopliteal or iliac to superficial femoral configuration. When technically feasible, many suggest that the autogenous saphenous vein graft may be preferable because it may be more resistant to reinfection than a synthetic graft. However, when recurrent infection does occur in an autogenous vein bypass graft, the consequences are disastrous. Infection of a saphenous vein graft results in irreparable deterioration of the wall of the graft, followed by hemorrhage. Although the risk of recurrent infection may be higher with a prosthetic graft, the risk of catastrophic hemorrhage is lower.

HIV Infection

HIV seropositivity is becoming increasingly common in surgical patients. In a recent series of femoral pseudoaneurysms related to drug abuse, 20% of patients were found to be HIV-seropositive. Several series of infected aortic aneurysms have been reported in patients known to be infected with the HIV virus.

In addition, *Salmonella* bacteremia is recognized as a common occurrence in patients with AIDS. It has been proposed that this could lead to a significant incidence of arterial infection, and reports are beginning to appear of vascular infections in AIDS patients. Repair of the aneurysms, particularly when ruptured and involve extensive aortic débridement and considerable blood loss, may prove to be a significant hazard not only to the patient but to the surgical care team as well. It is now estimated that HIV has been transmitted to more than 12 million people in the world; thus, this dilemma is likely to become more common.

Organ Transplants

Solid abdominal organ transplantation is rapidly increasing. More than 10,000 kidney transplantations, 3000 liver transplantations, and several hundred pancreas transplantations are performed annually in the USA. Because of the attendant immunosuppression, these patients are at increased jeopardy for infectious complications. Infectious complications that affect the arterial anastomoses produce breakdown and pseudoaneurysm formation if not frank rupture. An incidence in 1.2% of renal transplants, 2.2% with hepatic transplants, and 12% with pancreas transplants have been reported. The arterial anastomosis has been considered the Achilles heel of liver transplantation (Fig 21–5). The incidence has been high, particularly in the setting of biliary tract complications resulting in local sepsis. This allows infection of the adjacent hepatic artery anastomosis. The occurrence of hepatic artery complication has a significant deleterious effect on outcome in patients who have had liver transplantation. Pancreas transplantation has been associated with a remarkably high incidence of infection of the vascular

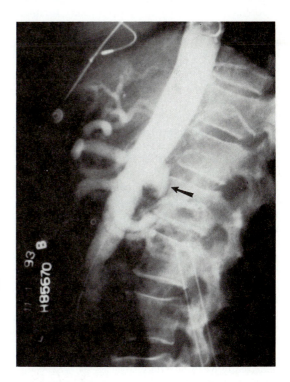

Figure 21–5. Large mycotic aneurysm of a liver transplant hepatic artery anastomosis. The wall of this aneurysm grew *Candida albicans,* which required ligation and hepatic artery reconstruction using a saphenous vein graft from the aorta to the uninvolved distal hepatic artery.

connections. Treatment of these infections often requires iliac artery ligation and extra-anatomic reconstruction to provide limb perfusion. The organisms involved in these cases have frequently been unusual. *Citrobacter, Bacteroides, Fusobacterium,* and *Enterobacter cloacae* have been found. These cases have proved to be difficult clinical challenges. Rupture is common and jeopardizes not only the graft but the patient as well. Graft function is usually lost. Occasionally, in liver transplantation, graft function has been preserved in the face of sacrifice of the hepatic artery, but the usual consequence of sacrifice of arterial perfusion is intrahepatic and extrahepatic bile duct stenosis and severe biliary obstruction with frequent sepsis.

MICROBIOLOGIC CONSIDERATIONS

For a number of years, it has been recognized that certain microorganisms have predilection for vascular infection. Among these are *Salmonella, Staphylococcus,* and *Streptococcus.* Although the relative incidence of these organisms has changed moderately in the decades since the introduction of effective antibiotic therapy, they remain the most frequently observed organisms in vascular infections. More recently, a number of bizarre organisms, such as *Aspergillus, S Arizona, Campylobacter, Histoplasma, Yersinia, Clostridia,* and *Candida* have been observed with vascular infection. Because of their frequency and importance in vascular infection, the 3 most common organisms will be described.

Salmonella

Salmonellae are motile, flagellated, gram-negative rods in the family Enterobacteriaceae. These organisms were first described by Salmon in swine in 1886 and are named for him. They are aerobic or facultative anaerobes and are related to other Enterobacteriaceae such as *Shigella, Proteus,* and *Escherichia.* Salmonellae are identified microbiologically by their inability to ferment sucrose and lactose and by their inability to metabolize urea. They have a wide distribution in nature and are found throughout the animal kingdom. More than 2000 serotypes have been identified. Salmonella frequently affects poultry, cattle, and swine. Human disease is most commonly attributed to oral-fecal contamination with the pathogen. The pathogens are rapidly killed by gastric acid but may survive passage through the stomach, which is buffered by food or water. Infection usually results in a self-limited gastroenteritis but may cause a fulminant enteric fever, particularly when infection is caused by *S typhi.* Infection may result in a chronic carrier state, which may or may not cause symptoms, or systemic bacteremia may occur. The carrier state may exist for many years and is sometimes not eradicated without cholecystectomy where the organisms may remain dominant for long periods of time. For reasons that remain unclear, 75% of aneurysms caused by *Salmonella* involve the abdominal aorta and the organism appears to have a predilection for atherosclerotic vessels, although it can attack normal vessels as well.

Patients with *Salmonella* bacteremia have a 6–25% chance of subsequently developing a vascular infection. Rupture of the vessel and pseudoaneurysm formation are very common. Recurrent infection, particularly with an in situ vascular prosthesis, is also very common. Mortality rate continues to be nearly 50% even in promptly treated patients.

Salmonella organisms may be cultured from 50% of commercially available chickens, and 20% of frozen egg whites, and a varying percentage of milk and ground beef. Another important clinical observation is that *Salmonella* infection is not only common in patients with AIDS, but it may be very severe. In terms of antimicrobial therapy, note that *Salmonellae* exhibit a high rate of plasmid-mediated resistance, particularly to such traditionally used drugs as ampicillin, trimethoprim sulfamethoxazole, and occasionally even to the new quinolones. The effective antimicrobials against *Salmonella* include chloramphenicol, ampicillin, amoxicillin, trimethoprim sulfamethoxazole, and third-generation cephalosporins such as cephtriaxone. The newer quinolone antibiotics such as ciprofloxacin also appear to have considerable efficacy against *Salmonella.*

Staphylococcus

The most common gram-positive organisms causing vascular infection are staphylococci. These strongly gram-positive cocci grow in grape-like clusters. *Staphylococcus aureus,* when grown on blood agar, produces opaque, golden-yellow colonies that are usually hemolytic. The production of coagulase distinguishes this species from *Staphylococcus epidermidis,* the other staphylococcal pathogen. *S epidermidis* is a major component of the normal flora of the skin and mucous membranes. Staphylococci are nonmotile and do not form spores. These organisms are important components of the normal flora of the body and self-contamination of intrinsic staphylococci carried by the patient is believed to be the most important event in infections of the vascular system. About 25% of adults are asymptomatic carriers of *S aureus,* usually in the nose or intertriginous areas. The treatment for *S aureus* and *S epidermidis* infections is becoming increasingly difficult because of the large numbers of organisms that have become resistant to all of the β-lactam antibiotics. Vancomycin resistance has not been reported but is expected to occur in the future. Recommended treatment for serious *S aureus* infections includes use of a penicillinase-resistant penicillin such as Methicillin, first-generation cephalosporins such as cefazolin, and then vancomycin. Vancomycin is the only available drug that is appropriate for methicillin-resistant *S aureus.*

Streptococcus

The third most commonly encountered microorganism is the *Streptococcus.* This heterogenous group of organisms has distinct clinical syndromes. They are strongly gram-positive, spherical or ovoid, and not larger than 2 µm in diameter. Cell division occurs in a single plane, resulting in the appearance of organisms in chains of variable length usually between 6 and 12. Group A streptococci (*S pyogenes*) are associated with laryngitis, pneumonia, pyoderma, lymphangitis, and the postinfectious sequelae of acute rheumatic fever and acute glomerulonephritis. Some secrete toxins, one of which (toxin A) may produce a toxic shock syndrome. The organisms are easily grown on sheep blood agar and produce a variable zone of β-hemolysis. The organisms may grow rapidly with division as frequently as every 20 minutes. Despite half a century of use, no strain of group A *Streptococcus* has been found to be resistant to penicillin. Group B streptococci are now referred to as *S agalactiae.* This organism is responsible for postpartum fever and can frequently be isolated from the vagina. It is also responsible for neonatal bacteremia and meningitis. *S agalactiae* is β-hemolytic and may be identified by its hydrolysis of sodium hippurate. Although somewhat less sensitive than group A, treatment of group B streptococci is also with penicillin. Vancomycin is the alternative in allergic patients. *S pneumoniae* (pneumococcus) microorganisms generally grow as single organisms or diplococci. This species is α-hemolytic and a component of the normal bacterial flora of the human nasopharynx. In times of local or systemic altered defense mechanisms, these organisms may invade the lung, middle ear, or other sites. They may also appear in the bloodstream as bacteremia even in the absence of a defined local infection.

Streptococci not in group A or group B are frequently labeled "miscellaneous." This group includes the *S viridans.* These organisms are non-β-hemolytic but may be α- or γ-hemolytic. At least 10 distinct species exist, although only a few appear to be important clinically. The clinical spectrum of infection by *S viridans* varies by species. The most pertinent is its propensity to cause bacterial endocarditis. It may also participate in abdominal abscesses, liver abscesses, cholecystitis, bone and joint infections, and skin and soft tissue infections, and *S viridans* may be more prevalent in patients with diabetes. A related organism is *S bovis.* Infection with this organism has a strong association with gastrointestinal malignancy. Penicillin is the recommended agent, although some recommend dual therapy with aminoglycoside for serious infections such as endocarditis or mycotic aneurysm.

Enterococci were formerly known as group D streptococci. Sophisticated microbiologic and DNA hybridization studies have demonstrated subtle differences between group D streptococci and Enterococci; thus, the enterococci are now classified as a separate genus. Nevertheless, irrespective of their taxonomy, these organisms are important causes of bacterial endocarditis and have been reported to be responsible for subsequent mycotic aneurysm development. Treatment of serious enterococcus infection requires vancomycin plus an aminoglycoside.

Summary

Infection in the wall of an artery reduces the tensile strength and may result in untreated cases in aneurysm formation or in vessel rupture. Most affected patients present with signs and symptoms of infection, and subsequently the arterial involvement with the infectious processes is identified. The most common organisms associated with mycotic aneurysm formation are *Salmonella, Staphylococcus,* and *Streptococcus.* More bizarre and unusual infections may be found in the setting of unhygienic vascular manipulation for purposes of illicit drug injection and in patients with immune depression associated with HIV or organ transplantation.

It is necessary to maintain a very high index of suspicion, since early diagnosis is mandatory for the best outcome. Uncontrolled infection inevitably leads to vascular rupture and loss of limb or life. Treatment involves organism-specific antibiotic therapy combined with resection of the infected vascular tissue with or without vascular reconstruction. Reconstruction is optimally performed through clean uncontaminated fields and often requires an extra-anatomic route. Even under optimal conditions, morbidity and mortality remain high emphasizing the difficult surgical challenge presented by arterial wall involved with infection.

REFERENCES

Akers DL, Jr, Fowl RJ, Kempczinski RF: Mycotic aneurysm of the tibioperoneal trunk: Case report and review of the literature. J Vasc Surg 1992;16:71.

Atnip RG: Mycotic aneurysms of the suprarenal abdominal aorta: prolonged survival after in situ aortic and visceral reconstruction. J Vasc Surg 1989;10:635.

Ben-Haim S, Seabold JE, Hawes DR, Rooholamini SA: Leukocyte scintigraphy in the diagnosis of mycotic aneurysm. J Nucl Med 1992;33.

Benoit G et al: Mycotic aneurysm and renal transplantation. Urology 1988;31:63.

Brown SL et al: Bacteriologic and surgical determinants of survival in patients with mycotic aneurysms. J Vasc Surg 1984;1:541.

Dean EH et al: Mycotic embolism and embolomycotic aneurysms: Neglected lesions of the past. Ann Surg 1986; 204:306.

Fichelle JM et al: Infected infrarenal aortic aneurysms:

When is in situ reconstruction safe. J Vasc Surg 1993; 17:635.

Gomes MN, Choyke PL: Infected aortic aneurysms: CT diagnosis. J Cardiovasc Surg 1992;33:684.

Gomes MN, Choyke PL, Wallace RB: Infected aortic aneurysms: A changing entity. Ann Surg 1992;13:435.

Gouny P et al: Human immunodeficiency virus and infected aneurysm of the abdominal aorta: Report of three cases. Ann Vasc Surg 1992;6:239.

Hollier LH et al: Direct replacement of mycotic thoracoabdominal aneurysms. J Vasc Surg 1993;18:477.

Katz SG, Andros G, Kohl RD: *Salmonella* infections of the abdominal aorta. Surg Gynecol Obstet 1992;175: 102.

McCann RL, Schwartz LB, Georgiade GS: Management of abdominal aortic graft complications. Ann Surg 1993; 217:729.

Moriarity JA, Edelman RR, Tumeh SS: CT and MRI of mycotic aneurysms of the abdominal aorta. J Comput Assist Tomogr 1992;16:941.

Oskoui R, Davis WA, Gomes MN: *Salmonella* aortitis. Arch Int Med 1993;153:517.

Oz MC, Brener BJ, Buda JA et al: A ten-year experience with bacterial aortitis. J Vasc Surg 1989;10:439.

Padberg F Jr, Hobson R II, Lee B et al: Femoral pseudoaneurysm from drugs of abuse: Ligation or reconstruction. J Vasc Surg 1992;15:642.

Pasic M et al: Treatment of mycotic aneurysm of the aorta and its branches: The location determines the operative technique. Eur J Vasc Surg 1992;6:419.

Patel KR, Semel L, Clauss RH: Routine revascularization with resection of infected femoral pseudoaneurysms from substance abuse. J Vasc Surg 1988;8:321.

Reddy DJ, Ernst CB: Infected aortic aneurysms: Recognition and management. Semin Vasc Surg 1988;1:174.

Reddy DJ et al: Infected femoral artery false aneurysms in drug addicts: Evolution of selective vascular reconstruction. J Vasc Surg 1986;3:718.

Taylor LM Jr, Deitz DM, McConnell DB, Porter JM: Treatment of infected abdominal aneurysms by extraanatomic bypass, aneurysm excision, and drainage. Am J Surg 1988;155:655.

Todo S et al: Hepatic artery in liver transplantation. Transplant Proc 1987;19:2406.

Tzakis AG et al: Arterial mycotic aneurysm and rupture. A potentially fatal complication of pancreas transplantation in diabetes mellitus. Arch Surg 1989;124:660.

Whimby E et al: Bacteremia and fungemia in patients with the acquired immunodeficiency syndrome. Ann Int Med 1986;104:511.

Mesenteric Ischemia Syndromes

22

Kimberley J. Hansen, MD

ACUTE MESENTERIC ISCHEMIA

Essentials of Diagnosis

- Acute abdominal pain with vague physical findings.
- Abdominal distention and gastrointestinal bleeding.
- Vomiting (especially after sudden onset of pain) and diarrhea.
- History of intestinal angina.
- Leukocytosis.

Acute mesenteric ischemic syndromes include a variety of clinical diseases, which challenge the skills of both the physician and the surgeon. Allowed to proceed undiagnosed and untreated, these syndromes culminate in intestinal infarction and patient death and therefore represent medical and surgical emergencies. Despite aggressive treatment, however, contemporary mortality rates for acute mesenteric ischemia (20–40%) remain unacceptably high.

General Considerations

Three main categories of acute visceral ischemia affect the small bowel and colon: (1) mesenteric artery occlusion resulting from either an embolus or a thrombosis; (2) mesenteric vein occlusion; (3) nonocclusive mesenteric ischemia (Table 22–1). When these 3 categories of acute ischemia are considered together, roughly 50% are secondary to mesenteric artery occlusion. The remaining 50% are equally divided between mesenteric vein occlusion and nonocclusive mesenteric ischemia. Arterial embolism and thrombosis are reported to occur equally as frequently in most series. However, Bergan and associates (1987) have reported a series in which embolism accounted for two-thirds of arterial occlusions.

Soon after the general acceptance of routine angiography in the diagnosis and management of acute visceral ischemia, the incidence of nonocclusive mesenteric ischemia first appeared to be increasing. However, more recent reports indicate that this condition may actually be decreasing. This apparent decline may reflect improved cardiovascular management of critically ill patients as well as widespread management of hypertension and ischemic heart disease with medications that induce arterial smooth muscle relaxation.

Etiology

The 3 major visceral arteries (celiac axis, superior mesenteric, and inferior mesenteric) that supply the mesenteric circulation are arranged in parallel fashion (Fig 22–1). Despite this parallel arrangement, 3 major collateral pathways may develop to bypass potential proximal arterial obstruction. First, the celiac and superior mesenteric arteries may communicate through pancreaticoduodenal arcades, whereas the superior and inferior mesenteric arteries may communicate through the "meandering mesenteric artery" (Fig 22–2). Finally, the inferior mesenteric artery and internal iliac arteries may communicate through sigmoidal and hemorrhoidal branches. Of these 3 collateral pathways, the radiographic demonstration of the meandering mesenteric artery is pathognomonic for preexisting obstruction of the superior or inferior mesenteric artery.

Under normal conditions, the 3 visceral arteries and their collaterals carry 25% of the total cardiac output, whereas the mesenteric venous system may harbor 30% of the total circulating blood volume. These figures reflect the high metabolic needs of the gastrointestinal tract and the capacitance function of the mesenteric venous system. Normally, blood flow through the major mesenteric arteries is controlled by the resistance of the vascular bed within the intestinal wall. This vascular bed consists of resistance vessels (arterioles, capillaries, and venules) arranged in series with little collateral potential. These resistance vessels control relative mesenteric blood flow such that the small intestine receives twice the blood flow per unit weight compared with that received by the colon and the stomach. Since the greatest metabolic activity is centered at the luminal surface of the intestine, the mu-

Table 22–1. Mesenteric ischemia syndromes.

I. Acute mesenteric ischemia
  A. Mesenteric artery occlusion
    1. Embolus
    2. Thrombus
  B. Mesenteric vein occlusion
  C. Nonocclusive mesenteric ischemia
II. Chronic mesenteric ischemia

(Adapted from Hansen KJ, Dean RH: Acute visceral ischemic syndromes. In: *General Surgery: Essentials of Practice.* Ritchie WP, Steele GD, Dean RH (editors). JB Lippincott [in press].)

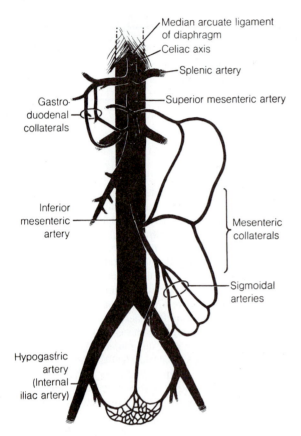

Figure 22–1. Schematic depiction of the major visceral vessels and their major collateral branches. The "meandering mesenteric artery" is a mesenteric collateral distinct from the marginal artery of Drummond. The former is seen deep within the mesentery; the latter is found at the colonic wall.

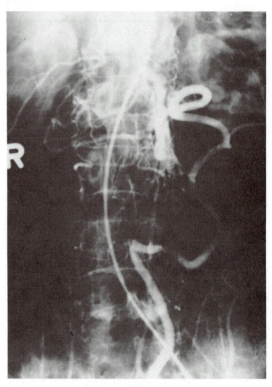

Figure 22–2. Anteroposterior aortogram demonstrating a large meandering mesenteric artery providing blood to the inferior mesenteric artery from its SMA origin. In this case, the pelvic branches of the inferior mesenteric artery also provide collateral flow to the lower extremities.

cosa and submucosa receive almost 70% of the entire mesenteric blood flow.

A. Embolic Occlusion: As medium-sized arterial branches of the anterior abdominal aorta, the mesenteric arteries may be occluded acutely by emboli. In fact, the superior mesenteric artery is the recipient vessel for 3–4% of all arterioarterial emboli. As with peripheral emboli in general, the recipient vessel is frequently free of preexisting occlusive disease, and the embolic phenomena signals serious underlying cardiac disease in most patients. Whereas atrial fibrillation secondary to mitral valve rheumatic heart disease predominated in the past, atrial fibrillation secondary to ischemic heart disease and transmural anterior myocardial infarction with mural thrombus are more frequently encountered today. Less common embolic sources that should also be considered are proximal aortic atheroma, left atrial myxoma, and paradoxical emboli from the systemic venous circulation.

B. Thrombotic Occlusion: Unlike embolic events, superior mesenteric artery thrombosis is most commonly superimposed on preexisting mesenteric atherosclerosis. The anatomic pattern is usually that of an atheroma of the anterior aortic wall encroaching upon the ostium of the superior mesenteric artery and occasionally extending 2–4 cm distally. Although the exact mechanism that precipitates acute thrombosis on this chronic atheroma is poorly understood, 50% of the patients presenting with acute mesenteric artery thrombosis have antecedent symptoms of chronic mesenteric ischemia and intestinal angina. Rheumatoid arthritis, polyarteritis nodosa, systemic lupus erythematosus, and Takayasu's arteritis may infrequently cause mesenteric artery thrombosis. In addition, fibromuscular dysplasia has been reported to underlie celiac axis and superior mesenteric artery thrombosis as well as intestinal angina.

C. Venous Occlusion: In mesenteric vein occlusion, an underlying disorder can be identified in only 50% of cases (Table 22–2). The remaining episodes fail to demonstrate any predisposing factors and have been termed "agnogenic" or idiopathic. Intraperitoneal sepsis resulting from appendicitis or diverticulitis seems to be the most common predisposing process causing pylephlebitis and subsequent venous throm-

Table 22–2. Mesenteric venous occlusion-associated conditions.

Hypercoagulable States

Neoplasms (particularly pancreatic or colonic)
Antithrombin III deficiency
Protein C or protein S deficiency
Polycythemia vera
Thrombocytosis
Thrombocytopenia (heparin-induced)
Oral contraceptives

Local Venous Congestion/Stasis

Portal hypertension
Congestive heart failure
Hypersplenism

Direct Injury

Postoperative state (particularly splenectomy)
Abdomninal trauma
Peritonitis (particularly appendicitis or diverticulitis)
Inflammatory bowel disease
Intra-abdominal abscess

(Adapted from Hansen KJ, Dean RH: Acute visceral ischemic syndromes: In: *General Surgery: Essentials of Practice.* Ritchie WP, Steele GD, Dean RH (editors). JB Lippincott [in press].)

bosis. In addition, a variety of hypercoagulable states may cause mesenteric vein occlusion, such as polycythemia vera and postsplenectomy thrombocytosis, antithrombin III, and protein C and S deficiencies. Oral contraceptives have been associated with a variety of venous and arterial thrombotic events, and a clear association with mesenteric venous thrombosis has been noted by several authors.

D. Nonocclusive Ischemia: Reactive arterial vasoconstriction is responsible for nonocclusive mesenteric ischemic. Central to the pathogenesis of this entity are underlying disease states that lead to systemic hypoperfusion. Most nonocclusive mesenteric ischemia is associated with either severe congestive heart failure or disease states culminating in dehydration. Although digitalis might be expected to improve intestinal perfusion through its myocardial effects, digitalis overdose has been implicated in several cases of nonocclusive mesenteric ischemic, perhaps secondary to its mesenteric arteriolar vasoconstriction.

Pathophysiology

The mechanism of injury following acute mesenteric artery occlusion is incompletely understood. It seems likely that a portion of the injury occurs during the period of ischemia, whereas a portion also occurs during the period of restored blood flow. This "reperfusion injury" results in local vascular damage as well as remote tissue damage mediating multisystem organ failure. The consequences of multisystem organ failure rather than local intestinal damage are responsible for most patient mortality.

Both local and remote injury following reperfusion appears to be related to leukocyte-endothelial cell interaction. After acute intestinal ischemia and reperfusion, leukocytes adhere to the postcapillary endothelium of the vesicle. Leukocyte adherence and activation seem to be dependent on the interaction of undesirable cell surface receptors (CD11/CD18 and ICAM-1). Activated leukocytes appear to mediate local and remote injury through reactive oxygen metabolites and complement activation.

In mesenteric venous occlusion, rapid loss of fluid occurs into the bowel lumen with hemoconcentration. As a result, the bowel wall becomes intensely hemorrhagic, causing separation of the mucosa and submucosa. As the thrombotic process extends to involve the mesentery, serosanguinous fluid weeps into the peritoneal cavity. Despite this sequence of events, occlusion of the major venous branches does not appear to lead to bowel infarction in every case; rather, the thrombosis of the vasa recti and intramural venous collaterals are the most important determinants of bowel infarction. Varying levels of venous involvement and unpredictable extension to involve these terminal venous branches may explain in part the variations in patient presentation with mesenteric venous occlusion.

Nonocclusive mesenteric ischemia most commonly reflects mesenteric vasospasm in response to systemic hypoperfusion in an attempt to shunt blood from the gut to the central circulation to maintain cerebral and cardiac perfusion. This mechanism appears to be mediated primarily through vasopressin and the renin-angiotensin axis. Although vasopressin induces vasoconstriction in a number of circulatory beds, this vasomotor effect is greatest in the mesenteric circulation. In a similar manner, an amplified vasoactive response within the mesenteric circulation is also seen with angiotensin II. The smooth muscle cells of the mesenteric arterioles appear to have increased angiotensin II receptors compared with other circulatory beds. Vasopressin and angiotensin II released in response to hypoperfusion states induce a powerful mesenteric vasoconstriction that is not reduced by local metabolic or myogenic reflexes. Even when systemic hypoperfusion is corrected and the production of vasopressin and angiotensin II decreases, mesenteric vasospasm may persist, further mediating intestinal ischemia, which may progress to frank infarction.

Clinical Findings

Successful treatment of patients with acute visceral ischemia requires prompt diagnosis and appropriate surgical intervention. An increase in patient mortality accompanies any delay in diagnosis and treatment. Even under ideal circumstances, aggressively treated acute visceral ischemia results in a 20–40% mortality rate. However, when delay in therapy results in extensive intestinal gangrene, the mortality rate approaches 95%. Early diagnosis requires recognition of patients at risk, recognition of characteristic abdominal complaints, and emergency angiography (Fig 22–3).

Prompt diagnosis of the acute visceral ischemic syndromes requires an awareness of the population at risk

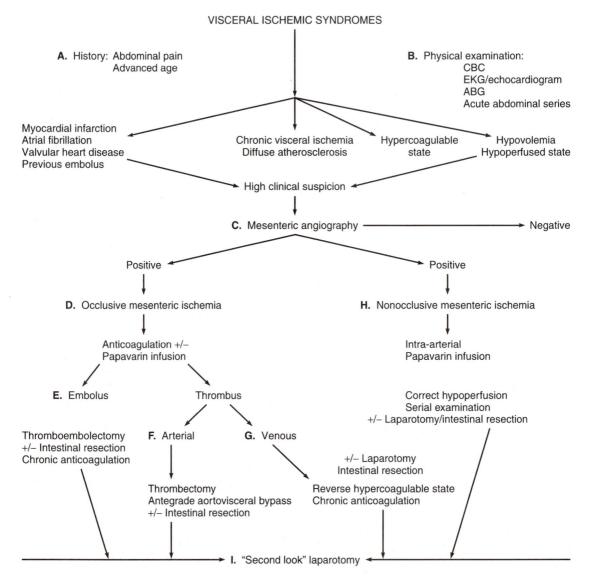

Figure 22–3. Algorithm for management of the acute visceral ischemic syndromes. Recognition of patients at risk followed by emergency angiography is crucial to successful management of each variety of mesenteric ischemia. CBC, complete blood count; EKG, electrocardiogram; ABG, arterial blood gas.

(see Table 22–2). Acute ischemia occurs most frequently in patients over 50 years of age; in one large series, 75% of patients were over 70 years. Ottinger reported a mean age of 60 years for all types of visceral ischemia and a mean age of 60 years for patients suffering from embolic arterial occlusion. Reflecting the high incidence of cardiac disease in this patient population, many patients present with longstanding congestive heart failure that is poorly controlled with digitalis and diuretics. Patients with a history of cardiac arrhythmias (especially atrial fibrillation), recent transmural myocardial infarction, or previous periph-

eral arterioarterial embolization are at increased risk for developing mesenteric artery embolus. Any disease process that leads to external and third-space fluid losses with hypovolemia and hypoperfusion predisposes to acute mesenteric ischemia in this elderly population. As previously mentioned, a variety of hypercoagulable states may also lead to arterial or venous mesenteric thrombosis.

A. Signs and Symptoms: Abdominal pain is the clinical hallmark of acute visceral ischemia (75–98%). Mesenteric artery occlusion typically produces sudden onset of severe periumbilical pain that initially is poorly localized and visceral. As the ischemia progresses, the pain becomes increasingly severe and frequently described as being out of proportion to objective physical findings. Vomiting (50–70%) and diarrhea (25–40%) reflect forceful gut emptying in response to continuing ischemia. Severe abdominal pain followed by forceful gut emptying in the absence of significant physical findings strongly suggests acute mesenteric ischemia and requires further evaluation.

1. Embolic occlusion–Embolic arterial occlusion produces a distinct clinical syndrome. The patient often demonstrates one or more of the cardiac risk factors previously described and does not relate premorbid history of weight loss or intestinal angina although one-third of patients may have suffered previous peripheral arterioarterial embolic episodes. Simultaneous with mesenteric embolization, the patient experiences sudden onset of severe abdominal pain, and shortly thereafter forceful gut emptying occurs. If this ischemic process progresses without intervention, abdominal distention, signs of peritoneal irritation, and gastrointestinal bleeding will occur in 75% of patients.

2. Thrombotic occlusion–In contrast to mesenteric embolization, mesenteric artery thrombosis usually follows a more insidious course. Thrombotic occlusion is characterized by a history of intestinal angina in 50% of cases and significant peripheral atherosclerotic disease in an additional one-third. Superimposed on the intermittent postprandial pain of intestinal angina, constant abdominal pain reflects uncompensated occlusion with critical, continuous ischemia. Pain may progress steadily until intestinal gangrene occurs, accompanied by physical findings of peritonitis.

3. Venous occlusion–Like mesenteric thrombosis, acute mesenteric vein occlusion and nonobstructive mesenteric ischemia are frequently characterized by vague abdominal findings and a subacute clinical course. The clinical course of this abdominal discomfort may be protracted sometimes lasting for weeks. Unexplained abdominal distention or gastrointestinal bleeding may be the only indication of these 2 varieties of visceral ischemia. In patients in both groups, the ill-defined abdominal complaints usually progress to colicky abdominal pain. Finally, frank intestinal gangrene may develop with its usual symptoms and physical findings.

B. Laboratory Findings: Laboratory findings are often characteristic of acute visceral ischemia but never diagnostic. A leukocytosis is present in more than 90% of patients, and in nearly 50% this exceeds 20,000 per cubic millimeter. A predominance of immature cells is characteristic, although in the elderly this occurs frequently without absolute leukocytosis. In addition, approximately 50% of patients are found to have significant uncompensated metabolic acidosis. Unfortunately, when leukocytosis and metabolic acidosis are recognized, it is late in the clinical disease course, and the ischemic bowel frequently progresses to frank infarction. A mild hyperamylasemia is noted in 25–50% of patients, and intestinal infarction routinely elevates the serum transaminases. Despite these characteristic laboratory findings, none of these tests provides the necessary sensitivity or specificity to guide further management of acute visceral ischemia.

C. X-Ray Findings: Almost all patients who are evaluated for acute or subacute abdominal pain will have abdominal plain films in the course of their evaluation. In the case of visceral ischemia, abdominal x-rays are useful to exclude other more common causes of acute abdominal pain. They may demonstrate the presence or absence of small bowel obstruction, renal or biliary calculi, chronic calcific pancreatitis, or perforated viscus. Although radiographic findings may be interpreted as abnormal in up to 75% of patients, abdominal radiographic accuracy in the diagnosis of acute visceral ischemia is low, ranging from 19% to 28%. Radiographic findings vary from "thumb printing," which represents intramural edema or hemorrhage to pneumatosis or portal vein gas, which represents bowel infarction with bacterial invasion. Nearly 50% of patients with acute visceral ischemia present with a pattern interpreted as consistent with mechanical small bowel obstruction.

In summation, patients with acute mesenteric ischemia frequently present with a marked dysparity between symptoms of severe abdominal pain and a paucity of physical findings. Laboratory and plain film radiographic findings are either nondiagnostic for visceral ischemia or diagnostic only after the onset of intestinal infarction. Suggestive symptoms in a patient at risk demand that acute mesenteric ischemia be excluded.

D. Angiographic Findings: Because routine diagnostic measures are nondiagnostic, emergency angiography should be performed once a diagnosis of acute mesenteric ischemia is considered. Additional therapy for acute visceral ischemia should begin while preparations are made for the angiogram. Anteroposterior and lateral midstream aortograms are obtained to delineate concomitant aortic disease and to evaluate collateral visceral circulation. These are usually followed by selective catheterization of the superior mesenteric artery to delineate an embolus or nonocclusive visceral ischemia. Angiography may also prove therapeutic by direct injection of vasodilators or thrombolytic agents through the arterial cannula.

A "meniscus" sign located 4–6 cm from the origin of the superior mesenteric artery is the classic angiographic finding in mesenteric arterial occlusion resulting from an embolus (Fig 22–4). Emboli of cardiac origin typically lodge just distal to the origin of either the middle colonic artery or the first jejunal branch. Proximal jejunal branches fill rapidly on the angiogram; however, the distal jejunoilial branches do not fill. These angiographic findings are in contrast to the characteristic findings of superior mesenteric artery thrombosis, which characteristically demon-

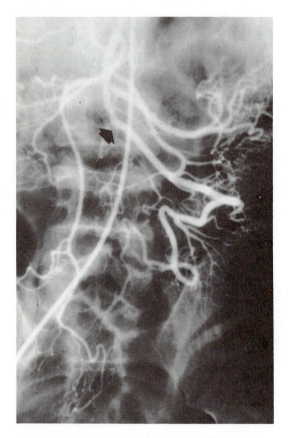

Figure 22–4. Embolic occlusion of the SMA defined by selective injection in the anteroposterior view. By lodging at SMA branch points, the proximal jejunal branches and jejunum are commonly spared, distinguishing an embolic from a thrombotic event.

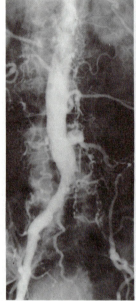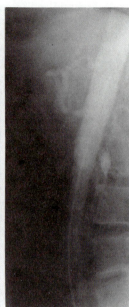

Figure 22–5. Aortogram demonstrating extensive mesenteric and left lower extremity collateralization with SMA thrombosis in the lateral projection. In this patient, critical celiac stenosis probably prevented effective collateralization of the SMA.

strates a sharp cut-off in the proximal 2 cm of the superior mesenteric artery without jejunal branch sparing. Extensive collateral circulation from the celiac or inferior mesenteric artery is often seen in patients with thrombotic mesenteric artery occlusion with preliminary symptoms of intestinal angina (Fig 22–5).

Unlike arteriography, the angiographic diagnosis of acute mesenteric ischemia secondary to venous occlusion is frequently made by inference (Fig 22–6). Angiographic findings consistent with mesenteric venous occlusion include reflux of contrast into the aorta, opacification of few peripheral arterial branches with prolongation of the remaining arterial phase, intense opacification of the thickened bowel wall, and no evidence of the mesenteric venous-portal system. Although no alternative screening test has proved capable of replacing angiography in arterial disorders, recent studies have suggested that computed tomography (CT) may demonstrate sensitivity to portal and main superior mesenteric venous thrombus equivalent to angiography. Although CT is not new, recognition of portal venous thrombosis and correlation with clin-

ical course and indications for management are just now evolving.

Nonocclusive mesenteric ischemia can be distinguished from embolic or thrombotic vascular disease, since the major mesenteric trunks are easily seen without proximal arterial obstruction. The angiographic abnormalities encountered in patients with nonocclusive mesenteric ischemia may be generalized arterial narrowing with slow filling of distal branches, regular abrupt tapering of arterial branches, and diffuse arterial spasm. The delineation of these anatomic findings requires selective superior mesenteric artery angiography when no proximal arterial occlusion is seen on aortography. After nonocclusive disease is defined, intra-arterial infusion of vasodilators (60 mg papaverine or 25 mg tolazoline bolus followed by 0.75–1.0 mg/min continuous infusion of papaverine) are begun with the hope of relieving regional mesenteric artery vasospasm. Although selective continuous arterial infusion has also been advocated in cases of mechanical arterial occlusion, I prefer to administer vasodilators as a single selective bolus to relieve associated branch vasospasm. The angiographic catheter is then removed, and the patient is taken immediately to the operating suite for correction of the arterial occlusion.

In summation, a visceral angiogram (anteroposterior and lateral aortogram with selective superior mesenteric artery injections) should be performed immediately whenever the diagnosis of acute visceral ischemia is considered. Angiography is the only reliable

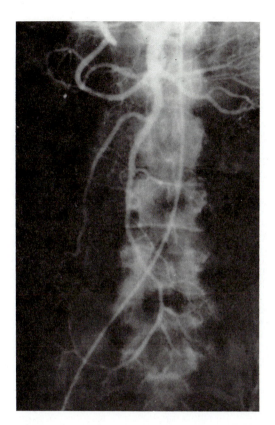

Figure 22–6. Features of mesenteric venous occlusion demonstrating stagnant flow within tapered intestinal branches with intestinal wall hyperconcentration of injected contrast on the arterial phase of the selective SMA angiogram.

method to define the pattern of occlusion in visceral branches and the adjacent aorta, as well as collateral arterial patterns. Although it may offer an option to treat certain patients with pharmacologic agents, angiography also requires transport of a critically ill patient with severe underlying cardiac disease to a remote radiology suite. Despite this unappealing scenario, immediate angiography is absolutely mandatory to properly diagnose and manage acute visceral ischemia. The 3 types of visceral ischemic syndromes are usually differentiated, thereby permitting appropriate surgical or nonsurgical management. In most reported series, the early introduction of emergency visceral angiography has decreased the incidence of intestinal gangrene and decreased associated mortality.

E. Other Imaging Studies: With the possible exception of CT in mesenteric vein occlusion, there are no diagnostic substitutes for emergency angiography in patients with suspected acute visceral ischemia. However, new diagnostic modalities may prove useful in the future as screening tests. Magnetic resonance imaging (MRI) is a powerful tool for defining soft tissue anatomy, obtaining sharp tissue contrast without

ionizing radiation or ingestion of contrast agents. MRI can delineate between vessels containing thrombus and free-flowing blood; however, the technique is limited by 24-hour availability and the acquisition time required for complete mesenteric arterial evaluation. With these limitations, the role of MRI seems most useful in areas of chronic visceral ischemic evaluation.

A new generation of CT known as Cine-CT provides rapid scanning with multiple simultaneous tomographic sections. The image of Cine-CT scanners can be reconstructed and played in series to provide calculations of mesenteric blood flow and total blood volume. Cine-CT scanning has a wide application in cardiac imaging and may prove useful in the future evaluation of both acute and chronic visceral ischemia.

Another imaging technique that may find further application in acute visceral ischemic syndromes is duplex scanning, which combines B-mode ultrasound images with spectral analysis of Doppler-shifted signals. Although the technique has found wide applicability and accuracy in the evaluation of superficial peripheral arteries, it has only recently been applied to the evaluation of the renal and visceral arterial systems.

Reports comparing duplex findings with those of conventional angiography have demonstrated high overall accuracy when the celiac axis or superior mesenteric artery is evaluated in a well-prepared patient. However, the examination with duplex scanning is limited by excessive bowel gas and lack of patient cooperation as well as its failure to evaluate reliably the inferior mesenteric artery and distal arterial branches. Although duplex scanning may prove useful as a screening test for chronic visceral disease, its role will probably remain limited in the evaluation of acute visceral ischemic syndromes.

Treatment

The goal of therapy in patients who suffer from acute visceral ischemia is restoration of mesenteric blood flow prior to intestinal gangrene. Patients require expedient evaluation and institution of therapy if they are to have any hope for a successful outcome. The urgency with which this is accomplished is dictated by the mode of onset of patient symptoms.

Embolic occlusion of the visceral arteries produces the most dramatic and abrupt onset of symptoms, since collateral blood vessels have not developed sufficiently to ensure bowel viability. In the person so afflicted, the goal of therapy is expeditious resuscitation and prompt operation. Throughout the course of the patient's initial evaluation (including angiography), resuscitation and monitoring are established to optimize end-organ function. Specific attention should be given to improving cardiac output and oxygen delivery, controlling cardiac dysrhythmias, and eliminating agents known to exacerbate mesenteric vasoconstriction. Appropriate volume resuscitation is critical because large volumes of fluid may be sequestered in the ischemic bowel. In elderly patients with underlying cardiac disease, volume resuscitation, cardiac performance and oxygen delivery are best guided by use of a pulmonary artery catheter.

Abdominal exploration is carried out through a midline incision. The operative findings are dependent on the site and duration of the occlusion. Most emboli lodge 5–7 cm from the origin of the superior mesenteric artery at a point distal to the first jejunal branches. This spares the duodenum in the first several centimeters of the jejunum, whereas the remainder of the small bowel and right colon show evidence of ischemia. The earliest signs of intestinal ischemia are vigorous tetanic bowel contraction and a pale to bluish-white appearance. With longer ischemic periods, the bowel begins to manifest evidence of infarction with bowel edema, dilatation, and hemorrhage into the mesentery. Despite these otherwise ominous findings, restoration of mesenteric blood flow may allow normal color and contractility to return to the revascularized bowel.

The arterial exposure is begun by elevating the transverse colon and incising the base of the transverse mesocolon overlying the superior mesenteric artery and vein. Frequently, the point of embolic obstruction can be identified by palpating a pulse at the origin of the superior mesenteric artery and noting its disappearance distal to the embolic occlusion. A transverse arteriotomy is made just distal to the middle colic artery, and bidirectional balloon catheter (No. 3 or 4) thromboembolectomy is then performed (Fig 22–7). Great care must be exercised since the distal superior mesenteric branches are fragile and easily damaged by improper balloon catheter technique. If no distal discontinuous thrombus is recovered on 1 or 2 catheter passes, the vessel is flushed with papaverine solution (60 mg papaverine added to 20 mL saline), and the arteriotomy is closed with fine interrupted sutures. The bowel is returned to its normal anatomic position, and viability is assessed after a 20-minute period carefully inspecting the bowel from the ligament of Trietz to midtransverse colon for color, spontaneous peristalsis, and pulsations within the distal mesenteric arcade.

When complete bowel revascularization is uncertain, assessment may be aided by a continuous-wave Doppler flow probe coupled to the vasa recti and the antimesenteric border to detect the presence of arterial flow signals. When arterial Doppler-shifted signals are present within the proximal superior mesenteric artery but demonstrate a "staccato" quality with absence of antimesenteric flow, a second 60-mg bolus of papaverine may be injected intra-arterially. Only obvious intestinal gangrene is resected at the time of initial revascularization. With evidence of complete revascularization and in the absence of intra-abdominal contamination, primary intestinal anastomosis should be considered safe.

Prior to the completion of the procedure, a decision should be made regarding the advisability of a second-look operation. The second-look laparotomy is generally favored by the author over intraoperative tests of

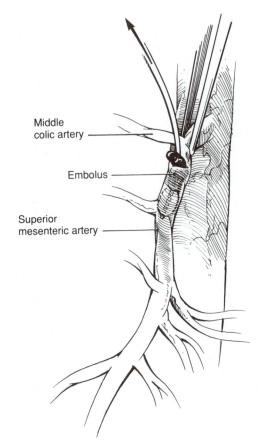

Middle colic artery

Embolus

Superior mesenteric artery

Figure 22–7. Balloon catheter thromboembolectomy with a Fogarty catheter (No. 3 or 4) performed through a transverse arteriotomy just distal to the middle colic branch of the SMA.

bowel viability or resection of marginal bowel at the initial exploration and intestinal revascularization. The second laparotomy is performed 48 to 72 hours after the first, inspecting all the abdominal contents and ensuring the patency of the vascular repair. Once the second laparotomy is planned, the subsequent clinical course should not alter this intraoperative decision.

Compared with embolic occlusion, thrombosis of the visceral vessels may have a more insidious onset. However, as the bowel ischemia becomes more severe, it may produce a picture of what may be best described as a "shocked bowel obstruction." Lateral aortography usually shows extensive occlusive disease involving the origins of the visceral vessels. While the radiographic diagnosis is being established, the patient is prepared for operation with volume resuscitation and correction of associated metabolic acidosis. Through a midline wound, attention is first directed at confirming the extent of visceral occlusion defined by angiography. Most frequently, the disease process begins as an aortic wall atheromatous plaque involving the anterior aortic wall encroaching on the visceral vessel orifice. The superior mesenteric artery, however, often has extensive plaque extending for several centimeters well beyond the radiographic disease.

In contrast to the superior mesenteric artery, the celiac axis usually demonstrates only orificial occlusion. After the vascular anatomy is confirmed, autogenous reconstruction using either a transaortic endarterectomy or an antegrade bypass from the supraceliac aorta is performed. For either mesenteric bypass or endarterectomy, the supraceliac aorta and the visceral vessels are best exposed through a left visceral mobilization (Fig 22–8). In this maneuver, the splenic flexure of the colon is first mobilized followed by the peritoneal attachments of the spleen. A retroperitoneal plane is developed between the left kidney and the left renal vein posteriorly and the pancreas anteriorly. A dissection proceeds medially, and the spleen, tail, and body of the pancreas and fundus of the stomach are retracted to the right. The left aortic crus is then divided along the left anterolateral aspect of the aorta. This approach allows exposure of the supraceliac aorta and descending thoracic aorta to the T9 or T10 level with easy access to the celiac axis and superior mesenteric artery after dissection of the periarterial neural plexus.

In the case of superior mesenteric artery thrombosis in combination with celiac axis stenosis, the author prefers antegrade revascularization of both vessels through this exposure (Fig 22–9). Given the frequent distal extension of atherosclerotic disease within the superior mesenteric artery, bypass procedures are frequently necessary. Autogenous tissue (reversed saphenous vein or hypogastric artery) is the preferred vas-

cular conduit unless intra-abdominal contamination is absent, in which case, a synthetic graft may be used. Prior to the completion of the reconstruction, balloon catheter thrombectomy is performed to clear the distal arterial tree of discontinuous propagated thrombus. The distal circulation is then flushed with papaverine solution. Following revascularization, the bowel is observed and its viability is assessed, followed by a decision for second-look laparotomy made in the manner just described for embolic occlusion.

Therapy for mesenteric venous thrombosis is directed primarily toward treating the underlying cause leading to the thrombotic event. Phlebotomy, anticoagulation, and antiplatelet agents have all been used to reduce the hypercoagulable states associated with mesenteric venous thrombosis. In 50% of the patients in whom no underlying precipitating cause can be identified early, continuous systemic heparin anticoagulation appears to decrease the immediate risk of intestinal gangrene and eliminate the short-term risk of recurrence. Surgical intervention is reserved for patients who show evidence of peritonitis and require exploration in anticipation of bowel resection.

Unless the underlying prothrombotic state can be clearly identified and eliminated, most authorities recommend long-term oral anticoagulation treatment after the acute phase of management. Venous thrombectomy has been attempted but rethrombosis of the mesenteric veins in all but a few patients has caused this procedure to be abandoned. Since 60% of recurrences of mesenteric venous thrombosis following resection occur at the site of re-anastomosis, extension of the thrombotic process at preestablished sites seems to be an important mechanism. As much as controlling

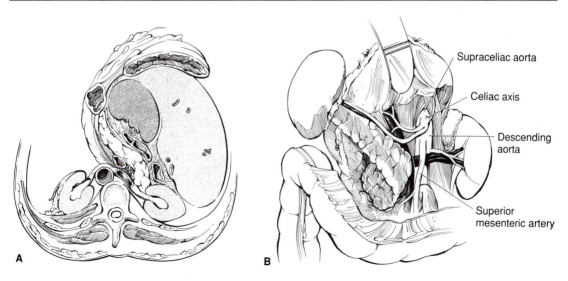

A **B**

Figure 22–8. Artist's depiction in cross-sectional (**A**) and sagittal (**B**) projections of a left visceral mobilization for exposure of the supraceliac and descending aorta, celiac axis, and superior mesenteric artery. For purposes of visceral revascularization, the left kidney remains posterior to allow access to the distal SMA.

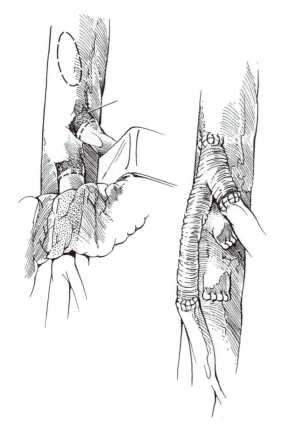

Figure 22–9. Artist's depiction of an antegrade aortomesenteric graft. The graft usually takes its origin from the supraceliac portion of the abdominal aorta. In the absence of frank intestinal gangrene or contamination, both the celiac axis and SMA may be revascularized using a 12- × 6-mm bifurcated prosthetic graft.

a generalized thrombotic potential, heparin probably acts to limit local extension of preexisting thrombus to the vasa recti and intramural veins, thereby decreasing the risk of subsequent venous gangrene.

Nonocclusive mesenteric ischemia may have a presentation similar to both embolic and thrombotic visceral ischemia, but it must be distinguished from these conditions. In the appropriate clinical setting, consideration of nonocclusive mesenteric ischemia should lead to the elimination of vasoconstricting agents and angiography to exclude obstruction of visceral vessels. Although the critical angiographic finding is an absence of major trunk obstruction, additional supportive evidence for nonocclusive visceral ischemia may be obtained by noting a beading pattern of the visceral vessels, poor peripheral perfusion, and proximal arterial dilatation. The delineation of these angiographic features requires selective superior mesenteric artery injections, which should always follow anteroposterior and lateral aortography. Having established the di-agnosis of nonocclusive mesenteric ischemia with selective angiography, the catheter may then provide a route for administration of selective intra-arterial vasodilators. Tolazoline (25-mg bolus) followed continuous papaverine infusion (0.75–1.0 mg/min) has been shown to interrupt angiotensin II- and vasopressin-mediated vasoconstriction and should be used in cases of nonocclusive mesenteric ischemia. Continuous papaverine infusion is continued for a least 24 hours and replaced by saline infusion 30 minutes prior to repeat angiography. If the patient's symptoms have resolved and the vasospastic angiographic features of vasospasm have abated, the catheter is removed. Otherwise, intra-arterial papaverine infusion is continued and the angiographic sequence repeated 24 to 48 hours later.

Surgical intervention is dependent on the patient's response to vigorous medical management and intra-arterial papaverine infusion. Exploration is reserved for therapeutic failures demonstrated by signs of intestinal gangrene. In patients requiring laparotomy and resection of gangrenous bowel as well as second-look laparotomy, continuous catheter infusion of papaverine should be continued 24–48 hours postoperatively. Selective superior mesenteric artery catheters have been maintained for up to 5 days without concomitant anticoagulation free of associated catheter thrombosis.

Summary

Acute visceral ischemic syndromes constitute a spectrum of disease that culminate in fatal intestinal gangrene unless clinically suspected, promptly detected, and aggressively treated. Although measures of general support and resuscitation are similar in each of these syndromes, the methods of surgical management are contingent upon accurate delineation of the ischemic mechanism. These problems are therefore emergencies both in diagnosis and treatment and require close cooperation among physician, surgeon, and angiographer.

Bergan JJ et al: Nontraumatic mesenteric vascular emergencies. J Vasc Surg 1987;5:903.

Boley SJ et al: Initial results from an aggressive angiographic and surgical approach to acute mesenteric ischemia. Surgery 1977;82:848.

Boley SJ et al: New concepts in the management of emboli of the superior mesenteric artery. Surg Gynecol Obstet 1989;153:561.

Harward TRS et al: Mesenteric venous thrombosis. J Vasc Surg 1989;9:328.

Hernandez LA et al: Role of neutrophils in ischemia-reperfusion-induced microvascular injury. Am J Physiol 1987; 253:H699.

Ottinger LW, Austen WG: A study of 136 patients with mesenteric infarction. Surg Gynecol Obstet 1967;124: 251.

Sachs SM, Morten JH, Schwartz SI: Acute mesenteric ischemia. Surgery 1982;92:646.

CHRONIC MESENTERIC ISCHEMIA

Essentials of Diagnosis
- Gnawing, dull abdominal pain 15–30 minutes after meals.
- Weight loss and food fear.
- Peripheral vascular or coronary artery disease.

In contrast to acute ischemia, chronic mesenteric ischemia often poses a diagnostic dilemma rather than a surgical emergency. Diagnosis requires the recognition of the clinical triad that typifies the syndrome. Successful mesenteric revascularization is required to relieve associated abdominal pain and weight loss and to prevent progression to intestinal infarction.

Etiology
In chronic visceral ischemia, atherosclerosis is responsible for mesenteric artery occlusion in over 95% of cases. As in mesenteric artery thrombosis, the "ostial" lesions represent atherosclerosis of the anterior aortic wall that encroaches on the mesenteric lumen. The proximal location of major visceral artery atherosclerotic occlusion allows a protective collateral network to develop, preventing intestinal infarction in most cases. Chiene recognized the efficiency of this collateral network over a century ago when he described occlusion of all 3 major mesenteric arteries without infarction. It is widely believed that at least 2 of the 3 major mesenteric vessels must be involved before symptoms of chronic visceral ischemia manifest.

Blood flow for this collateral network is provided by nonischemic parallel segments. The medium-sized mesenteric arteries do not limit flow; therefore, without decreasing their distal perfusion, the normal segments can also supply the ischemic segments. Reduced resistance within the ischemic segment favors its perfusion. Experimental data have shown that the resistance of the nonischemic segments remains unchanged, suggesting that vasoactive drugs given systematically might actually disrupt this protective collateral mechanism. This is in contrast to the selective intra-arterial infusion of vasodilators, which may overcome local mesenteric vasospasm in response to circulating vasopressin and angiotensin II.

Beside atherosclerosis, there are other less common causes of chronic visceral ischemia. The most common of these is celiac axis compression, also known as **median arcuate ligament syndrome.** Although Dunbar described celiac axis compression syndrome as a cause of intestinal angina 25 years ago, the significance of this syndrome remains controversial. The presumed basis for visceral ischemia in this syndrome is the external compression of the celiac axis by the median arcuate ligament. Occasionally, the superior mesenteric artery is involved as well. Although celiac axis compression is, at this time, associated with symptoms of chronic visceral ischemia, affected per-

sons are most frequently asymptomatic and often diagnosed on a lateral aortogram obtained for other reasons. Note that the rich collateral network between major mesenteric arteries that is present in atherosclerotic patients is often less evident in the celiac axis compression syndrome. External compression of the celiac axis may also occur in diseases that affect the surrounding autonomic neuroplexus, such as von Recklinghausen's neurofibromatosis.

Rather than involving the ostia of the major mesenteric branches, atherosclerosis may produce a localized obstruction of the suprarenal aorta, where it has been termed a **coral reef atheroma.** These lesions may diminish perfusion or undergo embolization to the visceral, renal, or lower extremity circulation. About 25% of these patients present with visceral ischemia, whereas most present with renovascular hypertension and lower extremity ischemia.

In addition to the celiac axis compression syndrome and the coral reef atheroma, spontaneous intimal dissection of the superior mesenteric artery has been reported as a rare cause of chronic visceral ischemia. The celiac axis and the superior mesenteric artery are also affected by fibromuscular dysplasia, but the disease is rarely responsible for intestinal angina. Visceral ischemic syndromes have also been described as a consequence of vasculitis secondary to rheumatoid arthritis, systemic lupus erythematosus, and external-beam irradiation.

Pathophysiology
Although an ischemic basis for intestinal angina is widely accepted, the pathophysiologic mechanism that mediates chronic mesenteric ischemia is poorly understood. Since severe pain occurs only with foot intake in this syndrome, the pain seems secondary to a discrepancy between increased postprandial oxygen demands and the failure of the collateral system to provide adequate compensation. Most patients experience pain within 15–20 minutes after foot intake, well before the food bolus has reached the small intestine. Researchers have suggested that food ingestion increases demand for gastric blood flow, thereby creating a "gastric steal" from the remaining gastrointestinal tract. Subsequent small intestinal acidosis may mediate the characteristic abdominal pain.

Clinical Findings
As in mesenteric ischemia secondary to arterial occlusion, chronic mesenteric ischemia produces a well-defined clinical syndrome in symptomatic patients. Likewise, successful treatment requires recognition of this clinical syndrome, confirmation of the diagnosis with arteriography, and appropriate visceral revascularization before severe nutritional depletion or intestinal infarction occurs with lethal sequelae. When recognized before the onset of these complications, chronic visceral ischemia may be successfully treated

by visceral artery reconstructions, with nearly all patients receiving long-lasting benefit.

A. Signs and Symptoms: The pain of chronic visceral ischemia is usually gnawing and dull in quality and either periumbilical or epigastric in location. Intestinal angina has its onset between 15 and 30 minutes after meals and may persist from 1 to 4 hours. As the occlusive disease progresses, smaller amounts of food result in more severe and persistent abdominal discomfort. Finally, the patient develops food avoidance (food fear), which leads to significant weight loss (loss of 15% of ideal body weight in 79%).

On evaluation, patients often exhibit the signs of weight loss, with the severity paralleling the duration of symptoms. Examination of the abdomen reveals an epigastric bruit in most patients (80–90%). Evidence of peripheral vascular disease (70–80%) and coronary artery disease (30–40%) is frequently present.

B. Imaging Studies: As with all mesenteric ischemic syndromes, diagnosis of chronic mesenteric ischemia depends on a high index of suspicion in any patient who demonstrates the triad of postprandial abdominal pain, food aversion, and weight loss. Definitive diagnosis requires aortography performed in both anteroposterior and lateral projections. The anteroposterior view best demonstrates the visceral collateral pathways. The lateral projection demonstrates the proximal visceral artery stenosis or occlusion. Intra-arterial digital subtraction arteriography may be performed with a very small amount of contrast agent in patients with preexisting renal dysfunction or contrast hypersensitivity. Selective visceral arteriography also provides the rare opportunity for percutaneous transluminal angioplasty in patients with distal mesenteric artery lesions.

In general, intravenous digital subtraction arteriography has been inadequate to define the mesenteric artery anatomy necessary for diagnosis and planning of a surgical strategy. The volume of contrast agent required for an intravenous digital subtraction arteriogram is equal to or greater than that required for a routine intra-arterial study.

Most commonly, aortography and visceral arteriography reveal obstructive lesions of both the celiac axis and superior mesenteric artery (90–95%). Fifty percent of all these patients have significant occlusive disease involving the inferior mesenteric artery as well. Additional atherosclerotic stenosis of one or both renal arteries is present in one-third of patients, whereas one-fourth have significant infrarenal aortic aneurysmal or occlusive disease. Visual duplex sonography has demonstrated accuracy sufficient to guide the management of a patient with suspected chronic visceral ischemia. The celiac axis and SMA are usually easily interrogated, however, failure to interrogate the IMA is obscured in roughly 50% of the studies.

Treatment

A patient with symptoms of chronic mesenteric ischemic does not require the same urgency of treatment as a patient with acute mesenteric ischemia. Prior to elective visceral reconstruction, nutritional repletion may be necessary and intravenous alimentation may be required. It is important to anticipate and avoid situations that can lead to dehydration to minimize the risk of a thrombotic occlusion and the precipitation of an acute ischemic event. Selection of the most appropriate operation for patients with chronic mesenteric ischemia depends on the disease pattern, the presence of associated arterial lesions, and the severity of associated systemic illness.

A. Aortovisceral Bypass Grafting: Prosthetic conduits are ideal for aortovisceral bypass. They can be oriented in an antegrade fashion by attaching the proximal end to the undiseased supraceliac aorta and the distal end to the divided visceral vessel. This technique ensures antegrade flow and provides a short unrestricted inflow to the mesenteric or celiac artery or both. Flanged knitted Dacron prostheses are preferred for single-vessel bypasses, and bifurcated grafts are used when both vessels are reconstructed.

The operation is conducted through a midline incision. The celiac artery and supraceliac aorta are exposed through the lesser omentum. The abdominal viscera are retracted laterally, and the crus of the diaphragm divided to provide circumferential control of the supraceliac aorta. Ganglionic tissue is excised from around the celiac and superior mesenteric arteries. A bifurcated prosthetic graft is anastomosed to the supraceliac aorta and the graft limbs individually anastomosed to the divided ends of the celiac and superior mesenteric arteries.

When extensive disease exists in the distal superior mesenteric artery, revascularization of the celiac artery alone may be sufficient. Intraoperative duplex scanning is used to visualize the reconstruction and confirm adequacy of visceral blood flow. Before the patient's discharge from the hospital, arteriography is obtained to confirm patency of the reconstruction.

B. Visceral Endarterectomy: Endarterectomy was the first procedure used to relieve symptomatic obstruction of the superior mesenteric artery. The original procedure was performed in a retrograde manner from the superior mesenteric artery into the aorta. Although the procedure successfully relieves the obstruction to flow, it fails to remove the aortic atheroma effectively, which progresses and is responsible for late failures. Transaortic visceral endarterectomy allows for the removal of both the aortic atheroma and the orifice disease that causes the obstruction to splanchnic blood flow.

Because of the location and direction of the visceral vessels, a left thoracoretroperitoneal or wide subaortal approach is preferred because it allows unrestricted access to the thoracoabdominal aorta and its major branches. With this approach, complete exposure of the involved upper abdominal aortic segment and its 4 major branches may be obtained. A left lateral aortotomy is performed in a trap-door fashion, and the aortic and orifice atheroma contained in the ventral aorta are removed by means of extraction endarterectomy. The visceral vessels are allowed to backbleed and are then flushed with a heparin-saline solution to confirm their patency. The aortotomy is closed with a running suture, and aortic continuity and flow are restored.

If the atheromatous obstruction in the superior mesenteric artery has already progressed to occlusion, the distal propagated thrombus at the level of the re-entry collateral may not be completely extracted through the aortotomy. A separate longitudinal arteriotomy is placed distally in the superior mesenteric artery, and the remaining thrombus is removed under direct visualization. The vessel is closed with a vein patch to prevent narrowing. Intraoperative patency is confirmed with duplex scanning of the upper abdominal aorta that has undergone endarterectomy and its branches.

Rapp JH et al: Durability of endarterectomy and antegrade grafts in the treatment of chronic visceral ischemia. J Vasc Surg 1986;3:799.

Stanton PE et al: Chronic intestinal ischemia: Diagnosis and therapy. J Vasc Surg 1986;195:554.

23

Renovascular Disease

Stanley B. Fuller, MD, & Richard H. Dean, MD

Although hypertension has been recognized for centuries, the importance of its identification and treatment has been appreciated only during the past 150 years. Usually, hypertension is a silent process and is manifested only by acceleration in the rate of atherogenesis and the frequency of cardiovascular morbidity and mortality rates. Occasionally, the hypertension may be so severe that the elevated pressure itself produces vessel wall injury and the clinical picture of malignant hypertension. Although most physicians appreciate the potentially lethal nature of the malignant type of hypertension and the importance of controlling it, physician apathy regarding the merits of aggressive diagnostic evaluation and management of asymptomatic patients with less severe hypertension continues to limit the impact of current knowledge on the success of treatment of this disorder.

In addition, flow-limiting lesions of a renal artery may lead to progressive excretory renal dysfunction, known as ischemic nephropathy. **Ischemic nephropathy** is a rapidly progressive form of renal insufficiency, which is more common than previously thought. The diagnosis and management of patients so affected are becoming increasingly important, since evidence suggests that renal artery stenosis may be a common and correctable cause of end-stage renal disease.

Traditionally, study of the sequelae of renovascular occlusive disease has centered on the pathophysiology and management of the resultant renovascular hypertension. Recently, the potential for simultaneous retrieval of excretory function in some patients with combined hypertension and renal insufficiency has been recognized.

General Considerations

A. Anatomy: The renal arteries are retroperitoneal structures. Most frequently, single right and left renal arteries arise from the abdominal aorta just below the superior mesenteric artery (SMA) at the level of the intervertebral disc between the first and second lumbar vertebrae. Nevertheless, about 25% of the population has more than 2 renal arteries, which may rise as high as the T12 vertebra and as low as the common iliac artery. Typically, the main renal artery branches into 5 extraparenchymal segmental arteries (apical, upper, middle, lower, and posterior), which supply each kidney. Each segmental artery gives rise to a lobar artery, which further branches into interlobar arteries that

travel between the pyramids. The interlobar artery terminates in the arcuate artery, which turns perpendicular and courses between the cortex and the medulla. The arcuate artery gives rise to the interlobular artery followed by the intralobular artery, which terminates in the afferent glomerular arteriole.

The renal veins course anterior to the arteries with the left renal vein longer as it passes between the aorta and the superior mesenteric artery to enter the inferior vena cava. The 3 major branches of the left renal vein are the gonadal, adrenal, and posterior lumbar veins. The posterior lumbar vein is the largest nonrenal branch of the renal vein. Mobilization of the renal vein requires control or ligation of all 3 tributaries. Awareness of the renal venous anatomy is equally important in measurements of renal vein renin activity because an improperly positioned renal venous catheter may result in incorrect test interpretation.

B. Pathogenesis: Atherosclerotic occlusive disease accounts for most (75%) renal artery occlusive lesions. Atherosclerotic lesions most frequently affect the renal artery orifices, but any segment of the artery is a potential site of involvement.

Fibromuscular dysplasia (FMD) is the other primary cause of renovascular disease (RVD). FMD consists of dysplastic and fibrosing lesions of intima, media, or adventitia. Medial FMD is most common and produces mural microaneurysms interspersed with "web-like" stenoses, which give an angiographic appearance of a "string of beads." Young women are characteristically affected, but FMD may be found in either sex at any age. The cause of FMD is unknown. FMD frequently occurs in multiple arteries and often extends into renal artery branches.

C. Pathophysiology: The kidney is a dominant site of blood pressure regulation because of its influence on circulating plasma volume as well as its activity in modulation of vasomotor tone. To examine the pathophysiology of renovascular hypertension, it is appropriate to first review the normal homeostatic activities of the kidney in the regulation of blood pressure.

The renin-angiotensin-aldosterone system is a complex feedback mechanism, which, in its normal state of activity, maintains a stable blood pressure and blood volume under varying conditions. Richly innervated, modified smooth muscle cells located along the afferent arterioles in juxtaposition to the renal glomerulus (juxtaglomerular apparatus) are sensitive monitors of perfusion pressure. Diminished perfusion pressure stimulates these cells to release renin, a proteolytic enzyme. Renin, in turn, interacts with an α_2-globulin (angiotensinogen) manufactured in the liver to produce angiotensin I. Angiotensin I, an inactive and labile decapeptide, is converted to the potent vasoconstrictor angiotensin II by a converting enzyme found primarily in the lungs. In addition to its potent vasoconstrictor properties, angiotensin II also increases blood pressure through its stimulation of aldosterone release from the zona glomerulosa of the adrenal cortex. This, in turn, increases plasma volume by increasing sodium and water resorption in the renal tubules. Through these actions of angiotensin II, blood pressure, plasma volume, and plasma sodium content are increased. In addition, the adjacent cells of the distal convoluted tubule (macula dens) may play a role by acting as a sensor of sodium concentration in the distal tubules and thereby exerting a positive feedback mechanism on renin release. As these mechanisms increase perfusion pressure to the juxtaglomerular cells, further renin production and release are suppressed, and blood pressure is modulated within a narrow range.

Potentially, 2 forms of hypertension may be produced by the development of RVD: renin-dependent hypertension and volume-dependent hypertension. Through the mechanisms just described, decreased perfusion activates the renin-angiotensin-aldosterone axis of vasoconstriction and volume expansion. Currently, information regarding the nature of renovascular hypertension suggests that a functionally significant unilateral renal artery stenosis activates both the angiotensin II-mediated increase in peripheral resistance and blood pressure as well as aldosterone-mediated volume expansion. When the contralateral renal artery and kidney are normal, the normal feedback mechanisms in the normal kidney produce an effective natriuresis and compensatory reduction in circulating plasma volume. In this scheme, an angiotensin II vasoconstrictive source of hypertension is created.

By contrast, when the contralateral renal artery or kidney is also diseased, this compensatory diuresis is lost and volume expansion occurs, producing an angiotensin-aldosterone-mediated volume-dependent hypertension. Modification and renal perfusion by renal revascularization can effectively diminish or abolish the underlying mechanism, producing either of these 2 varieties of renovascular hypertension.

Clinical Findings

The selection and appropriate sequence of diagnostic studies in the evaluation of hypertensive patients remain ill defined. Continued modifications of attitudes regarding the merits of evaluation and introduction of new techniques prevent a statement that defines which studies to use in all patients. The general evaluation of all hypertensive patients should include a careful medical history, physical examination, serum electrolytes and creatinine, and an electrocardiogram (ECG). ECG is important to gauge the extent of secondary myocardial hypertrophy or associated ischemic heart disease. Serum electrolytes and serial serum potassium determinations can effectively exclude patients with primary aldosteronism if potassium levels are greater than 3.0 mg/dL. Remember that hypokalemia is often due to salt-depleting diets and previous diuretic therapy. Finally, estimation of renal function is mandatory. Preexisting renal disease may reduce renal function and cause hypertension. Furthermore, hypertension from any cause may produce intrarenal arteriolar nephrosclerosis and subsequent depression of renal function.

A. Signs and Symptoms:

1. Renovascular hypertension (RVH)–Severe diastolic hypertension is the most important sign associated with RVH. Although RVH probably accounts for less than 5% of the about 60 million hypertensive persons in the USA, it is very common in the small severely hypertensive subgroup. Estimates suggest that RVH may be the cause of diastolic hypertension greater than 120 mmHg in 40% of white adult patients. Nevertheless, RVH appears to be uncommon (less than 10%) in similarly severely hypertensive black patients.

Characteristics such as recent-onset hypertension, young age, absence of family history, and abdominal bruit are characteristic of RVH. Unfortunately, these factors lack sufficient specificity to distinguish RVH from other much more common forms of hypertension (eg, essential hypertension). More important, absence of these factors should not preclude further diagnostic evaluation of the renal vasculature as a possible cause of a patient's severe hypertension.

2. Ischemic nephropathy–Most frequently, patients with ischemic nephropathy present with hypertension (ie, RVH) in conjunction with an elevated serum creatinine. Most patients are in the atherosclerotic age range and therefore have concomitant cardiovascular pathology. Current data suggest that as many as 20% of persons over 50 years of age entering dialysis dependence have renovascular occlusive disease as the cause of their end-stage renal disease. Since ischemic nephropathy results from globally reduced renal perfusion, it is more commonly due to bilateral disease or its equivalent (stenosis in a solitary kidney) and is considered the most rapidly progressive form of chronic renal insufficiency.

B. Screening Studies: Identification of a noninvasive screening test that will accurately identify all patients with RVD who might require interventional management remains an elusive goal. Prior methods such as peripheral plasma renin activity, rapid sequence intravenous pyelography, and saralasin acetate infusion are examples of such tests that have been abandoned. Isotope renography continues to be proposed as a valuable screening test, but the methods used are continuously modified with the hope of improving the sensitivity and specificity. The newest method of isotope renography consist of renal scans performed before and after exercise or captopril infusion. In these methods, a test is interpreted as positive when augmentation of derangements in renal perfusion occurs following exercise or following captopril infusion. Although these methods have improved the specificity of isotope renography, reliance on activation of the renin-angiotensin system with the captopril renogram leads to an unacceptable incidence of false-negative results.

Our bias is that screening tests that image the vascular anatomy and assess hemodynamics of renal flow are the most promising methods of widespread screening for RVDs. In this regard, vascular images using magnetic resonance imaging or positron-emission tomography may hold great promise. Current expense, lack of widespread availability, and limitations of patient selection criteria prevent its application as a screening tool except in the most unusual circumstances.

Renal duplex sonography (RDS) has been proposed by several authorities as a useful screening test with which candidates for arteriography can be identified. When single renal arteries are present, it can have an overall diagnostic accuracy greater than 95%. It does not accurately identify branch or accessory renal artery lesions causing hypertension alone, nor does it predict hypertension or renal function response after correction of RVD.

Because of the above-mentioned points, RDS is recommended as the screening tool of choice. Nevertheless, since it does not accurately identify accessory vessels or branch vessel disease, arteriography is recommended when hypertension is severe or difficult to control.

1. Renal arteriography–Controversy continues over the use of aortography and renal arteriography in the routine screening of hypertensive patients. Some clinicians feel arteriography should be reserved for selected groups of patients. However, this view is conservative and arteriography is recommended for any patient who would be a candidate for renal artery revascularization if a lesion were found, regardless of other screening tests. As a general rule, it is recommended that the patient have documented diastolic blood pressures higher than 120 mmHg.

Both aortography and selective renal arteriography using multiple projections are necessary to adequately examine the entire renal artery. The proximal third of the left renal artery usually courses anteriorly, the midthird transversely, and the distal third posteriorly, whereas the right renal artery pursues a more consistent posterior course. Previous review of these factors has underscored the necessity of oblique aortography and oblique selective renal arteriography to project these portions of the vessels in the profile and identify the stenosis.

Through the introduction of computer-assisted subtraction angiography, anatomic definition of the renal vasculature can be obtained as an outpatient screening procedure. Unfortunately, further technologic refinements are required before this type of angiography can replace conventional arteriography. Currently, it does not identify fibromuscular dysplastic lesions with accuracy and frequently provides a picture that erroneously exaggerates the severity of atherosclerotic lesions.

2. Renal venous renin assay (RVRA)–When an obstructive lesion is found by renal arteriography, its functional significance should be evaluated. RVRAs constitute the single functional study that can prove the causal relationship between the renal artery occlusive lesion and hypertension. Their value, however, is limited to assessment of unilateral lesions, because the results compare the involved with the uninvolved side.

Some clinicians have stressed the importance of expressing RVRAs in relation to the systemic renin activity rather than simply evaluating the ratio of renin activity in the 2 renal veins. In patients with RVH secondary to unilateral renal artery stenosis, hypersecretion of renin from the ischemic kidney and suppression of renin secretion from the normal kidney are generally found.

Nevertheless, if the decision for operative management is based solely on whether or not absolute cure is to be expected, then many patients who would receive the benefit of reduction in severity of hypertension to a mild easily controlled level would be dropped from consideration as operative candidates. Therefore, this method of RVRA interpretation should be considered only as an additional predictive tool and not an alternative to the evaluation of renal vein/renin ratios. A 1.5:1 ratio between the involved and uninvolved sides can be considered a positive test and as functional proof that the renovascular lesion is causing RVH.

Treatment

Identification of the optimal method of treating patients with RVH remains an elusive goal. Advocates of drug therapy, operative management, and, more recently, percutaneous transluminal angioplasty (PTA) defend their viewpoints with selective data from the literature to strengthen the validity of their argument. Unfortunately, most of the medical community still evaluates only patients for RVH when medications are not tolerated or hypertension remains severe and uncontrolled.

A. Percutaneous Transluminal Renal Angioplasty: The introduction of the alternative interventional modality, percutaneous transluminal angioplasty, by Grüntzig in 1978 has led to a new era in the management of hypertensive patients with renal artery stenosis. This technique uses the principle of coaxial dilatation of the vessel by inflation of a balloon-tipped catheter, which has been introduced across the stenotic renal artery lesion. The stenotic lesion is disrupted, and, by stretching the vessel wall itself, portions of the media are disrupted as well, leaving the vessel with a greater diameter than its dimension prior to dilatation. The increased luminal diameter is primarily created by disruption of the intima, the atherosclerotic or fibrodysplastic lesion, and portions of the media. Early reports of the results of this technique showed that stenotic renal arteries frequently could be dilated successfully with immediate improvement in levels of hypertension in patients with RVH.

By reviewing the reported experience with PTA and the observations from the operative management of unsuccessful PTA, indications for the preferential use of each procedure can be formulated in the treatment of patients with RVH. Reported experience with PTA in patients with fibrodysplastic lesions produces results similar to those for open surgical repairs. Beneficial blood pressure responses have been reported to be as high as 100% following PTA in properly selected cases. Moreover, although vessel perforation, hemorrhage, and branch occlusions have been reported, their incidence has been less than 5%. Such complications may be presumed as being most likely in patients with diffuse fibromuscular dysplasia affecting both the distal main renal artery and its branches.

The cure rate after PTA of fibromuscular dysplasia, even when the procedure is performed by experienced surgeons, varies from 37% to 51%. Similarly, about 60% of patients with fibrodysplastic lesions in one clinical experience have been cured of hypertension. Angiography has been routinely found to underestimate the distal extent of fibromuscular dysplasia; this difference in cure rates is believed to represent residual, inadequately managed disease in the PTA group. For this reason, fibromuscular dysplasia extending to the branch level is believed to be best managed primarily by an open operative approach, with PTA being reserved for the subgroup of medial dysplastic lesions that are clearly limited to the main renal artery.

Stenotic lesions occurring in children are usually discrete narrowings and therefore would appear ideal for PTA. However, the stenotic area is commonly a congenital narrowing of the entire vessel wall and is predominantly composed of elastic tissue. When such a vessel is submitted to PTA, the original diameter returns after dilatation or, if the vessel has been overdistended, rupture of the entire vessel wall is likely. Therefore, PTA is considered an inappropriate method of intervention in children with renal artery stenosis, and success is best achieved by operative correction.

Finally, review of results of PTA of bilateral ostial atherosclerotic lesions shows infrequent success with sustained benefit at 1 year, varying from 14% to 45%. Such results suggest that PTA has little value in the treatment of this variety of lesion, since the risks of cholesterol embolization, vessel thrombosis, and loss of renal function are present, accompanied by only a minimal chance for prolonged benefit.

In summation, experience with the liberal use of PTA has helped to clarify its role as one of the therapeutic options in the treatment of renovascular hypertension, but the data now accumulated argue for its selective application. In this regard, PTA of nonorificial atherosclerotic lesions and medial fibrodysplastic lesions limited to the main renal artery yields results comparable to those of operation when carried out by surgeons experienced in the technique. In contrast, the use of PTA for the treatment of congenital stenotic lesions, fibrodysplastic lesions involving renal artery branches, and ostial atherosclerotic lesions is associated with inferior results and increased risk of complications. For this reason, it is recommended that operation remains the initial treatment of choice for patients with the latter conditions and that the type of interventional therapy for RVH must always be individualized.

B. Surgical: A variety of operative techniques have been used to correct renal artery stenoses. From a practical standpoint, 2 basic operations have been most frequently used: aortorenal bypass and thromboendarterectomy. Aortorenal bypass, preferably with saphenous vein, has been found to be preferable and limits endarterectomy to orificial lesions of accessory renal arteries and to cases of severe bilateral orificial stenoses. Uncommonly, the renal artery may be redundant after it has been circumferentially mobilized. In such patients with orificial lesions, renal artery reimplantation also has been used with gratifying results.

1. Aortorenal bypass–Three types of graft are usually available for aortorenal bypass: autologous saphenous vein, autologous hypogastric artery, and synthetic prosthesis. The decision as to which graft to use depends on a number of factors. In one clinical experience, the saphenous vein is preferred. However, if the renal artery is small (less than 4 mm in diameter), the hypogastric artery or a synthetic prosthesis may be preferable. A 6-mm polytetrafluoroethylene graft is satisfactory when the distal renal artery is of large caliber (greater than 4 mm in diameter).

2. Thromboendarterectomy–Thromboendarterectomy is carried out only for atherosclerotic renal artery stenosis. It is not applicable for patients with fibromuscular disease. Preferred is a transverse aortotomy, carrying the incision across the stenoses and into each renal artery. By this method, the entire endarterectomy can be performed under direct vision. The transaortic route of thromboendarterectomy is recommended when multiple renal arteries arising at different levels from the aorta require management. Completion intraoperative duplex sonography is required when used to confirm the absence of distal intimal flaps or residual lesions in the distal renal artery.

3. Ex vivo reconstruction–Ex vivo management is necessary in patients with fibromuscular dysplasia and aneurysms or stenoses involving renal artery branches; patients with fibromuscular dysplasia and renal artery dissection and branch occlusion; patients with congenital arteriovenous fistulas of renal artery branches requiring partial resection; and patients with degeneration of previously placed grafts to the distal renal artery. Several methods of ex vivo hypothermic perfusion and reconstruction are available. The primary reason for removal of the kidney, hypothermic preservative perfusion, and ex vivo reconstruction is to allow prolonged safe ischemia times to reconstruct multiple branches. This technique provides several hours of safe renal ischemia.

4. Nephrectomy—Nephrectomy is a procedure that should be limited to a subgroup of patients with RVH in whom the kidney responsible for the hypertension has nonreconstructible vessels and negligible or no residual excretory function. In these circumstances of unretrievable renal function, nephrectomy can provide benefit in control of hypertension while not diminishing overall excretory function. In all other circumstances in which significant residual excretory renal function exists, the price of nephrectomy (loss of functioning renal mass) is greater than the potential benefit. Exception to this rule occurs only when hypertension is uncontrollable with the patient on maximal drug therapy and residual pressures consistently are severely elevated (greater than 120 mmHg).

This extreme conservatism for the role of nephrectomy is based on the knowledge that more than 35% of patients with atherosclerotic lesions develop contralateral severe lesions during follow-up. Such lesions place such a patient at risk for clinically severe renal failure and recurrent hypertension. This is of even greater importance in children, in whom 50% of those who initially present with a unilateral lesion subsequently develop contralateral disease.

Prognosis

Current results of operative intervention in centers experienced with management of RVH underscore the predictability of success. Although our experience spans over 25 years and includes the operative management of over 800 patients, review of the results of a recent series of 200 consecutive patients exemplifies current experience. The evolution of the patient population presenting for management is shown by comparing this group with a group of 122 patients reported by an author over 20 years ago (Table 23–1).

In the most recent experience, during a 54-month period, atherosclerotic RVD was the predominant pathologic condition, accounting for 78% of patients, 83% of renal artery lesions repaired, and 100% of the operative (3.1%) and follow-up patient mortality rates (17.1%). Despite the frequent need for extensive vascular repair (69%) superimposed on diffuse or extreme atherosclerotic disease (85%) and organ-specific damage (94%), beneficial hypertension response was observed in 90% of patients with atherosclerotic RVD. Note that the contemporary group is considerably older and more diffusely atheroscle-

Table 23–1. Comparison of surgical experience in renovascular hypertension.

	1961–1972*	1987–1991†
No. of patients	122	200
Mean age (yr)		
NAs-RVD	33	38
As-RVD	50	62
Duration hypertension (yr)		
NAs-RVD	4.6	11.2
As-RVD	5.1	15.0
Renal artery disease		
NAs-RVD	35%	21%
As-RVD	65%	79%
Renal artery repair		
Uniliteral	80%	60%
Bilateral	20%	40%
Combined‡	13%	32%
Renal insufficiency		
Not dependent on dialysis	8%	65%
Dependent on dialysis	0%	6%
Graft failure	16%	3%
Hypertension response§		
NAs-RVD		
Cured	72%[?]	43%[?]
Improved	24%[?]	49%[?]
As-RVD		
Cured	53%[?]	15%[?]
Improved	36%[?]	75%[?]

* Date derived from Foster et al (1973).
† Current series. Hansen et al (1992).
‡ Combined aortic repair for occlusive or aneurysmal disease.
§ Hypertension response excluding technical failures.
[?] As, atherosclerotic; NAs, nonatherosclerotic.

rotic than the patients treated in the earlier era (see Table 23–1).

Among patients with nonatherosclerotic RVD, 92% demonstrated a beneficial hypertension response; however, only 43% were considered cured, a figure below cure rates reported from earlier surgical series. This difference may be explained by the number of older patients, the number of patients with uncorrected contralateral lesions, and the duration of hypertension in many of these patients with nonatherosclerotic RVD. In contrast to the blood pressure results obtained in the entire group, patients less than 55 years of age who had all anatomic renal artery lesions corrected and had been hypertensive for less than 5 years had a cure rate of 68% and an improvement rate of 32%. This response is comparable to results from earlier reports.

Current published experience suggests that two-thirds of patients with bilateral revascularization and one-third of patients with unilateral revascularization will have at least a 20% improvement in their glomerular filtration rate. Even more encouraging is the recent recognition that over 60% of patients with ischemic nephropathy who have had revascularization after they have progressed to dialysis dependence have become dialysis independent after operation.

REFERENCES

Chiantella V, Dean RH: Basic data related to clinical decision making in renovascular hypertension. Ann Vasc Surg 1988;2:92.

Dean RH: Operative management of renovascular hypertension. In: *Surgery of the Aorta and its Body Branches.* Bergan JJ, Yao JST (editors). Grune & Stratton, 1979: 377.

Dean RH: Renovascular hypertension: An overview. In: *Vascular Surgery,* 3rd ed. Rutherford RB (editor). WB Saunders, 1989:1211.

Dean RH: Renovascular hypertension. Curr Probl Surg 1985;Feb;22:6.

Dean RH, Hansen KJ: Renal artery reconstruction. In: *Rob & Smith's Operative Surgery: Vascular Surgery,* 5th ed. Jamieson CW, Yao JST (editors). Chapman & Hall Medical, 1994:262.

Dean RH et al: Deceptive patterns of renal artery stenosis. Surgery 1974;76:872.

Dean RH et al: Evolution of renal insufficiency in ischemic nephropathy. Ann Surg 1991;213:446.

Foster JH et al: Ten years experience with the surgical management of renovascular hypertension. Ann Surg 1973; 177:755.

Hansen KJ, Reavis SW, Dean RH: Use of duplex scanning in renovascular hypertension. In: *Technologies in Vascular Surgery.* Yao JST, Pearce WH (editors). WB Saunders, 1991;174.

Hansen KJ et al: Contemporary surgical management of renovascular disease. J Vasc Surg 1992;16(3):319.

Harrison EG, McCormack LJ: Pathologic classification of renal artery disease in renovascular hypertension. Mayo Clin Proc 1971;46:161.

Meacham PW, Hollifield JW, Burko H, Dean RH: Predictable variation of plasma renin activity within the human left renal vein and correlation with anatomic study of left renal venous tributaries. Surg Forum 1980;31:220.

Meier GH et al: Captopril renal scintigraphy: A new standard for predicting outcome after renal revascularization. J Vasc Surg 1993;17:280.

Miller GA et al: Percutaneous transluminal angioplasty vs. surgery for renovascular hypertension. AJR 1985;144: 447.

Page IH, Helmes OM: A crystalline pressor substance (angiotensin) resulting from the reaction between renin and renin activator. J Exp Med 1940;71:29.

Pattison JM et al: Percutaneous transluminal renal angioplasty in patients with renal failure. Quart J Med 1992; 85(3007–308):883.

Robaczewski DL, Dean RH: Pathophysiology of renovascular hypertension. In: *Vascular Surgery: Basic Science & Clinical Correlations.* White RA, Hollier LH (editors). JB Lippincott,1994:263.

Sos TA et al: Percutaneous transluminal renal angioplasty in renovascular hypertension due to atheroma of fibromuscular dysplasia. N Engl J Med 1983;309:274.

Tegtmeyer CJ, Kellum D, Ayers C: Percutaneous transluminal angioplasty of the renal artery: Results and long-term follow-up. Radiology 1984;153:77.

Tobian L: Relationship of juxtaglomerular apparatus to renin and angiotensin. Circulation 1962;25:189.

Vaughn ED et al: Renovascular hypertension: Renin measurements to indicate hypersecretion and contralateral suppression, estimate renal plasma flow, and score for surgical curability. Am J Med 1973;55:402.

24 Acute Limb Ischemia

John Blebea, MD, & Richard F. Kempczinski, MD

Essentials of Diagnosis

- Pain, pallor, paresthesias, paralysis, pulselessness, poikilothermia (6 Ps).
- Severity of signs and symptoms depend on the adequacy of the preexisting collateral circulation and the duration of the ischemic insult.
- Decreased sensation on the dorsum of the foot and loss of great toe or ankle dorsiflexion in advanced ischemia.

General Considerations

Acute extremity ischemia may result from 1 of 5 pathologic processes:

- Arterial embolization
- Thrombosis of a diseased artery
- Acute occlusion of a vascular graft
- Atheroembolization
- Arterial trauma

These processes most often involve the lower extremities. However, the upper extremity is affected by cardiogenic emboli or iatrogenic trauma. Although the appearance and the secondary effects of acute arterial ischemia are similar regardless of the underlying cause, their treatment and prognosis are different. Therefore, establishing the correct diagnosis is important.

Arterial embolization is most frequently a complication of ischemic cardiac disease, with atrial fibrillation occurring in most of these patients. Emboli from the heart usually lodge at the bifurcation of large arteries. Axial limb vessels account for 60–80% of all clinically recognized emboli. Most arterial embolisms involve the lower-extremity arteries, with the common femoral artery being the most frequently affected. After the initial impaction of the embolus, fragmentation can occur with more distal embolization and occlusion of smaller vessels, resulting in many levels of obstruction. Extension of the thrombosis proximally and distally can develop because of cessation of blood flow both above and below the point of embolic occlusion. This may involve secondary thrombosis of important collateral vessels as well as discontinuous distal thrombosis.

A. Cardiac Causes: The incidence of arterial embolization has been increasing as the population has aged, and the number of patients with significant cardiac disease or dysrhythmias has grown. The incidence of arterial embolization has doubled from 23.1 per 100,000 admissions in the 1950s to 50.4 per 100,000 admissions in the 1970s. The heart is presumed to be the source in over 80% of all patients with peripheral emboli (Table 24–1). Although rheumatic heart disease was previously the most common cardiac disorder, **atherosclerotic heart disease** now accounts for more than 70% of all cardiac sources. **Atrial fibrillation** with presumed mural thrombus is present in up to 77% of patients with peripheral embolization. Transmural **myocardial infarction** precedes peripheral embolization in 24% of patients and is the second most common cardiac condition. Almost 50% of patients affected have suffered an acute infarct within 2 weeks prior to the event. Left ventricular mural thrombus develops after transmural myocardial infarction in 30–44% of patients, depending on the extent of the infarct. Although less than 5% of all acute infarcts result in distal emboli, the large number of patients who suffer myocardial infarction make it the responsible cause in up to one-third of all cases of peripheral embolization.

Cardiomyopathy, which produces dilatation of the cardiac chambers and the formation of secondary laminated thrombus, can also result in emboli. In a similar manner, **left ventricular aneurysms,** which can occur after myocardial infarction, have a laminated thrombus within them in more than 50% of cases. Embolization occurs, however, in only about 5%, and the total number of such events is relatively small. Overall, underlying atherosclerotic heart disease is the most common cause of mural thrombus and distal embolization.

Rheumatic heart disease, associated with mitral valve disease and atrial fibrillation, has declined steadily since 1950 and now accounts for less than 20% of all cardiac emboli. Cardiac valvular disease presently contributes to peripheral embolization primarily secondary to thrombus formation on **prosthetic valves.** This is especially problematic in patients who fail to comply with life-long anticoagulation. Secondary fungal and bacterial **endocarditis** developing on diseased aortic or mitral valves can also produce distal emboli. Valvular vegetations may develop after bacteremia or intravenous drug abuse. Left **atrial myxomas** are rare but, when present, portions may break off and undergo embolization to peripheral vessels.

Table 24–1. Cardiac causes of peripheral emboli.

Atrial fibrillation
Myocardial infarction
Cardiomyopathy
Left ventricular aneurysm
Valvular disease
  Rheumatic
  Prosthetic
  Endocarditis
Left atrial myxoma

Pathologic examination of retrieved emboli is thereby important to identify such an unsuspected cause.

B. Noncardiac Causes: A number of other sites need to be considered as potential sources of distal embolization, although they are much less common than the heart. The following are noncardiac sources of peripheral emboli:

- Abdominal aortic aneurysm
- Peripheral aneurysms
- Atherosclerotic ulcer/stenoses
- Prosthetic grafts
- Iatrogenic sources
- Paradoxical sources

Aneurysms are the most common noncardiac source of peripheral embolization. About 5% of distal emboli may originate from proximal unrecognized abdominal aortic aneurysms. Smaller peripheral aneurysms in the femoral or popliteal location may also produce distal arterial emboli, although they are infrequently large enough to induce complete extremity ischemia. Large proximal **atherosclerotic ulcerations** or **stenoses,** especially in the aorta or the common iliac artery, may form large thrombi that can occlude major distal arteries in another 5% of patients (Fig 24–1). More frequently, however, stenoses are associated with smaller atheroemboli. Proximal prosthetic **vascular grafts** can be the source of thrombotic vegetations and distal embolization in 1–4% of patients. **Iatrogenic embolization** may result from the formation of thrombus around a catheter or site of arterial puncture for diagnostic or therapeutic purposes. **Paradoxical arterial embolization** can occur, in the presence of an intracardiac defect, most frequently through a patent foramen ovale. Thrombus from deep vein thrombosis (DVT) in the leg can enter the left atrium of the heart through a right-to-left shunt and thereafter pass into a peripheral artery. This occurs in less than 0.5% of patients but should be considered in any patient with concurrent acute DVT. Finally, the exact source of emboli is never identified in 10–12% of cases.

C. Other Causes: Several variants of the basic processes of arterial embolization and thrombosis may induce acute limb ischemia. Macroscopic **atheroembolization** is the embolization of a portion of an atherosclerotic plaque from a large proximal arterial

ulcer. Distal arterial occlusion therefore is composed of atheroma rather than an organized embolus or large blood clot. Although usually composed of microscopic cholesterol emboli, such embolic plaque can occasionally give rise to an ischemic limb in the presence of underlying atherosclerotic stenosis in the extremity. Under these conditions, besides revascularization of the limb, resection of the proximal plaque source is required to prevent recurrent episodes.

Arterial thrombosis occurs in atherosclerotic vessels in which a narrow, irregular, or ulcerated lumen may develop an occluding clot. Thrombosis of a diseased vessel may be induced by hypotension, dehydration, congestive heart failure, polycythemia, hyperviscosity syndromes, or hypercoagulable states. Thrombosis may also take place because of decreased flow through a more proximal stenosis. After thrombosis occurs, clotting will extend proximally to a patent arterial branch and distally to a reentry point by collateral vessels. Longstanding arterial stenosis in such patients has stimulated the development of collateral pathways that may decrease the severity of the acute thrombosis compared with what happens in acute occlusion of a previously undiseased artery. The extremity may thus remain threatened for several days while alternative vessels provide blood flow beyond the occlusion. Because of an aging population with extensive atherosclerotic disease but prolonged survival, acute arterial thrombosis has now become as common as embolization as a cause of acute extremity ischemia.

Graft occlusion frequently induces acute limb-threatening ischemia. This diagnosis is more readily suspected because of the history of graft placement and the visible surgical scars. Treatment is similar to that for native but is usually more problematic because surgical bypass options may be more limited. Iatrogenic **arterial trauma** includes both embolic and thrombotic complications. Pericatheter thrombus during intra-arterial invasive procedures may undergo embolization down the extremity during catheter manipulation and induce acute ischemia. Local arterial trauma, in the form of intimal flaps, subintimal dissections, or extrinsic hematomas may induce local arterial thrombosis. The temporal relation of the acute ischemia to the arterial procedure readily identifies these complications and allows for speedy surgical repair. Traumatic arterial injury—either penetrating or blunt—generally necessitates immediate surgical intervention to restore arterial flow before irreversible ischemic injury occurs.

In addition to the potential pathophysiologic processes already described for the lower extremity, the upper extremity is subject to several additional processes inducing ischemia. Emboli into the arms can be caused by proximal subclavian thrombus and atherosclerotic aneurysms of the subclavian or axillary artery, as well as by a poststenotic arterial dilatation/aneurysm due to thoracic outlet compression (Fig

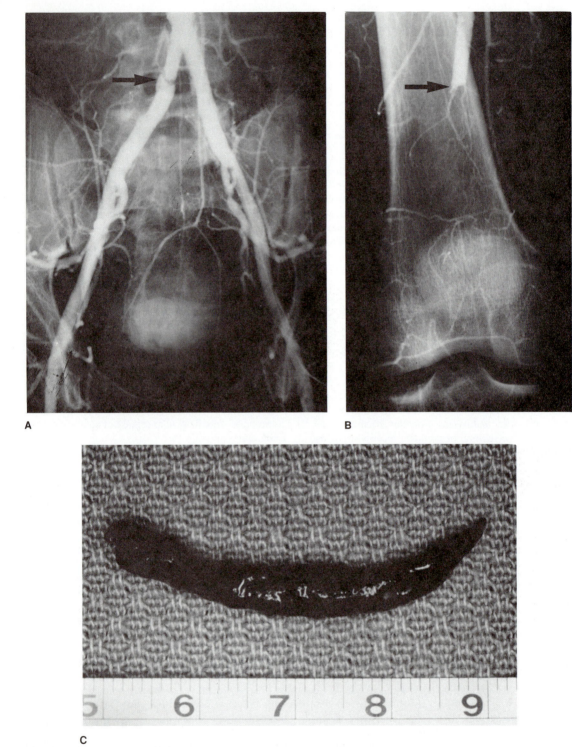

Figure 24–1. **A:** A focal atherosclerotic stenosis of the right common iliac artery. **B:** Associated occluding embolus of the proximal popliteal artery illustrating the abrupt cutoff (*arrow*) characteristic of embolic occlusion. **C:** The retrieved pathologic specimen with a proximal flattened end and distal tail.

24–2). A cervical rib or anomalous first rib fibrous band may traumatize the artery and produce a mural thrombus with distal embolization in patients too young to normally be considered for atherosclerotic disease. Improper use of crutches may occasionally lead to the same problem. Chronic extrinsic mechanical injury to the subclavian artery by a rib may cause its occlusion and upper-extremity acute ischemia.

Clinical Findings

A. Signs and Symptoms: During the initial stages of ischemia, the skin appears pale, waxy-white, and cadaveric. After 8–12 hours, the vessel spasm that normally accompanies acute vascular occlusion diminishes and areas of local stasis develop, reflected as a bluish mottling of the skin. With decreased inflow into the leg, there is poor capillary filling and the superficial veins are collapsed. Late signs of severe ischemia are the development of blebs and superficial skin necrosis. Dry gangrene and mummification in advanced cases may occur when the patient is comatose or does not feel the progressive ischemic pain. The leg is cold (poikilothermia).

The hallmarks of acute arterial ischemia are pain, pallor, paresthesias, paralysis, pulselessness, and poikilothermia. Although other pathologic entities may produce sudden onset of pain, pallor, and paresthesias of the foot or hand, arterial emboli have such a clear-cut onset that an exact time can often be elicited from the patient. The pain is constant but exacerbated by movement of the extremity. Paresthesias are a reflection of ischemia of the peripheral nerves and a sensitive sign of inadequate distal perfusion. They begin as a feeling of "pins and needles" in the foot and, if untreated, progress to loss of sensation to light touch. Complete loss of sensation to touch does not preclude persistent severe pain in the affected extremity. The leg or upper extremity will be cold and may also have associated muscular weakness. In patients with embolization, a history of previous embolism may be present. Patients may have stopped taking anticoagulation agents or have a subtherapeutic level of anticoagulation. In about 10% of patients, more than one embolism may be identified on presentation.

Absence of palpable pulses is a classic finding in patients with acute limb ischemia. Patients with an embolus to the common femoral artery may also have localized tenderness. The neurologic examination of the affected extremity is both an important prognostic indicator and the clinical parameter that will dictate the urgency of revascularization. Numbness with decreased sensation to touch may be demonstrable. Hypesthesia or anesthesia is first seen in the web space between the second and third toes. Ischemia of the deep peroneal nerve, located in the anterior compartment, leads to footdrop. Decreased motor function in toe and ankle dorsiflexion may occur and in advanced cases complete foot paralysis. Usually, patients with this finding eventually require an amputation, since most never regain motor function after revascularization. With prolonged ischemia, muscle rigor develops, which also indicates a nonviable extremity.

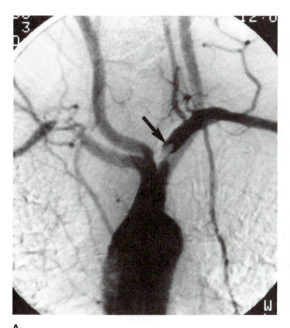
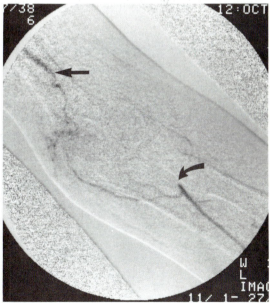

A   B

Figure 24–2. A: Proximal left subclavian floating thrombus (*arrow*) **B:** Associated embolization into the distal brachial artery (*straight arrow*) and reconstitution of the ulnar artery (*curved arrow*).

Arterial thrombosis produces symptoms similar to those in patients with embolization. However, with thrombosis, patients often have an antecedent history of claudication. There is also only a 4% incidence of associated atrial fibrillation compared with greater than 70% in patients with distal embolization. The onset of symptoms is less striking in arterial thrombosis, and the patient may have had progressive pain of a less severe nature.

Patients with local arterial thrombosis usually have evidence of preexisting atherosclerotic disease in the affected limb or the contralateral extremity, for example, trophic skin changes such as loss of hair on the dorsum of the foot or toes. Increased thickness of the toenails, and a dry scaly skin are also indicative of a chronic process. The contralateral side may also lack palpable distal pulses and may show the same chronic trophic skin changes.

B. Imaging Studies:

1. Duplex sonography–Peripheral arterial duplex scanning may localize and identify the presence of a common femoral artery thrombus or embolus and identify a patent proximal external iliac artery. Arterial scanning can additionally directly image the superficial femoral or popliteal artery occlusion, but it cannot distinguish between an embolus or thrombosis. It may also be very useful in documenting the presence of either a thrombosed femoral or a popliteal aneurysm, which might not be obvious on physical examination. Abdominal ultrasonic evaluation can also rule out the presence of an infrarenal abdominal aortic aneurysm or iliac artery aneurysm, which may have been the source of a distal embolus.

The diagnosis of phlegmasia cerulea dolens is suggested by an inappropriately high or normal ankle-brachial index. A concomitant venous duplex scan will establish the diagnosis.

2. Angiography–In patients with viable limbs, contrast angiography should be performed to provide a road map for surgical intervention. It will identify not only the site of occlusion but also potential proximal inflow sources and possible sites of distal anastomoses. If occlusion of the aorta and iliac vessels is found, the surgeon will be prepared for an abdominal procedure if catheter thromboembolectomy fails. Arteriography is especially helpful when arterial thrombosis is suspected. Thrombectomy in such patients is unlikely to be sufficient, and a knowledge of the arterial anatomy may be critical in planning a potential bypass. However, since angiography typically delays surgical intervention for 2–3 hours, patients with threatened limbs, such as those with decreased sensory and motor function, should not undergo angiography but should be taken directly to the operating room.

The presence of a normal femoral or axillary pulse usually excludes proximal inflow problems. Therefore, in such cases, intraoperative distal angiograms are usually adequate in planning the revascularization, and preoperative angiograms are unnecessary.

3. Arteriography–Diagnostically, arteriography can help to distinguish between an embolus and a thrombus. An embolus appears angiographically as a sharp cut-off of contrast or a reverse meniscus sign. It is usually seen in otherwise normal-appearing vessels (see Fig 24–1*B*). A thrombus usually demonstrates a tapering stenosis with vessels both proximally and distally showing evidence of diffuse atherosclerotic disease (Fig 24–3). However, peripheral vascular disease may also be present in patients with embolization. In

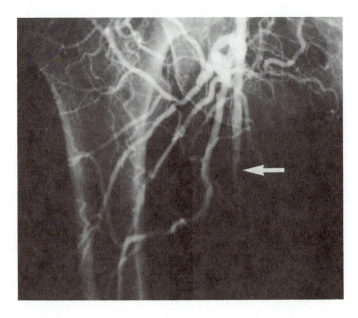

Figure 24–3. Thrombosis in situ of the proximal superficial femoral artery demonstrating tapered angiographic appearance (*arrow*).

the presence of an embolic event and no identifiable heart disease, biplanar angiography from the descending thoracic aortic to the foot vessels may identify an ulcerative atheromatous plaque with mural thrombosis in the aorta or iliofemoral vessels.

4. Echocardiography–In patients with distal embolization and no obvious arterial source of emboli, **echocardiography** should be performed, since the heart is the most common source of peripheral emboli. Although transthoracic echocardiography (TTE) is accurate in identifying thrombus in the left and right ventricles and left atrial myxomas, it misses 30–50% of thrombi in the left atrium and up to 85% in the atrial appendage. TTE also cannot evaluate the aortic arch and descending aorta. Because of these limitations, transesophageal echocardiography (TEE) should be performed in such patients. TEE provides a significantly improved sensitivity in detecting right and left atrial thrombi, in which it is up to 4 times as accurate as TTE. In addition, TEE can identify pedunculated mural thrombus in the descending thoracic aorta, which cannot be seen well with contrast angiography (Fig 24–4). Because TTE is technically less difficult, noninvasive, and widely available, it may be performed first. If no abnormalities are noted, it should be followed by a transesophageal echocardiogram.

5. Magnetic resonance angiography (MRA)– MRA may better define distal vessels available for bypass because it does not require that contrast reach areas distal to more proximal occlusions. Limited experience with MRA, however, suggests that visualization of the aorta or iliac vessels is less accurate than with standard contrast or digital subtraction angiography. Its future role is now undergoing a prospective multicenter evaluation.

The temporal sequence with iatrogenic trauma during arterial catheterizations, insertion of monitoring lines, or intra-aortic balloon pumps usually makes identification of the pathophysiology self-evident. If removal of the offending line does not restore distal perfusion, further diagnostic studies are generally not required, since the site of injury is known. A direct surgical approach can usually repair the arterial injury and retrieve distal thrombus. Patients with bypass grafts may present with limb ischemia secondary to graft thrombosis, although in a small number of cases the grafts themselves may be the source of distal emboli. Occluded grafts are managed in a manner similar to thrombosis in situ, but prior noninvasive and angiographic studies are frequently available as a frame of reference.

C. Laboratory Findings: Beyond the patient history and physical examination, further evaluation in patients whose clinical status does not preclude it should include a number of options. Information from the clinical laboratory may be helpful in assessing the severity of the ischemia and in preparing the patient for surgery. After several hours of ischemia, increases in hemoglobin, blood urea nitrogen, and creatinine often reflect fluid sequestration in the limb and intravascular hypovolemia. In the presence of extensive muscle necrosis, a dramatic increase in creatine phosphokinase, an elevation in white blood cell count (often over 20,000/mm^3), and systemic acidosis may occur. Thrombocytopenia may be due to disseminated intravascular coagulation. A 12-lead electrocardiogram may document the presence of cardiac dysrhythmias, especially atrial fibrillation and is also useful to rule out myocardial infarct or evolving cardiac ischemia. A chest radiograph should be performed to

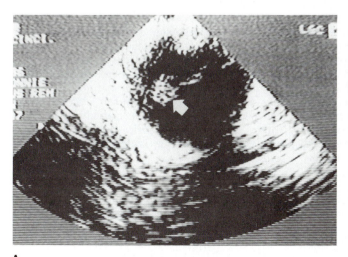

A

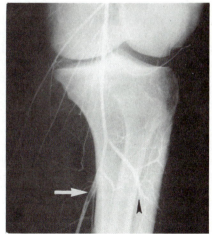

B

Figure 24–4. A: Transesophageal echocardiography showing descending thoracic aortic thrombus (*arrow*) with free-floating intraluminal tail. **B:** In the same patient, distal emboli from the aorta into the posterior tibial (*arrow*) and occluding the anterior tibial arteries (*arrowhead*).

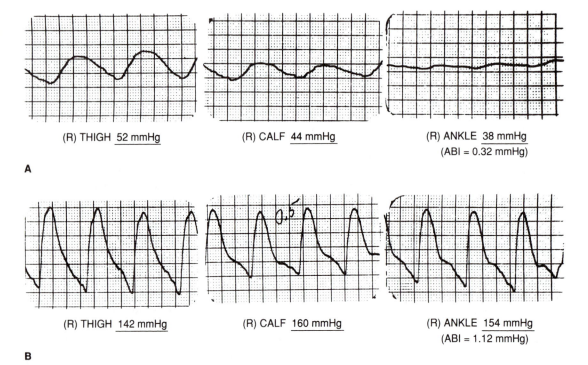

Figure 24–5. *A:* Segmental pressures and pulse volume recordings in a patient with aortic occlusion showing decreased pressures throughout the length of the leg and significantly diminished pulse volume recordings (PVR) amplitudes. *B:* Following revascularization, pressures are returned to normal, and the PVR waveforms have increased and have the characteristic normal dicrotic notch.

evaluate the presence of cardiomegaly or left ventricular aneurysm.

The **vascular noninvasive laboratory** is very useful both in documenting the severity of the extremity ischemia, the probable site of arterial occlusion, and the presence of contralateral atherosclerotic disease. Although Doppler arterial evaluation should be done and an ankle-brachial index should be determined as part of the initial physical examination, a formal examination by an experienced vascular technologist should also be performed if circumstances permit. Both segmental arterial pressures and pulse volume recordings can provide useful information as to the degree of ischemia along the length of the extremity and the probable site of occlusion (Fig 24–5). Such data are helpful in determining whether an infrainguinal procedure alone will be adequate or whether a femorofemoral, aortofemoral, or axillofemoral bypass may be needed. Noninvasive studies can also reveal the presence of chronic peripheral vascular occlusive disease in the contralateral leg. These date make the diagnosis of in situ thrombosis much more likely and will also establish whether the contralateral common femoral artery is suitable as a potential inflow source for revascularization. If the patient had previously been seen in the vascular laboratory, old records can provide a useful basis for comparison with the

acute event both in making the appropriate diagnosis and in providing insight into potential revascularization options.

Differential Diagnosis

In addition to differentiation between embolus and thrombosis, several other entities need to be considered. The most common of these is a low cardiac output state. In critically ill patients such as those with acute myocardial infarction or congestive heart failure, sepsis, dehydration or trauma, low cardiac output and the subsequent vasopressor support needed to maintain blood pressure may be associated with **low flow states.** Systemic vasoconstriction and decreased peripheral blood flow may cause patients to lose previously palpable distal pulses and even Doppler-detectable arterial flow. The legs may become cold and mottled. In such circumstances, all 4 extremities are usually similarly affected. The placement of a Swan-Ganz pulmonary artery catheter confirms a low cardiac output in association with increased systemic vascular resistance. Appropriate fluid resuscitation and cardiac support, with reversal of the primary underlying cause, ameliorates the appearance of the involved extremities and confirms the lack of an arterial occlusion.

Acute occlusion of a **popliteal** or **femoral aneurysm** is another potential cause of acute leg ischemia.

Often, a large mass, which may still be pulsatile, can be palpated at the appropriate anatomic locations. Duplex arterial scanning will confirm the presence of both an aneurysm and intraluminal thrombosis. Extensive iliofemoral vein thrombosis, **phlegmasia cerulea dolens,** can induce acute leg pain with cyanotic mottling and unilateral loss of palpable pulses. Unlike the pallor seen in those with arterial insufficiency, these patients have severe cyanotic mottling as the initial color change in the leg. The leg is usually swollen with visible venous distention rather than venous collapse. Also, the feet are not cold, even though palpable pulses are absent. Doppler arterial pulses are easily detectable. The most useful diagnostic test for phlegmasia cerulea dolens under these circumstances is a Doppler ankle-brachial index. This is usually greater than 0.50 and much higher than would be expected if the leg ischemia were due to arterial insufficiency. In less extensive DVT, pulses may still be palpable even though the leg is cyanotic.

Rarely, an **aortic dissection** may continue distally to occlude both the iliac arteries with resulting lower-extremity ischemia. In this circumstance, patients are usually hypertensive and have severe interscapular back pain or chest pain to suggest the diagnosis.

The most important initial determinations in managing patients with acute limb ischemia are the severity of the ischemia, the location and extent of arterial occlusion, and the underlying cause. The assessment of the severity of the ischemia is based on the clinical examination and determines the amount of time available for further investigation into the precise location of arterial occlusion and the probable underlying cause. If no motor or sensory deficits are found, a more complete evaluation can be performed, and one might consider with the use of thrombolytic agents or systemic anticoagulation alone.

Patients with advanced limb ischemia, which is documented by the presence of calf vein rigor or complete loss of motor and sensory function, require no further diagnostic evaluation, since these patients usually need emergency amputation. However, most patients fall between these two extremes. Although they may have some decreased sensation to light touch, their motor function is generally intact and the pain is tolerable. In such circumstances, a more complete evaluation is possible, and additional therapeutic alternatives are available. Under special circumstances such as occlusion of a known bypass graft or iatrogenic trauma, the underlying pathologic process is usually obvious. Therapeutic alternatives in these patients are more easily selected.

In most patients with advanced limb ischemia, the principal differential diagnosis is between arterial embolism and thrombosis. In older patients with evidence of both atherosclerotic peripheral vascular and cardiac disease, distinguishing between these two disorders can be very difficult. In fact, a precise diagnosis cannot be established in 10–15% of patients.

Treatment

The initial treatment of patients with acute limb ischemia is similar, regardless of whether the cause is an embolic or a thrombotic process. Historically, the maximum time period before irreversible extremity ischemic injury has been thought to occur is 6 hours. However, severity of ischemic injury varies from patient to patient and is not always proportional to the duration of ischemia because the extent of preexisting collateral circulation in any individual patient is usually unknown. The actual severity of the ischemic insult at time of presentation is much more important than the length of time that has evolved.

All patients who present with an acutely ischemic extremity should be immediately started on intravenous therapeutic doses of heparin unless a specific contraindication exists. Subsequent treatment is dictated by the degree of ischemia, the patient's general medical condition, and the underlying cause. Careful attention should be paid to local care of the affected extremity, especially if immediate intervention is not planned. The limb should be kept either in a horizontal position or slightly below the level of the heart. Heat may be injurious to the skin because of inadequate skin blood flow to dissipate it. Similarly, cold compresses should not be applied. The extremity should be placed on a soft surface such as an egg-crate mattress or sheepskin mat to prevent the development of pressure sores.

A. Embolus: Blaisdell (1978) has argued eloquently that administration of high doses of heparin in patients with acute ischemia is associated with less morbidity and mortality than surgical intervention. He recommends a 15,000–20,000 U intravenous bolus (300 U/kg) followed by 3000–5000 U per hour (50–70 U/kg) by continuous infusion, which subsequently may be increased according to the degree of clinical improvement. He reasons that much larger doses of heparin are required to prevent propagation of an ongoing thrombotic process compared with what is required when heparin is used prophylactically. The prevention of initial clot formation is easier because there is no induction of thrombin production by thrombus. However, this viewpoint has not been widely adopted, and most clinicians use an initial bolus dose of 10,000 U (100–150 U/kg), followed by a continuous infusion of 1500 U per hour (20–30 U/kg).

The partial thromboplastin time (PTT) should be checked 4 hours after beginning heparin and maintained at 2.5–3 times baseline levels (75–90 seconds). To attain a therapeutic level, initial maintenance doses as high as 2000–3000 U per hour may be required. A PTT greater than 100 seconds should not be particularly worrisome because it has not been shown to correlate with bleeding complications. Platelet counts, on the other hand, should be checked daily to identify potential heparin-induced thrombocytopenia and the white clot syndrome. In patients who will subsequently go on to surgical intervention, the PTT should be maintained at therapeutic levels and heparinization continued until immediately prior to surgery. When converting patients to oral anticoagulants, the therapeutic objective should be a prothrombin time (PT) target level of 1.5–2.0 times normal. Unlike heparin, bleeding while on warfarin is correlated with supratherapeutic levels.

Heparin therapy may be the only treatment used in patients with acute limb ischemia secondary to arterial emboli who have severe underlying medical conditions such as a recent major myocardial infarction or metastatic carcinoma or who were nonambulatory before the event. These patients should be started on heparin with the expectation that, if the limb remains viable, this therapy will be converted to oral anticoagulants. If the limb does not survive, amputation will subsequently be required. In patients with irreversible advanced ischemia, regardless of associated medical problems, anticoagulation is the proper initial therapy with urgent or elective amputation to follow as soon as is feasible.

1. Types—Patients with acute limb ischemia may be categorized into three groups to assist in deciding among therapeutic alternatives: (1) those with minimal ischemia, (2) those with moderate ischemia, and (3) those with advanced ischemia. Patients with **minimal ischemia** can usually be safely managed with an initial course of heparin therapy on which they will frequently show significant improvement. In good-risk patients without serious cardiopulmonary dysfunction, embolectomy can then be performed in a nonurgent manner after they have been fully evaluated. Patients with decompensated medical illnesses will have time for treatment of their illness prior to surgery. If the patient improves with heparin alone to either mild rest pain or severe claudication, delayed embolectomy can be performed. These patients often may not present for days or weeks after the embolic event, but they have a viable although ischemic leg. This usually means that the arterial occlusion is segmental and that distal vessels are patent. Delayed embolectomy will therefore be effective because irreversible muscle and nerve damage has not occurred. Patients who are medically unfit for surgery but whose limb ischemia does not improve on heparin can undergo planned thrombolytic therapy provided they do not have significant motor or sensory deficits.

Patients with **moderate ischemia** may have severe rest pain and some sensory dysfunction, but no irreversible muscle injury has occurred. In this group, heparinization and urgent embolectomy must be performed before irreversible injury occurs. Immediate embolectomy is thus the treatment of choice in almost all of these cases.

The last group of patients are those in whom significant ischemic injury has already taken place, as evidenced by mottling of the skin, total lack of sensation, muscle rigidity, motor dysfunction without ankle or toe dorsiflexion, and markedly elevated creatine phosphokinase. This group of patients should be considered for urgent primary amputation. Although there are circumstances in which early muscle rigor may still be associated with a salvageable leg, these are rare. Initial fasciotomy with inspection of the muscles can help the surgeon to decide whether limb salvage is still possible. However, revascularization with such advanced ischemia results in 50–75% mortality rate because of the reperfusion syndrome and is associated with a high risk of adult respiratory distress syndrome, renal failure and cardiac arrhythmias.

2. Procedure—After the decision has made been to proceed with embolectomy, local anesthesia with intravenous sedation is usually sufficient in most patients. In the lower extremities, a vertical groin incision is made to explore the common femoral artery. If it is unclear whether the occlusion is embolic or thrombotic, a longitudinal arteriotomy should be performed. This can later be closed with a vein patch to prevent stenosis. When the problem is clearly embolic, a transverse incision should be made on the common femoral artery just above its bifurcation through which proximal and distal embolectomies can be performed. The catheter should be passed until two successive passes yield no further clots. In the presence of an aortic saddle embolus (Fig 24–6), exposure of both femoral arteries is required and simultaneous iliac embolectomies performed using a 4Fr embolectomy catheter. However, in such circumstances, the patient should be prepared for a possible aortobifemoral or axillofemoral bypass if iliac embolectomy is unsuccessful. If arterial inflow is questionable after embolectomy, a retrograde angiogram should be performed to rule out a proximal arterial stenosis or retained thrombus.

An embolus localized to the common femoral artery and its bifurcation will permit direct removal. If the embolus is more distal along the leg, an embolectomy can be performed down the superficial femoral and popliteal arteries with a 3Fr embolectomy catheter. Embolectomy is repeated until two successive passes yields no further clots. After embolectomy, "good backflow" is not an adequate indicator of successful removal of all distal embolus. Intraoperative completion angiography should always be performed to confirm there is no retained distal embolus. If there is retained embolus and repeated embolectomies are unsuccessful, a popliteal exploration may be required.

Selective embolectomy into either the anterior or the posterior tibial arteries is rarely successful through a femoral approach. The catheter invariably goes down the peroneal artery. If all tibial arteries remain occluded without any direct run-off into the foot, a popliteal exposure will be required. With a medial below-the-knee incision, the popliteal artery is exposed to the origin of the anterior tibial and tibial-peroneal trunks so that the catheter can be selectively directed into all tibial vessels. For tibial embolectomy, a smaller 2Fr catheter should be used. Great care should

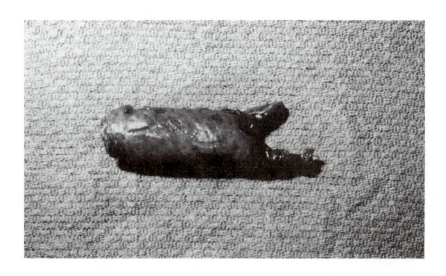

Figure 24–6. Aortic saddle embolus with forked extension into both iliac arteries.

be taken when passing an embolectomy catheter distally not to overinflate the balloon and injure the small distal vessels. Complications associated with balloon embolectomy include arterial perforation, intimal dissection, balloon fragment embolization, and the subsequent development of an arteriovenous fistula. Minimal residual clot may not require further embolectomy if the leg and foot are adequately perfused.

After embolectomy, a palpable pulse should be present. About 20% of patients have a good functional result despite failure to restore a distal palpable pulse. Because of arterial vasospasm immediately after embolectomy, some patients may have weak or absent pulses that improve during the postoperative recovery period. This is more likely to occur in normal vessels. Intra-arterial papaverine should be used in such circumstances.

If a distal tibial embolus cannot be removed by multiple passes of the embolectomy catheter, intra-arterial urokinase can be attempted. A dose of 100,000 U may be infused directly into the artery, then left in place for 15 minutes. Afterward, heparinized saline is flushed down the leg, and arteriography is repeated to document successful vessel clearance. A similar dose may be repeated twice. If still unsuccessful, some authors have advocated leaving a small intra-arterial catheter in place for continuous urokinase infusion during the postoperative period. Such therapy has been associated with bleeding complications in up to 17% of patients.

Intraoperative angioscopy permits more accurate detection of retained distal emboli after balloon catheter embolectomy. It allows clot removal under direct visualization and provides guidance for directed embolectomy from tibial arteries. In some circumstances, this may prevent the need for a separate distal popliteal exposure.

Although the surgical procedure can usually be limited to an embolectomy, a local endarterectomy, profundaplasty, patch angioplasty, or extra-anatomic femorofemoral bypass will be required in 21% of patients. Because concomitant cardiac disorders, particularly myocardial infarction and cardiac dysrhythmias, are common in these patients, more extensive distal revascularization procedures should be deferred until the patient has improved and more complete cardiopulmonary evaluations can be performed. If a patient would require an extensive initial revascularization procedure and his or her general medical condition is poor, primary amputation may be the most prudent course of action.

In patients with prolonged ischemia, especially in the presence of sensory or motor function loss, significant muscle swelling may occur after revascularization. Such edema within a closed fascial compartment can lead to skeletal muscle and neurologic ischemia despite successful revascularization. The associated increase in compartmental pressures occludes the small nutrient vessels with subsequent tissue ischemia. Under conditions of prolonged ischemia, prophylactic fasciotomies should be performed at the time of initial embolectomy (Fig 24–7). If there has been a long period of ischemia but no sensory or motor function has taken place, a subcutaneous fasciotomy is an acceptable alternative. Because of the increased probability that a more extensive compartment syndrome may develop, full open fasciotomies of all 4 muscular compartments in the lower extremity should be performed when the patient already has neurologic deficits preoperatively. If fasciotomies are not felt to be clinically indicated intraoperatively, compartment pressures

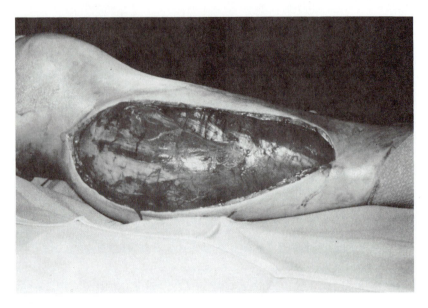

Figure 24–7. Compartment syndrome that developed following reperfusion required fasciotomy demonstrates underlying muscle swelling.

may be monitored postoperatively and a fasciotomy subsequently performed if intracompartmental pressures exceed 30 mmHg.

Postoperatively, intravenous heparin should be continued in the immediate postoperative period to prevent the recurrent embolization that occurs in 10–28% of patients. This also reduces the likelihood of rethrombosis in areas of intimal damage after embolectomy and in the presence of retained distal thrombi. Depending on the extent of the surgical dissection and the hemostatic control at the end of the operation, heparin may be restarted 4 hours postoperatively at a rate of 800 U per hour without an initial bolus. The dosage can subsequently be increased to achieve therapeutic anticoagulation. This dosage schedule carries a decreased risk of wound hematomas while still achieving 1.5–2 times normal PTTs. Very large doses of heparin are usually not required because the thrombotic load has been reduced and the ischemia ameliorated. When emboli have originated from the heart, warfarin is usually continued indefinitely to prevent recurrence.

Percutaneous aspiration embolectomy has also been reported in a small number of patients. However, aspiration alone of femoropopliteal emboli was successful in only 36% of patients. The others required additional interventions such as thrombus fragmentation, thrombolytic therapy, and percutaneous transluminal angioplasty of stenotic lesions. Aspiration embolectomy is a time-consuming procedure, which can remove only small amounts of thrombus during each pass. However, it may be useful as a way of avoiding amputation in high-risk patients in whom surgery is too risky. It also may have a useful role in retrieving

iatrogenic distal tibial emboli associated with interventional procedures.

In the upper extremity, emboli to the brachial, axillary, or distal subclavian arteries can be removed through a brachial arteriotomy. For axillary and subclavian occlusions, a longitudinal incision may be made in the upper third of the arm and a transverse arteriotomy in the proximal brachial artery. Thrombectomy can be accomplished with a 3Fr embolectomy catheter. Embolus or in situ thrombosis present at the brachial bifurcation can be approached using an S-shaped incision across the antecubital fossa. In this manner, the distal brachial and the proximal radial and ulnar arteries can be selectively controlled and catheter embolectomy appropriately directed into the respective vessels with a 2Fr embolectomy catheter.

B. Thrombosis: In patients with suspected thrombosis of native vessels or bypass grafts, an initial nonoperative approach is preferred because surgical revascularization usually requires a more extensive procedure than simple thrombectomy and the extremities are more able to tolerate the ischemia because of better of preexisting collateral circulation.

The clinical evaluation of patients with thrombosis in situ and the decisions about potential revascularization versus anticoagulation or primary amputation are similar to those described in patients with arterial emboli. However, patients who are candidates for revascularization present a greater operative challenge. They frequently require a much more extensive revascularization procedure. Unlike simple embolectomy, balloon catheter thrombectomy alone is rarely effective, since it fails to address the underlying cause of the thrombosis and a bypass graft or thromboendarterectomy is usually required to prevent rethrombosis (Fig 24–8). Therefore, preoperative angiography is more important in patients with thrombosis those with emboli. Angiography can usually define the responsible lesion and predict the type of revascularization procedure that will be required. In anticipation of the longer duration of these procedures, local anesthesia is rarely adequate, and better preoperative preparation of the patient is essential. Postoperatively, chronic anticoagulation has not been shown to be beneficial provided that the underlying lesion has been corrected with surgery, unless a specific hypercoagulable state has been identified.

C. Amputation: Primary amputation is the procedure of choice for patients with irreversible muscular injury of any cause or for those who require but cannot tolerate extensive reconstructive procedures for limb salvage. Motor paralysis or deep sensory loss indicates severe irreversible ischemia of the limb. Patients with an acute myocardial infarction, refractory congestive heart failure, or severe pulmonary insufficiency should probably have primary amputation rather than revascularization of a severely ischemic limb, which is likely to be poorly tolerated in such circumstances. The presence of severe extremity edema, muscle rigor, or gangrene requires emergency amputation to prevent secondary systemic effects. Limb amputation does not need to be performed urgently in the presence of paralysis or sensory loss, and time should be spent to optimally prepare the patient for surgery.

D. Thrombolytic Therapy: In patients whose limbs are not in immediate peril, intra-arterial thrombolytic therapy is a viable alternative to surgical intervention. Its potential advantages are especially evident in patients with significant concomitant cardiopulmonary disease, those with thrombosis of a previous bypass, or those with extensive underlying atherosclerotic peripheral vascular disease who would not be amenable to a simple revascularization procedure. Thrombolysis may also dissolve thrombi in the distal tibial vessels of the leg, which are less amenable to direct surgical thrombectomy. Thus, simplifying the revascularization that would be required and permitting it to be performed on a more elective basis.

Urokinase is usually given intra-arterially into the thrombus at a dose of 4000 U per minute for the first 4 hours and then at 1000–2000 U per minute for up to a total of 48 hours. Initial thrombolysis may begin within the first 12 hours, but it may take up to 48 hours for total dissolution to occur. If most of the thrombus has not been lysed by that time, the chance for significant lysis with additional infusion is small. Heparin is also given simultaneously at 500–1000 U per hour to reduce the risk of thrombus formation around the catheter but is associated with an increased risk of bleeding.

Thrombolytic therapy leads to successful lysis in 60–70% of patients and limb salvage in over 80%. However, it is associated with a mortality rate of 2–5% and major bleeding requiring transfusions in 4% of patient with an additional 15% rate of lesser complications. In cases of arterial stenoses discovered after successful thrombolytic therapy, balloon angioplasty can be performed to prevent rethrombosis or to allow for an elective surgical bypass to be undertaken at a later date (Fig 24–9). Because of the time generally required for successful thrombolysis, the ischemic limb must not be in such acute jeopardy that a delay of 24–48 hours would be critical to its survival.

Complications

The **reperfusion syndrome** is a recognized complication after revascularization of severely ischemic muscle regardless of the method used. The extremity may develop significant swelling with an associated compartment syndrome and superficial skin blistering (Fig 24–10). The systemic complications after reperfusion include metabolic acidosis, hyperkalemia, myocardial depression, pulmonary insufficiency, and renal failure secondary to rhabdomyolysis and myoglobinuria. Anaerobic metabolism that takes place in the ischemic extremity can lead to a sudden decrease in pH due to lactic acidosis and an increase in serum potassium, both of which have been measured in the venous blood from the affected limb. The acidosis and hyperkalemia can lead to cardiac arrhythmias. Acute

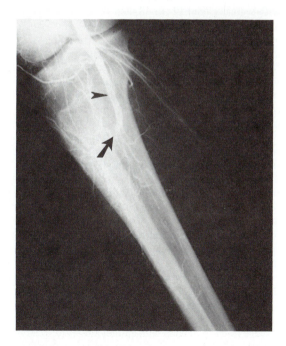

Figure 24–8. Remnant thrombus in the distal popliteal artery (*arrowhead*) and occluding the takeoff of the anterior tibial artery following successful surgical thrombectomy of an occluded femoropopliteal above-knee bypass. A distal bypass to the anterior tibial artery was required.

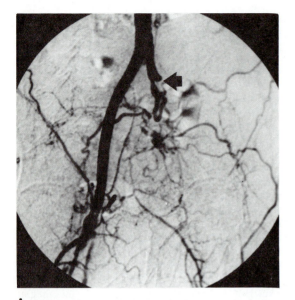

A

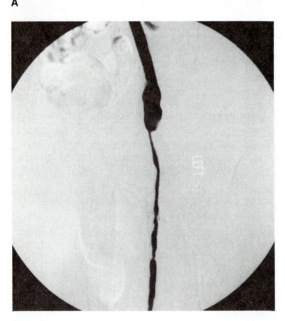

B

Figure 24–9. A: Occlusion of the left limb of an aorto-bifemoral bypass. **B:** After successful urokinase thrombolysis, occlusion of the profunda femoris artery and severe stenosis of the superficial femoral artery suggest the probable cause of thrombosis of the proximal prosthetic limb.

of the urine to prevent myoglobin precipitation. Mannitol acts as both an osmotic agent to induce diuresis and protect from renal failure as well as a scavenger of deleterious oxygen free radicals. Vigorous hydration and infusion of sodium bicarbonate and mannitol must be started before revascularization and continued periodically thereafter. Serum potassium levels are monitored and if they approach dangerous levels the patient is treated aggressively with glucose and insulin infusions.

Prognosis

After acute embolic occlusion of an extremity, the extremity is likely to survive if the collateral circulation is able to provide for the minimal resting requirement of the limb. Overall, in patients with acute extremity ischemia, the mortality rate ranges from 5% to 32% and amputation from 4% to 31%, regardless of treatment. Mortality results primarily from cardiopulmonary decompensation. Although the Fogarty embolectomy catheter greatly facilitated limb revascularization, mortality and limb salvage rates have not been significantly improved. Limb salvage is primarily influenced by the severity of ischemic injury at the time of presentation, whereas mortality depends on the patient's underlying medical condition.

Delay in treatment is a significant prognostic factor for both limb salvage and mortality. In patients with arterial emboli, if the duration of symptoms was less than 6–12 hours, mortality rate is only 19%. In patients with a greater than 12- to 48-hour delay in treatment, the mortality rate increases to over 31%. The associated limb salvage rates are 93% and 78% for the same intervals. The striking correlation between mortality rate and the patient's underlying medical condition is illustrated by the observation that patients with atherosclerotic heart disease have about a 50% mortality rate compared with 8–18% for patients without atherosclerotic disease.

In patients with atrial fibrillation, prognosis is better when fibrillation was of recent onset and transient rather than chronic. Similarly, emboli due to rheumatic valvular disease have a better prognosis. Increased mortality with lower-extremity embolectomy also correlates with older age, proximal vascular occlusion, and coexistent peripheral vascular disease. Emboli that involve the aorta or iliac arteries are much more dangerous than peripheral emboli. It is not surprising that multiple emboli have a worse prognosis than isolated episodes. Overall, perioperative mortality rates for patients with lower-extremity embolization ranges from 17% to 41% with an average of 27%. Heart disease is responsible for more than 50% of these deaths. Limb salvage rates associated with emboli ranges from 60% to 98% and averages 74%. Lifelong anticoagulation is the only effective long-term treatment.

Patients with arterial thrombosis generally have a lower mortality rate than patients with emboli because they are less likely to have acute myocardial infarction

renal tubular necrosis occurs from the precipitation of myoglobin released from ischemic muscle in an acidic environment.

Prevention of such reperfusion injury includes the infusion of sodium bicarbonate to counter the systemic metabolic acidoses and to induce alkalinization

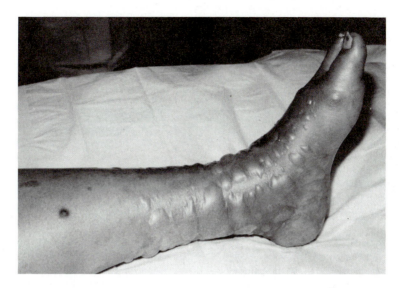

Figure 24–10. Leg swelling and skin blistering in the presence of advanced ischemia and reperfusion.

or severe cardiac disease. In the same series, mortality rates were 20% for patients with emboli compared with only 8% in those with arterial thrombosis. By contrast, limb salvage was possible in only 67% of patients with thrombosis compared with 85% of patients with emboli. This reflects the fact that patients with thrombosis have diffuse underlying atherosclerotic disease and require more complex procedures to provide adequate limb revascularization. The more proximal the thrombosis, survival of the limb is more likely, because more effective collateral vessels are available.

Acute upper-extremity ischemia is invariably due to emboli, and the prognosis for mortality and limb salvage is much better than lower extremity ischemia. The average mortality rate in collected series is 12% with a range of 7–25%. The limb salvage rate averages 97%, varying from 91% to 100%. The mortality rate is much lower because these patients with upper-extremity ischemia have less extensive coronary and pulmonary disease and the operative intervention is usually more limited. In addition, the skeletal muscle mass of the upper extremity is much less compared

with the legs, and the reperfusion syndrome is rarely seen (although a compartment syndrome can occur).

Unless a patient has untreatable concurrent medical illness that will invariably result in death within a few days, some type of therapy is indicated in all patients since the prognosis is otherwise grim. In patients with arterial embolization, three quarters of all those who survive the initial episode of hospitalization will have a good quality of life. However, recurrence can be expected in 6–45% of patients with progressively greater limb loss and mortality in the absence of continued treatment. Long-term anticoagulation can decrease this rate 3-fold to lower than 10%. Mortality rates for both embolic and thrombotic episodes have improved little over the past several decades. Limb salvage rates have improved but are consistently higher in embolic cases because those with thrombosis have extensive underlying peripheral vascular disease that can render limb salvage very difficult. Future advances in our understanding of the reperfusion syndrome and the prevention of progressive skeletal muscle injury after revascularization may help to improve both limb salvage and mortality.

REFERENCES

Blebea J, Kempczinski RF: Atheroembolism. In: *Vascular Surgery: Principles and Techniques,* 4th ed. Haimovici H (editor). Appleton & Lange, 1994.

Eglund R, Magee HR: Peripheral arterial embolism: 1961–1985. Aust NZ J Surg 1987;57:27.

Fowl RJ, Kempczinski RF: Arterial embolism. In: *General Surgery: Essentials of Practice.* Ritchie WP, Steele GD, Dean RH (editors). JB Lippincott, 1994.

Panetta T, Thompson JE, Talkington CM: Arterial embolectomy: A 34 year experience with 400 cases. Surg Clin North Am 1986;66:339.

IMAGING STUDIES

Karalis DG et al: Recognition and embolic potential of intraaortic atherosclerotic debris. JACC 1991;17:73.

Reeder GS et al: Transesophageal echocardiography and cardiac masses. Mayo Clin Proc 1991;66:1101.

TREATMENT

Arnold TE et al: Thrombolytic therapy of synthetic graft occlusions before vascular reconstruction procedures. Am J Surg 1992;164:241.

Blaisdell FW, Steele M, Allen RE: Management of acute lower extremity arterial ischemia due to embolism and thrombosis. Surgery 1978; 84:822.

Dale WA: Differential management of acute peripheral arterial ischemia. J Vasc Surg 1984;1:269.

Elliott JP et al: Arterial embolization: Problems of source, multiplicity, recurrence and delayed treatment. Surgery 1980;88:833.

Graor RA et al: Thrombolysis of peripheral arterial bypass grafts: Surgical thrombectomy compared with thrombolysis. J Vasc Surg 1988;7:347.

Haimovici H: Muscular, renal, and metabolic complications of acute arterial occlusions: Myonephropathic-metabolic syndrome. Surgery 1979;85:461.

Kempczinski RF: Lower-extremity arterial emboli from ulcerating atherosclerotic plaques. JAMA 1979;241:807.

McNamara TO, Bomberger RA, Merchant RF: Intra-arterial urokinase as the initial therapy for acutely ischemic lower limbs. Circulation 1991;83(Suppl I):I106.

Mills JR, Porter JM: Nonoperative therapy for arterial macroembolism in the extremities. In: *Current Therapy in Vascular Surgery,* 2nd ed. Ernst CB, Stanley JC (editors). BC Decker, 1991.

Segalowitz J et al: Angioscopy for intraoperative management of thromboembolectomy. Arch Surg 1990; 125:1357.

Turnipseed WD et al: Percutaneous aspiration thromboembolectomy (PAT): An alternative to surgical balloon techniques for clot retrieval. J Vasc Surg 1986; 3:437.

White GH et al: Angioscopic thromboembolectomy: Preliminary observations with a recent technique. J Vasc Surg 1988;7:318.

PROGNOSIS

Baxter-Smith D, Ashtib F, Slaney G: Peripheral arterial embolism: A 20 year review. J Cardiovasc Surg 1988; 29:453.

Cambria RP, Abbott WM: Acute arterial thrombosis of the lower extremity: Its natural history contrasted with arterial embolism. Arch Surg 1984;117:784.

Jivegard LE et al: Selective conservative and routine early operative treatment in acute limb ischemia. Br J Surg 1987;74:798.

Tawes RL et al: Acute limb ischemia: Thromboembolism. J Vasc Surg 1987;5:901.

The Diabetic Foot

25

Frank W. LoGerfo, MD

Essentials of Diagnosis
- Ulcers.
- Significant ischemia.

General Considerations

Problems of the diabetic foot are often encountered by vascular surgeons and are the most common reason for hospitalization in diabetic patients. These problems account for more than $1 billion in health care annually. About 10% of the population over the age of 65 years has diabetes mellitus. In this group, the risk of undergoing amputation is about 1% per year. Thus, for a patient with non-insulin-dependent diabetes mellitus (NIDDM) for 10 years, the risk is 10%. Among some groups, such as the Mexican Americans, the incidence of NIDDM is 30–40%, and among the Oklahoma Indians with diabetes mellitus the risk of amputation is nearly 2% per year overall and nearly 4% per year in men. Even though only 7–8% of the total population has diabetes mellitus, over two-thirds of all amputations are done in this group.

A. Pathogenesis: The magnitude of the clinical care and morbidity associated with the diabetic foot mirrors the severity and complexity of the underlying pathobiology. The three pathogenetic mechanisms involved are neuropathy, infection, and ischemia. Seldom do these mechanisms work in isolation; rather, most foot problems result from a complex interplay among all three. For the vascular surgeon, ischemia is the mechanism most often under consideration, but the basic concept of ischemia must be adjusted to the diabetic foot milieu. As will be described, many abnormalities in physiology, ultrastructure, and cellular metabolism lead to a generalized compromise in biology. This reality leads to a useful clinical rule that it takes greater tissue perfusion to maintain skin integrity in the presence of diabetes. Thus, arterial reconstruction and restoration of foot perfusion require a different perspective when applied to the diabetic foot in which neuropathy, infection, and metabolic abnormalities are also present.

The cause of ischemia in the diabetic foot is, as in the nondiabetic foot, atherosclerotic occlusive disease. The lesions are similar when examined histologically. The most notable difference is in the distribution of the occlusive lesions. With diabetes, there is a much greater propensity for the occlusive lesions to involve the distal popliteal and tibial arteries. Prospective stud-

ies of Conrad (1967) and Strandness and associates (1964) of amputation specimens using an arterial casting technique and blinded histology demonstrate clearly this pattern. It is surprising that in spite of the tibial and peroneal occlusive disease, these studies demonstrated a relative sparing of the arteries in the foot, especially the dorsalis pedis. Menzoian (1989), in a study of angiograms confirmed this observation. Thus, successful arterial reconstruction in patients with diabetes more frequently requires bypass to the distal tibial vessels or the dorsalis pedis. On the other hand, in many diabetics, especially nonsmokers, the superficial femoral artery may remain patent. This allows the possibility of using the superficial femoral or popliteal artery as an inflow source. Calcification of the arterial media is common in diabetics, but it does not correlate with arterial occlusive disease either in the periphery or the heart.

B. Microcirculation: The development and application of distal arterial reconstruction in the management of diabetic foot problems have been impeded by the misconception that there is an occlusive lesion in the microvasculature. This arose from an early histologic study describing periodic acid-Schiff (PAS)-positive material occluding arterioles in amputation specimens from diabetic patients. Subsequent prospective studies using arterial casting, blinded histology, vascular resistance, and plethysmography have not confirmed the existence of an arteriolar or microcirculatory occlusive process. If an occlusive lesion existed in the microcirculation, it would mitigate against arterial reconstruction, because both run-off and tissue perfusion would be limited. The concept of microcirculatory occlusion in diabetes has been tenacious and has led to a hopeless attitude in care of the diabetic foot. Fundamental to success in diabetic foot management is the elimination of the concept of a diabetic microcirculatory occlusive lesion.

Nonocclusive anatomic and physiologic abnormalities in the microcirculation are associated with diabetes. The most notable of these is thickening of the capillary basement membrane, which has been noted in several studies. This is not associated with a reduction in capillary luminal diameter. In fact, the capillary luminal diameter has been noted to be increased in diabetics in both skin and nerve, even in the presence of neuropathy. Increased glycation of basement membrane proteins occurs, with displacement of highly charged sulfur groups. This is one explanation for the frequently noted increase in albumin leak from the capillaries in diabetes. It is logical to assume, although it is not proven, that the capillary basement membrane thickening impairs the flux of nutrients and possibly the transmural migration of white blood cells. There is no evidence, however, of impairment of oxygen diffusion. In fact, the transcutaneous PO_2 of diabetics presenting with foot ulcers is higher than that of nondiabetics with foot ulcers. Thus, there seems to be no rationale for the use of hyperbaric oxygen in the management of foot ulcers that is specific to diabetes.

C. Neuropathy: Polyneuropathy involving the autonomic and somatic systems is a common complication of diabetes. The autonomic neuropathy may result in shunting of blood through arteriovenous connections in the microcirculation. This is one of several mechanisms that probably contribute to inefficient tissue perfusion, even in the presence of normal arterial supply. A potentially more harmful interplay between neuropathy and perfusion relates to the nociceptive reflex. When a sensory fiber is stimulated, the signal travels centrally to the nerve cell body and the spinal cord (orthodromic conduction). At the same time, antidromic conduction carries the signal to other axon branches, that is, the **axon reflex.** One function of this reflex is to release substance P from the nerve that triggers mast cells to release histamine. This is the mechanism leading to the wheal-and-flare response to a noxious stimulus that is greatly attenuated in patients with diabetes and may precede clinically apparent neuropathy. Its absence may contribute to the diminished inflammatory response to infection in the foot. These abnormalities in the microneurovascular physiology represent another area of compromised defense mechanisms, increasing the susceptibility of the foot to injury, ulceration, and infection.

Motor neuropathy leads to loss of function of the intrinsic muscles of the foot. Initially, the metatarsals are flexed and the toes are drawn up in the "claw" position. This creates pressure points beneath the metatarsal heads and also over the dorsum and tips of the toes. At the same time, the sensory component of neuropathy diminishes awareness of the pressure points, setting the stage for pressure-induced ulceration. The point at which external pressure halts blood flow in the overlying skin occurs at less external pressure in the presence of arterial occlusive disease and diminished intrinsic perfusion. When both neuropathy and ischemia are present, correction of ischemia can often lead to healing of the ulceration. Thus, the presence of neuropathy along with ischemia should not mitigate against arterial reconstruction. In fact, in a patient with neuropathy, restoration of arterial circulation is even more important in order to achieve and to maintain healing in the presence of the compromised defense.

Clinical Findings

A. Infection: Infection in the diabetic foot is usually a consequence of injury and is often polymicro-

bial. Because of the depressed nociceptive reflex, the usual inflammatory response is blunted with diminished erythema, induration, and edema. The patient often notes no pain and may become aware of the infection only through the present of drainage or a foul odor. These infections are usually well established and more extensive than would be predicted by the signs and symptoms. The masking of clinical signs of infection contributes to the axiom of diabetic foot care that infections must be drained promptly and completely. This often requires amputation of one or more toes combined with an incision along the entire course of the infected tract on the plantar or dorsal aspect of the foot. Concerns about subsequent closure of the foot are minor with adequate drainage being the single most important goal. Subsequently, the wound should be examined and probed on a daily basis, with prompt incision and débridement of additional, or overlooked, infection. Cultures should be taken from the depths of the wound, and initial treatment should be with broad-spectrum antibiotics with subsequent adjustment based on culture results.

B. Osteomyelitis: The diagnosis of osteomyelitis in the diabetic has been approached in several ways. The simplest and probably most effective diagnostic tools are the plain x-ray film and the metal wound probe. Osteomyelitis in the absence of any point of entry is most unusual. The presence of inflammatory signs along with an x-ray picture of bony degradation with intact skin should be regarded as Charcot osteoarthropathy. The simplest test being to put the patient at complete bed rest for 24–48 hours without antibiotics; if the inflammation resolves, proceed with the assumption that osteomyelitis is not involved. Many so-called cures of osteomyelitis with antibiotics alone probably represent the misdiagnosis of neuro-osteoarthropathy.

If an open wound is present, a probe should be inserted and if the hard surface of bone is encountered, the presence of osteomyelitis should be presumed. The use of these simple diagnostic methods to detect osteomyelitis should make unnecessary the use of bone scans and magnetic resonance imaging (MRI). Although these expensive diagnostic technologies have both advantages and shortcomings, they remain of minimal value in the context of the aforementioned approach to osteomyelitis.

C. Ischemia: Ischemia is best understood as a relative term. The point at which skin necrosis occurs as perfusing pressure drops depends on many local and systemic factors. As already mentioned, pressure point deformities, absent sensation, muted mechanisms of inflammation, and inefficient microcirculation add up to compromised biologic defenses in the diabetic foot. As perfusing pressure drops, ulceration occurs sooner in the patient with diabetes. This may explain the observation that diabetics presenting with foot ulcers actually have a higher transcutaneous PO_2 than nondiabetics; keep this in mind when using transcutaneous

PO$_2$ to assess the role of ischemia in diabetic foot ulcers.

The usual parameters for determining the significance of ischemia must be modified to the specific clinical conditions. A superficial ulcer in a patient with relatively intact defense mechanisms will heal at a transcutaneous PO$_2$ similar to that in nondiabetics. However, a deep ulcer with exposed bone, active infection, and compromised defense mechanisms requires normal perfusion to heal. Thus, the diabetic foot presents a spectrum of complex biologic conditions that compound the standard guidelines for assessment of ischemia.

The use of standard noninvasive testing for peripheral vascular disease is also compromised in the presence of diabetes. Calcification of the arterial media is a common feature of vascular pathology in diabetics. This is not part of the occlusive process and in fact does not correlate with the presence of atherosclerotic occlusion. When the tibial vessels are calcified, it is difficult or impossible to compress them with a blood pressure cuff, resulting in inaccurate or undetermined ankle blood pressures. The digital arteries are somewhat spared from calcification, and it is often possible to obtain toe pressures even when the ankle vessels are not compressible. Unfortunately in many patients with foot ulcers, the toe pressure may not be obtainable because of the proximity of the ulcer. Nonetheless it is a useful, if somewhat underutilized, tool for assessment of ischemia.

Pulse volume recordings are another alternative to ankle pressures. These are essentially a form of plethysmography using strain gauges encircling the thigh, calf, ankle, and forefoot. The output is not quantitative in the sense that the deflection is partially a function of initial strain and amplification. Nonetheless in a given laboratory, the technique can be well standardized. In addition, the quality of the derived waveform is useful, that is, whether it is monophasic, triphasic, and so on. Again, the limitation exists that the presence of foot ulcers can prevent placement of the forefoot cuff.

Continuous wave (CW) Doppler-derived pulse waveforms are helpful in the presence of noncompressible tibial vessels and, like pulse volume recordings, are not quantitative. However, useful information can be gained from the pulse waveform. The Doppler-derived technique is generally limited distally to the ankle level and has not found application at the toe or forefoot level.

The foregoing discussion shows that noninvasive vascular testing has significant limitations when applied to lower-extremity occlusive disease in diabetics. This, combined with the many biologic factors influencing the significance of a given level of ischemia, greatly reduces the value of noninvasive testing in the presence of a diabetic foot ulcer. Often, debate is centered around whether an ulcer will heal on its own or whether a minor amputation will heal based on noninvasive testing. However, the complex and variable pathobiology makes it difficult to have a standardized approach based on noninvasive testing alone.

In the patient presenting with ulceration or gangrene combined with deep infection, few, if any, noninvasive tests can be applied other than CW Doppler waveforms. Even palpation of pulses is compromised by the accompanying edema. As a result, many decisions regarding the role of ischemia in the diabetic foot must be guided primarily by clinical observations. Fortunately, in spite of the complexity of the underlying pathology, all this information can be applied in a stepwise clinical approach to the acutely infected diabetic foot, which can be defined as follows:

(1) All obviously necrotic tissue should be removed and all infected tissue planes opened to provide prompt, adequate drainage.

(2) Broad-spectrum antibiotics should be initiated until bacteriology is determined.

(3) Systemic evidence of sepsis, fever, and glycemia must be brought under control.

(4) The role of ischemia should be defined by noninvasive testing to the extent possible under the individual circumstances:

(a) In the presence of clearly normal circulation (palpable pulses with a triphasic signal), the problem may be assumed to be purely neuropathic.

(b) In the absence of a palpable pulse, ischemia may be assumed to be a significant contributing factor. (As a general rule, under the latter circumstance, arteriography should be performed.)

(5) The arteriogram must demonstrate the status of the foot arteries even when the more proximal femoral or tibial arteries are occluded. Digital subtraction arteriography is highly effective, although other techniques for enhancement of distal vessels may also be successful. The angiographer should understand that the foot arteries are often patent even when the tibial arteries are occluded.

Treatment

Arterial reconstruction should be designed to restore maximum perfusion to the foot. In diabetics, the choice is often between bypass to an isolated popliteal segment, the peroneal, or the dorsalis pedis. Bypass to an isolateral popliteal segment will result in a marginal improvement in foot perfusion. It may be effective in relieving rest pain and may result in healing of superficial ulcerations that do not involve the bone, joint, or tendon. Bypass to the peroneal artery results in much improved foot perfusion but may not be effective in achieving healing of deep ulcerations or sepsis of the forefoot. When adequate saphenous vein is available bypass to the dorsalis pedis artery is the preferred option and has proven to be effective and durable. It provides maximum possible perfusion to the forefoot and results in healing of even severe forefoot infections with minimum tissue loss. Because the operation is no more difficult than bypass to the isolated popliteal seg-

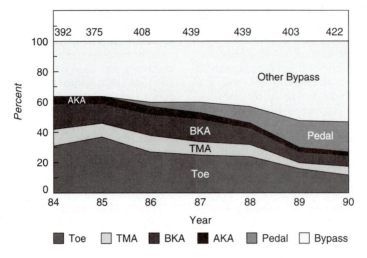

Figure 25–1. The rate of each operation as the primary procedures. All amputations occurring during an admission for a bypass procedure are also included. AKA, above-knee amputation; BKA, below-knee amputation; TMA, transmetatarsal amputation.

ment or peroneal and has an equivalent patency with maximum tissue salvage, it is the preferred option for most foot lesions.

Final wound closure, if necessary, should be accomplished under conditions of optimal perfusion. Further amputation, skin grafting, or local flaps may be used; free flaps have occasional application. In patients with severe neuropathy, foot ulcers, usually located over neuropathy-induced pressure points, may persist after arterial reconstruction. For ulcers directly under a metatarsal head, resection of the head or osteotomy often eliminates the pressure point and prevents recurrence. This approach has resulted in a

marked reduction of both major and minor amputations at the author's institution (Fig 25–1).

Probably the single most important factor in the achievement of reduction of amputations has been success in the application of the dorsalis pedis bypass, which is especially apparent in an analysis of major amputations (Fig 25–2). Vein bypass grafts to the dorsalis pedis may originate from the common femoral, superficial femoral, or popliteal artery. The conduit may be reversed, translocated, or in situ. None of these factors seems to influence outcome, providing a great deal of flexibility in the surgical technique. It is surprising that dorsalis pedis bypass has a patency and

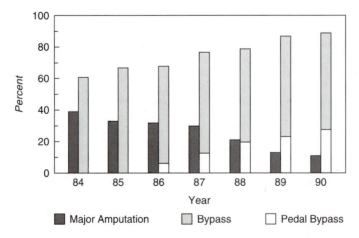

Figure 25–2. The ratio of major amputation to bypass procedures has declined. This correlates closely with the increasing use of bypass grafts to the dorsalis pedis artery. (Reproduced, with permission, from LoGerfo FW, Gibbons GW, Pomposelli FB Jr et al: Evolving trends in the management of the diabetic foot. *Arch Surg* 1992;127:617.)

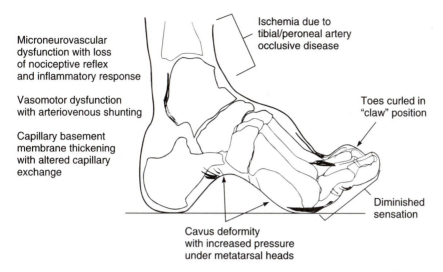

Microneurovascular
dysfunction with loss
of nociceptive reflex
and inflammatory response

Vasomotor dysfunction
with arteriovenous shunting

Capillary basement
membrane thickening
with altered capillary
exchange

Ischemia due to
tibial/peroneal artery
occlusive disease

Toes curled in
"claw" position

Diminished
sensation

Cavus deformity
with increased pressure
under metatarsal heads

Figure 25–3. Diabetic foot problems result from the combined pathology of neuropathy, ischemia, and infection.

limb salvage rate equal to that of femoropopliteal or femorotibial bypass, yet other investigators have reported similar experiences with extreme distal bypass.

In preparation for dorsalis pedis bypass, both anteroposterior and lateral views of the foot are helpful. When a choice exists between dorsalis pedis bypass and bypass to an equivalent posterior tibial artery at the malleolus, the decision should be based on the proximity of the ulcer to the specific run-off bed. Bypass to the most proximal artery with direct continuity to the ischemic territory is the desirable endpoint. However, the availability of adequate length of autogenous conduit may force compromise to an alternative run-off vessel. With distal reconstruction, the quality of the conduit is the key to long-term success. Angioscopy of the vein conduit provides an optimal means of assessment and is almost essential when preparing arm vein grafts because of the high incidence of preexisting abnormalities.

Summary

Overall success with diabetic foot management requires a comprehensive understanding of the complex underlying pathophysiology (Fig 25–3). The overall outcome of arterial reconstruction in the diabetic in terms of mortality, graft patency, or limb salvage, is equal to or better than that in nondiabetics. Even in the subgroup of diabetics presenting with ischemia and severe foot sepsis there appears to be no compromise in outcome when the clinical care plan described earlier is followed. Clinical care is enhanced by interdisciplinary team management incorporating specialists in infectious disease, podiatry, cardiology, and diabetology. In addition, specialized nursing care and thoughtful social service input are important for achieving the best patient care. The diabetic foot is a clinical problem that can be solved with a high degree of success; essential to this is the application of modern vascular surgical techniques.

REFERENCES

Barner HB, Kaiser GC, Willman VL: Blood flow in the diabetic leg. Circulation 1971;43:391.

Britland ST, Young RJ, Sharma AK, Clarke BF: Relationship of endoneurial capillary abnormalities to type and severity of diabetic polyneuropathy. Diabetes 190;39:909.

Brownlee M, Cerami A, Vlassara H: Advanced glycosylation end products in tissue and the biochemical basis of diabetic complications. N Engl J Med 1988;318:1315.

Chantelau E et al: Effect of medial arterial calcification on O_2 supply to exercising diabetic feet. Diabetes 1990;39:938.

Conrad MC: Large and small arterial occlusion in diabetics and nondiabetics with severe vascular disease. Circulation 1967;36:83.

Cronenwett JL et al: Limb salvage despite extensive tissue loss: Free tissue transfer combined with distal revascularization. Arch 1989;124:609.

Ctercteko GC, Dhanendran D, Hutton WC, Lequesne LP: Vertical forces acting on the feet of diabetic patients with neuropathic ulceration. Br J Surg 1981;68:608.

Direct and indirect costs of diabetes in the Unites States in 1992. American Diabetes Association, 1993.

Edmonds ME, Roberts VC, Walkins PJ: Blood flow in the diabetic neuropathic foot. Diabetologia 1982;22:9.

Goldenberg SG, Alex M, Joshi RA, Blumenthal HT: Nonatheromatous peripheral vascular disease of the lower extremity in diabetes mellitus. Diabetes 1959;8:261.

Huse DM et al: The economic costs of non-insulin-dependent diabetes mellitus. JAMA 1989;252:2078.

Irwin ST et al: Blood flow in diabetics with foot lesions due to "small vessel disease." Br J Surg 1988;75:1201.

Kacoyanis GP, Whittemore AD, Couch NP, Mannick JA: Femorotibial and femoropopliteal bypass vein grafts. Arch Surg 1981;116:1529.

Katz MA et al: Relationships between microvascular function and capillary structure in diabetic and nondiabetic human skin. Diabetes 1989;38:1245.

Lee JS et al: Lower extremity amputation: Incidence, risk factors, and mortality in the Oklahoma Indian Diabetes Study. Diabetes 1993;42:876.

Louie TJ, Bartlett JG, Tally FP, Gorbach SL: Aerobic and anaerobic bacteria in diabetic foot ulcers. Ann Intern Med 1976;85:461.

Maser RE et al: Cardiovascular disease and arterial calcification in insulin-dependent diabetes mellitus: Interrelations and risk factor profiles. Arterioscler Thrombos 1991;11:958.

Menzoian JO et al: Symptomatology and anatomic patterns of peripheral vascular disease: Differing impact of smoking and diabetes. Ann Vasc Surg 1989;3:22.

Miller A et al: Continued experience with routine intraoperative angioscopy for monitoring infrainguinal bypass grafting. Surgery 1991;109:286.

Parving HH, Rasmussen SM: Transcapillary escape rate of albumin and plasma volume in short- and long-term juvenile diabetics. Scand J Clin Lab Invest 1973;71:974.

Patel VG, Wieman TJ: Effect of metatarsal head resection for diabetic foot ulcers on the dynamic plantar pressure distribution. Am J Surg 1994;167:297.

Pomposelli FB Jr et al: A flexible approach to infra-popliteal vein grafts in patients with diabetes mellitus. Arch Surg 1991;161:724.

Ramsey DE, Manke DA, Sumner DS: Toe pressure: A variable adjunct to ankle pressure measurement for assessing peripheral arterial disease. J Cardiovasc Surg 1983;24:43.

Rosenblum BI et al: Maximizing foot salvage by a combined approach to foot ischemia and neuropathic ulceration in patients with diabetes mellitus: A five year experience. Diabetes Care, September 1994 (in press).

Ruderman N, Haudenschild C: Diabetes as an atherogenic factor. Progr Cardiovasc Dis 1984;26:373.

Seldin GW et al: Effect of soft-tissue pathology on detection of pedal osteomyelitis in diabetics. J Nucl Med 1985; 26:988.

Sidawy AN, Menzoian JO, Cantelmo NL, LoGerfo FW: Effect of inflow and outflow sites on the results of tibioperoneal vein grafts. Am J Surg 1986;152:211.

Siperstein MD, Unger RH, Madison LL: Studies of muscle capillary basement membranes in normal subjects, diabetic, and prediabetic patients. J Clin Invest 1968;47:1973.

Strandness DE Jr, Priest RE, Gibbons GE: Combined clinical and pathologic study of diabetic and nondiabetic peripheral arterial disease. Diabetes 1964;13:366.

Tannenbaum GA et al: Safety of vein bypass grafting to the dorsalis pedal artery in diabetic patients with foot infections. J Vasc Surg 1992;15:982.

Taylor LM Jr, Phinney ES, Porter J: Present status of reversed saphenous vein bypass grafting: 5 year results of a modern series. J Vasc Surg 1990;11:193.

Walmsley D, Wiles PG: Early loss of neurogenic inflammation in the human diabetic foot. Clin Sci 1991;80:605.

Wyss CR, Matsen FA, Simmons CW, Burgess EM: Transcutaneous oxygen tension measurements on limbs of diabetics and nondiabetics with peripheral vascular disease. Diabetes 1964;13:366.

Vasculogenic Impotence

26

Ralph G. DePalma, MD, FACS

Although no precise estimate can be made, impotence is a common complaint among middle-aged men. An estimated 10 million American men are impotent, and the incidence increases with age. Twenty-five percent of men are impotent by 65 years of age and almost 80% by age 80. It is not surprising that in the last 15 years, there has been increasing interest in the diagnosis and treatment of impotence. Sophisticated diagnostic tests have been developed, and effective forms of therapy can now be offered to many men. This chapter outlines the authors' current approach to diagnosis and treatment.

Penile erection requires adequate arterial inflow and closure of cavernosal outflow. The erectile process is mediated primarily by relaxation of the smooth muscle of the corporal bodies with a subsequent increase in corporeal arterial inflow. Closure of venous drainage occurs by compression of the veins against the tunica albuginea mainly by subalbugineal muscle. Venous leakage, therefore, can relate to inadequate arterial inflow. On the other hand, venous leakage is also seen in the presence of perfectly normal arterial inflow. A typical history of congenital venous leakage is that of a young man who has never experienced an adequate erection. Appropriate diagnostic tests reveal a large leak from the corpus cavernosum into the corpus spongiosum. Such cases are relatively rare. Acquired venous leakage can be associated with penile trauma such as fracture, Peyronie's disease, or other unknown causes, possibly related to aging factors in the corpora and the tunica albuginea.

It was initially assumed that aging contributed to decrements in arterial flow. However, examination of results of noninvasive screening reveals that the average age of men presenting with or without arterial insufficiency is 55 years. Significant risk factors predicting the detection of inadequate penile arterial flow on noninvasive screening are cigarette smoking and the presence of large vessel disease elsewhere.

Clinical Findings

A. Signs and Symptoms: The cause of impotence can be vasculogenic, neurogenic, endocrine, drug-induced, or psychogenic. Two or more factors may coexist, and psychogenic problems often complicate organic impotence. Inasmuch as erection is a dramatic vascular process, much attention has been paid to vasculogenic impotence in particular. A classifica-

tion of causes of vasculogenic impotence is offered in Table 26–1. Three general categories of vascular dysfunction exist: (1) arterial insufficiency due to large or small vessel occlusive disease, (2) cavernosal malfunction, and (3) venous leakage. The presenting signs and symptoms of each type of impotence overlap considerably and often cannot be distinguished from each other without more sophisticated examinations. In general, 2 large categories of patients with arterial disease can be defined: men with aortoiliac occlusive or aneurysmal disease and those with small vessel pudendal atherosclerosis or diffuse penile involvement.

Men with aortoiliac atherosclerosis usually present with the primary complaint of claudication, not impotence, although as noted by Leriche in 1923, impotence is often the first symptom of early aortoiliac occlusive disease. These men typically exhibit risk factors for atherosclerosis such as cigarette smoking, hypertension, hypercholesterolemia and, much less commonly, diabetes. Men with aneurysms also offer the complaint of impotence. Although the incidence of impotence is high in diabetics and sometimes relates to vascular occlusive disease, more often diabetic impotence is related to cavernosal malfunction due to a smooth muscle dysfunction with possible inadequate release of nitric oxide and also to neuropathy. Each of these etiologic factors often coexist in diabetics in varying combinations. Finally, men with predominantly small vessel occlusive disease involving pudendal or penile arteries or venous leakage, present with a complaint of impotence of gradual onset—first, the inability to maintain an erection and ultimately the inability to obtain an erection. This usually occurs in the absence of any traumatic life event and in the presence of an interested partner. The typical symptoms and signs of major aortoiliac atherosclerosis are usually absent as well as risk factors predisposing to this disease.

B. Physical and Laboratory Examinations: Men with the chief complaint of impotence are requested to visit the vascular laboratory for neurovascular penile noninvasive testing before their first office visit. Tests include measurement of penile brachial pressure indices, pulse volume recording, and neurologic evaluations. Neurologic evaluation involves measurement of pudendal-evoked potentials and bulbocavernosal reflex time. This testing is especially necessary in men with a past history of back injury or

Table 26–1. Vasculogenic impotence.

Cavernosal
  Arteriolar
    Functional or anatomic
    Helicine vessel abnormalities
    Blood pressure medication
  Fibrosis
    Postpriapic
    Drug injection
  Peyronie's disease
    Deformity invading cavernous smooth muscle
    Venous leakage through tunical
  Refractory smooth muscle
    Hormonal: prolactinemia, testosterone level
    Blood pressure medication
    Metabolic: diabetes, anemia
Venous Leakage
  Acquired
    Abnormal tunica albuginea trauma
  Congenital
    Isolated leakage from corpora spongiosum
Arterial
  Aortoiliac atherosclerosis
  Steal due to external iliac disease
  Occlusive disease of pudendal arteries
  Occlusive disease of penile arteries: atherosclerotic,
    idiopathic proliferative, atheroembolization

disk disease. The information gathered in this testing prior to the office visit is important to help determine a more efficient course of treatment and examination. For example, men with neurologic deficits, particularly those due to diabetes or spinal cord injury, are exquisitely sensitive to injection of intracavernosal vasoactive materials, which is an important aspect of assessment and treatment of vasculogenic impotence. Generally, if neurologic testing is foregone, initial doses of intracavernous agents should be very conservative. A neurologic deficit, with rare exceptions, makes the patient a less favorable candidate for a direct vascular surgical intervention.

On physical examination, the findings of aortoiliac disease are decreased femoral pulses and bruits. With small vessel or internal iliac disease, these findings cannot be discerned during physical examination. Sensory testing of the extremities, perineum, or glans occasionally reveal neuropathy. However, most of these abnormalities, often subtle, are disclosed only by neurovascular testing, using pudendal-evoked potentials and measurement of bulbocavernosal reflex time.

At the time of initial presentation, the prostate should be examined for nodules, and prostatic specific antigens (PSA) should be obtained as a screening measure. Examination is completed by (1) methodical palpation of the corpora cavernosa for Peyronie's plaques and (2) palpations of the scrotum for estimation of testicular size. In most men presenting with impotence, the physical examination is unrevealing.

After the initial examination, the erectile mechanism is tested in the office setting by intracavernous injection of 10–40 μg of prostaglandin E_1 (PGE). If an erection sufficient for intercourse results, arterial in-

flow is considered adequate and veno-occlusive mechanisms are considered functional in these circumstances. A rigid erection can occur in the presence of neurologic deficit and can be enhanced after intracavernous injections. Provided that aneurysmal disease is ruled out by careful palpation or, in men with cardiovascular risks, by sonography, cavernosal self-injection therapy can be selected at this point for treatment in many men.

Subsequent laboratory examinations need not be elaborate. At the time of office examination, prolactin, testosterone, and glucose levels are routinely drawn. A prevalent abnormality is very high glucose in the range of 300–400 mg/kL, seen in so-called "borderline diabetic" patients. Impotence in these men signal poor control of the diabetic state and must be reversed by meticulous treatment. Endocrinopathies with low testosterone levels are uncommon, affecting less than 3–4% of patients in the authors' experience. For example, 1 prolactinoma was found in screening over 1000 men; however, 9 aortic aneurysms were uncovered in men with the chief complaint of impotence with no other peripheral manifestations of vascular disease.

C. Imaging Studies: At the time of office examination or in the vascular laboratory, duplex ultrasonography can be used to scan the penile vessels and corpora at time intervals after the intracavernous injection of a vasoactive agent. Control values for normal erectile function in middle-aged men after PGE injection and visual sexual stimulation were reported to be a 70% increase in deep cavernosal artery diameter, a systolic peak blood flow velocity greater than 30 cm per sec, and more than 10 mL per minute of blood volume. Although color flow Doppler sonography measures cavernous artery blood flow velocity suggesting inadequate arterial inflow, its role in the assessment of penile venous leakage is less clear. Furthermore, any cause of inflow restriction more proximally is not demonstrated. Since our approach is to perform both dynamic infusion, cavernosometry, and cavernosography (DICC) and highly selective arteriography only in patients who are possible candidates for a small vessel reconstruction, ultrasonographic studies are not used routinely. The response to intracavernous injection, that is, an erection adequate for intercourse, will give the needed information as well as provide a means of treatment.

Ultrasonography is most useful in defining corporeal abnormalities such as extension of Peyronie's disease into the corpora and fibrosis due to drug injection It is also used for follow-up after microvascular reconstructions.

Cavernosal artery occlusion pressure (CAOP) is obtained by Doppler insonation of the penile base at the point of full erection. At some point during flow increase, the cavernosal artery signals disappear. While the intracavernous pressure is gradually reduced by stopping or slowing flow, Doppler signals in the cavernous arteries reappear and this pressure is recorded. CAOP is taken as normal at 90 mm or greater or with a gradient of less than 30 mm of mercury compared with simultaneously obtained brachial pressures. CAOP is a useful measure of the pressure available for erection from the cavernosal arteries. However, selective arteriography is recommended prior to any veno-ablative procedures, since 23% of men undergoing DICC exhibited proximal unsuspected arterial lesions when they were suspected of having primary venous abnormalities based on noninvasive screening.

A sharp, funnel effect is seen in the selection of men for the invasive tests as illustrated in Figure 26–1. For example, after screening 431 men with normal inflow noninvasively (mean age 54.8 years) and consequent exclusion of those with hypertension and hormonal, arteriogenic, or neurogenic abnormalities, 44 impotent men with a mean age of 48.8 years ultimately became candidates for and received DICC. Among these, 20 exhibited leakage amenable to operative intervention. It is believed that noninvasive screening sequences and even the invasive studies of DICC with CAOP are too imprecise to facilitate selection of patients for venous interruption, deep dorsal vein arterialization, or arterial bypass. Selective pudendal arteriography is needed before any of these procedures is considered.

D. Invasive Studies: In men failing to achieve erection with increasing intracavernous injections of PGE and in whom the suspicion of vasculogenic impotence based either on venous leakage or small vessel occlusion exists, the appropriate next steps in the workup are invasive. These procedures include DICC with measurement of CAOP, and highly selective pudendal arteriography.

DICC involves the injection of a standard and rather large dose of intracavernous vasoactive agents to ob-

tain maximal cavernosal smooth muscle relaxation. Presently, we use 60 mg papaverine hydrochloride and 2 mg phentolamine. Two fine needles are inserted into the corpora, one for injection of warm heparinized saline impelled by a calibrated roller pump and one for pressure monitoring. The most critical measure in DICC is the flow to maintain erection. This is taken normally to be 40 mL per minute or less to maintain a full erection with an intracavernous pressure of 80–90 mm of mercury.

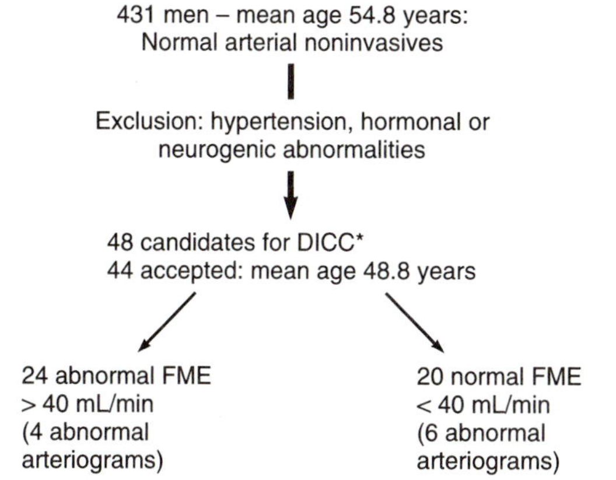

Treatment

A. Medical: Many men respond to the medical therapy that is first recommended. Medical therapy includes risk factor intervention, particularly smoking cessation, which provokes intense spasm of penile vessels and the cavernosal smooth muscle. This stimulus can be so intense that smoking 1 or 2 cigarettes immediately before treatment can obliterate a normal erectile response to intracavernous injection. Diabetes control and a blood pressure medication change to angiotensin-converting enzyme inhibitors are advisable, provided that no contraindications to the latter exist. Drugs found to be useful are isoxsuprine hydrochloride, as well as Yohimbine hydrochloride, which is thought to be useful in treating the psychogenic component of impotence.

Intracorporeal injections using PGE, 10–30 µg, prior to intercourse are effective. It has been observed that men have functioned up to 5–6 years with intracorporeal self-injections in a satisfying manner and without side effects using PGE. Vacuum constrictor devices are also available, although these are usually chosen less frequently by men with problems of impotence.

B. Surgical: Microvascular surgical interventions for impotence are evolving procedures. Several types of microvascular operations are available. One operation consists of microvascular bypass into the dorsal artery and another uses arterialization of the deep dorsal vein. Still another variant is epigastric artery bypass into a fistula between dorsal arteries and veins. The best source for inflow has been the inferior epigastric artery. This permits direct arterial reconstruction of the dorsal artery in appropriately chosen patients based on results of highly selective angiography. The ideal patient is a young man with a history of perineal trauma, pelvic fracture, or localized proximal disease. In one clinical setting, these procedures have been about 70% successful for up to 4 years. The oldest patient selected was 63 years of age; however, this patient's bypass, although patent, did not reverse the impotence, again demonstrating the importance of aging as a contributor to impotence. More work is needed to develop investigative methods that achieve better postoperative results.

Deep dorsal vein arterialization is an option used in younger men when the dorsal arteries are not suitable for bypass. The inferior epigastric artery is sutured into

---

431 men – mean age 54.8 years:
Normal arterial noninvasives

↓

Exclusion: hypertension, hormonal or
neurogenic abnormalities

↓

48 candidates for DICC*
44 accepted: mean age 48.8 years

↙   ↘

24 abnormal FME   20 normal FME
> 40 mL/min   < 40 mL/min
(4 abnormal   (6 abnormal
arteriograms)   arteriograms)

Figure 26–1. Selection of men to receive DICC. Asterisk indicates those who failed to erect in office setting with increasing dosages of intracavernous agents. DICC, dynamic infusion, cavernosometry, and cavernosography; FME, Flow to maintain erection.

an isolated segment of the deep dorsal vein. These procedures offer about a 70% prospect of success for up to 3 to 4 years. The physiology of this operation was initially thought to be reverse arterial flow via the emissary veins into the corpus cavernosum. However, it has been shown that the flow is largely into circumflex veins and into the corpus spongiosum. The physiologic reason why this operation works is not clear. A serious and specific complication of this procedure is glans hyperfusion, due to severe distal venous hypertension. Necrosis of the glans penis and distal urethra can occur if neglected. This complication has been noted by the author twice in a series of 28 patients. Urgent early distal venous ligation can avert the severe consequences of glans hypertension reported in the European literature.

Prognosis

Sexual dysfunction associated with aortoiliac disease and surgery is common. In a recently described series, 55% of men with aneurysms were preoperatively impotent, whereas 95% were postoperatively impotent. For occlusive disease, 31% were preoperatively impotent and 60% became postoperatively impotent. In contrast, a series of men operated on by the author using techniques previously described has been followed up for at least 3 years. The incidence of impotence as a result of emergency surgery or interventions for internal iliac artery aneurysms approximated 3%. Among 125 men, 53 men (average age 64.6 years) were impotent preoperatively and postoperatively, whereas 30 men (average age 57 years [39–71]) were potent preoperatively and remained so postoperatively. Thirty-nine men (average age 58 years [38–69]) were impotent preoperatively and regained function postoperatively.

Overall, technical modifications of conventional aortoiliac surgery make it possible to restore or maintain function in 54% of men. Note that the average age of men postoperatively potent in the authors' series is 57.5 years, compared with about 65 years for those postoperatively impotent. Figure 26–2 illustrates reconstruction of an abdominal aortic aneurysm in a 52-year-old man pre- and postoperatively potent, illustrating the use of bypass limbs to ensure prograde or retrograde pelvic flow. Men exhibit decreasing potency with aging, which does not appear to be related to arterial occlusions per se. Age-related decreases in nocturnal penile tumescence in frequency, duration, and degree have been reported. These correlate with desire, arousal, and coital frequency. Thus, patient age is a critical factor in determining sexual function both pre- and postoperatively. The decrement of sexual function associated with aging is not as previously believed simply related to arterial inflow compromise. More research is needed to separate arteriolar and cavernosal dysfunction from proximal occlusion.

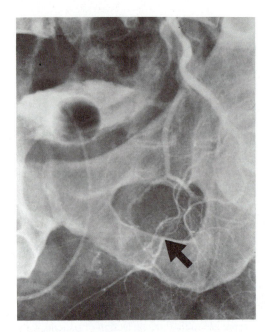

Figure 26–2. Fifty-two-year-old man with abdominal aortic aneurysm, preoperatively potent. Note reconstructive method to correct left external iliac stenosis by retrograde flow and extra graft limb to maintain dominant left internal iliac by prograde flow.

A segmental occlusion of the distal pudendal artery is shown in Figure 26–3. Most interesting are men in their late 20s to early 40s, who present with impotence due to diffuse arterial disease involving mainly the penile vessels and the distal pudendal vessels. The cause of this vascular disorder is not obvious; a few arterial sections obtained at the time of microvascular reconstruction reveal a thrombotic or proliferative process affecting the penile arteries themselves. On the other hand, venous leakage associated with cavernosal trauma, is obvious on cavernosography; this usually responds well to surgical intervention. However, the cause and pathogenesis of acquired venous leakage, for example, with aging is rather poorly understood. In a sense, in any form of erectile failure, venous outflow exceeds the capacity of arterial inflow. Therefore, caution is recommended before venous ablative procedures are done. Some treatment options require arterialization of the deep dorsal vein; this opportunity will be lost if an ill-considered resection of this venous structure is performed on inadequate diagnostic grounds.

Estimates of abnormal penile perfusion obtained in one clinical setting, based on noninvasive standards, are 85% specific and 70% sensitive when compared with pudendal arteriography as a gold standard. However, based on current screening data through March 1993, 635 of 1094 men had apparently normal arterial

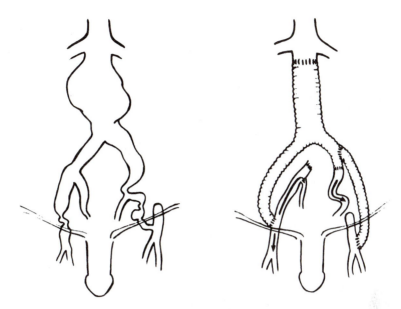

Figure 26–3. Selective pudendal arteriogram. Stenosis of internal pudendal artery at Alcock's canal in a 45-year-old man. Reconstructed using epigastric to dorsal artery microvascular bypass with good postoperative erectile function.

perfusion, whereas 459 exhibited abnormal arterial perfusion. The group with normal perfusion included many diabetics, particularly those receiving antihypertensive medications. Again, no relation appeared to exist between abnormal perfusion and age, with the age in either group being 55 years. About 17% of men with abnormal arterial perfusion had large vessel disease. As a result of careful screening and exclusion criteria, only 5–7% of impotent men ultimately have been considered to be good candidates for direct vascular intervention, either arterial or venous or both. This is an important group, however, since many of these men prefer revascularization over prosthetic implantation. The long-term results of penile vascular procedures need careful scrutiny, as was done in the initial evaluation of limb bypasses.

The success rates for venous ligation without bypass for leakage have been reported to vary from 28% to 73%. This wide range of results probably relates to cases in which arterial insufficiency was undetected when other contraindicating factors existed. The authors believe that the best procedure is excision of the dorsal vein when this appears to be the prominent leak point. Diffuse leakage (crural or spongiosal) does not respond well. Routine dynamic cavernosography and cavernosometry are recommended postoperatively after 3 months in all cases after venous ligation. This step rules out a sham effect, since abnormally elevated flow rates to maintain erection are most often found to be reduced to normal by the procedure. When venous collateral veins remain or recur, early results can be improved by coil embolization by the radiologist at the

time of DICC. Although many men achieve erection spontaneously early after these procedures, many subsequently respond only with intracorporeal injection of vasoactive agents. This need is gratefully accepted, since these men were completely unresponsive to intracavernous treatments preoperatively.

Summary

Current diagnosis and treatment of vasculogenic impotence are rapidly evolving. A well-disciplined multidisciplinary approach usually uses vascular surgical interventions rarely and medical treatment frequently. In all men with aortoiliac disease, careful attention to preservation of autonomic nervous system and restoration of flow to the internal iliac arteries are rewarding. Also, procedures directed at the internal iliac arteries themselves are useful. Finally, the option exists for the use of new improved prostheses, which are soft and allow normal erection around the device with minimal cavernosal disruption. The conventional prostheses in patients with severe neurologic disorder or other postoperative conditions can be gratifying for many men when the procedures are carried out by surgeons skilled in implantation of these devices. The treatment of men with vasculogenic impotence above all requires sensitivity to the patient's needs and aspirations as well as meticulous attention to detail. The outcomes are often satisfying, since increasingly effective modes of therapy are applied more precisely for the variety of conditions underlying this distressing complaint.

REFERENCES

DePalma RG: Vasculogenic impotence. In: *Vascular Surgery: A Comprehensive Review.* Moore WS (editor). WB Saunders, 1993:171.

DePalma RG et al: A screening sequence for vasculogenic impotence. J Vasc Surg 1987;5:228.

DePalma RG et al: Experience in the diagnosis and treatment of impotence caused by cavernosal leak syndrome. J Vasc Surg 1989;10:117.

DePalma RG et al: Noninvasive assessment of impotence. Surg Clin North Am 1990;70:119.

DePalma RG et al: Predictive value of a screening sequence for venogenic impotence. Int J Impot Res 1992;4:143.

Fredberg U, Mouritzen C: Sexual dysfunction as a symptom of arteriosclerosis and as a complication to reconstruction in the aortoiliac segment. J Cardiovasc Surg 1988;29:149.

Glina S et al: Impact of cigarette smoking on papaverine induced erection. J Urol 1988;140:523.

Krane RG, Goldstein I, DeTejada IS: Impotence. N Engl J Med 1989;321:1948.

Lee B et al: Standardization of penile blood flow parameters in normal men using intracavernous prostaglandin E_1 and visual sexual stimulation. J Urol 1993;149:49.

Leriche R: Des obliterations arterielle hautes (obliteration de la terminasion de l'aorte) comme cause de insuffances circularitoires des membres inférieurs. Bull Mem Soc Chif 1923;49:1404.

Lue TF et al: Vasculogenic impotence evaluation by high resolution ultrasonography and pulse Doppler spectrum analysis. Radiology 1985;155:777.

Quesada ET, Light JK: The AMS 700 inflatable penile prosthesis: Long-term experience with controlled expansion cylinders J Urol 1993;149:46.

Rajfer J al: Nitric oxide as a mediator of relaxation of the corpus cavernosum in response to nonadrenergic, noncholinergic neurotransmission. N Engl J Med 1992;326:90.

Saenz deTejada I et al: Impaired neurogenic and endothelium-mediated relaxation of penile smooth muscle from diabetic men with impotence. N Engl J Med 1989;320:1025.

Schiave RC et al: Healthy aging and male sexual function. Am J Psychiatr 1990;147:766.

Sohn MH et al: Objective follow-up after penile revascularization. Int J Impot Res 1992;4:73.

Stackl W, Hasun R, Marberger M: Intracavernous injection of prostaglandin E_1 in impotent men. J Urol 1988;140:66.

Subrini L: Restoration of erectile function using new soft penile implants. Int J Impot Res 1992;4:129A.

Yu GW et al: Preoperative and postoperative dynamic cavernosography and cavernosometry: Objective assessment of venous ligation for impotence. J Urol 1992;147:618.

Vascular Anomalies & Acquired Arteriovenous Fistulas

27

Hugh H. Trout III, MD, FACS, & Richard L. Feinberg, MD

VASCULAR ANOMALIES

Classification System

Essential to management of vascular anomalies is a rational classification system to accurately assess pathogenesis and prognosis and to plan treatments. A unified classification system has been slow to emerge for vascular anomalies. The plethora of different names describing similar lesions and, even more confusing, the same names used by different specialties (eg, pathology, radiology, general surgery, pediatrics, pediatric surgery, vascular surgery, otolaryngology, dermatology, and plastic surgery) to describe lesions has made a difficult field almost impossible to understand.

Previous classification systems have been descriptive (eg, port-wine stain, cherry angioma), anatomicopathologic (eg, capillary hemangioma, cavernous hemangioma), and embryologic (eg, angiomas subdivided into various groups and explained as arrests at various stages of embryonic developments). None of these classification systems has proved to be particularly useful because of a lack of agreement among specialties as to which lesions properly belong in which categories. Moreover, lesions within one group often tended to have different biologic behaviors, thus negating one of the purposes for having a classification system, that is, to plan effective treatment based on a knowledge of pathogenesis.

Out of this morass has emerged a classification system based on biologic behavior that seems to be gaining acceptance among professionals in the disparate specialties who see patients with vascular anomalies. This commonality of language has allowed a better understanding of the effectiveness of different forms of treatment and has also begun to stimulate more investigations into the molecular mechanisms of vascular morphogenesis. These investigations into angioneogenesis, although clearly important to those with vascular anomalies, have other even broader applications, since an appreciation of the methods by which blood vessels grow (angiogenesis) lead directly to an improved understanding of how all tumors grow.

Based on cell kinetics, vascular anomalies can be divided into 2 broad groups: hemangiomas (those demonstrating endothelial hyperplasia) and vascular malformations (those with normal endothelial turnover). **Hemangiomas** are proliferative lesions that enlarge by rapid cellular proliferation, stabilize, and then regress. **Vascular malformations** grow commensurate with the child and do not regress. Vascular malformations can be further subdivided into capillary, venous, lymphatic, and arterial abnormalities (Table 27–1).

A note of caution about treatment of patients with vascular anomalies is needed. Many such patients appear to need urgent treatment; others seem to be easily treated; still others obviously require a master interventional radiologist or surgeon. All 3 situations may be an incentive to intervention. For the last couple of decades, physicians in the USA generally have been much less inclined to intervene than our European counterparts, as inferred from publications about vascular anomalies. The reasons for this are unclear and speculative. However, 2 obvious explanations for different treatment philosophies are apparent.

First, physicians in the USA have not had a simple and common classification system for vascular anomalies; therefore, we cannot be confident that we are talking about the same entities. The classification system proposed by Mulliken and presented here is becoming widely accepted, and this problem should now be diminished. A second explanation is that few practitioners see enough of patients with vascular anomalies to be able to judge good results; this is compounded by an almost universal tendency to publish short-term results without sufficient long-term followup. The admonitions are to be sure of the pathogenesis of the lesion for which treatment is contemplated and to know the long-term results of the treatment modalities being considered. Patients with vascular anomalies are especially prone to respond well (as judged by the intervening physician) in the early posttreatment period, but the long-term result tends to be less than satisfactory and often worse than would be expected if no treatment had been given.

Table 27–1. Classification of congenital vascular anomalies.

Hemangiomas
Malformations
  Low flow
    Capillary (dermal)
    Lymphatic
    Venous
      Simple anomalies
        Absence
        Hypoplasia
        Duplications
        Valvular
        Enlargements
      Spongy growths
  Fast flow
    Arterial
      Simple anomalies
        Duplication
        Hypoplasias
        Stenoses
        Enlargements
    Arteriovenous fistula
      Single AV communication
    Arteriovenous
  Complex-combined (syndromes)

HEMANGIOMA

Essentials of Diagnosis

- Most common tumor of infancy.
- Proliferative, firm, rubbery, and dense upon palpation.
- Almost always involuted by age 12 years; possible residual scarring.
- Possible organomegaly in lower dermis lesions.

General Considerations

The term **hemangioma** should be restricted to the proliferative lesion of infancy. Hemangiomas are congenital lesions and are the most common tumor of infancy, occurring in 12% of whites and in 22% of preterm infants with a birth weight of less than 1000 g. The female-to-male ratio 3:1. In a neonate, these lesions are frequently not visible or may appear as a small lesion. They then commonly grow at a faster rate than does the infant. This rapid proliferative phase generally lasts 8–18 months. The hemangioma then slowly regresses (involution stage) for the next 5–8 years. Complete regression of hemangiomas by age 7 years occurs in over 70% of children, with continued improvement in the remainder until age 12. The rate of regression apparently is not related to the gender or age of the infant or to the duration of the proliferative phase, nor to the site, size, and appearance of the hemangioma.

A small or absent lesion at birth, a rapid proliferative phase for the next 8–18 months, and an inevitable, although slow, involution phase over the next 11 years are the hallmarks of a hemangioma. During the involutional phase, the tumor becomes softer and the color changes to a dark purple and then to a mottled gray, with the final result being pale, somewhat wrinkled skin with a few residual telangiectasias.

Most hemangiomas are small and singular and involve only the skin. They become involuted uneventfully leaving normal or slightly blemished skin. Less frequently, a hemangioma may proliferate to establish a large cell mass; these masses cause considerable clinical consternation, either because the lesion is cosmetically disfiguring or because it threatens one or more major organ systems.

Larger lesions have larger feeding and draining vessels surrounding them. This has given rise to the belief by some that the deeper lesions behave more aggressively. These larger vessels are not part of the hemangioma but are merely part of the support system that enables growth of the hemangioma. Biopsy of hemangiomas—superficial or deep—reveals a relatively uniform morphology throughout, thus confirming the impression of those that manage many patients with hemangiomas that biologic behavior of superficial lesions is similar to that of deep lesions.

A. Signs and Symptoms: Hemangiomas are usually not seen at birth, although some may manifest as a small macular red spot. Most appear between the 1st and 4th week of life as a red patch, a blanched spot, or a localized telangiectasia. About 80% of hemangiomas are single lesions. The head and neck region is the most frequent site of hemangiomas (60%), although there may be some selection bias because of cosmetic concerns of the parents. Other sites are the trunk (25%) and extremities (15%). If the lesion is in the superficial dermis, the skin is raised and usually has a bright scarlet color that gradually deepens by the end of the first year. Most hemangiomas remain well circumscribed, although they may be 5 cm or more in diameter. If the lesion is restricted to the lower dermis and subcutaneous tissue with little involvement of the superficial layer, it may be slightly raised with a bluish hue or the skin may appear normal. A hemangioma feels firm, rubbery, and rather dense; moreover, compression will not empty all the blood within it.

Diagnosis of a hemangioma can almost always be made on the basis of clinical signs and symptoms, particularly if the clinical situation (no platelet trapping, no massive organ involvement) allows several months for observation.

B. Imaging Studies: In those instances in which the diagnosis is in doubt and family concerns are high or treatment is necessary, computed tomography (CT) with contrast or magnetic resonance imaging (MRI) with or without gadopentetate dimeglumine is almost always successful in accurately distinguishing hemangiomas from venous, arteriovenous, and lymphatic malformations.

Arteriography is rarely indicated for evaluation, although it sometimes is necessary for treatment (see section on Treatment).

Differential Diagnosis

The lesion that most mimics a hemangioma is a vascular malformation. The differences between the 2 lesions are summarized in Table 27–2. Because of the differences in time of appearance and rate of growth, clinical examination, particularly if done on multiple occasions, usually allows differentiation between hemangioma and vascular malformation without the need for biopsy or arteriography. Because urgent treatment is rarely indicated, time to observe the behavior of the lesion is usually available.

Diagnostic uncertainty is most likely to occur between a deep hemangioma and a localized lymphatic malformation. The latter lesion is usually soft or cystic and can usually be transilluminated unless hemorrhage has occurred in which case it is dark blue and firm and does not transilluminate.

In rare instances, when an infant presents with a rapid-growing unusually firm subcutaneous mass, a sarcoma must be considered. CT or MRI may be diagnostic, although a biopsy may be necessary.

Treatment

Most hemangiomas enlarge modestly and regress completely, leaving little evidence of their existence. Family requests (often demands) for definitive treatment of larger hemangiomas or those that cause an obvious cosmetic deformity are frequent and understandable. Nonetheless, great efforts should be made to convince parents not to insist on treatment of infants and children with hemangioma except for specific and noncosmetic reasons. Chemotherapy, cryotherapy, radiation therapy, ligation of feeder vessels, and laser therapy in almost all instances have no apparent benefit and usually do harm.

The organ or life-threatening hemangiomas, as well as some specific lesions, may require intervention. A discussion of effective therapeutic options follows.

A. Corticosteroids: Although the mechanism by which corticosteroids accelerate the involution of hemangiomas is not known, some cortisone analogues have been observed to inhibit the growth of new vessels under certain circumstances. In addition, many hemangiomas have increased numbers of estrogen receptors, and cortisone has been observed to inhibit estrogen binding to hemangioma tissue. Corticosteroid therapy is effective (30–60% of the time) primarily during the proliferative phase but has little efficacy after the quiescent or involution phases have been reached. In most instances, corticosteroid therapy should be considered the treatment of choice for the proliferative phase for those with hemangiomas that require treatment.

Keep in mind that although the complications of short-term corticosteroid therapy are few and short-lived in most infants and children, tiny infants on prednisone are predisposed to otitis media, pneumonia, and sepsis.

B. Interferon alfa-2a: Interferon alfa-2a was developed as an antiviral agent. When tested in patients with acquired immunodeficiency deficiency syndrome (AIDS), Kaposi's sarcoma, the vascular tumor associated with the AIDS virus, regressed. Subsequent investigations revealed that interferon inhibits the movement of capillary endothelium in vitro. Moreover, interferon alfa-2a inhibits angiogenesis in mice. As a consequence of these observations, interferon alfa-2a has been used in a number of patients with life- or vision-threatening hemangiomas that have not responded to corticosteroids. To date, a high success rate of initiating regression has been observed, although the side effects of treatment have been substantial (fever, neutropenia, and skin necrosis). Because of these side effects, corticosteroids are generally tried before interferon alfa-2a.

C. Embolization: Embolization can occasionally be useful when steroids and interferon alfa-2a have failed and the infant has congestive heart failure.

D. Excision: Occasionally, removal of a hemangioma is necessary to prevent encroachment on a vital organ. If too much tissue is removed, however, a defect frequently results as the lesion becomes involuted.

E. Ineffective Treatments: Various treatments have been found to be generally ineffective and have few, if any, indications. Chemotherapy such as cyclophosphamide has been tried with some success prior to the availability of interferon alfa-2a. Cryotherapy

Table 27–2. Comparison of hemangiomas and vascular malformations.

Clinical	Hemangiomas	Malformations
At birth	Usually not visible	Present, but usually not visible
Growth	Rapid, faster than infant	Commensurate
Stimuli for growth	Not known	Trauma, sepsis, & hormonal modulation
Gender ratio	Female:male 4:1	Female:male 1:1
Cellular	Plump endothelium	Flat endothelium
	Increased turnover	Slow turnover
	Increased mast cells	Normal mast cell count
	Multilaminated basement membrane	Thin unilanellar basement membrane
Hematologic	Platelet trapping	Venous stasis
	(Kasabach-Merritt syndrome)	Localized consumptive coagulopathy
Angiography	Well-circumscribed staining with	Low flow: ectatic channels
	equatorial vessels	High flow: large arteries with A-V shunting
Skeletal	Hypertrophy rare	Distortion, hypoplasia, or hypertrophy

(Adapted from Mulliken JB: Cutaneous vascular anomalies. Semin Vasc Surg 1993;6:204.)

causes tissue damage and scarring but does not appear to retard growth of hemangiomas. Radiation therapy is accompanied by long-term consequences (radiation burns, bone atrophy, and later malignancy), although proliferating hemangiomas, with their rapid endothelial turnover, are exquisitely sensitive to radiation. Radiation therapy should be avoided except for massive hepatic life-threatening hemangiomas that have been unresponsive to corticosteroids and interferon alfa-2a. Ligation of feeder vessels is usually ineffective at controlling growth and results in loss of angioaccess for subsequent study or embolization; moreover, the goal of reducing flow to the hemangioma can almost always be achieved with embolization techniques.

Laser therapy of superficial hemangiomas, in contradistinction to capillary dermal malformations (portwine stains), does not hasten involution but appears to increase subsequent scarring. There is no evidence that laser therapy, at least as delivered by current methods, results in a better cosmetic result. Much evidence suggests that the results after involution are worse.

As previously stated, most hemangiomas should not be treated and will become involuted with little to modest residual scar. Certain specific lesions, however, should be treated: (1) rapidly growing facial lesions that are causing marked facial distortion, (2) lesions that have recurrent bleeding, ulceration, or infection, (3) lesions that are interfering with normal physiologic function (vision, breathing, eating, hearing), (4) large hemangiomas causing congestive heart failure or bleeding secondary to thrombocytopenia (Kasabach-Merritt syndrome).

Special Presentation

A. Hemangioma of the Upper Eyelid: Hemangiomas of the upper eyelid frequently disturb vision (compared with lesions of the cheek or lower lid, which rarely do, even when large). If the lesion on the upper lid is small and seems limited, excision may be curative. Normally, these lesions have extended into the periorbital tissues, and excision is not possible. Corticosteroid therapy—usually by 1 or 2 intralesional injections—is effective 60–80% of the time. Because corticosteroid injection into lesions that extend into the retrobulbar tissues can cause complications and permanent visual disturbances, systemic corticosteroids are probably the best approach when the lesion is at all extensive.

B. Subglottic Hemangiomas: Subglottic hemangiomas that cause modest respiratory compromise should be treated with systemic corticosteroids. Infants with tight lesions should have a tracheostomy and CO_2 laser excision, although those with circumferential hemangiomas should not be treated with the laser because of the high risk of permanent subglottic stenosis from circumferential scarring.

C. Congestive Heart Failure: Infants who develop congestive heart failure secondary to a massive hemangioma or a hemangioma that has a large amount of arteriovenous shunting possess what has been termed an "alarming hemangioma." Since mortality rate for infants untreated for this lesion is about 80%, aggressive life-saving efforts are warranted. These treatments are, in order, digoxin, diuretics, corticosteroid therapy, interferon alfa-2a, embolization (particularly of the hepatic artery in those with a massive hepatic hemangioma), and, as a final effort to control growth, consideration of a short course of radiation or attempts at resection. The reported mortality rate of infants with congestive heart failure associated with large hemangiomas treated aggressively has been about 50%, although the current rate is probably substantially lower with the recent availability of interferon alfa-2a.

D. Coagulopathy: Hemangiomas can cause thrombocytopenia secondary to platelet trapping (Kasabach-Merritt syndrome). Although thrombocytopenia itself is not generally an indication for treatment, when bleeding occurs careful consideration needs to be given regarding whether to institute corticosteroid therapy. If corticosteroids are not successful, interferon alfa-2a has been reported to be efficacious. Untreated infants with recurrent bleeding secondary to platelet trapping have a mortality rate of about 40%. Current aggressive therapy with corticosteroids or interferon alfa-2a can lower this to under 20%.

Prognosis

Occasionally, hemangiomas ulcerate or bleed. Ulceration usually occurs at the time of most rapid proliferation and can be effectively managed by topical measures during the several weeks necessary for re-epithelialization. Ulceration itself is not an indication for excision. Moreover, recurrent ulceration is rare. Bleeding can be managed by direct pressure on the bleeding site, although occasionally a suture may be required for control. Bleeding can also reflect an underlying coagulopathy that mandates further evaluation and treatment.

Small hemangiomas occasionally threaten vision or the airway, and larger ones may threaten vital organs or cause a thrombocytopenic coagulopathy (Kasabach-Merritt syndrome). These are called "alarming hemangiomas" and mandate treatment. Untreated, patients with giant hemangioma have a mortality rate of about 50%; those with Kasabach-Merritt syndrome have a mortality rate of about 35%.

MALFORMATIONS

Vascular malformations are congenital lesions. Some are clinically apparent at birth, but most appear later, usually by the 4th decade and some even later. Nonetheless, even with a late appearance, they are not considered acquired lesions but are thought to have developed from a dormant analogue, present since birth.

Many different hypotheses have been advanced as to the cause of vascular malformations. Chemical, physical, biochemical, hormonal, and premature arrest of vascular development in utero have been postulated. Unfortunately, persuasive confirming evidence supporting any hypothesis is lacking. To date, the cause of vascular malformations is unknown.

The category of vascular malformations is subdivided into capillary, venous, lymphatic, and arterial (see Table 27–1). Usually, 1 type of vascular malformation is markedly predominant, but different combinations of the 4 types also occur frequently. It is not important to identify all components of a malformation, but it is clinically very important to distinguish a malformation (which will not regress) from a hemangioma (which will regress as outlined above). Moreover, it is clinically important to distinguish a low-flow malformation from a high-flow malformation, because the former gives rise to clinical difficulties primarily by virtue of the organ structures it involves. In contrast, a high-flow malformation tends to be more debilitating locally, can cause cardiac strain because of substantial arteriovenous shunting, and can be much more difficult to extirpate.

Capillary malformations are best exemplified by the port-wine stain familiar to all because of the obvious cosmetic disfigurement when the malformation involves the face. These malformations may be combined with an arterial, venous, or lymphatic abnormality but, by themselves, present no clinical problem, only a cosmetic problem. Obviously, this alone can have profound consequences.

Lymphatic malformations are low-flow lesions and cause difficulties because of their location and size but are rarely life-threatening. **Venous and arterial malformations,** singly or in combination with other malformations (such as a lymphatic malformation), are more difficult to classify because of their myriad presentations. A clinically useful way to think about venous and arterial malformations is to view them as a spectrum going from a simple venous aneurysm or single dilated vein extending to a highly complex and large lesion, primarily composed of tortuous veins with or without lymphatics (still low-flow). This then moves into simple arterial anomalies (the beginning of the high-flow end of the spectrum) and extending to the complex arterial lesions (arteriovenous malformations) that create major clinical difficulties.

CAPILLARY MALFORMATIONS (Low-flow)

Essentials of Diagnosis
- Discoloration (almost always present at birth).
- Mucous membranes often involved with facial stains.
- Possibly accompanied by other vascular anomalies.

General Considerations
The port-wine stain and other telangiectasias are examples of capillary dermal malformations. When they are associated with deeper and more extensive vascular anomalies, the other associated anomaly determines prognosis and treatment. When these capillary lesions, characterized by ectatic vessels in the upper dermis, are present without other associated lesions, treatment is designed solely to reduce the cosmetic defect, since these capillary anomalies themselves have no clinical consequences.

Clinical Findings
Signs and Symptoms: The stains or other telangiectatic lesions of capillary malformations are readily apparent. When not accompanied by other vascular or neural anomalies, they cause no symptoms. Capillary malformations require no diagnostic evaluation unless other anomalies are suspected.

Differential Diagnosis
The diagnosis of capillary malformation is almost always readily apparent, although a lesion of infancy, nevus flammeus neonatorum (salmon patch, angel's kiss, and others), is often misdiagnosed as a port-wine stain. In contrast to a port-wine stain, a nevus flammeus neonatorum usually involves the nuchal region, blanches when compressed, becomes more apparent when the infant cries, and tends to regress uneventfully within a few years. Occasionally, a hemangioma can also be confused with a port-wine stain. Usually, the hemangioma is darker and raised. Moreover, when the hemangioma either enlarges or becomes involuted, the differentiation from a capillary dermal malformation is established because the latter remains essentially unchanged. Capillary malformations do not regress, expand, or cause symptoms.

Treatment
Treatment for capillary malformation is carried out for cosmetic reasons. In instances of facial lesions, treatment becomes important, although therapy has often made the cosmetic appearance worse rather than better. Cryotherapy, scarification, radiation therapy, and tattooing all have been used extensively with uneven and generally unfavorable results. Excision has been carried out, but the skin grafts—whether full or partial thickness—have frequently resulted in only modest improvement over the lesion itself. Skin expansion with subcutaneous balloons prior to excision offers substantial promise for small-to-moderate-sized lesions that involve areas in which this approach is applicable.

Laser therapy appears to have potential for marked improvement in many, particularly young, persons and those with light stains. Argon and tunable dye lasers both have been useful and have achieved good results. Which laser and what technique produces the best long-term results has not been determined.

Make-up with opaque waterproof cream covers is useful for lesions not deemed appropriate for excision or laser treatment.

Prognosis

Laser treatment during infancy for capillary malformation provides the best opportunity to maximally reduce the cosmetic defect. Whether the current promising results will persist over a prolonged period remains unanswered, but early reports are encouraging.

VENOUS MALFORMATIONS (Low-flow)

Essentials of Diagnosis
- No pulsation.
- No palpable thrill.
- Minimal or no bruits.
- No major feeder vessels by arteriography.

General Considerations

On rare occasions, **venous malformations** can be lethal because of massive size or massive involvement of an organ, most frequently the liver. Venous malformations usually cause problems because of their cosmetic appearance, bulk, overlying skin ulceration, the organ or organs they involve, and their association with other anomalies, especially the Klippel-Trénauney syndrome.

Included in the category of venous malformations are the simple venous anomalies such as absence or hypoplasia of named veins, duplications, valvular anomalies, abnormal venous enlargements (either single or multiple), and spongy growths, previously erroneously referred to as "cavernous hemangiomas." These spongy venous malformations may occur as isolated lesions, or they may occur in conjunction with other anomalies (see section on Complex-Combined Malformations). They most often give rise to debate as to prognosis and appropriate treatment. For this reason, most of the remaining discussion about venous malformations is restricted to these isolated spongy mass lesions, with further mention under the category of syndromes.

Clinical Findings

A. Signs and Symptoms: Primary varicose veins associated with a paucity or absence of venous valves is an example of a venous malformation. Likewise, the left renal vein can pass behind the aorta or it can divide into 2 veins: one going anterior to the aorta and the other passing posteriorly. Numerous other examples abound. Except for those situations in which the venous anomaly gives rise to varicose veins or to swelling of an extremity, most go undetected until discovered serendipitously on an imaging study, during an operation, or at autopsy.

As previously mentioned, the venous anomaly that often elicits attention is the spongy mass type. This mass lesion can be seen as a cosmetic defect with pain from compression of surrounding tissues or with bleeding from erosion of skin overlying the mass. Spongy venous malformations do not pulsate, have a thrill, or have a bruit. They are somewhat soft and compressible, but the mass cannot be made to disappear completely with compression.

B. Imaging Studies: New and more sophisticated imaging technologies are rapidly becoming available. As a consequence, the best study to characterize spongy venous malformations may change as these imaging techniques evolve. The diagnostic tests that probably best help to delineate the size and extent of these lesions are computed tomography (CT) and magnetic resonance imaging (MRI). Vessel enhancement can be used with either. Formal invasive imaging with venography is usually not particularly helpful in characterizing the lesion because it will rarely be well visualized. If excision of a large mass or a mass that intimately involves critical structures is contemplated, it may be advantageous to obtain a venogram or arteriogram, depending on the clinical presentation. For diagnostic purposes, arteriography can demonstrate the absence of large arterial feeder vessels and thus distinguish between venous and arterial malformations, although this difference can usually be made on clinical examination or with noninvasive imaging with CT or MRI.

Differential Diagnosis

The vascular lesion that may be confused with a spongy venous malformation is the arterial malformation (see Table 27–2). Other benign soft tissue masses may also be confused, but a history of a mass that has been present for a long period and physical examination that reveals a soft spongy partially compressible mass with a consistent feel throughout are usually sufficient to differentiate venous malformations from other benign processes. Similarly, malignant lesions have usually recently enlarged and are firmer. If uncertainty persists, CT or MRI is generally diagnostic, and, if necessary, biopsy will be confirmatory.

Treatment

Many venous malformations do not require treatment. If the lesion is in an extremity and produces mild to moderate symptoms, well-fitting support stocking or socks may provide sufficient relief. Low-dose antiplatelet therapy (aspirin) may reduce the incidence of symptomatic phlebitis in those with a prior history of thrombosis within the redundant or dilated veins.

Sclerosing agents such as hypertonic saline, sodium tetradecyl sulfate, and Ethiblock (in Europe) can be used percutaneously. Ethyl alcohol can also be used but is so toxic to tissues that great caution should be exercised before deciding to use this agent. As a general rule, sclerosing agents should be infrequently used, since most patients with venous malformations have few symptoms. The risk of causing permanent damage to normal tissues and the low probability that an entire venous malformation can be obliterated with sclerosing techniques mitigate against their use.

If more extensive treatment for venous malformations is necessary because of bleeding, chronic ulceration, or pain from compression, excision is effective and recurrence is low. If cure rather than palliation for a local problem is the goal, the lesion should be completely excised. For this reason, preoperative MRI is most likely to delineate the full extent of tissue involvement by the venous malformation.

Cryotherapy, radiation therapy, and laser therapy have little, if any, benefit and usually are detrimental.

Prognosis

Spongy venous malformations grow commensurate with the growth of the individual. The malformations are usually present at birth, although some may first appear in the second or third decades of life and sometimes even later. They do not become involuted. The malformations may grow in response to trauma, menarche, pregnancy, or hormonal manipulation such as birth control pills.

Venous malformations that are composed of a preponderance of dilated veins periodically develop thrombi in some of these dilated channels, presumably on the basis of sluggish blood flow. These thromboses can be painful, analogous to the symptoms of patients with superficial phlebitis.

Venous malformations that are completely excised do not recur. Those that are extensive and are not amenable to complete excision may persist and enlarge after incomplete excision. As previously indicated, most venous malformations do not require treatment and remain relatively quiescent.

ARTERIAL MALFORMATIONS (High-flow)

Essentials of Diagnosis

- Pulsation.
- A palpable thrill.
- Bruits present and extensive.
- Large feeder vessels by arteriography.

General Considerations

At the least extensive end of the spectrum of arterial malformations are the abnormalities of position or structure such as duplications, hypoplasias, stenoses, aneurysms (congenital, not atherosclerotic), and arterial ectasias. Next are the arteriovenous malformations that have only one arteriovenous communication. These are currently called **arteriovenous fistulas,** although this is probably an unfortunate designation because the lesion is congenital and rare and is often confused with the more common arteriovenous fistulas that are acquired (see final section of this chapter), usu-

ally after trauma. Such a congenital lesion is indistinguishable, except by history, from an acquired arteriovenous fistula. The clinical relevance of this entity is that a malformation (congenital) that consists of only a single arteriovenous communication is amenable to treatment by nonexcisional techniques that obliterate that communication, just as with an acquired arteriovenous fistula. Finally, in increasing clinical complexity are those lesions with multiple arterial and venous communications, usually referred to as **arteriovenous malformations** (AVMs). These lesions range from those with many small arteriovenous communications with relatively high resistance to those with either few or numerous large arteriovenous communications. These abnormal congenital arteriovenous communications can be divided into localized, truncal, and diffuse AVMs.

The localized lesions most resemble venous malformations in that they are composed of a mass of very small communications between arteries and veins. The resistance within this mass is high, the feeder arteries are small, and shunting of blood is modest. These localized lesions are probably at the transition between the low-flow venous malformation and the high-flow AVM. The clinical importance lies in whether they are low flow or high flow, not whether they are called venous malformations with numerous tiny arteriovenous communications or AVMs with high resistance.

Truncal AVMs have large inflow arteries and dilated outflow veins. The multiple arteriovenous communications tend to involve the head, neck, and upper limb. They are discrete, demonstrable by arteriography, usually involve major arteries, and are high flow.

Diffuse AVMs have large inflow arteries with rapid filling of the surrounding venous tree on angiography. The communications involve the lower limb more than the upper limb. The communications are extensive and are themselves difficult to demonstrate by arteriography, although the overall shunting is high.

Clinical Findings

A. Signs and Symptoms: AVMs pulsate, have a palpable thrill, and have loud and extensive bruits. They may cause symptoms by compression of surrounding structures, by ulcerating, by "stealing" or shunting blood away from distal tissues, or rarely by causing congestive heart failure. AVMs may be relatively circumscribed and accessible to embolization or excision, or they may be diffuse and involve one or more vital structures extensively. If ulceration is present, the cause is either a shunting of blood away from the ulcerated area or an increase in venous pressure near the area of the ulceration, almost identical with that seen in patients with chronic venous insufficiency.

B. Imaging Studies: The diagnosis of an arterial malformation almost always can be made on clinical criteria of a pulsatile mass of long duration in the absence of a history of trauma. The extent of this highly vascular mass is probably best determined by CT or

MRI. If therapy is contemplated or if the possibility of an arteriovenous fistula is present, an arteriogram is necessary.

Differential Diagnosis

The lesion most likely to be mistaken for an AVM is an arteriovenous fistula. If a history of trauma is present, an arteriogram is necessary to look for the distinguishing characteristic of a single arteriovenous communication, which is the hallmark of an acquired arteriovenous fistula. An AVM can possess a single arteriovenous communication, but this is exceedingly rare, as already discussed. Also, AVMs can coexist with other abnormalities, the most common being Parkes Weber syndrome (see following section on Complex-Combined Malformations).

Treatment

For those who are asymptomatic or have minimally symptomatic lesions, no treatment is probably best.

Excision may be necessary for symptomatic lesions that are relatively localized or have overlying non-healing or recurrent ulcerations. If the ulceration is thought to be secondary to venous hypertension, local excision of the tissues beneath the ulceration, skin grafting, and long-term external support may prevent recurrent ulceration.

Embolization in an effort to decrease blood flow may be helpful in situations in which excision is planned 2 or 3 days later. Also, embolization can be useful in those moderately to severely symptomatic patients in whom excision is not possible because of the extent or location of the lesion.

Many different embolic agents have been used for AVMs. Wires or coils are easy to insert but usually are positioned too proximal in the feeder arteries. As a consequence, collateral vessels develop and little, if any, benefit is derived. Polyvinyl alcohol foam (Ivalon particles) are permanent and have been popular in the past. It is difficult to inject the correct size because some of the particles pass through the malformation and go to the lung, whereas others occlude the small feeder vessels and do not fill the nidus of the malformation.

Isobutylcyanoacrylate (super glue) has been used successfully to fill AVMs that are not excisable, and excellent long-term palliation has frequently been attained. Unfortunately, this substance is exceedingly difficult to work with because the catheters used to inject the isobutylcyanoacrylate tend to become glued to the lesion; few invasive radiologists are true masters of this medium. Another disadvantage is that use of isobutylcyanoacrylate is restricted by the Food and Drug Administration (FDA) because chemical analogues have been shown to have carcinogenic potential in animals.

Ethibloc is a vegetable protein mixed with alcohol that stimulates autolysis of tissue. It is biodegradable and cleared by phagocytosis, although occasionally it provokes a considerable inflammatory response soon after injection. It is used in Europe but has not been approved for use in the USA by the FDA.

Ethyl alcohol is a highly toxic sclerosing agent, which is easy to inject but difficult to control. It is painful, can cause thrombosis as it passes into the venous system, and can damage normal tissues if they are exposed to high concentrations. Nerves and the central nervous system are particularly susceptible to injury. Notwithstanding all these caveats, administration of ethyl alcohol by an experienced radiologist can be effective in controlling some of the more extensive and complex malformations.

A word of caution: Short-term results of embolization may appear exceedingly promising, especially when compared with other treatments. Good long-term follow-up studies, however, are sparse. Of these, most imply that embolization is a temporizing therapy at best and that the indications for treatment should be carefully considered before initiating treatment.

Prognosis

AVMs are rarely observed in infancy. They can lie dormant for many years, sometimes becoming obvious as late as the third or fourth decade, but most become apparent in childhood or adolescence. Some remain fairly quiescent, cause few symptoms, and require no treatment. Increased cardiac output is common due to shunting of blood from the arterial tree to the venous system without passing through a capillary bed. This increased cardiac work is generally well tolerated for many years.

Other AVMs cause moderate symptoms because of their size or the compression of surrounding tissues. Still others cause ulceration of overlying skin, either by diversion of arterial blood or by increasing local venous pressure. AVMs can also cause considerable pain owing to shunt-induced distal ischemia or to compression of surrounding structures. Although it is unusual, large malformations can cause marked increases in cardiac output and symptomatic congestive heart failure. Finally, massive AVMs, usually seen in infancy or childhood, can cause death—either from cardiac failure or from organ failure—usually hepatic.

Outcome of management of AVM patients depends almost entirely on the extent and degree of involvement of the AVM with vital structures. Embolization will be deleterious if the major arterial feeders are obstructed, because this promotes dilatation of collateral vessels and does not reduce lesion size or the amount of shunting. If the embolization is effective in obliterating the major portion of the arteriovenous communications (the nidus of the AVM), it sometimes reduces the shunting and may reduce the size of the mass. Even with highly successful embolization with alcohol or glue-like substances, excellent long-term control is unlikely. Embolization should be thought of as a temporizing modality, which may be all that is necessary for controlling mass size or pain, but by itself should not be considered curative except in the rare instance when the AVM consists of a single arteriovenous communication (lesions with a single arteriovenous communication are almost always acquired arteriovenous fistulas).

Excision of AVMs is curative if the entire mass is removed. Excision should never be undertaken lightly because of the possibility of massive blood loss or damage to critical structures, even in the hands of highly skilled and experienced surgeons. Moreover, because these masses are often extensive and involve essential organs or structures, complete excision is frequently not possible. Partial excision may be successful as palliation, but can also result in promoting dilatation of collaterals or in rendering adjacent or distal tissue ischemic. As a consequence, thorough preoperative assessment, careful planning of the operation, meticulous operative technique, and modest expectations should be hallmarks of excisional therapy of AVMs.

COMPLEX-COMBINED MALFORMATIONS

Vascular malformations can be combined with a variety of other congenital abnormalities. The use of eponyms has generally confused rather than clarified, especially in the field of congenital vascular lesions. Nevertheless, until our understanding of many of the syndromes that have been described increases, eponyms are a convenient shorthand for purposes of discussion. Many vascular malformation syndromes have been described (Bannayan, Barker-Kausch, Bean, Beckwith-Wiedemann, Bloom, blue rubber bleb nevus, Boder-Sedgwick, Bonnett-Dechaume-Blanc, Brushfield-Wyatt, Cobb, Cockett, Divry-Van Bogaert, Esau-Bensaude, Fabry, Foix-Alajouanine, Gorham, Haferkamp, Jahnkhe, Kaijser, Lawford, Louis-Bar, Maffucci, Martorell-Servelle, Milles, Paine-Efron, Proteus, Rendu-Osler-Weber, Riley-Smith, Roberts, Rothmund-Thomson, Rubinstein-Taybi, Schirmer, Storino-Engel, Sturge-Weber, Van Lohuizen, von Hippel-Lindau, Klippel-Trénaunay, Parkes Weber). For the most part, the conditions are rare or have little relevance to vascular surgeons. The last 2 are not rare and occasionally are seen by vascular surgeons. The following discussion of vascular malformations combined with other congenital lesions is restricted to the 2 syndromes, Klippel-Trénaunay and Parkes Weber.

Klippel-Trénaunay & Parkes Weber Syndromes

A. Clinical Findings: Klippel-Trénaunay syndrome is characterized by a capillary (dermal) malformation and one or more venous malformations involving an extremity (usually lower) with limb hypertrophy and congenital varicose veins. Parkes Weber syndrome is characterized by a capillary (dermal) malformation and an arterial malformation or malformations involving an extremity with limb hypertrophy and congenital varicose veins. The difference between the 2 syndromes is the type of malformation. Because the malformation is venous, patients with Klippel-Trénaunay syndrome have near-normal blood flow to the affected extremity and generally have an excellent prognosis. In contrast, patients with **Parkes Weber syndrome** have increased blood flow to the involved extremity due to arterial malformations. Pain, ulceration, and increased cardiac output with associated cardiac enlargement are often encountered in patients with the Parkes Weber syndrome.

Lymphatic abnormalities may be associated with both syndromes, as can deep venous abnormalities. Some investigators believe almost all patients with Klippel-Trénaunay syndrome have deep venous abnormalities; others think deep vein abnormalities are common but by no means universal. This issue appears to have modest clinical relevance.

B. Treatment: Treatment of patients with Klippel-Trénaunay syndrome consists primarily of educating patients and their families as to the favorable prognosis and of counseling about external support garments. Occasionally, venous ulcers may develop secondary to venous hypertension at the level of the ankle. Local measures (scleropathy, removal of underlying veins) designed to reduce this venous hypertension may be necessary if the compressive therapies usually used for venous ulcers are not successful.

Treatment of patients with Parkes Weber syndrome can be much more complex than that of patients with Klippel-Trénaunay syndrome. Because the limb-length disparity is usually much more severe in patients with Parkes Weber syndrome than in those with Klippel-Trénaunay syndrome, epiphyseal arrest procedures may be necessary. In patients with extensive arteriovenous involvement, it may be necessary to advise amputation to control pain caused either by distal ischemia or by involvement of nerves by the mass of the AVM. In general, despite heroic and often ingenious attempts to control the arteriovenous component, efforts to do so, either by embolization or by an operation, have been notoriously unsuccessful and have often seemed to hasten the need for amputation.

Belov S: Correction of lower limbs length discrepancy in congenital vascular-bone diseases by vascular surgery performed during childhood. Semin Vasc Surg 1993;6:245.

Bilyk JR, Adamis AP, Mulliken JB: Treatment options for periorbital hemangioma of infancy. Int Ophthalmol Clin 1992;32:95.

Brem H, Folkman J: Analysis of experimental antiangiogenic therapy. J Pediatr Surg 1993;28:445.

Calligaro KD et al: Congenital pelvic arteriovenous malformations: Long-term follow-up in two cases and a review of the literature. J Vasc Surg 1992;16:100.

Enjolras O, Mulliken JB: The current management of vascular birthmarks. Pediatr Dermatol 1993;10:311.

Ezekowitz RA, Mulliken JB, Folkman J: Interferon alfa-2a therapy for life-threatening hemangiomas of infancy. N Engl J Med 1992;326:1456.

Fishman SJ, Mulliken JB: Hemangiomas and vascular malformations of infancy and childhood. Pediatr Clin North Am 1993;40:1177.

Hurvitz CH et al: Cyclophosphamide therapy in life-threatening vascular tumors. J Pediatr 1986;109:360.

Jackson IT, Carreno R, Potparic Z: Hemangiomas, vascular malformations and lymphovenous malformations: Classification and methods of treatment. Plast Reconstr Surg 1993;91:1216.

Meyer JS, Hoffer FA, Barnes PD, Mulliken JB: Biological classification of soft-tissue vascular anomalies: MR correlation. AJR 1991;157:559.

Morad AB, McClain KL, Ogden AK: The role of tranexamic acid in the treatment of giant hemangiomas in newborns. Am J Pediatr Hematol Oncol 1993;15:383.

Mulliken JB: A plea for a biologic approach to hemangiomas of infancy. (Editorial). Arch Dermatol 1991;127:243.

Mulliken JB: Capillary (port wine) and other telangiectatic stains. In: *Vascular Birthmarks: Hemangiomas and Malformations.* Mulliken JB, Young AE (editors). WB Saunders, 1988:170.

Mulliken JB: Cutaneous vascular anomalies. Semin Vasc Surg 1993;6:204.

Mulliken JB: Diagnosis and natural history of hemangiomas. In: Mulliken JB, Young AE (editors). *Vascular Birthmarks: Hemangiomas and Malformations.* WB Saunders, 1988:41.

Mulliken JB: Treatment of hemangiomas. In: *Vascular Birthmarks: Hemangiomas and Malformations.* Mulliken JB, Young AE (editors). WB Saunders, 1988:77.

Patrice SJ, Wiss K, Mulliken JB: Pyogenic granuloma (lobular capillary hemangioma): A clinicopathologic study of 178 cases. Pediatr Dermatol 1991;8:267.

Riding K: Subglottic hemangioma: A practical approach. J Otolaryngol 1992;21:419.

Rutherford RB: Congenital vascular malformations: Diagnostic evaluation. Semin Vasc Surg 1993;6:225.

Strauss RP, Resnick SD: Pulsed dye laser therapy for port-wine stains in children: Psychosocial and ethical issues. J Pediatr 1993;122:505.

Silverman RA: Hemangiomas and vascular malformations. Pediatr Clin North Am 1991;38:811.

Tan OT: Lasers for vascular lesions in pediatric dermatology. Pediatr Dermatol 1992;9:358.

Young AE: Arteriovenous malformations. In: *Vascular Birthmarks: Hemangiomas and Malformations.* Mulliken JB, Young AE (editors). WB Saunders, 1988:228.

Young AE: Venous and arterial malformations. In: *Vascular Birthmarks: Hemangiomas and Malformations.* Mulliken JB, Young AE (editors). WB Saunders, 1988:196.

Young AE, Ackroyd J, Baskerville P: Combined vascular malformations. In: *Vascular Birthmarks: Hemangiomas and Malformations.* Mulliken JB, Young AE (editors). WB Saunders, 1988:246.

ARTERIOVENOUS FISTULAS

Essentials of Diagnosis

- Acquired lesion; may be traumatic or "spontaneous."
- Usually seen in the extremities.
- Audible bruit or palpable thrill overlying involved vessels.
- Warmth of overlying skin.
- Prominent regional superficial veins.
- Venous congestion with edema formation.
- Increased limb size.
- Distal end-organ ischemia.
- Systemic hypervolemia.
- High-output cardiac failure.

General Considerations

A. Cause: First described by William Hunter in 1761, arteriovenous fistulas remain a relatively uncommon clinical entity compared with other forms of vascular pathology more commonly encountered by vascular surgeons. For purposes of discussion in this chapter, arteriovenous fistulas (AVFs), as distinguished from congenital arteriovenous malformations (AVMs), represent a form of acquired abnormal connection between the arterial and venous sides of the circulation and have the effect of short circuiting the normal anatomic pathway of blood flow away from the peripheral vascular bed. Most such acquired AVFs occur in the extremities and are the sequelae of penetrating vascular injury. However, AVFs can and do occur anywhere in the body where an artery and vein lie in close proximity. As a result, the occurrence and behavior of pelvic, thoracic, intra-abdominal, and intracranial AVFs have been amply documented.

In the absence of a history of localized trauma, other causes that may underlie the development of an AVF include erosion of an aneurysm (either atherosclerotic or pseudoaneurysm) into an adjacent vein, invasion by neoplasm or abscess into local vessels, and iatrogenic injury of an adjacent artery and vein, either by operative trauma or, with increasing frequency, by percutaneous catheter-based manipulations. This chapter does not discuss the therapeutic arteriovenous anastomoses constructed for hemodialysis access or as adjuncts to infrainguinal bypass procedures.

B. Pathophysiology: The abnormal short-circuiting of blood flow through an AVF results in several characteristic hemodynamic, anatomic, and systemic alterations associated with these lesions. The primary determinants of the pathophysiologic changes attendant to an AVF are the location of the fistula and the magnitude of flow through the fistula. As an aid to better understanding these changes, think of an AVF in schematic terms as an H-type communication between an adjacent artery and vein (Fig 27–1). In such a configuration, several discrete components of the abnormal circuit can be seen, including (1) the proximal (afferent) artery, (2) the distal (efferent) artery, (3) the proximal (efferent) vein, (4) the distal (afferent) vein, (5) the arteriovenous communicating channel, (6) the collateral arteries and veins, and (7) the peripheral vascular bed.

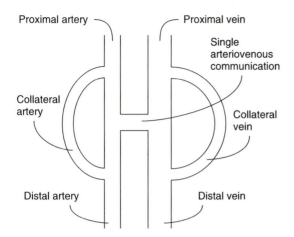

Proximal artery

Proximal vein

Single arteriovenous communication

Collateral artery

Collateral vein

Distal artery

Distal vein

Figure 27–1. Schematic depiction of the vessels contributing to an arteriovenous fistula.

Note that the degree of the physiologic effect produced by an AVF is inversely proportional to the resistance inherent in the fistulous circuit; that is, the lower the resistance through the abnormal fistulous communication, the more pronounced will be the local and systemic physiologic aberrations resulting from it. The resistance of the fistulous circuit, in turn (as predicted by Poiseuille's law), is primarily governed by the diameter of the communicating channel and the length of the channel.

Many, if not most, of the clinically important AVFs consist of an artery and vein immediately juxtaposed one to another, in which the length of the communicating channel is essentially negligible. Therefore, the diameter of the opening between artery and vein emerges as the dominant factor determining the intrinsic resistance of a given AVF. As a consequence, a fistula with a very small diameter opening between artery and vein has a relatively high intrinsic resistance to flow and, as such, will exert relatively weak effects on both regional and systemic hemodynamics. As the diameter of such a fistulous opening increases, approaching the diameter of the parent artery (as is often the natural history of these lesions), the resistance of the circuit rapidly diminishes, and the resulting physiologic derangement increases abruptly, producing significant consequences for local, regional, and systemic flow patterns.

Several characteristic flow patterns have been observed in the vessels participating in the fistulous circuit, and a number of distinct anatomic changes have been described as occurring in these vessels, presumably as a consequence of the altered flow dynamics:

1. Proximal artery–Flow in the proximal artery is always increased in an AVF of significant size. Much of this increased flow occurs during the diastolic phase and often results in loss of the typical diastolic flow reversal that ordinarily characterizes medium-sized peripheral arteries. Accompanying this augmentation

of diastolic flow is a decreased pulsatility in the proximal artery. The direction of flow in the artery proximal to the AVF is always toward the fistula. Concomitant with the dramatic augmentation in flow, the artery proximal to an AVF characteristically undergoes progressive elongation and dilatation, resulting in considerable tortuosity of the vessel. In addition, the wall of the proximal artery often becomes thinned and friable as a result of atrophy of the medial smooth muscle layer, and an increased tendency toward atherosclerotic changes may be seen.

2. Distal artery–Flow within the distal artery may remain antegrade, become reversed (retrograde flow), or be stagnant, depending on the relative resistances to flow offered by the fistulous tract, the collateral arterial pathways, and the distal arterial bed. As the diameter of the fistulous tract increases and the resistance to flow through the fistula decreases, a tendency to develop a "pressure sink" occurs within the artery just distal to the fistulous opening, and the likelihood increases that retrograde flow will occur. With increasing magnitude of flow through the fistula, the pressure within the distal artery diminishes. This can be partially compensated as flow through the collateral arterial channels increases over time. The degree to which such compensation occurs determines the degree of distal ischemia produced by the AVF. Because of the variability of flow patterns that can occur in the distal artery, no predictable anatomic change is seen, although this vessel tends to become atrophic as more and more flow is diverted through the fistulous tract at the expense of the distal arterial bed.

3. Proximal vein–Flow within the proximal vein is always increased in the presence of an AVF, and the direction of flow in the proximal vein is always toward the heart. Despite the massive increases in flow seen within the proximal vein in even the largest AVFs, pressure within the vein generally remains unchanged, owing to the tremendous capacitance of the venous system. As in the proximal artery, the dramatically increased flow within the proximal vein usually results in marked dilatation, tortuosity, and friability of this vessel (**arterialization**).

4. Distal vein– Flow within the distal venous limb may remain in the normal antegrade direction (toward the heart) when the fistula is relatively small. As flow through the fistula increases, the direction of flow within the distal vein reverses itself, as the normally low pressure within the distal vein is overcome by the arterialized flow through the fistula. As the valves within the distal vein are sequentially rendered incompetent by the distending effect of the retrograde transmission of arterialized flow down the distal vein, progressive dilatation of the distal venous bed follows, resulting ultimately in progressive distal venous hypertension, with its potential sequelae of edema and ulceration.

5. Fistulous channel–Most fistulous openings increase in diameter over time. This region is the locus of maximal turbulence as high-pressure arterial flow creates a jet stream directly into the low-pressure venous circuit.

6. Collateral vessels–The presence of an AVF is a very strong stimulus for the development of collateral blood vessels, with both arterial and venous collaterals undergoing tremendous dilatation and proliferation as the fistula matures.

In addition to the local alterations in blood flow patterns that occur as a result of an AVF, fistulas also produce significant regional and systemic effects as a consequence of the altered hemodynamics.

7. Regional effects–Depending on the proportion of total blood flow that is diverted through the fistula, ischemia of the distal arterial bed may develop. This ischemia may become clinically manifest in a variety of ways, depending on the location of the fistula. In AVFs of the visceral circulation, for example, symptoms of ischemia involving the particular end-organ may develop (eg, progressive renal insufficiency in the case of renal AVFs, intestinal angina in the case of mesenteric AVFs). AVFs involving either the carotid or subclavian arteries may occasionally result in symptomatic cerebral ischemia, particularly when more distal obstructive lesions are present as well.

When an extremity AVF begins to siphon enough blood flow through the fistulous circuit at the expense of distal extremity perfusion, the hallmark findings of critical limb ischemia (pallor, rest pain, ischemic ulceration, gangrene) may then develop. In addition, the regional consequences of venous hypertension may take on clinical importance, as in the gastrointestinal hemorrhage seen in some patients with portal hypertension resulting from hepatic arterioportal fistulas, or in the venous engorgement, limb hypertrophy, edema, and stasis dermatitis seen in the lower extremity of a person with a traumatic femoral AVF. In the case of an extremity AVF occurring before epiphyseal closure has been completed (during childhood or adolescence), a significant increase in limb growth can be seen on the involved side.

During the early stages of the development of the AVF, significant stealing of distal blood flow through the fistula may be compensated for by reactive vasodilatation of the peripheral arterial bed. Nevertheless, over time this compensation will be inadequate relative to the amount of flow siphoned away through the fistulous circuit. At this point, distal ischemia becomes manifest. Additionally contributing to the loss of distal arterial perfusion pressure is the obligate energy loss dissipated as a result of increased turbulence at the site of the fistula.

8. Systemic effects–The systemic hemodynamic effects produced by an AVF are different in the acute compared with the chronic setting. Although most AVFs, when brought to the attention of the managing clinician, have had sufficient time to "mature," several clinically important AVFs commonly present as an acute event (eg, the spontaneous rupture of an athero-sclerotic aneurysm of the infrarenal abdominal aorta into the inferior vena cava, producing an aortocaval fistula).

Acute systemic changes. The immediate systemic consequence of the opening of an AVF is always a decrease in total peripheral resistance perceived by the left side of the heart as a result of the diversion of a portion of the cardiac output away from the regulators of the systemic resistance, the arterioles, directly into the low-resistance venous circuit. A concomitant effect is an elevation of the central venous pressure, which results from the increased flow being siphoned directly into the venous system. This lowering of total peripheral resistance results in a drop in systemic arterial blood pressure, the immediate physiologic response to which is an increased cardiac output by means of increases in both the stroke volume and the heart rate. Stroke volume is initially augmented as a result of the functionally increased "preload" (Starling's myocardial stretching) created by the elevated central venous pressure. The reflex tachycardia occurs as a baroceptor-mediated sympathetic response to decreased systemic arterial blood pressure. The abolition of this reflex tachycardia by means of compression of the fistula or the artery proximal to it, with a resulting bradycardic response, is known as Branham's sign and is pathognomonic of AVFs.

The net effect of these physiologic responses in the acute setting is the reestablishment of homeostasis, with a normalization of central venous pressure, due to the increased stroke volume and heart rate, and a return of systemic arterial pressure toward, although slightly below, prefistula levels. In the event of a large, acute AVF, as in the case of an aortocaval fistula resulting from massive rupture of an abdominal aortic aneurysm, the ability to augment cardiac output may be inadequate to compensate for the massive fistula flow, with the result that the systemic arterial pressure may remain depressed well below baseline levels.

Chronic changes. After the initiation of the acute physiologic responses just enumerated, systemic arterial pressure is usually restored to normal or near normal levels. In the well-compensated person (without intrinsic underlying myocardial disease), a tendency is for the initial tachycardia to diminish somewhat, in view of the adequate restoration of systemic arterial pressure. In patients with preexisting intrinsic cardiac disease, however, a failure to reestablish equilibrium initially leads to persistent systemic hypotension and presents an ongoing stimulus for further pathophysiologic adaptation. Even in those without underlying cardiac abnormalities, such a stimulus often arises as the fistula matures and the magnitude of fistula flow increases over time, resulting in further decreases in peripheral resistance. In such situations, additional physiologic adaptations occur in response to the persistently reduced systemic arterial pressure.

Activation of the renin-aldosterone-angiotensin axis provides a stimulus for both expansion of plasma volume (sodium and water retention) and peripheral vaso-constriction in an attempt to restore the blood pressure toward normal. With time, the chronic high cardiac output leads to cardiac hypertrophy and subsequently dilatation and congestive cardiac failure. Although even these advanced changes may be completely reversed after fistula repair in young, healthy patients, such decompensation in patients with preexisting underlying cardiac disease usually results in death.

Clinical Findings

A. Physical Examination: The diagnosis of acquired AVF is usually straightforward and can most often be made on the basis of characteristic historical information and physical findings alone. Because most acquired fistulas are a consequence of trauma, a history of previous injury to the area in question can usually be obtained. Remember that the antecedent trauma can be relatively recent or may predate the patient's presentation by many months or even years. In addition to classic forms of external trauma, note any history, either recent or distant, of iatrogenic catheter-based intra-arterial manipulation, which may represent a potential source of injury. The presence of an audible bruit or a palpable thrill overlying an area of previous injury is highly suggestive of an AVF. Bruits are characteristically loud and holosystolic and often occupy much of diastole as well. A local increase in the temperature of the overlying skin or the presence of prominent dilated superficial veins in the affected area are additionally supportive of the diagnosis. Such history and physical findings in an extremity leave little doubt as to the diagnosis.

In the case of intracavitary AVFs (eg, mesenteric or renal AVFs), the diagnostic trail may be more subtle, with merely a history of previous abdominal surgery and the finding of an abdominal bruit to suggest the presence of a fistula. As mentioned previously, the physical findings associated with specific types of visceral AVFs may be protean (eg, gastrointestinal bleeding, intestinal angina, progressive renal dysfunction, focal cerebral ischemia) and are related to the particular end-organ involved.

B. Diagnostic Studies: In the typical case of acquired AVF, the clinical presentation is straightforward, and objective diagnostic testing is not required to make the diagnosis. In cases in which the diagnosis remains in question, a variety of noninvasive tests are available from which supportive or confirmatory information may be obtained in selected circumstances.

1. Segmental blood pressure testing–A cornerstone in the screening of patients with lower extremity arterial occlusive disease, segmental blood pressure recordings from an extremity (upper or lower) with a suspected AVF may provide indirect data in support of this diagnosis. When flow diverted through the parasitic fistulous circuit exceeds the capacity of the arterial collaterals to provide compensatory flow to the distal arterial bed, distal ischemia develops. This may be exacerbated during the latter stages of the compensatory changes, which occur in response to the physiologic derangements induced by the fistula, when peripheral vasoconstriction supervenes in an attempt to maintain central arterial blood pressure. In such an extremity, a decrease in blood pressure recorded distal to the site of the suspected AVF will be observed.

Although a segmental drop in blood pressure is hardly pathognomonic of AVF, occurring much more frequently in the setting of atherosclerotic occlusive disease, it may provide additional support when the clinical circumstances point toward AVF (eg, a 30-year-old with an audible bruit over the right femoral vessels 1 month after a stab wound to that thigh). Further substantiation of the diagnosis of AVF may be obtained when there is a substantial increase in the distal segmental pressures and a decrease in heart rate following manual compression of the fistulous site.

2. Segmental plethysmography–Similarly, the volume of plethysmographically determined segmental pulse waveforms in an extremity distal to a suspected AVF may be diminished. As a diagnostic maneuver, compression of the fistula may result in a return of the recorded pulse volume to normal, confirming the presence of a hemodynamically significant AVF. Obviously, both segmental pressure measurements and plethysmography are applicable only to extremity lesions and hold no usefulness in the assessment of central AVFs.

3. Duplex ultrasonography–Duplex scanning, the combination of B-mode ultrasonic vascular imaging with pulsed Doppler spectral waveform analysis, may be helpful in providing direct information useful for establishing the diagnosis of an AVF. Anatomic findings on B-mode imaging may include the characteristic dilatation and tortuosity of the proximal feeding artery and of the veins emerging from the fistula. Also, because pseudoaneurysm formation is a common companion anomaly seen in many traumatic AVFs, the ultrasonographic demonstration of a pseudoaneurysm, with its circumscribed cavity and turbulent internal eddy currents, may provide additional circumstantial support for the presence of a traumatic fistula. In addition to such anatomic evidence provided by B-mode imaging, Doppler spectral analysis of the flow waveforms within the vessels contributing to an AVF reveals several distinct patterns. Among these are (1) a loss of the typical triphasic arterial flow pattern usually seen in medium-sized peripheral arteries, with a loss of diastolic flow reversal and an increased peak flow velocity within the proximal artery; (2) arterialization of the venous flow signals with increased pulsatility and increased velocity of flow within the proximal veins emerging from the fistula; (3) reversal of flow within the distal artery possibly observed in patients in whom distal arterial steal has developed; and (4) finally, in rare cases, a discrete high-velocity "jet," with severely disordered, turbulent flow detectable at the precise site of fistulous communication between the parent artery and vein.

Although the duplex ultrasonographic detection of AVFs has been most reliably described in extremity fistulas, in which the relatively superficial location of the involved vessels renders them most easily accessible, advances in probe technology allowing for better imaging of the deep abdominal vasculature have recently facilitated the noninvasive diagnosis of visceral AVFs as well.

4. CT and MRI–Although both CT and MRI are effective in demonstrating the enhanced soft tissue mass surrounding AVFs, the value of routinely using these imaging modalities in the diagnostic evaluation of acquired AVFs is uncertain. Because of the ability of MRI to demonstrate blood flow patterns as well as to delineate anatomic tissue interfaces, an increasing role for this technology is likely in the future.

5. Angiography–Biplanar contrast arteriography remains the standard for the precise delineation and characterization of AVFs, regardless of their cause or location within the body. The typical arteriographic findings suggestive of an AVF include the demonstration of dilated, tortuous axial and collateral arteries and veins in the vicinity of the lesion and early venous opacification, suggesting a direct fistulous communication between artery and vein. Additionally supportive of the diagnosis of AVF may be the demonstration of a pseudoaneurysm in proximity to the area in question. Rarely, the precise fistulous channel may be directly visualized during arteriography, although this is seldom required to establish the presence or location of the fistula. Because of its reliability in establishing the diagnosis, ability to provide a complete characterization of the tributary vessels, applicability in both peripheral and central AVFs, and usefulness in enabling access for subsequent catheter-based interventional treatment, angiography remains the single most valuable diagnostic tool in the evaluation and therapy of AVFs.

Treatment

Because the natural history of most AVFs is believed to involve progressive enlargement of the fistula, with consequently increasing flow through the parasitic circuit resulting ultimately in advanced local, regional, and systemic anatomic and hemodynamic aberrations, observational management is seldom advisable. Therefore, an aggressive policy of early intervention is usually warranted. Although reports of spontaneous regression or closure of small peripheral AVFs have been made, such biologic behavior cannot be reliably expected; thus, with rare exceptions, expectant management should not be advocated.

The earliest attempts at treating AVFs relied on simple ligation of the feeding artery. Because of the complex network of collateral vessels involved in most mature fistulas, however, such an approach is usually doomed to failure inasmuch as new collateral inflow tributaries are likely to develop and mature. In addition to allowing for persistence of the fistulous connection, ligation of the main inflow artery severely compromises the opportunity for direct endovascular access to the fistula in the future, if a subsequent attempt at catheter-based evaluation or therapy is desired. As a result, simple arterial ligation is contraindicated in the management of AVFs.

The main tenets underlying the current surgical approach to the treatment of AVFs consist of (1) complete vascular control of all of the major afferent and efferent arteries and veins contributing to the fistula; (2) direct dissection and separation of the fistulous channel between the involved artery and vein; (3) complete obliteration of the fistulous communication; and (4) vascular reconstruction, if necessary, to restore circulatory continuity. Any operative endeavor that does not address these points is likely to result in persistence of the fistula, which will hamper subsequent attempts at repair and may possibly aggravate ischemia of the distal vascular bed.

Because of the nature of mature AVFs, with the presence of numerous dilated and friable collateral vessels often intimately involved in a generalized inflammatory local tissue reaction, the actual operative implementation of the principles of repair previously enumerated is often tedious and fraught with potential hazard. Points of technique that are often useful are control of venous backbleeding by means of manual compression (by fingertip, sponge sticks, or intraluminal balloon occlusion rather than by clamp application); avoidance of ligation of major veins, if possible; reconstruction of major veins if ligation becomes necessary; and preferential use of autogenous material if vascular reconstruction is required.

Depending on the extent of vessel wall injury, options for repair of arterial defects at the site of the fistula may include lateral arteriorrhaphy with fine monofilament suture, patch angioplasty with a segment of autogenous vein, or formal autogenous vein bypass. In view of the large blood losses that may occur during repair of large mature AVFs, the use of autotransfusion devices is advisable. In repairing extremity AVFs, the application and use of a sterile pneumatic tourniquet may be a useful adjunct to prevent excessive operative hemorrhage.

A. Endovascular Therapy: Transcatheter embolization has played an increasingly important role in the treatment of AVFs. With the advent of superselective catheterization techniques, as well as improvements in the transcatheter delivery of embolic materials such as detachable balloons, steel coils, and liquid acrylic adhesive agents, the ability to control many AVFs without incurring the risks of operative repair has developed. Particularly effective for relatively small fistulas, percutaneous catheter embolization has become the first line of therapy for treating small- to medium-sized AVFs, especially in areas where surgical exposure may be expected to be relatively difficult and associated with excessive morbidity.

In certain types of AVFs (eg, carotid-cavernous sinus fistulas), percutaneous catheter embolization represents the only practical method of treatment. Catheter-based techniques are less effective in treating large AVFs, in which the high flows and large communication predispose toward a significant risk of migration of the embolic agents into the venous circulation. The reliable performance of percutaneous embolization of AVFs requires sophisticated angiographic equipment and highly skilled interventional radiologists, either of which may not be readily available where patients with these lesions are treated. As experience with these techniques grows, they can be expected to play an increasing role in the management of AVFs.

B. Therapy for Specific AVFs:

1. Aortocaval AVFs–Most aortocaval fistulas represent the spontaneous rupture of an atherosclerotic aortic aneurysm into the inferior vena cava. The remaining few cases occur as a result of trauma, either from penetrating abdominal injury or as a complication of lumbar disk surgery. The presentation of such cases, usually as a result of aneurysm rupture, is most often acute, often with profound hemodynamic derangement. The most consistent findings are a palpable pulsatile abdominal mass and a continuous harsh abdominal bruit. In addition, less consistent findings that have been reported are lower extremity cyanosis and edema, scrotal edema, priapism, hematuria, gastrointestinal bleeding, and distal lower extremity ischemia. Because of the high incidence of associated cardiac disease in patients with atherosclerotic abdominal aortic aneurysms, the acute hemodynamic decompensation created by this complication is usually poorly tolerated. Attempts at preoperative visualization of aortocaval fistulas are seldom indicated: the acute deterioration seen in these patients ordinarily mandates prompt operative repair. Percutaneous catheter-based therapy has no role in these patients.

The surgical treatment of spontaneous aortocaval fistulas consists of expedient proximal aortic control, transaortic closure of the fistula (usually by direct suture repair), and direct aortic reconstruction with prosthetic graft material. Care must be taken during initial mobilization of the aneurysm to avoid excessive manipulation, because this may produce paradoxical embolization of aneurysmal debris through the fistula resulting in life-threatening pulmonary embolism. When the aneurysm is opened, venous backbleeding from the vena cava through the fistula may be fierce. Control of venous bleeding is best provided by sponge stick compression of the vena cava both above and below the fistula. Insertion of balloon-tipped catheters through the fistula into the vena cava provides an alternate means of obtaining venous control and may be lifesaving. After successful repair, a prompt reversal of the hemodynamic derangements and a brisk diuresis usually ensue. Operative mortality in various series ranges from 20% to 50%. Although similar in many respects, other distinct patterns of aortovenous fistulization after aneurysm rupture have been reported, including aorta-left renal vein fistula and aortoiliac venous fistula.

2. Renal AVFs–Acquired fistulas of the renal vasculature most frequently occur as a result of iatrogenic injury after percutaneous renal biopsy. These fistulas are usually intrarenal and often are small. Many have been shown to undergo spontaneous closure, although the natural history of such injuries is far from established. Other causes of renal AVFs are external trauma (either penetrating or blunt), operative injury (usually after mass ligation of the renal pedicle), and rarely invasion by tumor (malignant or inflammatory) into adjacent renal arteries and veins. When symptomatic, patients with these lesions often present with evidence of renal dysfunction, hypertension, hematuria, and an abdominal or flank bruit. Because of the high proportion of blood flow received by the kidney, renal AVFs are often accompanied by systemic cardiovascular complications including high-output cardiac failure. Although selected, small asymptomatic renal AVFs may be successfully observed, definitive treatment is indicated in the presence of hypertension, increased cardiac output, or persistent hematuria. In addition, in a solitary kidney the indication for treatment must be considered on an individual basis.

The optimal strategy for treating a symptomatic renal AVF is a function of its location, size, and the status of the involved kidney. Options for treatment are nephrectomy (partial or complete), fistula excision and vascular reconstruction, or percutaneous embolization.

3. Gastrointestinal AVFs–AVFs of the gastrointestinal tract are extremely rare and may involve the splenic artery and vein, the hepatic artery and portal venous system, or branches of the mesenteric arteries and veins. Splenic AVF usually arises as a consequence of either splenic aneurysm rupture or penetrating trauma. Effective treatment is accomplished with splenectomy. Hepatic arterioportal fistula (HAPF) occurs most often as an iatrogenic complication after percutaneous transhepatic procedures such as liver biopsy, percutaneous transhepatic cholangiography, or biliary tract interventions. Much less frequently, rupture of an atherosclerotic aneurysm of the hepatic artery may lead to fistulization into the portal venous system. Symptoms are most often a result of the development of portal hypertension, primarily as gastrointestinal bleeding and less commonly as ascites.

Systemic cardiovascular complications are infrequent, probably as a result of the buffering effect of the intervening hepatic sinusoids, which serve to dampen the transmission into the systemic circulation of the portal hyperdynamic state. Treatment for extrahepatic arterioportal fistulas is primarily by operative excision with or without vascular reconstruction. For intrahepatic arterioportal fistula, percutaneous embolization has been demonstrated to be highly effective and is the procedure of choice.

AVFs of the mesenteric vessels occur after penetrating or operative trauma. During small bowel resective procedures, mass ligation of mesenteric arterial and venous branches may lead to the development of a U-type fistula, a functional end-to-end arteriovenous communication in which there is no bowel distal to the fistula. In such cases, symptoms result from portal hypertension and not from ischemia of distal bowel. Simple resection of such fistulas is curative. Mesenteric AVFs following penetrating trauma usually occur as classic H-type fistulas. In such cases, symptoms of small bowel ischemia are likely to predominate during the acute phase, whereas portal hypertension and its complications dominate in chronic cases. For peripheral mesenteric AVFs, simple excision is satisfactory, whereas excision and vascular reconstruction are required for fistulas involving the proximal portion of the superior mesenteric artery and vein.

Percutaneous embolization may be useful as an adjunct to the surgical repair of selected proximal mesenteric AVFs.

Alexander JJ, Imbembo AL: Aorta-vena cava fistula. Surgery 1989;105:1.

Anda S et al: Anterior perforations in lumbar discectomies: A report of four cases of vascular complications and a CT study of the prevertebral lumbar anatomy. Spine 1991;16:54.

Batt M et al: Traumatic fistula between the aorta and the left renal vein: Case report and review of the literature. J Vasc Surg 1989;9:812.

Calligaro KD, Savarese RP, DeLaurentis DA: Unusual aspects of aortovenous fistulas associated with ruptured abdominal aortic aneurysms. J Vasc Surg 1990;12:586.

Courtheoux P et al: Postnephrectomy arteriovenous fistula of the renal pedicle treated with detachable balloons: A case report. Cardiovasc Intervent Radiol 1988;11:340.

Crotty KL, Orihuela E, Warren MM: Recent advances in the diagnosis and treatment of renal arteriovenous malformations and fistulas. J Urol 1993;150:1355.

Donell ST, Hudson MJ: Iatrogenic superior mesenteric arteriovenous fistula: Report of a case and review of the literature. J Vasc Surg 1988;8:335.

Gilling-Smith GL, Mansfield AO: Spontaneous abdominal arteriovenous fistulae: Report of eight cases and review of the literature. Br J Surg 1991;78:421.

Gregoric ID, Jacobs MJ, Reul GJ, Rochelle DG: Spontaneous common iliac arteriovenous fistula manifested by acute renal failure: A case report. J Vasc Surg 1991;14:92.

Guglielmi G: Successful embolization of a spontaneous carotid cavernous fistula fed only by the external carotid artery: Case report and literature review. J Neurosurg Sci 1988;32:83.

Halldorsson A, Hunter GC, McIntyre KE, Bernhard VM: Internal mammary artery subclavian vein fistula following internal jugular vein catheterization: A case report and review of the literature. J Cardiovasc Surg (Torino) 1991;32:376.

Hoballah JJ et al: Aortic aneurysm rupture into a retroaortic left renal vein. Ann Vasc Surg 1993;7:363.

Hubsch P, Schurawitzki H, Traindl O, Karnel F: Renal allograft arteriovenous fistula due to needle biopsy with late onset of symptoms: Diagnosis and treatment. Nephron 1991;59:482.

Johansen K: Management of acquired arteriovenous fistulas. In: Current Therapy in Vascular Surgery. Ernst CB, Stanley JC (editors). BC Decker, 1991.

Kato S, Nakagawa T, Kobayashi H, Arai E: Superior mesenteric arteriovenous fistula: Report of a case and review of the literature. Surg Today 1993;23:73.

Lanne T, Bergqvist D: Aortocaval fistulas associated with ruptured abdominal aortic aneurysms. Eur J Surg 1992;158:457.

Levy PJ et al: Rare presentation of anastomotic iliac artery false aneurysm: Rupture with formation of ilio-iliac arteriovenous fistula. Am Surg 1993;59:713.

Lumsden AB et al: Hepatic arterioportal fistula. Am Surg 1993;59:722.

Mansour MA, Rutherford RB, Metcalf RK, Pearce WH: Spontaneous aorto-left renal vein fistula: The abdominal pain, hematuria, silent left kidney syndrome. Surgery 1991;109:101.

Mateo AM et al: Postnephrectomy arteriovenous fistula. J Cardiovasc Surg (Torino) 1988;29:491.

Matsubara J, Nagasue M, Nakatani B, Shimizu T: Aortocaval fistula resulting from rupture of an abdominal aortic aneurysm: Report and review of Japanese reported cases. Eur JR Vasc Surg 1991;5:601.

Morrow C, Lewinstein C, Ben-Menachem Y: Spontaneous iliac arteriovenous fistula. J Vasc Surg 1987;6:524.

Osmundson PJ: Arteriovenous communications. Cardiovasc Clin 1992;22:127.

Pabst TS III et al: Subclavian artery-to-innominate vein fistula: A case caused by subclavian venous catheterization. Surgery 1989;105:801.

Redmond PL, Kumpe DA: Embolization of an intrahepatic arterioportal fistula: case report and review of the literature. Cardiovasc Intervent Radiol 1988;11:274.

Rosenthal D et al: Traumatic superior mesenteric arteriovenous fistula: Report of a case and review of the literature. J Vasc Surg 1987;5:486.

Saunders MS, Riberi A, Massullo EA: Delayed traumatic superior mesenteric arteriovenous fistula after a stab wound: Case report. J Trauma 1992;32:101.

Sonmez B et al: Ruptured abdominal aortic aneurysm with fistula into the right iliac vein. J Cardiovasc Surg (Torino) 1988;29:486.

Strodel WE et al: Presentation and perioperative management of arterioportal fistulas. Arch Surg 1987;122:563.

Sumner DS: Hemodynamics and pathophysiology of arteriovenous fistulas. In: Vascular Surgery. Robert B. Rutherford (editor). WB Saunders, 1989.

Tarazov PG, Prozorovskij KV: Intrahepatic spontaneous arterioportal fistula: Duplex ultrasound diagnosis and angiographic treatment. Am J Gastroenterol 1991;86:775.

Thompson RW, Yee LF, Natuzzi ES, Stoney RJ: Aorta-left renal vein fistula syndrome caused by rupture of a juxtarenal abdominal aortic aneurysm: Novel pathologic mechanism for a unique clinical entity. J Vasc Surg 1993;18:310.

Extra-Anatomic Bypass Grafting   28

F. William Blaisdell, MD, & William C. Pevec, MD

The first successful extra-anatomic bypass graft was reported in 1952 by Norman Freeman and Frank Leeds (Fig 28–1). Subsequently, McCaughan and Kahn carried out an external iliac contralateral femoral bypass. A series of successful operations described by Vetto are credited for giving impetus to the femorofemoral bypass being adopted for general use.

The next major advance occurred when Lewis bypassed a dissecting aneurysm of the thoracic aorta with a 10-mm Dacron tube, carrying it from the proximal subclavian artery retroperitoneally to the ipsilateral common iliac artery. This procedure proved that a smaller conduit could furnish adequate circulation for the lower half of the body.

Another major advance in the use of extra-anatomic grafts was reported by Shaw and Baue in 1963. Their procedure entailed routing a graft from the common iliac artery to the femoral artery through the obturator foramen to bypass a graft groin infection. This resulted in salvage of the limb and permitted removal of the infected graft with adequate drainage of the groin.

General Considerations

For all practical purposes, prosthetic grafts are required for extra-anatomic bypass because the high flow rates required for the lower half of the body cannot be met in most instances by a 4- to 5-mm vein. Eight- to 10-mm grafts usually can provide sufficient flow for the lower extremities. Although we favor knitted Dacron as the prosthetic material, the literature suggests that polytetrafluorethylene (PTFE) grafts are equally satisfactory.

A. Issues of Concern: The issue of steal was a major consideration in the initial use of grafts. However, the demonstration that high flow rates were possible in the axillary artery provided reassurance that this would not be a problem.

Another early concern in the use of grafts was the superficial placement of long grafts and whether the weight of the body would compress the graft and result in thrombosis. However, the advent of externally supported grafts provides protection against compression thrombosis or compression impairment of flow, which is believed to be the factor responsible for graft thrombosis in the absence of proximal or distal disease.

When ischemic arm symptoms occur, they are more likely to be the result of acute technical problems that produce thrombosis of the axillary artery.

Ischemic symptoms are extremely rare in our personal experience.

B. Indications for Bypass: Absolute indications for extra-anatomic bypass are infection along the route of a conventional graft, intra-abdominal or retroperitoneal inflammatory disease, and high-risk patient (recent myocardial infarction, cardiac pulmonary obstructive disease, congestive heart failure). Relative indications are previous abdominal vascular procedures, mechanical factors such as previous radiation therapy, multiple abdominal operations, elderly patient, extensive aortic disease, and extreme obesity.

C. Preoperative Assessment: The primary risk factors for major operative procedures are chronic obstructive pulmonary disease and arteriosclerotic coronary artery disease. The former is easily assessable by appropriate pulmonary function tests. Although patients with marginal pulmonary function can still have conventional procedures with acceptable risk, extra-anatomic bypass offers a low-risk alternative. However, when a patient has chronic bronchitis with moist secretions and marginal pulmonary function, he or she represents an unacceptable risk for subsequent pulmonary problems with conventional major thoracic or abdominal incisions.

The primary risk factor for mortality is myocardial infarction. Most patients with peripheral vascular disease have some degree of coronary artery involvement. We have found that electrocardiogram stress tests or Persantine (dipyridamole)-thallium scans are effective screening methods for latent myocardial dysfunction. Patients with occlusive disease rarely can be subjected to an exercise stress test and usually require a dipyridamole-thallium scan. If unstable myocardium is demonstrated, the alternatives are either extra-anatomic bypass or myocardial revascularization followed by a conventional operation if the former lowers the cardiac risk acceptably.

The final phase of workup of patients usually involves aortography. Although indirect noninvasive procedures are being used more frequently, the most certain way to anticipate potential technical problems with inflow or run-off is by aortography. In most instances, visualization of the femoral arteries and their run-off is all that is needed.

The absence of bruits along the course of the subclavian axillary artery, the absence of a blood pressure differential in the arms, and the presence of good dis-

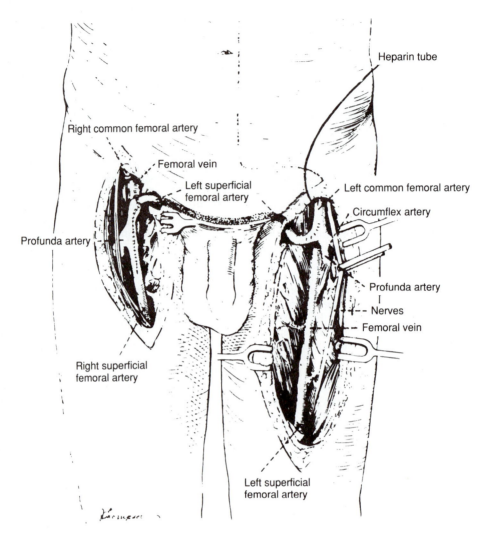

Figure 28–1. The first extra-anatomic bypass. (Reproduced, with permission, from Freeman NE, Leeds FH: Operations on large arteries. Calif Med 1952;77:229.)

tal pulses usually are sufficient to ensure that the feeding vessel will have adequate flow to support both the arm and the lower half of the body. When the left axillary artery is being considered for the inflow site, it is especially important to ensure patency because the left axillary artery is much more commonly involved with disease than the right.

TYPES OF EXTRA-ANATOMIC BYPASS

Thoracic Aorta-to-Femoral Bypass

A. Indications: Thoracic aorta-to-femoral bypass has been receiving increased attention in recent years. Its usefulness is the greatest when the patient has a "hostile" abdomen. This may result from a previous abdominal vascular operation, aortic thrombosis ex-

tending to the level of the renal arteries, infrarenal or suprarenal atherosclerotic disease that makes aortic cross-clamping hazardous, and infection in the abdominal cavity either as the result of previous vascular surgery or nonvascular disease such as diverticulitis. Another justification for extra-anatomic bypass is the irradiated abdomen following treatment of prostate, bladder, or uterine cancer. Compared with other procedures, thoracic aorta-to-femoral bypass should be limited to patients with good pulmonary and cardiac reserve who are able to tolerate thoracotomy.

B. Operative Technique: The patient should be positioned in semioblique position with the left chest rotated upward about 45° and the hips supported only by a pad under the left buttock.

The thoracic incision is optimally made in the left 7th–8th interspace as an anterolateral or lateral thoracotomy incision. The aorta can be exposed in any convenient location, but the optimal location is just above the diaphragm. Although the aortic dissection can be limited to its anterior portion and the clamp used without complete mobilization, for safety the aorta is best encircled above the location of an occluding clamp. A partial occluding Satinsky-type clamp is then placed to isolate a generous portion of the anterior wall of the aorta and still ensure distal flow. A longitudinal arteriotomy is made, and a 8- or 10-mm graft is sutured side to end to the aorta.

The left common femoral artery is exposed simultaneously or subsequently in conventional fashion, and a dissection plane is developed lateral to the femoral artery into the retroperitoneum. A small hole is made in the diaphragm at its attachment to the 12th rib at a convenient posterior medial location. A tunneler can then be passed downward in the retroperitoneum just lateral to the kidney until it can be palpated by a finger placed in the retroperitoneum from the groin incision and guided for the remaining distance. The graft is pulled down the retroperitoneal tunnel and anastomosed in conventional fashion to the common femoral artery or at the femoral bifurcation, depending on the presence or absence of disease. If a simultaneous femorofemoral bypass is done, a separate incision is recommended in the femoral artery either proximal or distal to the thoracic aortofemoral graft rather than placement of an anastomosis on the graft itself.

C. Complications: Experience has shown that thoracofemoral bypasses compare very favorably with conventional anatomic grafts. This is not unexpected, since the thoracofemoral grafts are almost anatomic and lie in a protected position.

D. Prognosis: The largest reported series of thoracic aortofemoral artery bypasses is that of McCarthy and associates. In their series of 21 patients, there were (1) no operative deaths, (2) a 4-year primary patency of 100%, and (3) a 5-year primary patency of 86%.

Axillofemoral Bypass

A. Indications: Axillofemoral bypass is the most useful in high-risk patients who have aortoiliac occlusive disease, infection within the abdominal cavity, or previous multiple vascular procedures. It is useful for the same group of patients who would have had thoracofemoral bypass. Axillofemoral bypass also has been used to simplify management of abdominal aneurysms in high-risk patients; it permits a staged procedure in which the aneurysm is bypassed initially. Subsequently, the intra-abdominal aneurysm is ligated.

B. Operative Technique: The patient is positioned supinely on the operating table. The arm being used for the operation is placed on an arm board at a right angle to the body. The skin should be prepared from the supraclavicular area to the upper thigh and to the table line on the ipsilateral side. An infraclavicular incision is made from just lateral to the sternum to the midclavicle, parallel with and 1 fingerbreadth below that bone. The pectoral fascia is opened, and the fibers

of the pectoralis major muscle are spread by blunt dissection. Exposure is maintained with an automatic retractor. The subpectoral fascia is opened, and the axillary vein is identified and mobilized downward, dividing any venous branches coming into the superior portion of the vein. The artery is then identified and exposed posterior and superior to the axillary vein. The axillary artery is mobilized from where it passes under the clavicle to the pectoralis minor muscle and encircled with a tape. The only branch in the first portion of the axillary artery is the highest thoracic, a 1-mm vessel that comes off the posterior inferior portion of the artery. This is easily identified and ligated.

At this point—if not done simultaneously—the ipsilateral common femoral artery should be exposed in conventional fashion. A small incision is made in the inferior portion of the inguinal ligament just lateral to the femoral artery, and a plane of dissection is developed under the external oblique fascia. A tunneler is then passed obliquely upward in the subfascial plane, carefully passing over, not under, the costal margin. The tunneler is curved laterally to the mid- or posterior axillary line, at or near the level of the 8th or 9th rib, where a counter incision is made and the tip of the tunneler is passed out through the skin. An umbilical tape is then drawn down the tunnel as the tunneler is extracted. The tunneler is passed downward in the plane under the pectoralis major and minor muscles to the previously made counterincision. The umbilical tape is then passed through the entire length of the incision. This tunnel is placed in the midaxillary line so that the graft will be stressed minimally with flexion of the trunk.

At this point, the axillary artery is isolated and a side-to-end anastomosis done with an 8- to 10-mm externally supported graft. We use a graft that has external support over its entire length, although a few rings are removed at the anastomotic sites. The graft is then pulled down the tunnel using the umbilical tape and anastomosed to the femoral artery.

C. Complications: Complications relating to axillofemoral grafts are surprisingly few. An apparent increased thrombosis rate occurs with axillofemoral grafts in contrast to what occurs with conventional grafts. The longer length and the subcutaneous position of the extra-anatomic bypasses may render them more vulnerable to compression thrombosis or kinking.

The unique complications of axillofemoral grafts are related to the axillary artery—either false aneurysms or axillary artery thrombosis. Most of the reported problems with the axillary artery appear to result from placing the anastomosis too far distally on the artery. When the anastomosis is placed on the proximal portion of the axillary artery, there is very little motion of the artery with motion of the shoulder. If the proximal anastomosis is placed in the first portion of the axillary artery, collateral flow is excellent, and if local thrombosis occurs, it will not produce ischemia of the arm. The greatest advantage in using the first portion of the axillary artery is that stress on the anastomosis is minimized. When the anastomosis is placed on the third portion of the artery, considerable stress can be exerted with elevation of the shoulder.

D. Outcome: The following are factors that are considered important for optimizing patency rates.

- Anastomosis to the proximal axillary artery to minimize stressing the graft with motion of the shoulder.
- Placement of the graft in axis of flexion of the trunk.
- Use of externally supported grafts.
- Use of axillofemorofemoral grafts to increase outflow, wherever possible.
- Avoidance of parallel flow in native arteries.

A list of all the axillofemoral graft series in the English literature that have reported follow-up for 5 or more years is provided in Table 28–1. Axillofemoral grafts on the whole had a 1-year patency rate of 48 to 95% and a 5-year patency rate of 9–80%. The axillobifemoral grafts had a 1-year patency rate of 58–93% and a 5-year patency rate of 30–80%. Review of these reports does reveal any significant difference between the series using PTFE grafts and those using Dacron grafts. However, one report suggested that the former were superior. In addition, no differences were apparent as to whether 8- or 10-mm Dacron grafts were used, although we found a difference in long-term patency between woven and knitted Dacron that markedly favored the latter. Unquestionably, technical factors influence the immediate and long-term patency of axillofemoral grafts.

Ultimately, the patency of axillofemoral grafts appears to relate directly to flow. Ray and associates and LoGerfo and associates did studies of blood flow in patients and found that axillofemorofemoral grafts had a much higher patency rate than unilateral grafts, with an average flow rate of more than 600 mL/min compared with half that for unilateral grafts. In LoGerfo's series, a 74% 5-year patency of axillobifemoral grafts was found, compared with a 37% 5-year patency with axillounifemoral grafts. The combined series also demonstrates the superiority of the bilateral grafts with higher flow rates. The reason for this probably relates to neointimal changes within the graft itself. When flow rates are high, it has been our observation that the neointima is thin, in contrast to grafts with lower flow rates in which there is a thick neointima. A thick neointima does not in itself compromise patency, but when there is kinking or trauma to the graft, the thicker intima is more vulnerable to sloughing or flap elevation, which is believed to be one of the factors that accounts for graft thrombosis. If a difference in longevity of axillofemoral grafts is seen compared with conventional grafts, it is because of the vulnerability of the former to external trauma,

since progression of proximal and distal disease should be similar.

Femorofemoral Bypass

A. Indications: Femorofemoral bypass can be the procedure of choice for a patient with disease limited to one iliac system or a patient with a patent aortofemoral bypass on one side either as the result of a unilateral procedure or more commonly a thrombosis of one limb of a bifurcated graft. It is particularly useful in high-risk patients and is generally much less stressful to the patient than redoing one limb of an aortobifemoral bypass using the abdominal route.

B. Operative Technique: When a femorofemoral graft is to be carried out, the anastomosis for the axillofemoral graft is placed at the femoral bifurcation, well distal to the inguinal ligament. After completion of this anastomosis, which favors either the superficial femoral or the profunda femoral artery depending on which will provide the best outflow, the common femoral artery is divided at the level of the inguinal ligament and the proximal artery is oversewn. The distal end of the divided artery is then anastomosed end to end to a femorofemoral graft. The graft is then passed through a subcutaneous tunnel to the exposed common femoral artery on the contralateral side. An end-to-end or end-to-side anastomosis is done, depending on whether or not back perfusion is indicated. To ensure maximal flow rates through all portions of the reconstruction, the distal femorofemoral anastomosis is carried out end to end in patients with patent ipsilateral iliac arteries and end to side in patients with complete common iliac occlusion.

C. Prognosis: The operative mortality for femorofemoral bypasses is low, ranging from 2.4% to 6.4% in several recent series (Table 28–2). However, long-term patency is variable in those series, ranging from 4% to 87% at 5 years.

Obturator Bypass

A. Indications: The obturator bypass can consist of an aortotransobturator distal superficial femoral bypass or an iliac transobturator superficial femoral or profunda bypass. It is used optimally when there is a hostile inguinal region, which is the result of infection or multiple previous operations. The obturator bypass is an underused procedure with few large series in the literature documenting its efficacy. However, our experience with it has been uniformly good. A major advantage is that the obturator bypass lies in the axis of flexion of the hip and therefore is less subject to flexion trauma at the groin than are other bypass procedures.

B. Operative Technique: The key factor in carrying out obturator bypass is deciding on the optimal location for the proximal and distal anastomosis. Because this bypass is often done using a retroperitoneal incision, the proximal anastomosis is most easily placed on the lowest convenient location proximal to

Table 28–1. Axillofemoral grafts.

Year	Author		Mortality			Graft Patency		
		N	30-days (%)	5-yr (%)	Type	N	1-yr (%)	5-yr (%)
1971	Moore et al.[11]	52	8	70	AF(F)*	52	62	9
1977	Eugene et al.[12]	59	8	73	AF	35	62	30
					AFF	24	62	30
1977	Lo Gerfo et al.[13]	130	8	23	AF	64	64	37
					AFF	66	89	74
1977	Johnson et al.[14]	56	2	37	AFF	56	82	76
1978	Sheiner[15]	45	2	32	AF	25	60	51
1979	Ray et al.[16]	84	3.7	32	AF	33	75	67
					AFF	21	90	77
1982	Kenney et al.[17]	92	–	–	AF	58	85	66
1982	Courbier et al.[18]	220	3.6	24	AF	220	87	64
1985	Ascer et al.[19]	56	5.3	57	AF	34	68	44
1985	Allison et al.[20]	109	6.4	44	AF	87	48	16
					AFF	25	58	45
1986	Chang[21]	88	2	47	AF	47	–	33
1986	Christenson et al.[22]	85	3.6	45	AF(F)	85	74	68
1986	Foster[23]	52	12	60	AF(F)	52	60	32
1986	Donaldsen et al.[24]	100	8	31	AF(F)	72	78	48
1986	Savrin et al.[25]	33	18	59	AF(F)	96	91	75
1986	Schulz, Sauvage[26]	41	–	–	AF(?)**	41	95	80
1987	Rutherford et al.[27]	42	12	50	AF	15	48	19
					AFF	27	78	62
1987	Pietri et al.[28]	167	7.2	–	AF(F)	167	–	35
1988	Hepp et al.[29]	124	4.9	40	AF	102	60	46
					AFF	22	83	80
1989	Mason et al.[30]	37	2.8	–	AF(F)	37	–	80‡
1990	Naylor et al.[31]	38	11	56	AF	21	–	50
					AFF	17	–	80
1990	Harris et al.[32]	76	4.5	–	AFF	76	93	85‡‡
1991	Dé & Hepp[33]	131	5.3	–	AF	107	–	44
					AFF	24	–	73
1992	Bacourt et al.[34]	98	24	55	AFF	98	–	65
1992	Wittens et al.[35]	117	12	–	AFF†	58	38‡‡‡	–
					AFF‡‡	59	84‡‡‡	–
1993	El-Massry et al.[36]	79	5	79	AF	50	–	79
					AFF	29	–	76
1994	Taylor et al.[10]	184	5	48	AF(F)	184	–	71
Weighted average (%)								
Overall			6.9	44			75	55
Axillounifemoral							71	49
Axillobifemoral							83	68

[AF = Axillounifemoral graft; AFF = axillobifemoral graft.]

* AF(F) = Combined AF and AFF.

** AF(?) = AF or AFF not specified.

– = No data.

† = Femorofemoral limb at 90 degree angle from axillofemoral graft.

†† = Bifurcated graft with symmetrical "flow splitter."

‡ = 3-yr (%) graft patency.

‡‡ = 4-yr (%) graft patency.

‡‡‡ = 2-yr (%) graft patency.

any iliac artery disease. The retroperitoneum is exposed by an oblique incision carried upward from 2 fingerbreadths above the pubic tubercle running parallel with the inguinal ligament, then curving upward medial to the anterior iliac spine. The incision can be carried out into the flank as necessary, depending on whether the distal aorta or common iliac artery is to be used.

The proximal anastomosis is done in conventional side-to-end fashion. The obturator membrane is ex-

Table 28–2. Femorofemoral grafts.

			Mortality		Graft Patency		
Year	Author	N	30-days (%)	5-yr (%)	1-yr (%)	3-yr (%)	5-yr (%)
1975	Brief et al.[38]	57	–	33	93	–	81
1978	Sheiner[39]	73	4	22	82	–	73
1978	Flanigan et al.[40]	71	4	24	88	–	74
1979	Livesay et al.[41]	36	5.6	17	82	–	56
1979	Ray et al.[42]	67	–	–	93	–	86
1980	Dick et al.[43]	133	6	19	89	–	73
1981	Raithel & Meier[44]	81	–	–	90	–	75
1982	Lamerton et al.[45]	54	4	16	85	–	60
1982	Hill et al.[46]	50	2	20	89	–	74
1983	Subram et al.[47]	85	2.4	–	90	–	63
1987	Pietri et al.[28]	50	–	–	–	–	71
1989	Mason et al.[30]	40	2.5	–	–	78	–
1989	Fahal et al.[48]	150	4.0	–	–	–	–
1990	Ghilardi et al.[49]	62	6.4	–	–	77	–
1991	Dé and Hepp[33]	42	2.4	–	92	–	87
1991	Self et al.[50]	68	4.4	45	83	–	42
1992	Harrington et al.[51]	162	6.2	32	72	–	57
Weighted average (%)			4.5	26	86	77	68

– = no data.

posed in its upper inner corner, and the obturator artery and nerve are identified. The obturator membrane is then opened sharply in its upper corner adjacent to but carefully avoiding the neurovascular bundle. The index finger is passed through the membrane followed by a tunneler. The tunneler, normally passed in the plane of the adductor muscles, usually meets the superficial femoral artery in the lower portion of Hunter's canal, which is the optimal location if this artery is free of disease.

If the profunda femoral artery is to be used for the distal anastomosis, the surgeon's index finger must be inserted through the incision exposing the profunda femoral artery and passed upward toward the obturator membrane. The index finger then guides the tunneler to the profunda.

When the superficial femoral artery is to be the outflow after completion of the proximal anastomosis, the graft is passed down the tunnel to the superficial femoral or profunda femoral artery and is anastomosed in an appropriate end-to-side fashion. Alternatively, in

a patient with superficial femoral occlusive disease, the graft can be tunneled down to the popliteal space for bypass to that artery.

C. Complications: The only other complication unique to obturator bypass is injury to the obturator nerve. As indicated, the obturator bypass minimizes stress on the femoral anastomosis, so that the graft is not stretched with flexion of the body. This is also true of thoracofemoral bypass grafts.

D. Prognosis: Only 2 series with significant numbers of patients and long-term follow-up have been reported for obturator bypass (Table 28–3). In one series, the patency at 4 years was 33%; in the other, the patency at 5 years was 37%. It is not surprising that patients with suprageniculate distal anastomoses fared better than those with infrageniculate anastomoses: 71% versus 45%, respectively, at 3 years.

Conclusion

Comparison of the results of extra-anatomic grafts with conventional grafts is difficult because extra-

Table 28–3. Obturator grafts.

			Mortality		Graft Patency		
Year	Author	N	30-days (%)	5-yr (%)	Type (%)	1-yr (%)	5-yr (%)
1987	Pietri[28]	7	29.0	–	–	–	–
1987	Nevelsteen et al.[51]	55	9.5	42	All*	86	37
					AK*		71
					BK*		23
1989	Kretschmer et al.[52]	21	–	48	–	–	33‡

‡ 4-yr (%) graft patency.
* AK = above-knee outflow, BK = below-knee outflow, All = entire series.
– = no data.

anatomic bypasses are usually selected for use in high-risk patients or those with some local complication that increases the risk of the operation. Since the advent of externally supported grafts, the overall difference in thrombosis rates would probably be very slight if similar patients were compared in a randomized fashion.

In our personal experience, false aneurysms have been rare. This may relate to the proximal placement of the anastomosis and to the fairly uniform use of Dacron, which is considerably stronger than PTFE. The only large series with long follow-up that shows a significant incidence of proximal anastomotic problems is the series of Taylor and associates in which 10 proximal anastomotic disruptions occurred in 202 cases in which PTFE grafts were used. This may be related to anastomotic technique, distal placement of the grafts on the axillary artery, or failure to curve the graft tract laterally in the axis of flexion of the body on the graft material.

REFERENCES

Allison HF, Terblanche J, Immelman EJ: Axillofemoral bypass: A 2-decade experience. S Afr Med J 1985;68:559.

Ascer E et al: Comparison of axillounifemoral and axillobifemoral bypass operations. Surgery 1985;97:169.

Bacourt F et al: Axillobifemoral bypass and aortic exclusion for vascular septic lesions: A multicenter retrospective study of 93 cases. Ann Vasc Surg 1992;6:119.

Blaisdell FW, DeMattei GA, Gauder PJ: Extraperitoneal thoracic aorta to femoral by-pass graft as replacement for an infected aortic bifurcation prosthesis. Am J Surg 1961;102:583.

Blaisdell FW, Hall AD: Axillary-femoral artery bypass for lower extremity ischemia. Surgery 1963;54:563.

Blaisdell FW, Hall AD, Thomas AH: Ligation treatment of abdominal aortic aneurysms. Am J Surg 1965;109:560.

Blaisdell FW, Stuart FP, Hall AD: The effect of diameter and angulation on blood flow through plastic arterial substitutes. Am J Surg 1964;106:192.

Brief DK et al: Crossover femorofemoral grafts followed up five years or more. Arch Surg 1975;110:1294.

Chang JB: Current state of extra-anatomic bypasses. Am J Surg 1986;152:202.

Christenson JT et al: The late results after axillo-femoral bypass grafts in patients with leg ischaemia. J Cardiovasc Surg (Torino) 1986;27:131.

Courbier R, Jausseran JM, Bergeron P: Axillo-femoral bypass material of choice. In: *Extra-anatomic Secondary Arterial Reconstruction.* Greenhalgh RM (editor). Pitman Press, 1982.

Dé P, Hepp W: Present role of extraanatomic bypass graft procedures for aortoiliac occlusive disease. Int Angiol 1991;10:224.

Dick LS et al: A 12-year experience with femorofemoral crossover grafts. Arch Surg 1980;115:1359.

Donaldson MC, Louras JC, Buckham CA: Axillofemoral bypass: A tool with a limited role. J Vasc Surg 1986;3:757.

El-Massry S et al: Axillofemoral bypass with externally supported, knitted Dacron grafts: A follow-up through twelve years. J Vasc Surg 1993;17:107.

Eugene J, Goldstone J, Moore WS: Fifteen-year experience with subcutaneous bypass grafts for lower extremity ischemia. Ann Surg 1977;186:177.

Fahal AH, McDonald AM, Marston A: Femorofemoral bypass in unilateral iliac artery occlusion. Br J Surg 1989;76:22.

Flanigan DP et al: Hemodynamic and angiographic guidelines in selection of patients for femorofemoral bypass. Arch Surg 1978;113:1257.

Foster, MC: A review of 155 extra-anatomic bypass grafts. Ann R Coll Surg Engl 1986;68:1.

Freeman NE, Leeds FH: Operations on large arteries. Calif Med 1952;77:229.

Ghilardi G, Bortolani EM, D'Armini A: The femorofemoral bypass graft: Report of a 11-year experience. Panminerva Med 1990;32:71.

Harrington ME et al: Iliofemoral versus femorofemoral bypass: The case for an individualized approach. J Vasc Surg 1992;16:841.

Harris EJ et al: Clinical results of axillobifemoral bypass using externally supported polytetrafluoroethylene. J Vasc Surg 1990;12:416.

Hepp W, deJonge K, Pallua N: Late results following extra-anatomic bypass procedures for chronic aortoiliac occlusive disease. J Cardiovasc Surg 1988;29:181.

Hill DA, Lord RSA, Tracy GD: Haemodynamic consequences of cross femoral bypass. In: *Extra-anatomic and Secondary Reconstruction.* Greenhalgh RM (editor). Pitman Press, 1982.

Johnson WC et al: Is axillo-bilateral femoral grafts an effective substitute for aortic-bilateral iliac-femoral graft? Ann Surg 1977;186:123.

Kenny, DA et al: Comparison of noncrimped, externally supported (EXS) and crimped, nonsupported Dacron prostheses for axillofemoral and above knee femoropopliteal bypass. Surgery 1982;92:931.

Kretschmer G et al: Groin infections following vascular surgery: Obturator bypass (BYP) versus "biologic coverage" (TRP): A comparative analysis. Eur J Vasc Surg 1989;3:25.

Lamerton A et al: Selection for long-term results of femorofemoral bypass. In: *Extra-anatomic and Secondary Reconstruction.* Greenhalgh RM (editor). Pitman Press, 1982.

Lewis CD: A subclavian artery as a means of blood supply to the lower half of the body. Br J Surg 1961;48:574.

Livesay JJ et al: Late results of extra-anatomic bypass. Arch Surg 1979;114:1260.

LoGerfo FW et al: A comparison of the late patency rates of axillobilateral femoral and axillounilateral femoral grafts. Surgery 1977;81:33.

Mason RA et al: Alternative procedures to aortobifemoral bypass grafting. J Cardiovasc Surg 1989;30:192.

McCarthy WJ et al: Descending thoracic aorta-to-femoral artery bypass: Ten years' experience with a durable procedure. J Vasc Surg 1993;17:336.

McCaughan JJ Jr, Kahn SF: Crossover graft for unilateral occlusive disease of the iliofemoral arteries. Ann Surg 1960; 151:26.

Moore WS, Hall, AD, Blaisdell FW: Late results of axillary-femoral bypass grafting. Am J Surg 1971;122;148.

Naylor AR, Ah-See AK, Engeset J: Axillofemoral bypass as a limb salvage procedure in high risk patients with aortoiliac disease. Br J Surg 1990;77:659.

Nevelsteen A et al: Obturator bypass: A sixteen year experience with 55 cases. Ann Vasc Surg 1987;1:558.

Pietri P et al: Long term results of extra anatomical bypasses. Int Angiol 1987;6:429.

Raithel D, Meier H: Analysis and follow-up of 186 alternative bypasses. J Cardiovasc Surg (Torino) 1981;22:281.

Ray LI et al: Axillofemoral bypass: A critical reappraisal of its role in the management of aortoiliac occlusive disease. Am J Surg 1979;138:117.

Rutherford RB, Patt A, Pearce WH: Extra-anatomic bypass: A closer view. J Vasc Surg 1987;6:437.

Savrin RA, Record GT, McDowell DE: Axillofemoral bypass: Expectations and results. Arch Surg 1986;121:1016.

Schulz GA, Sauvage LR, Mathisen SR: A five to seven year experience with externally supported Dacron prostheses in axillofemoral and femoropopliteal bypass. Ann Vasc Surg 1986;1:214.

Self SB et al: Utility of femorofemoral bypass: Comparison of results with indications for operation. Am Surg 1991; 57:602.

Shaw RS, Baue AE: Management of sepsis complicating arterial reconstructive surgery. Surgery 1963;53:75.

Sheiner NM: Peripheral vascular surgery: Alternate anatomical pathways and the use of allograft veins as arterial substitutes. In: *Current Problems in Surgery: Arterial Infection.* Wilson SE, van Wagenen P, Passaro E Jr (editors). YearBook Medical Publishers, 1978.

Subram AN et al: Femorofemoral bypass: Prognostic factors. Tex Heart Inst J 1983;10:257.

Taylor LM et al: Acute disruption of PTFE grafts adjacent to axillary anastomoses. Presented at the Western Vascular Society Meeting, January 1994 (in press).

Taylor LM et al: Axillofemoral grafting with externally supported polytetafluoroethylene (PTFE). Presented at the Western Surgical Association Meeting, November 1993 (in press).

Vetto RM: The treatment of unilateral iliac artery obstruction utilizing femoro-femoral graft. Surgery 1962;52:342.

Wittens CHA, van Houtte HJKP, van Urk H: European prospective randomised multi-center axillo-bifemoral trial. Eur J Vasc Surg 1992;6:115.

Femoropopliteal Occlusive Disease **29**

William D. Suggs, MD, Frank J. Veith, MD, & Kurt R. Wengerter, MD, RVT, FACS

Essentials of Diagnosis

- Intermittent calf claudication.
- Rest pain.
- Disabling claudication.
- Gangrene.
- Ulcerations in diabetics.

General Considerations

Femoropopliteal occlusive disease most frequently results from atherosclerotic narrowing of the superficial femoral and popliteal arteries. Stenoses usually develop gradually and are accompanied by the formation of extensive collaterals between the deep femoral and the popliteal arteries. As a result, most patients with femoropopliteal occlusive disease are asymptomatic; thus, the prevalence of the disease in the general population is difficult to evaluate. Intermittent claudication occurs in 3–5% of men over the age of 50 years. These figures clearly underestimate the true prevalence of femoropopliteal occlusive disease. More accurate estimates are obtained by using noninvasive tests, which have found disease in 12–36% of the population, depending on the type of test performed and the age of the patient.

Intermittent calf claudication is the most common symptom associated with femoropopliteal occlusive disease, and it generally represents a short segmental occlusion of the superficial femoral artery. Rest pain, disabling claudication, and gangrene are evidence of more extensive occlusions with hemodynamically significant lesions at the aortoiliac and femoropopliteal levels or either of these occlusions combined with infrapopliteal disease.

Surgical intervention is indicated for limb-threatening ischemia or severe claudication. As the average age of the population increases, the incidence and manifestations of femoropopliteal disease can be expected to increase unless there is a decrease in risk factors such as smoking, hypertension, hyperlipidemia, and diabetes mellitus.

Clinical Findings

A. Signs and Symptoms:

1. Claudication–Because the reserve of the human arterial system is extensive, hemodynamically significant stenoses can exist in the arterial tree with no or only minimal symptoms. This is particularly true when collateral pathways are normal or the patient's activity level is limited by other disease processes. **Intermittent claudication** is defined as a pain or a cramp in the calf with ambulation that is relieved by rest. Mild calf claudication occurring at several blocks is usually associated with a segmental occlusion of the popliteal or superficial femoral artery. Claudication can also be described as a sense of pressure, heaviness, or fatigue, and it may be mistakenly diagnosed as a neuromuscular disorder.

Claudication-like symptoms can be produced by spinal stenosis or by lesions compressing the spinal cord or cauda equina. Neurologic problems can coexist with arterial occlusive disease, making it difficult to determine the cause of a patient's pain. In such circumstances, angiography, computed tomography (CT), or magnetic resonance imaging (MRI) and even myelography of the lumbar spine may be necessary.

2. Rest pain–Ischemic rest pain is experienced as an ache in the distal portion of the foot, which becomes severe at night when the patient is supine. Significant rest pain is associated with decreased pulses as well as other signs of ischemia such as atrophy, decreased temperature, marked rubor, and pain relief with dependency. Many patients with significant arterial lesions have pain at rest from other causes, such as neuritis or arthritis.

3. Gangrene–Gangrenous lesions usually occur in the distal portion of the foot, but they may occur anywhere. These lesions frequently arise after minor trauma and can be found in areas subject to pressure, such as the heel or the skin overlying the metatarsophalangeal joint. Other causes of these lesions must also be considered. Venous ulceration is characterized by lesions that are relatively painless and that typically occur on the ankle; they are associated with other evidence of venous stasis such as hyperpigmentation and dermatitis. Decubitus lesions caused by pressure may give rise to ulceration or gangrene in the presence of good perfusion of the foot. These lesions occur on the heel posteriorly or laterally, and they can be expected to heal with proper wound care, which includes complete avoidance of pressure on the affected area.

4. Ulcerations–Neurotrophic ulcerations are most commonly seen in diabetics. Typically, their location is over pressure points, that is, the plantar surface at the metatarsal head and the dorsum of toes with flexion contractures. Such ulcerations can be difficult to heal unless the pressure causing the ulceration is completely relieved. Local infection may be the sole or contributing cause of lesions of the foot, including gangrene. This can occur when local effects of the infection cause small vessel thrombosis; this is particularly true in diabetics. Local treatment of the infection with excision and drainage of all involved tissues is necessary for a successful outcome and in most cases should precede attempts at revascularization.

5. Ischemic toes–Ischemic black or blue toes may occur as the result of an embolic event. Such emboli can originate from the heart, a proximal aneurysm, or any proximal atherosclerotic lesion. In the latter circumstance, small cholesterol, platelet, or fibrin emboli may lodge in interosseous or digital arteries. Peripheral pulses may be normal, and spontaneous improvement of the resulting blue toe often occurs. This sequence of events has been termed the **blue toe syndrome.** If a single, dominant arterial lesion can be identified by angiography, it should be treated by endarterectomy or an appropriate bypass. These source lesions are most common in the larger proximal arteries, although they may also occur in the superficial femoral or popliteal arteries.

6. Embolus–Major emboli from the heart or a proximal aneurysm may cause varying degrees of ischemia, depending on where they lodge and the amount of existing atherosclerosis and collateral circulation. These emboli frequently lodge at sites in which the vessel caliber decreases due to a bifurcation or atherosclerotic disease. These locations include the common femoral bifurcation, the distal superficial femoral artery in the adductor canal, and the distal popliteal artery at the anterior tibial occurrence. The common occurrence of significant peripheral vascular disease makes the diagnosis and treatment of embolic disease difficult. The only certain diagnostic feature of embolus is multiplicity.

Furthermore, the location of the embolus may be atypical, and the vascular surgeon treating a presumed embolus in the presence of widespread atherosclerosis must be prepared to perform an extensive arterial reconstruction or bypass even if the operation is undertaken soon after the acute event. For these reasons and because acute thrombosis cannot always be differentiated from embolus, complete preoperative angiography should be mandatory in any suspected embolic occlusion of the lower extremity in a patient who could have arteriosclerosis.

Exploration of the distal popliteal artery is usually the best surgical approach for patients with severe ischemia due to an acute occlusion of the popliteal or distal superficial femoral arteries. This allows for removal of clot from the proximal vessels as well as complete embolectomy of the 3 calf vessels.

B. Physical Examination: The findings on physical examination of the involved extremity contribute to the staging of the atherosclerotic process and provide a rough guide as to whether or not diagnostic or therapeutic intervention is needed. Discoloration and swelling should provide evidence of the presence and extent of infection in the involved foot. As a general rule, the extent of infection and necrosis deep to the skin is greater than might be expected from an examination of the skin. Exploration of suspicious areas can sometimes be carried out without anesthesia if the patient has diminished sensation from diabetic neuropathy. Otherwise, such exploration and necessary débridement should be performed in the operating room under anesthesia.

In the initial examination of a patient with suspected arterial disease, careful inspection for operative scars is essential because patients may be unaware of the nature and extent of previous arterial surgery. The site of scars can provide clues as to whether the arteries below the knee were violated, whether ipsilateral saphenous vein was used, and, if so, how much is left.

Physical examination can also reveal associated chronic disease. In evaluating an ischemic limb, particular attention must be given to careful inspection of the heel and between the toes where unsuspected ischemic ulcers or infection may be present. A flashlight is extremely helpful in this regard. The uninvolved extremity must also be carefully examined. Because of the symmetry of atherosclerosis, the opposite extremity may harbor unsuspected ischemic lesions. Moreover, findings such as coolness and bluish discoloration are far more meaningful if they are asymmetric, since cool or dusky extremities may sometimes be present without major arterial disease.

C. Pulse Examination: Pulse examination of the lower extremities in a patient with suspected ischemia is extremely important. This requires considerable experience and must be performed carefully and with proper technique. The strength of a pulse as assessed by an experienced examiner is a valuable semiquantitative assessment of the arterial circulation at that level.

In examining a patient with diminished pulses, it is extremely helpful to count the pulse to an assistant who is palpating the patient's radial pulse to ensure that the examiner is not feeling his or her own pulse or spurious muscular activity. Before describing a pulse as being absent, considerable time and effort must be expended and ectopic localization of pulses such as the lateral tarsal artery pulse must be examined. In this era of too frequently performed noninvasive arterial tests, the value of a carefully performed and recorded pulse examination cannot be overemphasized. It provides a basis for comparison if subsequent disease progression occurs, and it is a simple way of accurately assessing the arterial circulation in the lower extremities at a given point in time. Pulse examination also provides an indicator of the type of approach that will be required to save a threatened foot.

D. Noninvasive and Imaging Tests:

1. Segmental pressures and plethysmography–Segmental arterial pressures and pulse-volume (plethysmographic) recordings are the 2 noninvasive modalities most commonly used for the initial evaluation of lower extremity ischemia. Segmental arterial pressure measurements use standard pressure cuffs as well as a continuous-wave Doppler probe to determine systolic pressure at various levels, including the thigh, knee, calf, and ankle. These tests are useful since they provide an objective, semiquantitative measure of the circulation and help to confirm the diagnosis made by the history and physical examination. In some instances, they can also provide an estimate of the level of the occlusive lesion, identifying infrainguinal disease in addition to the femoropopliteal disease. Segmental arterial pressures and plethysmography are unreliable, however, for localization of lesions above the inguinal ligament, since decreased thigh pressures and pulse-volume waveforms may be associated entirely with disease below the inguinal ligament as well as with aortoiliac disease.

Noninvasive testing can also be helpful in predicting the likelihood of healing foot lesions. Pressures below 55 mmHg and pulse-volume recording amplitudes less than 5–10 mm are frequently associated with poor healing, and in most cases a revascularization procedure is required. In rare cases, healing has occurred in association with poor pressures and pulse-volume recordings. However, the risk of extension of the necrosis makes prolonged observation risky in such cases. Because segmental arterial pressures and plethysmography do not evaluate the severity or extent of infection, the opposite is not always true. Good forefoot pulse waves and ankle pressures do not guarantee healing of foot wounds, although they suggest that it will occur if infection can be eliminated. Furthermore, there is a gray zone of intermediate values in which the noninvasive tests are of little predictive value, and a therapeutic trial with a local procedure such as a débridement or toe amputation is appropriate.

Not infrequently, results of noninvasive tests are normal at rest in patients with claudication. This occurs when the flow past mild-to-moderate stenoses is able to meet the demands of muscles at rest but not during exertion when the metabolic demands of the calf muscle cause a marked vasodilatation and increase in flow, which produce a decrease in pressure and pulse-volume amplitude. This effect can be induced by having the patient walk with or without the use of a treadmill. Alternatively, temporary application of a tourniquet for 3–7 minutes, which induces hyperemia on release, can also produce a drop in ankle pressure that correlates with stress testing results.

Arterial calcification frequently exists in diabetics, especially those on hemodialysis, and it is common at the crural level. When calcification is thick and circumferential, these vessels are difficult to compress with the external pressure cuff, and falsely high segmental pressure measurements result. Air plethysmography (pulse-volume recording) remains accurate under these circumstances, since it does not depend on compression of the vessel for its measurement; therefore, it is the preferred method for assessing diabetic patients.

2. Duplex scanning–Duplex scanning has been used increasingly to assess disease in iliac, femoral, and popliteal arteries prior to more invasive studies. These studies have been aided by the introduction of color Doppler imaging of flow, which allows more rapid intonation of the vessels, and by the availability of deep probes, which allow visualization of the iliac vessels. The information obtained from these studies can be used to determine the suitability of the arteries for iliac or superficial femoral angioplasty.

The duplex scanner has also been used to evaluate the greater saphenous as well as other veins prior to bypass surgery. Information obtained from this study includes anatomic definition of the course of the vein, determination of its size and data on vein quality, including wall thickness and patency. The scan is especially helpful for finding usable vein—including arm and lesser saphenous—prior to secondary operations. Duplex scanning can also be used to map the course of the vein on the skin with a marking pen to aid in the operative dissection.

E. Angiography: As in other areas of vascular surgery, proper high-quality arteriography is essential to make an assessment of the extent of arteriosclerosis and to determine whether therapeutic intervention is possible. It also allows planning of the optimal form that this intervention should take. In addition, adequate arteriography defines the localization and extent of arteriosclerotic involvement in the infrarenal aorta and iliac arteries, which can be supplemented by direct pressure measurements taken at the time of arteriography to assess the hemodynamic significance of isolated stenoses.

To provide adequate information about the infrainguinal arterial system, the arterial tree from the groin to the forefoot should be well visualized in continuity, preferably by the transfemoral route. Oblique views may be required to completely visualize the origin and proximal portion of the deep femoral artery. Good preoperative distal artery visualization is the key to performing optimal bypass surgery to arteries in the foot and lower leg. Reactive hyperemia, digitally augmented views, and delayed films may be necessary to achieve the needed visualization, although in our recent experience these measures were rarely required. Although others have advocated intraoperative arteriography to achieve this end, we have found it less effective and very rarely necessary.

Magnetic resonance angiography has provided preoperative evaluation of patent distal leg and foot arteries without the need for dye injection. However, these techniques are not widely available.

F. Evaluation of Systemic Factors: In addition to evaluation of the involved extremities, the assessment of systemic factors is essential in the candidate for invasive treatment of femoropopliteal occlusive disease. These factors include all those in the history, physical examination, and routine laboratory tests that might indicate major organ failure. Most important is evidence of heart disease, diabetes, renal insufficiency, hypertension, chronic pulmonary, and cerebrovascular disease. These intercurrent diseases, which are frequently present in this group of patients, require appropriate medical management before, during, and after diagnostic and therapeutic intervention so that the risks will be minimized.

Because most patients with infrainguinal arteriosclerosis also have some degree of coronary involvement and because myocardial infarction is the principal cause of early and late postoperative mortality in this patient group, evidence of myocardial ischemia and congestive failure must be sought. Clinical risk factors, including a history of myocardial infarction, congestive heart failure, unstable angina, abnormalities on electrocardiogram (ECG), diabetes mellitus, and advanced age (over 70 years), have been shown to pinpoint the patient at increased risk for postoperative cardiac events. Patients with at least 2 of these risk factors should undergo a noninvasive preoperative test such as dipyridamole-thallium scintigraphy or continuous portable ECG monitoring for evaluation of significant coronary artery disease. These tests serve to identify those who should be subjected to coronary arteriography and considered for aortocoronary bypass prior to being treated for limb ischemia.

Patients with recent myocardial infarctions, congestive heart failure, low ventricular ejection fractions, or severe renal dysfunction should receive a Swan-Ganz catheter and have their fluid and volume replacement optimized before, during, and after operation on the basis of appropriate cardiac output and pressure measurements. Renal function should also be repeatedly monitored after any angiographic procedure, because transient renal failure is not uncommon. If detected and appropriately treated, transient renal failure is almost always reversible and is rarely a serious problem, although it may delay operative intervention.

G. Inflow Disease: Disease of the aortoiliac vessels is often concomitantly present and must be addressed if reconstruction of the occluded femoropopliteal segment is to be successful. When symptoms of claudication or rest pain are the indication for the procedure, it is advisable to correct the aortoiliac obstruction first, even in the presence of a superficial femoral artery or popliteal occlusion. The extremity is then observed for relief of the symptoms before treatment of the femoropopliteal occlusion is attempted, since correction of the more proximal disease may be sufficient. However, when more extensive lesions such as infection and gangrene are present, both the aortoiliac and femoropopliteal level occlusions should be corrected without delay.

Evaluation for Type of Treatment

Patients presenting with femoropopliteal stenosis or occlusion who are asymptomatic do not require intervention other than to modify their risk factors such as smoking, diet, and exercise. Those presenting with minimal symptoms or intermittent claudication (after walking more than 1 block) should be treated conservatively. A cautious approach appears to be clearly justified in light of the numerous reports of the benign nature and slow progression of disease to more advanced stages in this group of patients. Without treatment, 10–15% of patients with claudication will improve over 5 years, and 60–70% will remain stable. Those who do worsen are best treated with a primary operation after their disease progresses.

Patients with disabling claudication (after walking 1/2 block) should be considered for intervention except in the presence of severe surgical risk factors such as severe pulmonary or cardiac disease. The presence of ischemic rest pain, a nonhealing ulcer, or gangrene is usually sufficient indication for arteriography and surgical intervention. When the patient has reached these stages, it is likely that a significant segment of the superficial femoral artery is involved, probably with other segments of disease proximally in the iliac arteries or distally in the crural vessels.

The presence of gangrene deep in the tarsal region or destruction of more than two-thirds of the plantar surface of the foot indicates that the foot cannot be salvaged. An above-knee femoropopliteal reconstruction or profundoplasty may still be advised if deemed necessary for healing of a below-knee amputation. Patients with severe organic mental syndrome resulting in inability to ambulate, communicate, or provide self-care also are not candidates for reconstruction and should undergo primary above-knee amputation.

If a patient with a gangrenous toe lesion has a pedal pulse, local treatment without reconstructive arterial surgery is usually the correct approach to achieve a healed foot, although there are rare exceptions. If a patient with an ischemic foot lesion has a normal popliteal pulse but no pedal pulses, some form of infrapopliteal or small vessel bypass is almost always the correct approach to obtain a healed foot. If a patient with an ischemic foot lesion has a normal ipsilateral femoral pulse without distal pulses, some form of infrainguinal arterial reconstruction, probably a femoropopliteal bypass, would be the correct approach to achieve a healed foot. When such a patient has a diminished femoral pulse, often with an associated bruit, some form of proximal arterial reconstruction or angioplasty above the inguinal ligament is almost certainly required.

Often, occlusive disease of the iliac vessels can be successfully treated with percutaneous angioplasty, in most cases at the time of the initial angiography. Five-year patency results with iliac angioplasty range from 59% to 85%, and the best results occur with discrete, single, short lesions (smaller than 3 cm); these results are similar to those for surgical treatment (>85% 5-year patency). The results are usually worse with multiple, more extensive lesions or occlusions. The recent availability of stents may further improve results, especially when redilatation of a lesion is needed.

When disease of the aortoiliac segment is more extensive and treatment with percutaneous transluminal angioplasty is not appropriate, a surgical procedure to provide inflow to the femoral level becomes necessary. Surgical procedures to treat the aortoiliac disease include aortobifemoral, aortoiliac, and axillofemoral bypasses. Patency rates for the aortobifemoral bypass far exceed those for the axillofemoral bypass (>80% compared with <50% at 5 years). However, when the patient is a poor medical risk, the axillofemoral bypass is a reasonable alternative.

Another option when simultaneous bypass of aortoiliac and femoropopliteal disease is necessary is an aortounifemoral bypass. Frequently, disease of the contralateral iliac artery is not extensive. In this situation, an aortounifemoral bypass can provide inflow to the femoral level with excellent patency results. Also, since this bypass involves less extensive surgery, it facilitates the performance of the femoropopliteal procedure at the same sitting.

Conservative Treatment

Conservative therapy is usually used for patients with intermittent claudication. It consists primarily of 3 components: cessation of smoking, exercise, and, in some cases, a trial of pentoxifylline.

A. Smoking Cessation: The relation between cigarette smoking and femoropopliteal disease, and more specifically claudication, is well recognized and is likely to be related to a variety of effects. At a chronic level of disease, smoking is known to stimulate atherogenesis and affect platelet function, lipid metabolism, and endothelial function. At an acute level, it is known to increase vasoconstriction and carbon monoxide blood levels. The clinical benefits of cessation of smoking not only are related to a decrease in intermittent claudication symptoms demonstrated by an increased walking distance but are also associated with improved graft patency and improved limb salvage.

B. Exercise: In patients with intermittent claudication, exercise is an effective means of improving the pain-free walking distance. Most patients report an improvement in walking distance after a regular exercise program is followed. The assumption that such improvement is a result of an increase in the collateral circulation around the obstruction may not be correct. Most studies indicate that exercise training leads to adaptive changes within the muscle, such as more effective extraction of oxygen from the blood.

C. Drug Therapy: The third conservative modality for the treatment of intermittent claudication is pharmacologic therapy. Vasodilator drugs, including prostaglandins, have not consistently been shown to be effective in the management of lower extremity obstructive disease. Only pentoxifylline, a hemorrheologic agent, has demonstrated some ability to reduce claudication symptoms. Its major effect is decreased platelet aggregation and increased red cell deformability. Although pentoxifylline has been shown to be effective in reducing the symptoms of claudication in a number of trials, it usually improved the symptom-free walking distance by only 50%. In most cases, this level of improvement is not perceived as a satisfactory endpoint by the patient and by the physician. A reasonable approach to the use of this drug is to reserve its application until after an adequate trial of smoking cessation and exercise therapy. If there is no improvement or only minimal improvement after a 6–8-week trial, pentoxifylline should be discontinued. Remember that pentoxifylline has not been demonstrated to be effective for the treatment of rest pain, ischemic ulcerations, or gangrene, and it cannot be recommended for these indications until adequate randomized trials have clearly demonstrated its efficacy.

Invasive Treatment

A. Angioplasty: Percutaneous transluminal angioplasty (PTA) is now recognized as an important tool in the management of patients with lower extremity peripheral vascular disease, especially in the iliac arteries, where the results achieved with treatment of selected lesions approaches the results achieved with aortobifemoral bypass. The results with femoral and popliteal artery angioplasty have been less promising, and 5-year patency rates ranging from 17% to 68% have been reported. However, improved long-term patency rates can be obtained with proper selection of cases, and 5-year patency rates as high as 70% can be expected with the dilatation of short (<3 cm) lesions with good run-off. The advantages of PTA over surgery include shorter hospital stay, lower morbidity and mortality, and lower cost. The implications of a failed angioplasty are also less ominous than those of a failed bypass graft, since few patients are rendered worse than their preintervention level. Thus, angioplasty can be useful for the treatment of symptomatic short lesions in the femoropopliteal vessels.

Although surgery clearly yields better results than PTA in patients with more extensive disease, especially when the limb is at risk, PTA is an alternative that can be used cautiously when the risk of surgery is prohibitive.

B. Femoropopliteal Bypass: Patients with disabling claudication, gangrene, or rest pain or those whose limbs are clearly threatened should undergo a femoropopliteal bypass when the superficial femoral or popliteal artery is continuous with any of its 3 terminal branches. This is true even if one or more of these branches ends in an occlusion more distally in the leg. Even if the popliteal artery segment into which the graft is to be inserted is occluded distally, femoropopliteal bypass with vein to this isolated segment should be considered. If the isolated popliteal segment is less than 7 cm in length or if there is extensive gangrene or infection in the foot, a femorodistal artery bypass should be considered. All femoropopliteal artery bypasses can be classified on the basis of their relation to the knee joint and run-off from the popliteal artery as determined radiographically (Fig 29–1).

Femoropopliteal Bypass Technique

A. Grafts:

1. Upper extremity veins–The cephalic and basilic veins from the upper extremities have been advocated for use as a graft when lower extremity autologous vein is unavailable. Although the work of Schulman and Badhey suggests that arm veins are inferior to the saphenous vein in infrainguinal bypasses, more recent observations indicate that the cephalic vein can be used with good success in lower extremity arterial reconstructions. However, arm veins are typically thinner walled and more difficult to work with than the saphenous vein. Moreover, arm veins can have frequent fibrotic, recanalized segments from previous trauma and venipunctures. When several healthy segments are joined to form a composite graft, poorer patency results.

Based on these observations as well as the high degree of symmetry in infrainguinal arteriosclerosis, use of a prosthetic graft in the femoropopliteal position is presently justified if the ipsilateral saphenous vein is unsuitable or unavailable.

2. Umbilical vein–Although we believe that polytetrafluoroethylene (PTFE) grafts are the best currently available alternative arterial prosthetic if the ipsilateral autologous saphenous vein is not available for femoropopliteal bypasses, other grafts have also been used with some success. The tanned umbilical vein graft has received the greatest attention, and patency rates similar to those of PTFE grafts have been reported in both the femoropopliteal and the infrapopliteal positions. However, no adequate randomized comparison of the 2 grafts has been completed. The reports of a high incidence of aneurysmal degeneration occurring in umbilical vein grafts after even a few years are worrisome and suggest that this graft be used with caution even though the manufacturers have recently strengthened the external Dacron mesh.

3. PTFE graft–The exact role of PTFE in infrainguinal arterial bypass surgery remains controversial. For patients who require a bypass to the above-knee popliteal artery, some surgeons preferentially use PTFE grafts to preserve the saphenous vein for potential later use. On the other hand, some have adhered to a policy of using only autologous vein for infrainguinal bypasses. For the last decade, our attitude about choosing an infrainguinal graft has tended to be intermediate between these 2 positions. Autologous vein can generally be used for most infrainguinal arterial reconstructions if the patient has a good ipsilateral greater saphenous vein. However, we perform a primary femoropopliteal bypass with PTFE when the ipsilateral saphenous vein is diseased or has been previously harvested. Elderly or debilitated patients with limited life expectancies may benefit from a less complex operation and are candidates for a bypass using PTFE.

The patency of infrainguinal PTFE bypass grafts is clearly related to the location of the distal anastomosis. In 1986, a large, randomized, prospective trial comparing autologous saphenous vein to PTFE grafts in all infrainguinal bypass operations was completed. Equivalent patency rates at 2 years were noted for autologous vein and PTFE grafts to the popliteal artery at the same level; thereafter, patency diverged and the difference became significant after 4 years with a patency of 68 plus/minus 8% for autologous vein versus 47 plus/minus 9% for PTFE. The differences in the 4-year patency rates were not statistically significant for above-knee grafts, but they were for below-knee grafts as illustrated in Figure 29–2.

In a large, retrospective review reported by the surgical group from UCLA, primary femoropopliteal bypasses done preferentially with PTFE had a 5-year patency rate of 61.5%. These investigators base their recommendations to use PTFE grafts on their superior patency results with autologous veins for secondary femoropopliteal bypasses and their poor results with PTFE grafts in this setting. In general, femoropopliteal

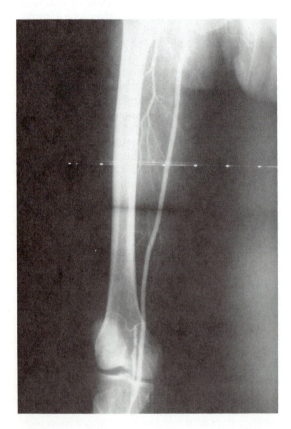

Figure 29–1. Angiogram of a common femoral to below-knee popliteal artery bypass performed with 6-mm PTFE.

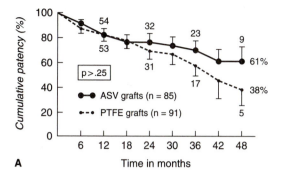

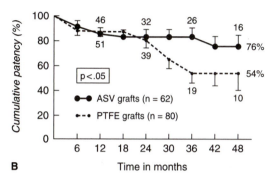

Figure 29–2. Cumulative life-table primary patency rates for all randomized autologous saphenous vein (ASV) and expanded polytetrafluoroethylene (PTFE) bypasses performed to the popliteal artery. **A:** Above knee. **B:** Below knee. Number with each point indicates number of patent grafts observed for that length of time. Standard error of each point is shown. (Reproduced, with permission, from Veith FJ et al: Six-year prospective multicenter randomized comparison of autologous saphenous vein and expanded polytetrafluoroethylene grafts in infrainguinal arterial reconstructions. J Vasc Surg 1986;3:109.)

bypasses should be performed preferentially when a patient's ipsilateral greater saphenous vein is of good quality.

B. Procedure: All operations are performed with the patient under general or epidural anesthesia. Intraoperative monitoring includes intra-arterial pressure measurements, digital pulse oximetry, and selective use of pulmonary artery wedge pressure measurement.

If the proximal superficial femoral artery is patent as documented on angiography (including oblique views of its origin), it is considered a satisfactory inflow site. This allows for the incision to be made in the thigh rather than in the groin and can result in a shorter bypass graft. When the common femoral artery is used as inflow, a vertical incision is made in the groin. Dissection is carried down to the artery directed by palpation, and proximal and distal control of the vessel are obtained. Exposure is optimized by the use of mechanical retraction.

For the above-knee popliteal artery bypass, the distal incision is made medially in the thigh, posterior to the adductor magnus muscle and anterior to the sartorius. Dissection is carried through the fascial layer into the popliteal fossa. Care must be taken to avoid injury to the greater saphenous vein when prosthetic material is being used. The neurovascular bundle is found just lateral in the popliteal fossa. The above-knee popliteal artery down to the mid- or upper patella level, as viewed on the angiogram, can easily be approached through this incision.

The below-knee incision is also made on the medial aspect, and the gastrocnemius muscle is retracted posteriorly so that the popliteal fossa can be entered (Fig 29–3). The neurovascular bundle containing the popliteal artery is readily identified as it passes behind the soleus muscle. Grafts placed to the below-knee popliteal artery are tunneled anatomically through the popliteal fossa between the heads of the gastrocnemius muscle. From the above-knee popliteal fossa, the graft is tunneled through a subsartorial plane into the groin.

Anastomoses are meticulously constructed with continuous 6-0 polypropylene sutures, with particular care to take small, evenly spaced bites of *all* layers of the vessel wall. As a rule, the distal anastomosis is performed first to permit the greatest freedom of movement and positioning of the graft during the more technically demanding anastomosis.

The proximal anastomosis is placed into the common femoral, superficial femoral, or deep femoral artery. Intraoperative angiographic examination is performed only when there is concern regarding the graft quality, the anastomosis, or the outflow tract. It is especially important when the graft pulse is decreased or when an expected distal pulse, based on the preoperative angiogram, is absent.

Harvest of the greater saphenous vein is usually begun in the groin or at its junction with the common femoral vein. Multiple skin incisions are made directly over the vein, and care is taken not to develop skin flaps. Branches are ligated 1–2 mm from the vein to prevent constricting adventitial bands. The vein is handled gently, and the desired length is excised and placed in a cold buffered physiologic solution. It is then carefully inspected and gently dilated to note the external diameter. A catheter is passed through the lumen to ensure continuous patency. Veins with calcified intraluminal plaques, scars, or occlusions or with an external diameter of less than 3.0 mm do not provide reliable patency, and a prosthetic graft such as PTFE should be used instead.

Graft Surveillance

Over the last 10 years, we have been able to detect about 190 failing grafts and have corrected the lesions before graft thrombosis has occurred. Invariably, the corrective procedure is simpler than the secondary operation that would be required if the bypass went on to become thrombosed. Vein grafts tend to fail as the re-

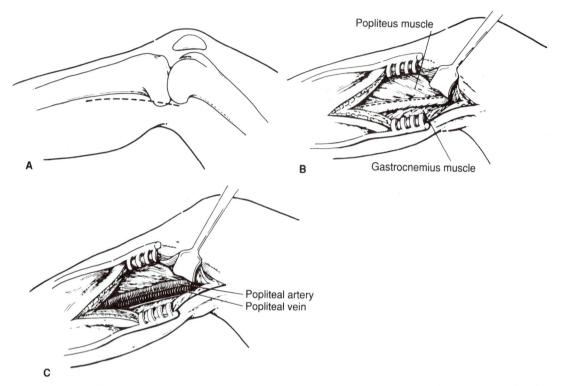

Figure 29–3. **A:** Medial incision for exposure of the below-knee popliteal artery. **B:** The crural fascia are incised and the medial head of the gastrocnemius is separated from the tibia and popliteal muscles to open the popliteal space. **C:** The popliteal vein is freed from the posterior aspect of the tibia exposing the popliteal artery.

sult of hyperplastic lesions associated with the body or anastomotic areas of the graft. By contrast, PTFE grafts tend to fail as the result of proximal or distal progression of atherosclerotic disease.

Solitary vein graft lesions of 15 mm or less can be treated by PTA. Longer or multiple vein graft lesions should be treated by an interposition graft or a proximal or distal graft extension, depending on the lesion location. Some PTAs of these lesions have failed, necessitating a second intervention; others have remained effective in correcting the responsible lesion, as documented by arteriography more than 2–5 years later. If the failing graft is a vein bypass, detection of the failing state permits accurate localization and definition of the responsible lesion by arteriography as well as salvage of any undiseased vein.

In contrast, if the graft is allowed to become thrombosed, the responsible lesion may be difficult to identify; the vein may be difficult or impossible to thrombectomize; and the patient's best graft, the ipsilateral greater saphenous vein, may have to be sacrificed, rendering the secondary operation even more difficult and more likely to fail with associated limb loss. More important, the results of reinterventions for failing grafts, in terms of both continued cumulative patency and limb salvage rates, have been far superior

to the results of reinterventions for grafts that have thrombosed and failed.

The inflow and outflow arterial lesions responsible for the failing state of PTFE grafts can be treated with PTA when they are short occlusions (3–5 cm) or stenoses. Longer or more complex lesions require a graft extension to either above or below the responsible lesion.

The improved results associated with reintervention for failing grafts mandate that surgeons performing bypass operations follow up their patients closely in the postoperative period and indefinitely thereafter. Ideally, noninvasive laboratory tests, including duplex studies, should be performed just as frequently. If the patient has any recurrence of symptoms or if the surgeon detects any change in the peripheral pulse examination or other manifestations of ischemia, the circulatory deterioration must be confirmed by noninvasive parameters and urgent arteriography.

Reoperation

Early graft failure (within 30 days of operation) is generally due to a technical flaw in the operation or poor choice of inflow or outflow sites. Vein grafts that fail immediately after operation may require replacement with PTFE, although in our experience an occasional thrombectomized vein graft remains patent when no causal lesion is present. However with PTFE, early graft thrombosis is not always related to easily defined anatomic problems and may be related to the inherent thrombogenicity of the PTFE graft itself or to a transient fall in cardiac output. An aggressive treatment of these early occlusions is justified. After an early graft thrombosis, the patient should be returned promptly to the operating room for graft thrombectomy and intraoperative arteriogram for examination of the distal anastomosis for technical problems or distal stenotic or occlusive lesions that were not appreciated on the original arteriogram. These reoperations with correction of any technical problems or residual lesions can result in good long-term patency and limb salvage.

As already noted, failed grafts may be secondary to either progression of atherosclerotic disease or anastomotic intimal hyperplasia. If late failure is accompanied by a threatened limb, reintervention should be undertaken. Prior to operation, a new complete arteriogram should be performed to examine for progression of inflow or outflow disease. If this reveals the cause of graft failure, the appropriate angioplasty or graft extension can be combined with graft thrombectomy to preserve graft function. This strategy of graft salvage may be used for failed femoral to above-knee popliteal PTFE grafts, and acceptable incremental 3-year patency rates have been reported. However, other strategies may be used, such as performance of a totally new vein or PTFE secondary bypass using virginal patent arterial segments.

Alternatively, the administration of catheter-directed thrombolytic therapy may be used to lyse the clot and reveal the cause of failure, which can then be corrected by the appropriate endovascular or operative procedure. In addition, if the distal circulation appears occluded on arteriography after graft failure, treatment with thrombolytic agents may restore distal run-off vessels, thereby improving the results of any subsequent intervention.

Thrombectomy of failed PTFE bypasses to the below-knee popliteal artery has not yielded results comparable with those from totally new secondary procedures. Therefore, secondary procedures should be performed in preference to graft thrombectomy whenever possible. These secondary procedures should be performed using unusual approaches to previously undissected segments of artery for the origin and insertion of the graft, and autologous vein should be used for the graft if it is available. These approaches include direct approach to the distal zones of the deep femoral artery and lateral approaches to the popliteal artery above and below the knee (Figs 29–4 through 29–6). A greater than 40% 2-year patency can be expected with this strategy.

Prognosis

The successful performance of a femoropopliteal artery bypass or angioplasty uniformly relieves symp-

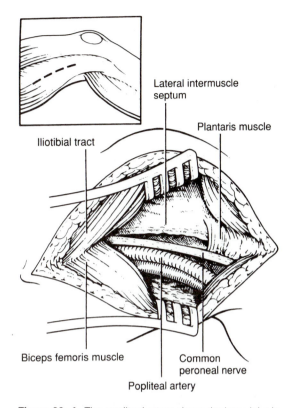

Figure 29–4. The popliteal artery above the knee joint is approached with a lateral incision between the iliotibial tract and the biceps femoris muscle. By deepening the incision in the lateral intermuscular septum, the popliteal space is entered and the neurovascular bundle can be palpated within the popliteal fat. The popliteal artery is easily isolated from the adjacent popliteal vein or veins, taking care not to injure the common peroneal nerve. After the popliteal artery has been dissected from these structures, gentle traction with silicone vessel loops can elevate it to close to the skin level, where surgical manipulation and anastomosis can be carried out with the same ease as is usual through the standard medial approach. (Reprinted, with permission, from Veith FJ: Reoperations for failed bypass grafts below the inguinal ligament. In: *Vascular Surgery,* 5th ed. Jamieson CW, Yao JST, [editors], Chapman & Hall Medical, 1994:350.)

toms such as claudication and rest pain if the revascularization is hemodynamically effective and if there are no additional obstructions in the remainder of the extremity circulation. If the symptoms are not relieved, other causes of the pain are likely, such as spinal stenosis causing pseudoclaudication or infection, ulcerations, or neuropathy causing foot pain.

A. Limb Salvage: Femoropopliteal bypass grafts have been demonstrated to achieve healing of ischemic lesions in 80% of patients or more. However, as with all revascularization procedures for limb salvage, multiple local operations on the foot over a 2–4-month period may be required in a small percentage (7%) of

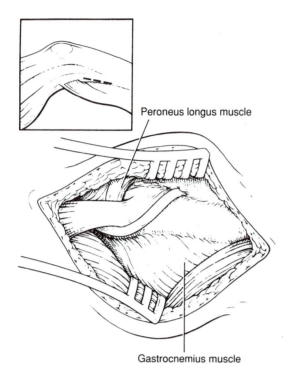

Figure 29–5. Below-knee popliteal artery. This is approached by a lateral incision over the head and proximal fourth of the fibula. The incision is deepened through the subcutaneous tissue and superficial muscular attachments to the fibula, taking care to identify the common peroneal nerve as it courses around the neck of this bone. This nerve is dissected free so that it can be retracted and protected from injury. The biceps femoris tendon is divided. The ligamentous attachments of the fibula head are incised, and the upper fourth of the fibula is freed bluntly from its muscular and ligamentous attachments, staying as close to the bone as possible. (Reprinted, with permission, from Veith FJ: Reoperations for failed bypass grafts below the inguinal ligament. In: *Vascular Surgery,* 5th ed. Jamieson CW, Yao JST [editors], Chapman & Hall Medical, 1994:351.)

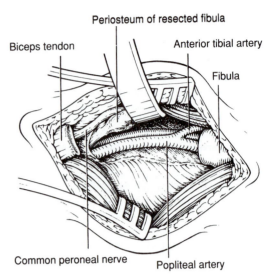

Figure 29–6. A retractor is placed deep to the fibula to protect the underlying structures, and 1 or 2 holes are drilled in this bone at its proposed site of transection. With such holes, a rib shears can cleanly transect the bone without leaving sharp spicules. After the bone has been divided, any remaining deep attachments can be exposed and cut. With the upper fibula removed, the entire below-knee popliteal artery, tibioperoneal trunk, anterior tibial artery, and the origins of the peroneal and posterior tibial arteries lie just deep to the excised bone and can easily be dissected from their adjacent veins. After mobilization, these arteries are more superficial in the wound than by way of standard medial approaches, and surgical manipulation and anastomotic suturing can be performed with greater ease. (Reprinted, with permission, from Veith FJ: Reoperations for failed bypass grafts below the inguinal ligament. In: *Vascular Surgery,* 5th ed. Jamieson CW, Yao JST, [editors], Chapman & Hall Medical, 1994:351.)

patients. Even when the initial revascularization procedure fails early, the extremity often can be saved by performing a secondary procedure, either to the same or more distal outflow. This is true not only for bypasses, but also when PTA is technically unsuccessful or fails to improve the arterial supply to the foot.

When attempts at reconstruction fail and ischemia progresses, amputation becomes necessary (see Chapter 30). The preferred site is the below-knee level, because an appropriate prosthesis requires much less exertion to walk than with the above-knee prosthesis, and the patient is more likely to learn to ambulate with it. In our experience, a below-knee amputation was performed in 90% of patients requiring amputation after femoropopliteal graft closure.

B. Patient Survival: Survival after femoropopliteal bypass procedures is good in the short term; the reported operative mortality rate is less than 4% in most series. However, these patients have a very poor long-term survival with less than 50% surviving more than 5 years.

REFERENCES

Ascer E et al: Reoperation for polytetrafluoroethylene bypass failure: The importance of distal outflow site and operative technique in determining outcome. J Vasc Surg 1987;5:298.

Bandyk DF, Cato RF, Towne JB: A low flow velocity predicts failure of femoropopliteal and femorotibial bypass grafts. Surgery 1985;98:799.

Bandyk DF et al: Durability of vein graft revision: The outcome of secondary procedures. J Vasc Surg 1991;13:200.

Boucher CA et al: Determination of cardiac risk by dipyridamole-thallium imaging before peripheral vascular surgery. N Engl J Med 1985;312:389.

Boyd AM: The natural course of arteriosclerosis of the lower extremities. Proc Roy Soc Med 1962;55:591.

Brewster DC: Direct reconstruction for aortoiliac occlusive disease. In: *Vascular Surgery,* 3rd ed. Rutherford RB (editor). WB Saunders, 1989:667.

Bylund AC et al: Enzyme activities in skeletal muscles from patients with peripheral arterial insufficiency. Eur J Clin Invest 1976;6:425.

Calligaro KD, Veith FJ: Proper technique of lower extremity pulse examination. Contemp Surg 1992;40:49.

Cooperman M, Pflug B, Martin EW Jr, Evans WE: Cardiovascular risk factors in patients with peripheral vascular disease. Surgery 1978;84:505.

Coran AG, Warren R: Arteriographic changes in femoropopliteal arteriosclerosis obliterans: A five year follow-up study. N Engl J Med 1966;274:643.

Cranley JJ, Karkow WS, Hafner CD, Flanagan LD: Aneurysmal dilatation in umbilical vein grafts. In: *Reoperative Arterial Surgery.* Bergan JJ, Yao JST (editors). Grune & Stratton, 1986:343.

Criqui MH et al: The prevalence of peripheral arterial disease in a defined population. Circulation 1985;71:510.

Cutler BS, Hendel RC, Leppo JA: Dipyridamole-thallium scintigraphy predicts perioperative and long term survival after major vascular surgery. J Vasc Surg 1992;15:972.

Dahlloff AG et al: Peripheral arterial insufficiency: Effect of physical training on walking tolerance, calf blood flow and blood flow resistance. Scan J Rehabil Med 1976;8:19.

Dardik H et al: Morphologic and biophysical assessment of long term human umbilical cord vein implants used as vascular conduits. Surg Gynecol Obstet 1982;154:17.

Eagle KA et al: Combining clinical and thallium data optimizes preoperative assessment of cardiac risk before major vascular surgery. Ann Intern Med 1989;110:859.

Ekroth R et al: Physical training of patients with intermittent claudication: Indications, methods and results. Surgery 1978;84:640.

Flanigan DP et al: Prebypass operative arteriography. Surgery 1982;92:627.

Gallino A et al: Percutaneous transluminal angioplasty of the arteries of the lower limbs: A 5 year follow-up. Circulation 1984;70:619.

Goodreau JJ et al: Rational approach to the differentiation of vascular and neurogenic claudication. Surgery 1978;84:749.

Greenhalgh RM et al: Progressing atherosclerosis following revascularization. In: *Complications in Vascular Surgery.* Berhard VM, Towne JB (editors). Grune & Stratton, 1980:21.

Gupta SK, Samson RH, Veith FJ: Embolectomy of the distal part of the popliteal artery. Surg Gynecol Obstet 1981;153:254.

Gupta SK, Veith FJ: Three year experience with expanded polytetrafluoroethylene arterial grafts for limb salvage. Am J Surg 1980;140:214.

Haimovici HC, Moss CM, Veith FJ: Arterial embolectomy revisited. Surgery 1975;78:409.

Harris RW et al: Successful long-term limb salvage using cephalic vein bypass grafts. Ann Surg 1984;200:785.

Hertzer NR et al: Coronary artery disease in peripheral vascular patients: A classification of 1000 coronary angiograms and results of surgical management. Ann Surg 1984;199:223.

Hobson RW II et al: Results of revascularization and amputation in severe lower extremity ischemia: A five-year clinical experience. J Vasc Surg 1985;2:174.

Hughson WG, Mann JI, Garrod A: Intermittent claudication: Prevalence and risk factors. Br Med J 1978;1:1379.

Imparato AM et al: Intermittent claudication: Its natural course. Surgery 1975;78:795.

Jamieson WR, Janusz MT, Miyagishima RT, Gerein AN: Influence of ischemic heart disease on early and late mortality after surgery for peripheral occlusive vascular disease. Circulation 1982;66(Suppl I):I92.

Johnston KW et al: Five-year results of a prospective study of percutaneous transluminal angioplasty. Ann Surg 1987;206:403.

Karmody AM, Powers SR, Monaco VJ, Leather RP: "Blue toe" syndrome: An indication for limb salvage surgery. Arch Surg 1976;111:1263.

Kavanaugh GJ, Svien HJ, Holman CB, Johnson RM et al: "Pseudoclaudication" syndrome produced by compression of the cauda equina. JAMA 1968;206:2477.

Kent KC, Whittemore AD, Mannick JA: Short term and mid term results of an all-autogenous tissue policy for infrainguinal reconstruction. J Vasc Surg 1989;9:107.

Kram HB et al: Unilateral aortofemoral bypass: A safe and effective option for the treatment of unilateral limb-threatening ischemia. Am J Surg 1991;162:155.

Leopold PW et al: Initial experience comparing B-mode imaging and venography of the saphenous vein before in situ bypass. Am J Surg 1986;152:206.

Lithell H, Hedstrand H, Karlsson R: The smoking habits of men with intermittent claudication. Acta Med Scand 1975;197:473.

Mannick JA, Jackson BT, Coffman JD et al: Success of bypass vein grafts in patients with isolated popliteal artery segments. Surgery 1967;61:17.

Murray RR et al: Long-segment femoropopliteal stenoses: Is angioplasty a boon or a bust? Radiology 1987;162:473.

Nunez A et al: Direct approaches to the distal portions of the deep femoral artery for limb salvage bypasses. J Vasc Surg 1988;8:576.

Panetta TF et al: Unsuspected preexisting saphenous vein disease: An unrecognized cause of vein bypass failure. J Vasc Surg 1992;15:102.

Pasternack PF et al: The value of silent myocardial ischemia monitoring in the prediction of perioperative myocardial infarction in patients undergoing peripheral vascular surgery. J Vasc Surg 1989;10:617.

Porter JM et al: Pentoxifylline efficacy in the treatment of intermittent claudication: Multicenter controlled double-blind trial with objective assessment of chronic occlusive arterial disease patients. Am Heart J 1982;104:66.

Quick CRG, Cotton LT: The measured effect of stopping smoking on intermittent claudication. Br J Surg 1982;69:S24.

Quinones-Baldrich WJ et al: Long-term results of infrainguinal revascularization with polytetrafluoroethylene: A ten-year experience. J Vasc Surg 1992;16:209.

Rivers SP, Scher LA, Veith FJ: Indications for distal arterial reconstruction in the presence of palpable pedal pulses. J Vasc Surg 1990;12:552.

Sanchez L et al: A ten-year experience with one hundred fifty failing or threatened vein and polytetrafluoroethylene arterial bypass grafts. J Vasc Surg 1991;14:729.

Sanchez LA et al: Is surveillance to detect failing polytetrafluoroethylene bypasses worthwhile? Twelve-year experience with ninety-one grafts. J Vasc Surg 1993;18:981.

Sanchez LA et al: Is percutaneous balloon angioplasty appropriate in the treatment of graft and anastomic lesions responsible for failing vein bypasses? Am J Surg 1994;168:97.

Schneider E, Gruntzig A, Bollinger A: Long-term patency rates after percutaneous transluminal angioplasty for iliac and femoropopliteal obstructions. In: *Percutaneous Transluminal Angioplasty Technique: Early and Late Results.* Dotter CT et al (editors). Springer-Verlag, 1983:175.

Schulman ML, Badhey MR: Late results and angiographic evaluation of arm veins as long bypass grafts. Surgery 1982;92:1032.

Sesto ME et al: Cephalic vein grafts for lower extremity revascularization. J Vasc Surg 1992;15:543.

Smith CR, Green RM, DeWeese JA: Pseudoocclusion of femoropopliteal bypass grafts. Circulation 1983;68(Suppl II):II–88.

Sprayregen S: Principles of angiography. In: *Vascular Surgery. Principles and Techniques.* Haimovici H (editor). McGraw-Hill, 1976:39.

Stokes KR et al: Five-year results of iliac and femoropopliteal angioplasty in diabetic patients. Radiology 1990;174:977.

Strandness DE: *Duplex scanning in vascular disorders.* Raven Press, 1990:121.

van Andel GJ et al: Percutaneous transluminal dilatation of the iliac artery: Long term results. Radiology 1985;156:321.

Veith FJ, Gupta SK: Femoral-distal artery bypasses. In: *Operative Techniques in Vascular Surgery.* Bergan JJ, Yao JST (editors). Grune & Stratton, 1980:141.

Veith FJ, Gupta SK, Daly V: Femoropopliteal bypass to the isolated popliteal segment: Is polytetrafluoroethylene graft acceptable? Surgery 1981;89:296.

Veith FJ et al: Changing arteriosclerotic disease patterns and management strategies in lower-limb-threatening ischemia. Ann Surg 1990;212:402.

Veith FJ et al: Diagnosis and management of failing lower extremity arterial reconstructions. J Cardiovasc Surg 1984;25:381.

Veith FJ et al: Lateral approach to the popliteal artery. J Vasc Surg 1987;6:119.

Veith FJ et al: New approaches in limb salvage by extended extraanatomic bypasses and prosthetic reconstructions to foot arteries. Surgery 1978;84:764.

Veith FJ et al: Progress in limb salvage by reconstructive arterial surgery combined with new or improved adjunctive procedures. Ann Surg 1981;194:386.

Veith FJ et al: Six year prospective multicenter randomized comparison of autologous saphenous vein and expanded polytetrafluoroethylene grafts in infrainguinal arterial reconstructions. J Vasc Surg 1986;3:104.

Wengerter KR, Veith FJ: Self-retaining retraction techniques for vascular surgery: Use of a mechanical robot arm. J Vasc Surg 1988;8:14.

Wengerter KR et al: Prospective randomized multicenter comparison of in situ and reversed vein infrapopliteal bypasses. J Vasc Surg 1991;13:189.

Lower Extremity Amputations

30

Richard H. Dean, MD

Although amputations might be considered an orthopedic procedure, more than 80% of such operations are performed as a consequence of complications of vascular disease and are undertaken by general or vascular surgeons. Frequently considered the ultimate failure to a vascular surgeon, issues surrounding the proper selection and performance of amputations have a major impact on cost-effective treatment and determination of the magnitude and duration of disability associated with such procedures. Considering that more than 50,000 amputations may be performed each year, the importance of timely and successful amputations as well as effective rehabilitation after operation should be self-evident.

The following are indications for amputation: acute ischemia, chronic ischemia, complications of diabetes, trauma, infection, and miscellaneous conditions (eg, frostbite, tumor). This chapter primarily considers amputations for vascular-related conditions. Since diabetes is a common comorbidity in vascular patients, special comment on the impact of its presence on management decisions in these patient also is included.

ACUTE ISCHEMIA

General Considerations

Several factors influence the need for amputation in patients with acute limb ischemia: the extent of limb involvement by acute ischemia, the severity and duration of ischemia, and the potential for restoration of tissue perfusion by limb revascularization. Understanding these important features of the clinical presentation of acute ischemia is important for accurate decision making and treatment of affected patients.

Acute embolic digital artery occlusion creates ischemia only to the distal end of the digit. In this circumstance, subsequent tissue death and gangrene are limited to the end of the digit. Observation alone in such a patient allows new tissue growth to occur underneath the gangrenous eschar, and no amputation is required. In contrast, when a large percentage of the leg has acute nonreversible severe ischemia, emergency amputation is necessary to prevent the absorption of the toxic byproducts of tissue death into the circulation.

Clinical Findings

A. Signs and Symptoms: Clinical findings of extreme acute ischemia include loss of sensation and motor function of the involved muscle groups. The skin temperature of the involved segment is cooler than the proximal viable level. After 12–24 hours, skin demarcation between the dying level and the viable skin also is visible. After such tissue death occurs, revascularization becomes inappropriate even when technically feasible. In this circumstance, amputation is required to salvage the patient's life. In addition, when muscle necrosis is extensive, large quantities of myoglobin are released into the circulation leading to acute renal failure. Therefore, emergency amputation may be required to interrupt this progressive cause of renal failure.

B. Determination of Amputation Level: Determination of the appropriate amputation level for the acutely ischemic and nonsalvageable limb should take into account several features of the patient's evaluation. All nonviable tissue must be removed. When the skin has been without adequate circulation to maintain cellular viability for several hours, it becomes mottled with a bluish hue and then gangrenous. Gangrenous skin that is present for several days may even develop bullae or black eschars. The amputation site must not only remove all dead tissue but also be at a site where the degree of perfusion is adequate to sustain healing of the wound after amputation. Skin temperature and pinprick sensation are useful tools to identify the level of adequate perfusion. If there is diminished temperature of the skin or loss of light touch and pinprick discrimination, then healing at that site is unlikely and a higher site should be chosen.

The presence of calf tenderness or marked elevation of lactate dehydrogenous isoenzymes in the serum of a patient with a nonviable calf are important signs that muscle necrosis is present, and urgent amputation is needed to prevent systemic side effects of myonecrosis. If myoglobinuria is present, institution of measures to promote diuresis and alkalinization of the urine by administration of intravenous fluids, osmotic diuretics, and sodium bicarbonate are important to abort the toxic effect of myoglobin on the renal tubular cells.

Finally, the presence of infection in the severely ischemic extremity increases the risk of limb loss. Careful observation for signs of systemic sepsis or ascending infection are mandatory while instituting appropriate antibiotic treatment. Development of systemic sepsis or progression of the infection should prompt urgent débridement of all infected tissue. This may require a guillotine amputation to adequately protect against recurrence of the infection in a closed amputation stump. Subsequent revision of the guillotine amputation at a standard level with closure of the wound after the infection has been cleared allows rehabilitation and consideration of prosthetic fitting.

CHRONIC ISCHEMIA

General Considerations

Consideration of amputation in patients with chronic ischemia is primarily focused on patients with severe rest pain, nonhealing ulcerations, or gangrenous lesions in which tissue revascularization through vascular reconstruction is not possible. Usually, the decision for amputation in patients with chronic ischemia is based on the absence of an alternative treatment that will resolve the clinical presentation (eg, pain, nonhealing ulcer) and the premise that the presenting clinical condition requires correction. In other words, a decision has been made that the clinical problem is of such magnitude that it must be resolved and no other solution is feasible.

Clinical Findings

Among the indications for amputation in patients with chronic ischemia, rest pain from ischemia is the most compelling. When tissue perfusion is below a critical level for normal neurologic function, the patient has inappropriate discharge of sensory nerve endings and this creates severe pain in the affected area. The patient seeks relief from the pain by keeping the limb in a dependent position to improve tissue perfusion. Unfortunately, below a threshold level of perfusion, nothing provides relief from such pain. Patients frequently describe a boring sharp pain, which is the worst pain they have ever experienced. Ultimately, a patient can become addicted to progressively stronger analgesics in a vain attempt to control the pain.

When pain alone is the indication for amputation, the patient can determine the timing of amputation. In this way, the patient has a more positive outlook on his or her status after amputation because of having accepted amputation as a therapy designed to eliminate the debilitating pain.

Nonhealing ischemic ulcers of the lower extremity requiring amputation most frequently have associated pain at the site of ulceration. The surface of an ischemic ulcer has exposed sensory nerve endings and frequently is exquisitely sensitive. In this circumstance, control of pain may be the primary reason for amputation. In contrast, observation and local treatment alone for prolonged periods without amputation

are appropriate when the ischemic ulcer is small, non-painful, and noninfected.

Although frank gangrene is an indication for amputation, the procedure can be delayed for prolonged periods when such tissue death is limited to digits and no pain or infection is present to require immediate removal. When gangrene has secondary infection, immediate institution of intravenous antibiotics and débridement/amputation of the necrotic tissue is important to control the extent of progressive tissue death and the potential for systemic sepsis.

SPECIAL CONSIDERATIONS IN DIABETICS

The presence of diabetes creates several special considerations in the management of patients presenting with gangrene or nonhealing lesions of the foot. Diabetic neuropathy alters the sensory integrity of the skin and can lead to ulcerations at pressure points on the heel or under the 1st metatarsal head. Since discomfort is not perceived during prolonged pressure, secondary pressure necrosis occurs producing a **neurotrophic ulcer.** Such tissue necrosis from chronic pressure can occur in the face of palpable pedal pulses. In addition, secondary infection in a neurotrophic or ischemic ulcer may not produce pain in the diabetic patient and progressive tissue destruction may occur with the patient being unaware of the deteriorating situation.

When evaluating the diabetic patient with an infected gangrenous digit or neurotrophic ulcer, assume that tissue destruction is more extensive than such physical findings as tenderness to palpation suggests. For this reason, early operative débridement and amputation of all gangrenous and infected tissue constitute a basic principle of management of these patients. Since infectious complications at the site of amputation of infected gangrenous tissue may go unrecognized in the diabetic, it is important to leave the amputation site open to minimize the risk of further tissue loss from ascending infection. Secondary closure after a period of dressing changes of the amputation site increases the probability of success in these circumstances.

DETERMINATION OF AMPUTATION LEVEL

Three basic principles must be satisfied when determining the appropriate level of amputation: (1) all nonviable and infected tissue must be removed; (2) perfusion at the level of the proposed amputation must sustain healing of the wound; and (3) the amputation stump, where necessary, must easily be able to be fitted with a standard type of prosthesis. In addition to these considerations, the amputation should to be performed as distally as possible. Conceptually, each major joint that is removed by the amputation increases the level of disability and difficulty in mastering ambulation with a prosthesis.

Methods to determine the adequacy of perfusion to ensure healing at a proposed amputation site continue to evolve. Table 30–1 lists several methods and lower limits of perfusion compatible with amputation site healing. The reader is directed to other sources (Barnes et al, Burgess et al, Cheng, Holloway & Burgess, Raines et al) to gain more knowledge regarding the principles and techniques used in these and other treatments.

Digit Amputations

Digit amputations are most frequently performed in patients with diabetes because diabetics are susceptible to subungual infections, digital ulcerations, and osteomyelitis. Patients presenting with distal digital gangrene secondary to atheroembolism to the digit are initially best managed by observation. As long as the gangrenous toe is dry, maturation of the gangrene and partial re-epithelialization under the dead tissue can be allowed, which in turn allows a more distal amputation. Autoamputation and complete epithelialization under the gangrene are allowed when only the digital tip is involved.

Figure 30–1 schematically demonstrates the technique of digital amputation. We prefer the fishmouth skin lesion. Other kinds of incisions may also be appropriate, however. The most important point is to have adequate skin and soft tissue to cover the end of the amputated bone without tension. Amputation through the joint space should be avoided. If the entire phalangeal bone must be removed, then removing the head of the proximal phalanx or metatarsal head should be done to avoid leaving a synovial lining at the end of the amputated bone.

When the gangrene extends to the proximal phalanx, a "ray amputation" of the single metatarsal head is indicated (Fig 30–2). If the dorsal skin incision is extended proximally, the metatarsal head can be removed to allow soft tissue coverage at the toe web-space level.

Forefoot Amputations

Transmetatarsal amputation is indicated for treatment of gangrenous lesions that extend proximal to the skin crease of the metatarsal phalangeal joint. This procedure also is used to treat diabetic or neurotrophic ulcers at the site of the first metatarsal head. The skin incision is carried around the plantar ulcer to include it with the metatarsal head in the amputated specimen. In this circumstance, the dorsal flap of skin is used to close the wound (Fig 30–3).

When gangrene involves more than two toes to a point proximal to the metatarsal-phalangeal crease, amputation of all toes in the form of a forefoot amputation is indicated. A single skin incision is used to accomplish this with the plantar skin used as a flap to close the skin (Fig 30–4).

Occasionally, closure of the transmetatarsal amputation may not be feasible because of the proximal extent of excised gangrene or infection. Therefore, institution of dressing changes on the open wound surface until all infection is eradicated and until a healthy granulating surface is present can allow subsequent split-thickness skin grafting of the soft tissue. This is appropriate only when the grafted skin is not on the weight-bearing surface of the foot.

Ankle Disarticulation

Disarticulation of the ankle is most commonly called a **Syme's amputation**, named after its original advocate. Although a well-healed Syme's amputation is less disabling than a below-knee amputation, it is a technically difficult procedure. In my experience, this procedure is rarely indicated in the patient undergoing amputation for ischemia. When a forefoot amputation is not feasible because of local ischemia or proximal infection, the more proximal foot wound for a Syme's amputation frequently does not heal or breaks down later secondary to the insensate skin. In all such instances, a well-vascularized below-knee amputation provides a more durable stump for prosthetic rehabilitation.

Below-Knee Amputations

After limb removal above the midfoot is required for ischemia, a standard below-knee (BK) amputation is the preferred procedure. Since BK protheses are designed for a standard length of tibial segment, more distal amputation and length salvage increase the difficulty for prosthetic fitting. Therefore, distal BK amputation increases disability, decreases soft tissue coverage available over the bone, and increases the chance of nonhealing from diminished perfusion. BK amputation is contraindicated in the debilitated, bedridden patient with knee contractures. In this patient, the

Table 30–1. Predictors of amputation healing.

Level	Test	Criteria
Digit/metatarsal	Doppler ankle systolic pressure	>70 mmHg
	Xenon skin clearance	>2.6 mL/100 g tissue/min
Below knee	Doppler calf systolic pressure	>70 mmHg
	Doppler thigh systolic pressure	>80 mmHg
	Transcutaneous partial pressure of oxygen	>35 mmHg
	Xenon skin clearance	>2.6 mL/100 g tissue/min

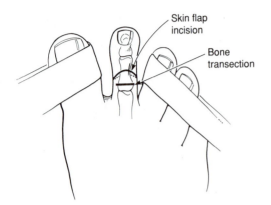

Figure 30–1. Skin incision and level of bone transection for digital amputation.

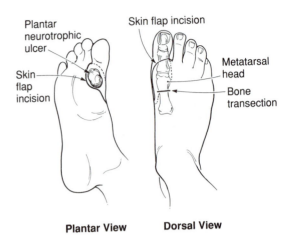

Plantar View   **Dorsal View**

Figure 30–3. Skin incision and bone transection for amputation of 1st metatarsal head in a patient with a neurotrophic ulcer at that site.

stump beyond the knee contracture may create more disability, and its removal may facilitate nursing care.

Principles important in the performance of BK amputation include creation of a long posterior gastrocnemius and soleus muscle flap to cover the transected tibia, division of the tibia about 10 cm below the tibial tuberosity, and beveling of the anterior portion of the transected tibia (Fig 30–5). Although soft tissue drains are usually not necessary in amputations for ischemia, meticulous soft tissue hemostasis is mandatory to prevent the development of a stump hematoma. A bulky modestly compressive dressing, which extends well above the knee to ensure maintenance of the knee joint in extension, is important to prevent the development of a knee contracture prior to prosthetic fitting. Occasionally, a rigid plaster-of-Paris covering of the dressing is used to accomplish this goal.

Above-Knee Amputations

Amputation at the above-knee (AK) level is indicated when ischemia of the calf makes healing of a lower amputation level unlikely, when the patient has

knee flexion contracture and is not expected to walk again, and when emergency limb removal is required to handle life-threatening sepsis from gangrene and infection, which would preclude lower amputation. Although AK amputation is easier to perform than BK amputation, the loss of the knee joint significantly increases the level of disability and the difficulty with prosthetic ambulation. For these reasons, sound judgment should be used to select the more proximal AK site. In addition, bilateral AK amputations increase the level of disability for the nonambulating patient. The presence of one BK stump for use as a lever to push off in turning and moving is of significant valve to the bilateral amputee.

Technical aspects of AK amputations are relatively simple. A wide "fish-mouth" skin and muscle incision based medial and lateral facilitates easy closure after amputation (Fig 30–6).

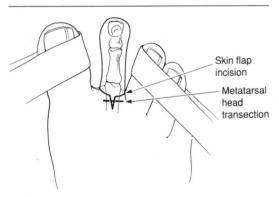

Figure 30–2. Skin incision and level of bone transection for ray amputation of digit.

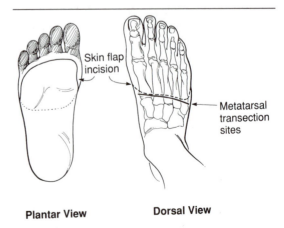

Plantar View   **Dorsal View**

Figure 30–4. Transmetatarsal amputation showing plantar-based skin flap.

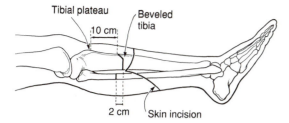

Figure 30–5. BK amputations showing posterior skin and muscle flap, transection point of tibia and fibula, and beveling of the anterior tibia.

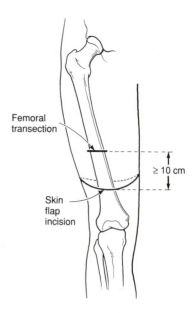

Figure 30–6. Skin incision and femur transection for AK amputation.

Remember to transect the femur well above (10–15 cm) the skin incision site. The transected muscle mass and skin must be closed over the femoral stump easily without tension. Revision of the femoral stump length is appropriate to facilitate this approximation when any tension is present on attempted wound closure.

COMPLICATIONS AFTER AMPUTATION

Since major lower extremity amputations for ischemia are usually performed in extremely debilitated patients with multiple cardiovascular risk factors, it is not surprising that the incidence of morbidity and mortality is significant. Depending on the clinical circumstances, the postoperative death rate can be expected to range from 0% to greater than 30%. Likewise, pulmonary complications are seen in about 10% of patients. Postoperative deep venous thrombosis may develop in the proximal deep venous system of the amputated leg in up to 35% of patients. Pulmonary emboli have been noted in 1–3% of patients. Healing of the amputation site depends on the adequacy of perfusion, the absence of infection, and the technical precision of the surgeon. Breakdown of the amputation stump has been noted in 12–28% of contemporary series.

Postoperative pain syndromes warrant special mention. Although pain in the incision site is expected in all patients, many patients experience pain syndromes in the amputated part (phantom pain). **Phantom pain** can best be described in most patients as phantom sensations, not pain, because they describe the feeling of the limb being present even when true pain is absent. Obviously, the phantom pain originates from stimulation at the site of the transected nerve that originated from the amputated limb. Phantom pain syndromes seem to be more severe and to last longer during the postoperative period in the patient group with extreme rest pain as an original reason for amputation. Although many therapies have been suggested for the treatment of phantom pain, none has been successful. Fortunately, such syndromes ultimately dissipate in almost all patients.

REFERENCES

Barnes RW, Shanik GO, Slaymaker EE: An index of healing in below-knee amputation: Leg blood pressure by Doppler ultrasound. Surgery 1976;79:13.

Bell ET: Atherosclerotic gangrene of the lower extremities in diabetic and non-diabetic persons. Am J Clin Pathol 1957; 28:27.

Burgess EM, Matsen FA, Wyss CR, Simmons CW: Segmental transcutaneous measurements of PO_2 in patients requiring below the knee amputation for peripheral vascular insufficiency. J Bone Joint Surg 1982;64A:378.

Cheng EY: Lower extremity amputation level using noninvasive hemodynamic methods of evaluation. Arch Phys Med Rehabil 1982;63:475.

Fearon J et al: Improved results with diabetic below-knee amputations. Arch Surg 1975;120:777.

Gibbons GW: Management of pre- and postoperative infection in the diabetic patient. Host Pathogen News 1983;1:1.

Haimovici H: Amputation of lower extremity. Vasc Surg 1984;68:1087.

Holloway GA Jr, Burgess EM: Cutaneous blood flow and its relation to healing of below knee amputation. Surg Gynecol Obstet 1978;146:750.

Malone JM, Moore WS, Goldstone J, Malone SJ: Therapeutic and economic impact of a modern amputation program. Ann Surg 1979;189:798.

Malone JM, Moore WS, Leal JM, Childers SJ: Rehabilitation for lower extremity amputation. Arch Surg 1981;116:93.

McKittrick LS, McKittrick MB, Risby TS: Transmetatarsal amputation for infection of gangrene in patients with diabetes mellitus. Ann Surg 1949;130:825.

Raines JK et al: Vascular laboratory criteria for the management of peripheral vascular disease of the lower extremities. Surgery 1976;79:21.

Roon AJ, Moore WS, Goldstone J: Below-knee amputation: A modern approach. Am J Surg 1977;134:153.

Sherma RA, Tippens JK: Suggested guidelines for treatment of phantom limb pain. Orthopedics 1982;5:1595.

Sizer JS, Wheelock FC: Digital amputations in diabetic patients. Surgery 1972;72:980.

White GH: Amputations in the dysvascular patient. Vasc Surg 1987;71:898.

Varicose Veins & Superficial Thrombophlebitis

31

William A. Marston, MD, & George Johnson, Jr., MD

VARICOSE VEINS

Essentials of Diagnosis
- Telangiectasias—small spider-like clusters of venules that usually extend outward from a feeder vessel.
- Fatigue and aching heaviness, exacerbated by prolonged standing.
- Chronic venous stasis (frequently).
- Occasionally no symptoms.

General Considerations
The treatment of lower extremity varicosities has been a concern of physicians throughout recorded history, with advice to avoid surgical treatment being offered as early as 1550 BC in the Ebers papyrus. Hippocrates, Galen, and Celsus all devoted passages to the treatment of varicose veins and lower extremity ulcers. Ambroise Paré reported the association of varicose veins with pregnancy, and in 1976 Richard Wiseman described the use of a leather stocking to apply compression to an ulcer associated with varicose veins. A proliferation of interest in the surgical treatment of varicose veins occurred in the late 19th and early 20th centuries, with Trendelenburg, Tavel, Mayo, Babcock, and others describing methods of ligating or stripping for treatment of varicose veins. Recently, the development of noninvasive techniques of diagnosis of venous insufficiency has led to increased efforts to scientifically treat this common, often debilitating disease.

Varicose veins (VVs) are defined by the World Health Organization as abnormally dilated saccular or cylindrical superficial veins, which can be circumscribed or segmental. This includes tiny spider telangiectasias as well as grossly dilated saphenous varicosities. VVs are usually divided into the more common primary VV, in which the deep venous system is normal, and secondary VV, in which the deep or perforator venous systems are incompetent. This distinction is important because patients with secondary VVs respond poorly to therapeutic efforts aimed at the superficial venous system while the abnormality in the deep or perforator venous systems is neglected. This can lead to a high incidence of recurrence.

In most reports, such as the Basle study, VVs are divided into 3 groups:

- Dilated saphenous veins (stem veins).
- Dilated tributaries of the saphenous veins (reticular veins).
- Dilated venules (hyphen-webs or telangiectasias).

This classification scheme is useful in communicating and documenting patient information and in comparing studies that comprise patients with a wide range of severity of disease.

Incidence & Risk Factors
The incidence of VVs is difficult to define precisely because various definitions have been used. The disease appears to be most common in Europe and the USA, with an estimated 24 million adults in this country affected by varicose disease. Nearly 50% of the population over the age of 40 has some form of varicosity or telangiectasia of the veins. Between 10% and 20% of adults have significant VVs, and 0.5% have superficial varicosities associated with chronic venous stasis and ulceration.

Risk factors associated with an increased risk of varicose disease are a family history of VVs, age (50 years or over), female sex, multiparity (2 or more pregnancies), oral contraceptive use, standing vocation (>6 hr/day), and obesity. The incidence of VVs increases with age; the peak incidence occurs in the 6th decade of life. Less than 1–2% of adults report varicose disease in their 20s, compared with up to 72% of women over 60 in one study. In the Basle study III comprising over 4500 subjects, the association of age was strongest in persons with VVs only, without telangiectasias or reticular veins or both (Fig 31–1). VVs are rarely seen in childhood and, if seen, are usually associated with congenital vascular syndromes such as Klippel-Trénaunay syndrome.

VVs are not only more common in women, but also occur earlier in life, leading to a female:male ratio of 5–6:1 in the 3rd and 4th decades of life. However, this ratio decreases as the population ages to a ratio of 1–2:1 after the 6th decade.

A family history of varicose disease is associated with development of the disease in 70–85% of first-degree relatives, compared with 10% of those with no family history. However, heredity is only one factor in the cause of VVs. The association between pregnancy

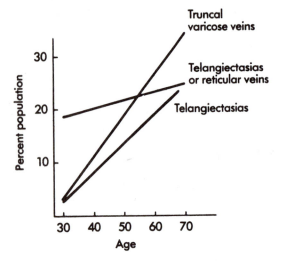

Figure 31–1. Association of age with telangiectasis, telangiectasias or reticular veins, and varicose veins. (Reproduced, with permission, from Widmer L: Peripheral venous disorders: Prevalence and socio-medical importance observations in 4529 apparently healthy persons. Basle Study III. Hans Huber Publishers, 1978.)

superficial venous system of the lower extremity comprises 3 systems: the greater saphenous vein, the lesser saphenous vein, and the perforating or communicating veins.

The **subcuticular thin-walled vessels** or venules form a plexus just under the skin. Usually, these vessels are not visible, but when abnormally dilated, they may form telangiectasias or other subcuticular abnormalities. These venules combine to form a network of moderate-sized subcutaneous veins, which are the tributaries of the main trunks of the superficial venous system, the greater (long) saphenous vein, and the lesser (short) saphenous vein. The subcutaneous tributaries of the GSV and LSV are usually the veins that form prominent varicosities.

The **greater saphenous vein** (GSV) is the longest vein in the human body. It is formed by the union of the veins draining the medial side of the sole of the foot with the medial dorsal veins (Fig 31–2). Usually, 4–6 tributaries join the GSV just prior to its entry into the common femoral vein. The numerous variations in the anatomy of these tributaries must be carefully identified and ligated to ensure the best results of high ligation and stripping procedures.

and venous disease is strong in some populations, with 10–20% of pregnant females developing VVs and up to 70% developing telangiectasias. However, the varicosities spontaneously resolve in most patients within 3–6 weeks postpartum, and the number of these women who develop persistent varicosities later in life is not well known.

Chronic differences in posture may be related to the development of varicosities as well. Prolonged standing at work (more than 6 hr/day) has been associated with the development of varicosities, but only in retrospective interview studies. Chair sitting, due to the addition of the force of gravity, results in increased ankle pressures compared with ground sitting, which may be a factor in the increased incidence of varicosities in Western industrialized countries. Oral contraceptive use and obesity have been associated with an increased risk of VVs in some studies.

Anatomy

Varicose conditions may be due to an abnormality of the superficial system alone, but are often the result of damage or dysfunction of the deep or perforator veins also. The selection of an appropriate form of therapy depends on identifying the site of dysfunction within the venous system and specifically correcting it. A solid understanding of the normal anatomy of the superficial, deep, and perforator venous systems in the lower extremity is essential to the physician making clinical decisions on the diagnosis and treatment of VVs.

Cadaveric studies have revealed marked diversity in the anatomy of the superficial venous system. The

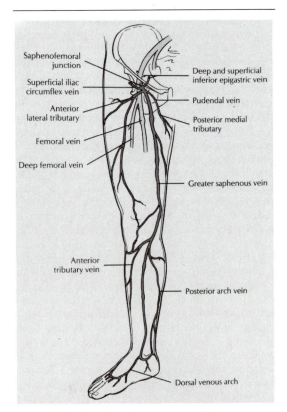

Figure 31–2. Anatomy of the greater saphenous vein and its major tributaries. (Reproduced, with permission, from Bergan JJ, Goldman MP [editors]: *Varicose Veins and Telangiectasias: Diagnosis and Treatment.* Quality Medical Publishing, 1993.)

The saphenous branch of the femoral nerve pierces the deep fascia at the level of the knee and joins the GSV, lying just posterior to it. The saphenous nerve then descends in close relation to the GSV, giving off several cutaneous branches, which cross over the GSV in the distal two-thirds of the leg. This relation may result in injuries to the nerve during stripping procedures manifested by sensory deficits as depicted in Figure 31–3. Duplication of the GSV occurs in 5–10% of patients. The **lesser saphenous vein** (LSV) arises at the outer border of the foot behind the lateral malleolus of the ankle. It is formed by the union of the lateral portion of the dorsal venous arch and the lateral marginal vein. It ascends straight up the middle of the calf to empty into the popliteal vein (in about 60%) in the popliteal fossa (Fig 31–4), into the GSV by way of the superficial thigh veins (in about 20%), and into other numerous sites (in about 20%)—most frequently the superficial femoral and deep femoral veins. In the lower third of the leg, the LSV is in close proximity to the sural nerve, which must be protected from injury during surgical procedures.

The **perforator veins** link the deep and superficial systems and usually function to carry blood from the superficial system to the deep veins. Valves in these veins, when competent, prevent reflux of blood from the deep to superficial veins. Incompetence of the per-

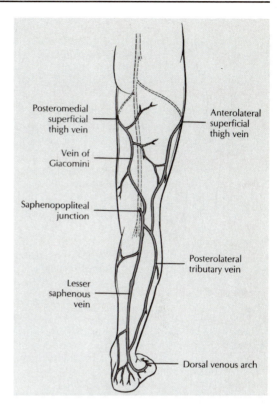

Figure 31–4. Anatomy of the posterolateral superficial leg drainage illustrating the course of the lesser saphenous vein and its important tributaries. The junction of the lesser saphenous with the popliteal vein is variable. (Reproduced, with permission, from Bergan JJ, Goldman MP [editors]: *Varicose Veins and Telangiectasias: Diagnosis and Treatment.* Quality Medical Publishing, 1993.)

forator veins is an important cause of VVs and venous ulceration and also a common cause of recurrent varicosities after ligation or stripping procedures. Figure 31–5 illustrates the location of the important groups of perforator veins. There are more than 100 in each leg, but only a few are large enough to be clinically significant.

Valve dysfunction due to a number of factors is the primary cause of varicosities and venous insufficiency. Valves prevent reversal of flow in the venous system, particularly on standing, to protect the lower extremities from the deleterious effects of a continuously elevated hydrostatic pressure. In general, deep veins have valves every 1–2 cm, and superficial veins have valves every 3–4 cm. These valves are usually located just distal to the entrance of a tributary vein. Perforator veins almost always have at least one valve, located deep to the muscular fascia. Valves are present in tributaries and smaller venules, even postcapillary venules.

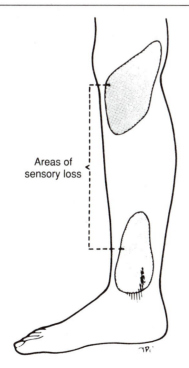

Figure 31–3. Potential areas of sensory loss after saphenous nerve injury during stripping of the greater saphenous vein. (Reproduced, with permission, from Ramasastry SS et al: Anatomy of the saphenous nerve: Relevance to saphenous vein stripping. Am Surg 1987;53.277.)

Pathophysiology

There are several conflicting theories of the etiology of primary VVs. Incompetence of the saphenous vein

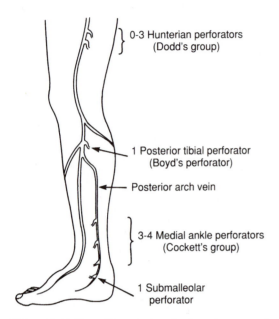

} 0-3 Hunterian perforators
    (Dodd's group)

1 Posterior tibial perforator
  (Boyd's perforator)

Posterior arch vein

} 3-4 Medial ankle perforators
    (Cockett's group)

1 Submalleolar
  perforator

Figure 31–5. Sites of important perforator veins connecting the deep and superficial venous systems. (Reproduced, with permission, from Criado E, Johnson G Jr: Venous disease. Curr Prob Surg 1991;28:335.)

valves, an inherent weakness of the walls of the veins, and the presence of arteriovenous (AV) fistulas are popular examples. The common pathway of these hypotheses is an increased pressure in the superficial veins with dilatation and incompetence of the valves, but the exact cause of the phenomenon remains unclear.

A. Arteriovenous Communications: This theory is based on studies reporting an increased PO_2 in blood within VVs compared with that in normal veins. If AV anastomoses are present, localized turbulence and increased pressure may lead to wall dilatation and valvular incompetence. There is evidence of the presence of AV communications based on early filling of VVs on arteriograms and suggestive Doppler flow measurements. However, examination of the microcirculation surrounding VV with macroaggregates revealed no evidence of increased AV shunting in the area of VVs. Also, in pathologic studies, no consistent association was found between VVs and the presence of significant AV communications. Others suggest that VVs are associated with peripheral vasodilatation including the venous capillaries, which may result in the opening of the capillary bed leading to a functional AV shunt as a result—not a cause—of VVs. Currently, controversy surrounds the contribution of AV communications to the cause of VVs.

B. Valvular Incompetence: This concept, first suggested by Trendelenburg, was supported by the reported absence of iliofemoral venous valves in up to

40% of normal cadavers. The theory postulates that the absence or incompetence of proximal valves transmits an increased hydrostatic pressure to the distal segment of vein leading to dilatation and further valvular incompetence. This concept led to the theory that high ligation of the saphenous vein would correct distal VVs. However, cadaveric studies have shown that patients with VVs frequently have varicosities distal to competent valves and that 40% of cadavers with no valve proximal to the saphenofemoral junction had no distal varicosities. Also, VVs are typically segmental and saccular. If incompetence of the valves allowing increased pressure were the cause, the entire distal vein would be expected to dilate down to the next competent valve. Although primary valvular incompetence or absence may be involved in the cause of VVs in some patients, it is difficult to explain the development of most cases of VVs by valvular incompetence alone.

C. Incompetence of Perforating Veins: Cockett reported that VVs are frequently associated with large incompetent perforating calf veins and suggested that these may be the cause in some cases. Patients occasionally present with VVs, venous ulceration, and incompetent perforators on duplex scan. In this situation, ligation of the incompetent perforators and local avulsion of the varicosities have resulted in resolution of the venous ulcers and a low incidence of recurrent VVs or ulceration. Other studies have found incompetent perforating veins to be associated with superficial varicosities in a minority of cases.

D. Defect in Structure of Vein Wall: Several observations led to the hypothesis that a structural defect of the vein wall was involved in the cause of VVs. First, VVs are typically saccular and usually begin peripherally in the tributaries of the GSV or LSV, not in the proximal main trunks. Second, normal saphenous veins exposed to pressures above 85 mmHg, with the pressure generated in an upright subject from the right atrium to the ankle without venous valves, showed no dilatation or loss of tone. Finally, there is a family history of VVs in patients with the disease in 43–80% of cases.

A combination of 2 theories proposes that a generalized vein wall weakness may exist, but does not result in varicosities unless associated with localized valvular incompetence of perforator veins. The transmission of an increased pressure to the abnormally weak vein segments results in varicosities only in the area near an incompetent perforator or proximal vein.

The cause of VVs is important in determining treatment, and the lack of agreement has led to a variety of procedures to treat VVs, depending on the practitioner's belief concerning the cause of a patient's varicosities. If incompetence of the valves of the GSV is believed to be the problem, high ligation of the GSV is considered the best treatment. If a primary vein wall defect or AV communications is considered to be the explanation, ligation and stripping would not be expected to result in a cure; stab avulsion and removal of each varicose tributary would be a more fitting treatment. If incompetent perforators are the likely cause, perforator ligation and individual VV removal are considered the best treatment.

E. Secondary Varicose Veins: Secondary VVs are usually the result of changes in the deep venous system secondary to deep vein thrombosis. The fibrotic response during recanalization and healing of the deep venous system after deep venous thrombosis frequently results in damage to the valves of the vein leading to reflux in the deep venous system. Frequently, perforator veins are also damaged and become incompetent, allowing reflux from the deep venous system into the superficial veins. This may lead to an increase in venous flow and pressure in the superficial system, which becomes the primary outflow tract for the extremity, resulting in secondary VVs. It is again critically important to diagnose deep or perforator venous incompetence, if present in a patient with varicosities.

Stripping of the superficial venous system in a patient with deep venous abnormalities may actually lead to a worsening of the patient's chronic venous stasis and result in ulcerations or other complications that were not present initially.

F. Congenital Vascular Malformations: VVs are associated with several congenital syndromes such as Klippel-Trénaunay syndrome and Parkes Weber syndrome. **Klippel-Trénaunay syndrome** is a condition characterized by limb hypertrophy, VVs, and capillary port-wine stains; this syndrome appears to be the most common of the congenital abnormalities associated with VVs. Patients with **Parkes Weber syndrome** have a similar presentation with limb hypertrophy, VVs, and AV malformations. Some authors believe that these syndromes are varied expressions of the same genetic defect.

The management of patients with these congenital malformations has centered on the surgical treatment of associated AV malformations or angiomas, but little has been done to address the limb hypertrophy or VVs, which is partly due to the controversy over the cause. Some have considered the primary cause to be deep venous obstruction. Thus, treatment of the varicose superficial system with surgical removal could lead to a further obstruction to outflow and increased limb swelling. Compression therapy has been the mainstay of treatment, along with sclerotherapy in some cases. However, some authors such as Servelle feel that surgical treatment of deep venous abnormalities diagnosed on duplex scan can lead to marked improvement in venous outflow in some patients. Perforator vein incompetence is frequently found in patients with these congenital malformations (100% of patients in Villavicencio's series) and should be treated surgically if the deep venous system is confirmed as being patent.

Clinical Findings

A. Signs and Symptoms: On physical examination, VVs are seen as usually dilated, tortuous superfi-

cial veins in the distribution of the tributaries of the GSV or LSV (Fig 31–6). Examination of the patient should be performed in the standing position with the leg in question unweighted and slightly flexed at the knee. Telangiectasias are seen as small spider-like clusters of venules, which blanch with pressure and appear to extend outward from a single feeder vessel (Fig 31–7). Signs of chronic venous insufficiency such as swelling, pigmentation, and edema localized in the gaiter area of the lower extremity may also be present. This is more common in secondary VVs associated with prior deep venous thrombosis. VVs and superficial venous reflux may also be associated with venous ulceration and may be the only venous abnormality. In a study of 59 patients with venous ulceration, Shami and associates found isolated deep venous reflux in 15%, a combination of deep and superficial reflux in 32%, and isolated superficial venous reflux in 53%.

Patients with VVs commonly present with symptoms of pain, fatigue, and aching heaviness, which may be exacerbated by prolonged standing. Elevation of the legs may provide relief. On the other hand, patients with significant VVs may be asymptomatic, with the primary complaint being the cosmetic appearance

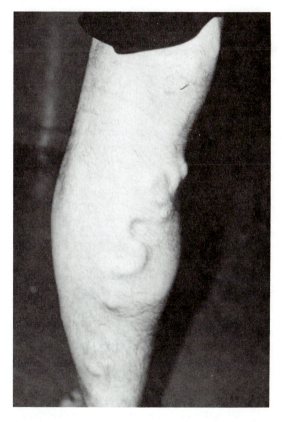

Figure 31–6. Patient with truncal varicosities of greater saphenous vein and tributaries.

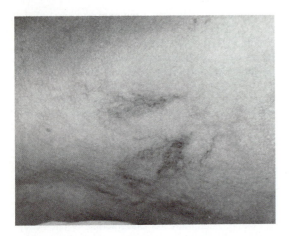

Figure 31–7. Patient with typical telangiectasia. (Reproduced, with permission, from Goldman MP [editor]: *Sclerotherapy: Treatment of Varicose and Telangiectatic Leg Veins.* Mosby-Yearbook, 1991.)

of the dilated, tortuous veins. Patients with telangiectasias are usually asymptomatic, but may complain of aching pain after prolonged standing.

B. Laboratory Findings: Identification of the distribution of varicosities and the source of venous hypertension is of great importance in developing a rational plan of treatment for each patient. Also, appropriate use of noninvasive diagnostic tests aid in differentiating between primary and secondary VVs and in helping to ensure that the therapy chosen is likely to correct the patient's varicosities with a minimal chance of recurrence. Of the common patterns of VVs, some involve the GSV, some the LSV, and some neither. Frequently, clusters of VVs arise in tributaries of the GSV or LSV, based on an incompetent perforator.

Goren and Yellin found the GSV or LSV to be diseased in 71% of limbs, with nearly 90% of these being GSV varicosities. In 22%, isolated perforator incompetence with no saphenous disease was found. In patients with isolated perforator incompetence, treatment would be possible without ligation of the main trunks of the saphenous veins, leaving them intact for later use in coronary artery bypass or lower extremity bypass, if needed.

Many noninvasive diagnostic modalities have been used to evaluate patients with VVs including photoplethysmography, air plethysmography, portable Doppler ultrasonography, and duplex ultrasonography. Air plethysmography is recommended to assess the physiologic significance of varicosities and duplex ultrasonography to carefully document the anatomic abnormalities in the venous system. Portable Doppler examination can be helpful to quickly assess the competence of veins in the clinic.

1. Air plethysmography–The air plethysmograph (APG) measures volume changes in the lower extremity during various maneuvers to quantitate physiologic function of the venous system. A 14-inch tubular air chamber is fitted around the lower leg and calibrated using a second air chamber placed against the leg. The patient is placed supine with the leg supported at the heel and elevated about 1 foot. A baseline lower leg volume is obtained and a second cuff around the proximal thigh is inflated to 80 mmHg prohibiting venous outflow. After the limb has filled to a plateau, the proximal cuff is rapidly deflated, and the venous volume leaving the leg over 1 second is measured. This outflow fraction is a measure of proximal venous obstruction.

The patient is then placed upright in the standing position. The change in leg volume is recorded until a plateau is reached. This represents the functional venous volume where the leg veins are full. The venous filling index (VFI) is obtained by dividing 90% of the venous volume by the time taken for the leg to reach this point. This represents the rate of venous filling, which should be relatively slow in normal limbs with competent valves. Limbs with incompetent venous valves have an increased VFI because the venous filling time is shorter. To differentiate between reflux in the deep and superficial venous systems, a tourniquet is placed around the upper leg occluding the GSV but not the deep system. The test is repeated with the superficial system occluded. If the VFI corrects, the reflux is likely related to superficial venous incompetence. If it does not correct with superficial occlusion, the reflux is located in the deep or perforator systems. If incompetence is suspected in the LSV, the tourniquet may be placed lower to occlude the LSV distal to the saphenopopliteal junction.

The patient is then asked to perform one vigorous tiptoe movement to determine the calf muscle pump ejection fraction. Ten successive tiptoe movements allow calculation of the residual volume fraction, which is a measure of the ability of the calf muscle pump to empty the limb. The residual volume fraction has been found to correlate with ambulatory venous pressure.

Using these maneuvers, an assessment of the function of the deep and superficial venous systems can be obtained. This is particularly useful in assessing the physiologic improvement after surgical or other interventions using the preoperative study as a baseline. Unfortunately, there are sources of error with use of the APG such as the difficulty in correctly occluding superficial veins with the tourniquet. Also, reflux from the ankle into the foot may affect measurements of reflux adversely. Until better methods of noninvasive assessment of venous function are developed, correlation of APG with anatomic evaluation of the limb using Doppler or duplex examinations probably provides the most reliable information to aid in selecting appropriate treatment for patients with VVs.

2. Portable Doppler ultrasonography–Handheld continuous-wave Doppler probes can be used to assess the competence of the saphenous veins and to determine the patency of the deep venous system. Interrogation of normal veins with the Doppler ultrasound probe while the limb is compressed distally results in increased venous flow in the absence of proximal obstruction. Incompetence of a segment is best assessed with the patient in the standing position. The vein segment to be studied is compressed and emptied and is then interrogated with the Doppler probe. Release of the segment results in a retrograde flow signal in incompetent segments. Valsalva's maneuver may also be used to promote reversed flow and to assess the competence of the saphenofemoral junction. Systematically, the superficial and deep vein systems can be examined as well as individual varicosities to determine the site of incompetence.

The site and competence of perforator veins also can be assessed. However, the entire examination is subjective and depends greatly on the experience of the examiner. The GSV can be easily mistaken for the superficial femoral vein near the saphenofemoral junction, and all veins may be difficult to locate in obese persons. At best, the ability of most examiners to correctly identify incompetent perforators is no better than 60–80%. In the hands of a skilled practitioner, information gained with the Doppler probe may be sufficient to support clinical decisions without requiring duplex scans or venograms.

3. Duplex scan–Duplex scanners combine the imaging capabilities of B-mode ultrasound with the velocity capabilities of pulsed Doppler to allow anatomic examination of the veins as well as a determination of the direction and velocity of blood flowing within. The ultrasound probe images the vessel, and the pulsed Doppler device may be set to examine the velocity of flow at any depth within the vessel. An automatic cuff inflator is placed distal to the vein being examined and is inflated. When equilibrium is reached, the cuff is rapidly deflated to assess for reflux within the vein. In normal limbs, van Bemmelen reported the median duration of reflux to be 0.19 seconds. Ninety-five percent of popliteal veins had reflux lasting less than 0.66 seconds. This may be repeated for any veins in question to determine the sites of incompetence in the limb. The valves of incompetent veins can be imaged closely to determine the presence of an abnormality in function. Also, the flow pattern in the deep veins can be examined with duplex scanning and is very suggestive of deep venous thrombosis, if present.

Perforator veins may be mapped with a similar procedure, although the sensitivity for identifying incompetent perforators is not as good as in the deep or superficial systems. This technology currently offers the most reliable assessment of the anatomic status of the venous system, but it is also highly dependent on the ability and experience as well as patience of the examiner and patient. A thorough examination can provide solid information on the site of incompetence to aid in the selection of a treatment plan.

4. Venography–The improvement of the noninvasive testing modalities previously described has led to a decreased reliance on venograms in diagnosis of venous disease. However, in situations in which noninvasive tests are not sufficiently diagnostic, a venogram is often helpful.

In **ascending venography,** contrast medium is injected into a superficial foot vein and allowed to ascend into the leg veins to define anatomy. Placing a tourniquet around the ankle prevents contrast from flowing directly up the superficial system. Thus, any contrast entering the superficial system above must do so via incompetent perforators aiding in their identification. Observation of the flow of contrast in the proximal direction identifies the venous anatomy and should reveal obstruction, thrombus, or other abnormalities.

In **descending venography,** contrast is injected in the retrograde direction into the common femoral or popliteal vein and the extent of retrograde flow is identified. The treating clinician should be present during the performance of venograms because the dynamic nature of the study is such that most information is obtained from watching the flow of contrast, not static images. Valvular insufficiency is graded as reflux as outlined in Figure 31–8.

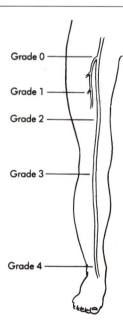

Figure 31–8. Categories of deep venous reflux on descending venography: Grade 0, no reflux below junction of superficial and profunda femoris veins; grade 1, reflux into superficial femoral vein but not below midthigh; grade 2, reflux into superficial femoral vein below midthigh but not into popliteal vein; grade 3, reflux into popliteal vein past level of knee; grade 4, reflux to the ankle level. (Reproduced, with permission, from Goldman MP [editor]: *Sclerotherapy: Treatment of Varicose and Telangiectatic Leg Veins.* Mosby-Yearbook, 1991.)

Differential Diagnosis

Patients with symptomatic VVs may have symptoms based on arterial, not venous, insufficiency, particularly elderly patients. Therapeutic attempts to correct VVs may lead to complications such as poor healing, thrombophlebitis, and VV recurrence if the arterial disease is not recognized and treated first. Digital or Doppler examination or both of distal extremity pulses should be performed and, if any abnormality exists, further evaluation with segmental pressures should be performed.

Patients with AV malformations may develop dilated superficial veins similar to varicosities. A palpable thrill or bruit on auscultation as well as a history of trauma are suggestive of this diagnosis. Doppler or duplex examination of the dilated vein should reveal a velocity pattern with an arterial character in an AV malformation or fistula.

Congenital venous malformations such as Klippel-Trénaunay syndrome must also be differentiated from primary VVs.

Treatment

A. Nonsurgical Treatment:

1. Compression therapy–Compression bandages or stockings are primarily indicated for patients with chronic venous insufficiency, which may develop with superficial venous incompetence alone. VVs associated with insufficiency and leg ulcerations would be treated with compression therapy as an aid to ulcer healing, but should not be expected to improve the chronic venous insufficiency, which should be managed surgically to prevent ulcer recurrence after healing. Compression stockings may help patients with VVs associated with symptoms by preventing reflux in the superficial system and reducing swelling while standing, which may lead to a reduction in leg fatigue and pain. Compression is unlikely to be effective in symptomatic VVs not associated with saphenous incompetence.

The most important factor in the use of compression stockings or bandages is patient compliance. Poor-fitting stockings or high-compression stockings are unlikely to be tolerated by most patients. Thigh-high stockings are probably worn less often than knee-high stockings, and they should be worn whenever the patient is not supine to be most effective. Thus, efforts aimed at providing the patient with a good-fitting stocking of the minimum compression and length necessary will result in the best chance for long-term use.

Compression is also important in minimizing the incidence of complications after sclerotherapy or surgery for VVs such as hemorrhage, recanalization, pigmentation, and thrombophlebitis and in reducing edema formation and enhancing wound healing. Most clinicians use compression bandages for 3–14 days after treatment of VVs and follow this with a variable length of treatment with compression stockings for optimum results. Compression therapy should not be used, or at least used cautiously, for patients with arterial insufficiency, severe congestive heart failure, or acute deep venous thrombosis.

2. Sclerotherapy: Injection of a sclerosing agent results in an injury to the endothelium followed by sloughing and a transmural injury. The vessel reacts with spasm, inflammatory changes, and thrombosis acutely, followed by chronic thickening and fibrosis leading to permanent occlusion of the varix. Differences in type and strength of sclerosant are a balance between efficacy and potential to induce complications. Compression after sclerosis is important to limit the incidence of complications and enhance endothelial fibrosis.

Excellent results have been reported after sclerotherapy of VVs of all sizes and in all locations, including the main saphenous trunks and incompetent perforator vessels. However, most authors agree that sclerotherapy should not be performed in the main saphenous trunks unless combined with ligation of the saphenofemoral or saphenopopliteal junction. In a randomized trial comparing sclerotherapy and surgery for treatment of VVs, after 1 year, 82% of patients were cured by sclerotherapy, but by 6 years, the cure rate was only 7%. The results in sclerotherapy of the main saphenous trunks were particularly poor. However, the results with sclerotherapy in treatment of smaller varicose branch veins were better than the results with surgical treatment (>75% cured or improved at 6 years after sclerotherapy compared with 40% cured or improved at 6 years after surgery). Bishop and associates evaluated the results of sclerotherapy using duplex ultrasonography and found a high incidence of recurrence of reflux into the previously sclerosed saphenous vein.

Sclerotherapy may be particularly effective in removal of residual varicosities after surgical treatment of a limb. The results obtained are highly dependent on the clinician, which should caution inexperienced practitioners from expecting similar results to those reported in the literature by experts in the field.

Telangiectasias are frequently associated with VVs and may also be treated by sclerotherapy. Complications that can occur after sclerotherapy of telangiectasias include pigmentation, cutaneous necrosis, superficial thrombophlebitis, folliculitis, and allergic reaction. Recurrence of telangiectasias is unusual if sclerotherapy is complete, but appearance of new lesions at different locations is common.

B. Surgical Treatment: Numerous surgical procedures are designed to treat varicosities, including high ligation, ligation and stripping, stab avulsion, perforator ligation, and others. Selection of the best procedure for each patient should be based on a careful preoperative evaluation of the anatomy involved. Assessment of surgical procedures and all forms of treatment for VVs is difficult because of several factors: relatively few well-designed prospective randomized trials comparing forms of treatment; comparison of studies is often difficult because of variations in definitions of treatment failure or VV recurrence; and, most important, most studies have evaluated results based on subjective impressions. Only recently have studies appeared using objective criteria generated from duplex scanning to evaluate the results of surgery for VVs. In addition, follow-up of patients in studies must extend 5–10 years to assess the true incidence of recurrence. In several long-term studies, the early results of a procedure were excellent, but the late results were poor.

1. High ligation with stab avulsion–Ligation of the saphenous vein at the saphenofemoral junction was conceived as a method of interrupting reflux down the incompetent saphenous vein, thereby limiting pressure on the distal saphenous vein and its tributaries that might lead to further valvular incompetence and distal varices. A transverse incision in the groin of 6–10 cm should be placed as near to the inguinal ligament as possible. The incision should be large enough for good exposure of all venous branches at the saphenofemoral junction. One study found a correlation between a smaller incision and an increased incidence of incomplete saphenofemoral ligation. Usually, several tributaries drain into the GSV near its junction with the femoral vein. The GSV must be ligated proximally at the saphenofemoral junction and these tributaries ligated as well to prevent recurrence due to collateral flow (Fig 31–9). No stripping of the main saphenous trunk is performed. Individual VVs are treated by stab avulsion through 2–4-mm incisions.

Recurrence of symptoms after this procedure is common, with over 50% of patients requiring further treatment at 5 years in several studies. The cause of recurrence of varicosities is multifactorial. The opera-

tion is not as simple as many believe because of the variation in venous anatomy at the saphenofemoral junction. In the report of McMullin and associates, 2 of 54 patients undergoing high ligation were found to have a patent saphenofemoral junction on postoperative duplex scan. In this study, 46% of the ligated GSVs were patent distally with reflux identified on duplex scan distal to the saphenofemoral junction. In 2 of these, reflux was identified through incompetent midthigh perforators, and, in the remainder, small tortuous veins appeared to be arising from the femoral vein at the groin distal to the site of ligation, which was the source of reflux.

Rutherford found that the distal saphenous vein remained patent in 85% of patients after ligation or proximal stripping. Bradbury reported 73% of 71 reoperated patients with recurrent VVs had an intact GSV in the thigh, and only 28% had a ligated GSV at the saphenofemoral junction. It is clear that simple high ligation is inadequate treatment for the patient with an incompetent GSV or LSV, because it frequently leaves a diseased vein with a high chance of recurrence.

2. High ligation and stripping with stab avulsion–Patients with preoperative noninvasive studies localizing incompetence to the superficial system with an incompetent diseased GSV or LSV are prime candidates for ligation and stripping procedures. Patients with deep or perforator disease should be evaluated carefully for correction of these systems first to avoid a high risk of recurrence. Patients with a competent, normal main saphenous trunk may be better candidates for stab avulsion or sclerotherapy.

The addition of stripping of the main saphenous trunk has the advantage of leaving no potentially dis-

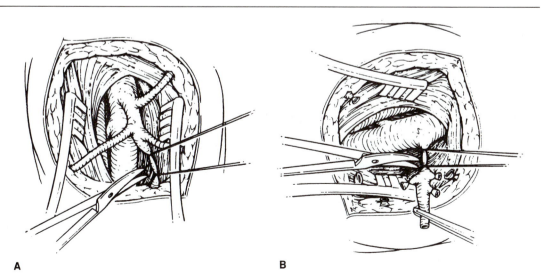

A   **B**

Figure 31–9. ***A:*** Exposure of saphenofemoral junction and multiple branches entering greater saphenous near junction. ***B:*** Flush ligation of GSV with tributary ligation. (Reproduced, with permission, from Bergan JJ, Kistner RL [editors]: *Atlas of Venous Surgery.* WB Saunders, 1992.)

eased saphenous vein behind to become incompetent. It also interrupts all perforators that connect directly to the saphenous trunk and theoretically should have a decreased long-term recurrence rate. Disadvantages are the loss of the saphenous vein, which may be needed at a later time for cardiac or vascular procedures, and the increased morbidity of a larger operation. The saphenous nerve is in close proximity to the GSV in the leg below the knee, and stripping operations may cause an injury to this nerve or to the sural nerve in stripping of the LSV, manifested by anesthesia or pain in the distribution of each nerve.

To perform high ligation and stripping of the main saphenous trunks, a high ligation is performed first, as previously described. The saphenous vein is also identified at the distal extent of the segment to be stripped through a small transverse incision. The stripper is passed through this distal incision proximally to the groin incision where the divided saphenous vein is secured to the stripper. It is then withdrawn distally, avulsing the saphenous trunk from its branches. A gauze pack may be placed in the tunnel by attaching it to the stripper to provide compression during the remainder of the procedure (Fig 31–10). Otherwise, strong compression with elastic bandages is used over the dressings after wound closure to compress any

bleeding from the avulsed branches. The LSV can be avulsed in similar fashion, but may be difficult because of the variable site of termination of the LSV in or above the popliteal space. Identification of the saphenopopliteal junction preoperatively with duplex scanning can be very helpful.

Methods to decrease the incidence of injury to the saphenous nerve include stripping in the proximal to distal direction and using the small olive on the stripper. In many cases, it may not be necessary to strip the GSV distal to the upper calf, the area of greatest risk to the saphenous nerve. In the calf, Cockett's perforator veins usually connect to branches of the GSV, not directly to the GSV. Therefore, if the distal GSV is not varicose, stripping to the upper calf would remove the hunterian, Dodd's, and upper Boyd's perforators, while reducing the risk of injury to the saphenous nerve.

Negus followed up 73 patients for 3–7 years after high ligation and stripping procedures, reporting a 13% recurrence rate, and a 4% rate of injury to the saphenous nerve. A combination of 4 prospective, randomized studies comparing saphenofemoral ligation with ligation plus stripping of the GSV yielded 573 patients with recurrence rates of 40.0% for high ligation and 17.2% for ligation plus stripping. The incidence of saphenous injury was significantly higher after GSV

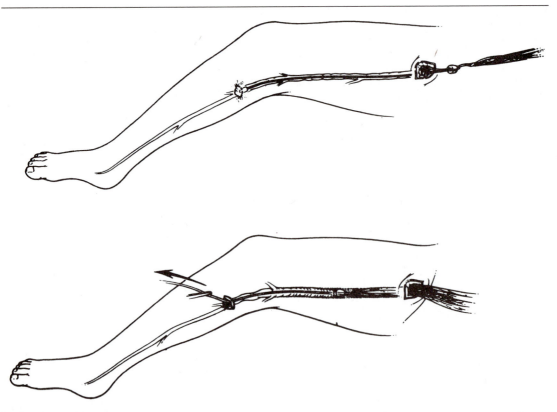

Figure 31–10. Stripping of GSV from saphenofemoral junction to upper calf. See text for details of technique. (Reproduced, with permission, from Bergan JJ, Kistner RL [editors]: *Atlas of Venous Surgery.* WB Saunders, 1992.)

stripping in one study, but not in another. In well-selected patients, this procedure results in a low risk of recurrence and a relatively low incidence of morbidity.

3. High ligation and sclerotherapy–The use of high ligation of the GSV or LSV combined with sclerotherapy of individual varices has also been proposed with advantages in cosmesis and postoperative morbidity cited. This procedure may be performed using local anesthesia and may be considered as an option for medically compromised patients. Unfortunately, long-term results have been mediocre, with only 40% having a satisfactory outcome in Neglen's study at 5 years and 65% at 3 years in Jakobsen's series. These results were significantly worse than the results achieved with ligation and stripping in both authors' reports.

4. Stab avulsion alone–Patients with VVs who have no evidence of GSV or LSV incompetence or disease may not need stripping of these main trunks. This situation occurred in 29% of patients in Goren and Yellin's study of 230 limbs with VVs. If the deep venous system is normal, suspicion of perforator incompetence should be high, and duplex studies, venography, or both should be performed to evaluate these veins. If perforator incompetence is diagnosed, perforator ligation should be performed along with stab avulsion of the individual varices.

Stab avulsion of varices has been well described in several articles. The varices to be treated are carefully marked with indelible ink prior to surgery. Small 2–4-mm incisions are made along the previously marked varices. The varix is exposed by minimal dissection with a mosquito hemostat and captured with a vein hook or similar instrument (Fig 31–11). The vein is teased from the subcutaneous tissue and drawn into the wound (Fig 31–12). It is then divided, and each end is avulsed using a rocking motion to gain as much length as possible (Fig 31–13). Compression is placed on the area to control bleeding, and the procedure is repeated until all marked varices are removed. The wounds may be closed with subcuticular sutures or adhesive tape. Compression therapy is important acutely to prevent hemorrhage or excessive bruising and is maintained for several weeks postoperatively.

Prognosis

The results with stab avulsion of VVs usually depend on the procedures with which it is combined, since most patients also undergo ligation, stripping of the main saphenous trunk, or perforator ligation. Complications are rare, but include superficial phlebitis, recurrent bleeding, nerve injuries (usually transient), and keloid formation.

The results of all forms of treatment for VVs depend on anatomic and physiologic information. As advances in the ability of noninvasive techniques to identify the abnormalities in the venous system have occurred, our understanding of the pathophysiology has increased, as has our ability to rationally select procedures to correct each patient's abnormalities. Much is still not known about the therapy of VVs, and well-designed randomized studies using objective criteria to assess pre- and postoperative venous function will help greatly to improve treatment results of patients with venous disease.

SUPERFICIAL THROMBOPHLEBITIS

Essentials of Diagnosis

- Painful, indurated vein in area of intravenous catheter or varicose vein.
- Erythema surrounding involved vein.
- Vein palpable as a tender, linear cord.

General Considerations

Thrombophlebitis of the superficial veins may occur at any location in the body, but it is most common in

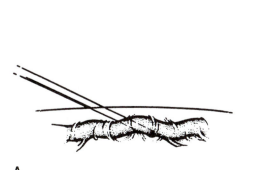
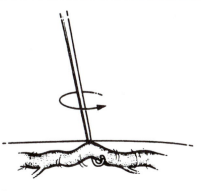

| A | B |

Figure 31–11. A: Through a small incision (2–3 mm), a hook, mosquito, or similar instrument is inserted. **B:** The varicosity is captured and freed from the surrounding subcutaneous tissue.

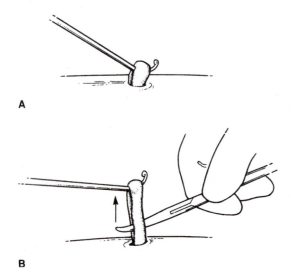

A

B

Figure 31–12. A: The vein is elevated through the incision. **B:** The loop is separated. (Reproduced, with permission, from Goren G, Yellin AE: Ambulatory stab avulsion phlebectomy for truncal varicose veins. Am J Surg 1991;162:166.)

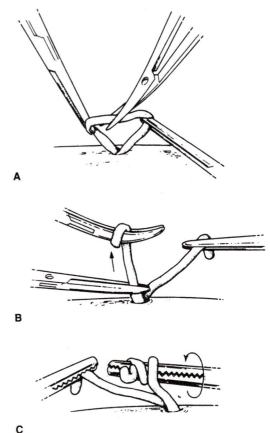

A

B

C

Figure 31–13. A: Hemostats are placed on each arm and the varicosity is divided. **B** and **C:** Using traction and rocking and twisting motions, the segments of vein are extracted to the fullest extent and avulsed. Compression is applied to limit bleeding. (Reproduced, with permission, from Goren G, Yellin AE: Ambulatory stab avulsion phlebectomy for truncal varicose veins. Am J Surg 1991; 162:166.)

the upper extremities, where it is associated with intravenous catheters or intravenous drug abuse, and in the lower extremities, where it is associated with VVs. Other causes include hypercoagulable states, pregnancy, oral contraceptives, and local trauma. Superficial thrombophlebitis (STP) was previously thought to be a self-limiting condition except in patients with systemic infection associated with septic thrombophlebitis. However, several recent studies have reported an incidence of subclinical deep venous thrombosis (DVT) of 12–23% in patients with STP. In one report, 4% of patients with STP developed evidence of a significant pulmonary embolus, emphasizing the need to treat these patients with greater suspicion for DVT and its sequelae.

Clinical Findings

A. Signs and Symptoms: The presentation of STP is usually relatively straightforward, since patients develop a painful indurated vein in an area of intravenous catheter therapy or varicosity. The vein can frequently be palpated as a thick, tender cord, and the previous site of access may still be visible. The area is usually surrounded by a variable amount of erythema. The diagnosis may be more difficult in the intensive care unit, where patients frequently have a compromised mental status. The only symptom may be an unexplained fever or septic picture. Routine surveillance of intravenous access sites should be performed in all patients to allow removal of catheters at the earliest sign of phlebitis and to prevent progression to septic thrombophlebitis.

The important decision at the time of examination of patients with STP concerns the severity of the lesion and whether operative incision and débridement of the vein should be performed. Most cases resolve with conservative therapy, but if STP is associated with severe induration, erythema, or a septic picture with chills and high fever, excision and débridement are usually recommended.

B. Adjunctive Testing: STP is best diagnosed by history and a thorough physical examination, and adjunctive tests are rarely needed. The main role for testing concerns the potential association of STP with DVT. Skillman, using venography, found STP to be associated with DVT in 12% of patients with no symptoms of DVT. Jorgensen and associates, using duplex scans to study patients with STP, found evidence of DVT in 23% of patients. Lutter reported STP to be followed by pulmonary embolus in 4% of 186 patients, and only 50% had evidence on duplex scan of an associated DVT. Location of the thrombus in the GSV was more likely to be associated with DVT or pulmonary embolus, as was bilateral STP or a history of prior DVT.

STP was previously believed to lead to DVT by propagating up the GSV or LSV to cause thrombosis in the femoral or popliteal veins, respectively. The previously mentioned studies revealed that this was true in only a minority of cases. STP was associated with extension to the deep system through perforators as well and with no evidence of direct contact with the DVT in other cases. Noninvasive evaluation of the deep venous system should be performed in all patients with lower extremity STP to identify patients with DVT who should be treated with anticoagulation therapy. In the upper extremity, this is probably not necessary unless some indication such as swelling suggests the presence of DVT. Although DVT of the upper extremity has been reported to cause pulmonary embolus, it is probably much less common than in the lower extremity.

Differential Diagnosis

In 1939, Mondor reported a case of STP of the breast. **Mondor's disease** is an uncommon condition of questionable etiology, which may lead to diagnostic confusion with other breast diseases and result in unnecessary biopsy. It is associated with pain and tenderness in 90% of patients, and a cord-like vein is frequently palpable, which should help in the differential diagnosis. The lesion usually involves a vein in the upper outer quadrant or in the submammary fold. Mondor's disease has been related in some cases to prior trauma or breast surgery and is usually self-limiting, resolving with conservative therapy in several weeks.

Treatment

Conservative therapy consisting of intravenous catheter removal, hot compresses, elevation, and nonsteroidal anti-inflammatory medications should lead to resolution in most patients. Antibiotics are not necessary unless septic thrombophlebitis develops. The affected vein should be examined frequently to assess the response to therapy and ensure that progression to

septic thrombophlebitis is not occurring. In the lower extremity, progression of the phlebitic process toward the saphenofemoral or saphenopopliteal junction has been treated with saphenous ligation and stripping of the affected vein to prevent the risk of deep venous extension and of potential complications. However, no randomized studies are available that show the superiority of surgical treatment to conservative treatment or anticoagulant therapy.

Heparinoid creams or nonsteroidal ointments for local treatment have been reported to increase the speed of symptom resolution. However, in a randomized trial comparing placebo with heparinoid cream and piroxicam gel (nonsteroidal anti-inflammatory ointment), Bergqvist and associates reported no difference in disease course among the 3 groups.

After resolution of the acute induration and erythema, compression may be particularly helpful in further resolution, especially in the lower extremity when associated with VVs. When STP is associated with varicosities, definitive treatment of the varicosity with excision or sclerotherapy can be performed to minimize the incidence of recurrence after resolution of the acute thrombophlebitis.

Patients who develop septic thrombophlebitis should have immediate operative excision of the affected vein with local débridement of infected tissue. The wound should be left open to granulate, and systemic antibiotics should be administered to cover skin flora (most frequently *Staphylococcus*) or indigenous opportunistic pathogens if in the intensive care setting. If blood cultures are positive, antibiotic therapy should continue 7–10 days.

In patients with no history of injecting drugs, of catheterization, or of varicosities, other sources of STP must be sought. A screen for hypercoagulability should be performed, since cases of migratory thrombophlebitis have been reported to be associated with abnormalities in antithrombin III, protein C and protein S, lupus anticoagulant, and factor XII levels. Occult malignancy should also be considered in patients with spontaneous migratory thrombophlebitis, an association known as **Trousseau's syndrome.**

REFERENCES

Beaglehole R: Incidence and risk factors: Epidemiology of varicose veins. World J Surg 1986;10:898.

Bejanga BI: Mondor's disease: Analysis of 30 cases. J R Coll Surg Edinb 1992;37:322.

Bergan JJ: Clinical application of duplex testing in treatment of primary venous stasis, varicose veins.

Bergan JJ: The current management of varicose and telangiectatic veins. Surg Annu 1993;25(Pt 1):141.

Bergan JJ: Surgical procedures for varicose veins: Axial stripping and stab avulsion. In: *Atlas of Venous Surgery,* Bergan JJ, Kistner RL [editors]. WB Saunders, 1992.

Bergan JJ, Goldman MP (editors): *Varicose Veins and*

Telangiectasias: Diagnosis and Treatment. Quality Medical Publishing, 1993.

Bergqvist D et al: Treatment of superficial thrombophlebitis: A comparative trial between placebo, hirudoid cream and piroxicam gel. Ann Chir Gynaecol 1990;79:92.

Bishop CCR et al: Real-time color duplex scanning after sclerotherapy of the greater saphenous vein. J Vasc Surg 1991;14:505.

Blumoff RL, Johnson G Jr: Saphenous vein pO2 in patients with varicose veins. J Surg Res 1977;23:35.

Clarke GH et al: Venous wall function in the pathogenesis of varicose veins. Surgery 1992;111:402.

Dindelli M et al: Risk factors for varicose disease before and during pregnancy. Angiology 1993;44:361.

Dodd H: The varicose tributaries of the popliteal vein. Br J Surg 1965;52:350.

Eger SA, Casper SL: Etiology of varicose veins from an anatomic aspect based on dissections of 38 adult cadavers. JAMA 1943;123:148.

Gandhi RH et al: Analysis of the connective tissue matrix and proteolytic activity of primary varicose veins. J Vasc Surg 1993;18:814.

Gillespie DL et al: The role of air plethysmography in monitoring results of venous surgery. J Vasc Surg 1992;16:674.

Goldman MP (editor): *Sclerotherapy: Treatment of Varicose and Telangiectatic Leg Veins.* Mosby-Yearbook, 1991.

Goren G, Yellin AE: Ambulatory stab evulsion phlebectomy for truncal varicose veins. Am J Surg 1991;162:166.

Goren G, Yellin AE: Primary varicose veins: Topographic and hemodynamic correlations. J Cardiovasc Surg 1990;31:672.

Haynes DF et al: Increased prostacyclin and thromboxane A2 formation in human varicose veins. J Surg Res 1990;49:228.

Hobbs JT: Surgery and sclerotherapy in the treatment of varicose veins: A random trial. Arch Surg 1974;109:793.

Jorgensen JO et al: The incidence of deep venous thrombosis in patients with superficial thrombophlebitis of the lower limbs. J Vasc Surg 1993;18:70.

McMullin GM et al: Objective assessment of high ligation without stripping the long saphenous vein. Br J Surg 1991;78:1139.

Papadakis K et al: Number and anatomical distribution of incompetent thigh perforating veins. Br J Surg 1989;76:581.

Prountjos P et al: Superficial venous thrombosis of the lower extremities co-existing with deep venous thrombosis: A phlebographic study on 57 cases. Int Angiol 1991;10:63.

Pulliam CW et al: Venous duplex scanning in the diagnosis and treatment of progressive superficial thrombophlebitis. Ann Vasc Surg 1991;5:190.

Raymond-Martimbeau P: Advanced sclerotherapy treatment of varicose veins with duplex ultrasonographic guidance. Adv Semin Dermatol 1993;12:123.

Ruckley CV: Does venous reflux matter? Lancet 1993;341:411.

Sadick NS: Predisposing factors of varicose and telangiectatic leg veins. Phlebology 1992;18:883.

Samlaska CP, James WD: Superficial thrombophlebitis I. Primary hypercoagulable states. J Am Acad Dermatol 1990;22:975.

Sarin S et al: Assessment of stripping the long saphenous vein in the treatment of primary varicose veins. Br J Surg 1992;79:889.

Scott HJ et al: Reappraisal of the oxygenation of blood in varicose veins. Br J Surg 1990;77:934.

Shami SK et al: Venous ulcers and the superficial venous system. J Vasc Surg 1993;17:487.

Shouler PJ, Runchman PC: Varicose veins: Optimum compression after surgery and sclerotherapy. Ann R Coll Surg Engl 1989;71:402.

Skillman JJ et al: Simultaneous occurrence of superficial and deep thrombophlebitis in the lower extremity. J Vasc Surg 1990;11:818.

Sumner DS: Venous dynamics: Varicosities. Clin Obstet Gynecol 1981;24:743.

Thomson H: The surgical anatomy of the superficial and perforating veins of the lower limb. Ann R Coll Surg Engl 1979;61:198.

van Bemmelen PS et al: Quantitative segmental evaluation of venous valvular reflux with duplex ultrasound scanning. J Vasc Surg 1989;10:425.

Widmer LK: *Peripheral Venous Disorders: Prevalence and Socio-medical Importance: Observations in 4529 Apparently Healthy Persons.* Basel Study III. Hans Huber Publishers, 1978.

Chronic Venous Insufficiency

32

Ralph G. DePalma, MD, FACS, & John J. Bergan, MD

Venous dysfunction in the lower extremities may manifest itself in a number of ways, such as (1) spontaneous appearance of telangiectatic blemishes; (2) increased prominence of the blue-green, subdermal, reticular network of veins; (3) development of protuberant, saccular varicosities; or (4) production of disabling pain, eczematoid dermatitis, brawny ankle induration, and intractable cutaneous ulceration. The latter condition has occupied the interest of many historically prominent surgeons including Ambrose Paré, Thomas Vicary, John Hunter, Thomas Brodie, Frederick Trendelenburg, and John Homans of Boston. Homans in particular tied the development of the severe sequelae of venous insufficiency to prior deep venous thrombosis.[25] Because of his influence, the condition has been referred to as the postphlebitic or post-thrombotic state. Now it is known that the disability and the advanced skin changes do not depend solely on a prior episode of deep venous thrombosis.[10] Realization of this fact has opened the door to a variety of effective treatments based on knowledge derived from physiologic and anatomic diagnostic testing. These methods of diagnosis and treatment are the subject of this chapter.

Essentials of Diagnosis
- Changes in skin pigmentation.
- Itching, weeping dermatitis.
- Ulceration.

General Considerations
Skin and subcutaneous tissues are the ultimate targets of chronic venous insufficiency (CVI), and the skin changes produced by venous hypertension are predictable. Early in the course of CVI, the skin pigmentation is caused by hemosiderin deposition. This develops in the lower third of the leg on the medial aspect. Pigmentation may be followed by an itching, weeping dermatitis. If left untreated, the dermatitis may progress to ulceration. In certain patients, progression of skin changes is accelerated by vigorous scrubbing with water, soap, or detergents in misdirected efforts to clear the condition. In others, application of medications triggers a contact dermatitis.

The skin changes are related to venous pressure, but the magnitude of cutaneous pathology does not depend on a linear relationship.[36] Identical venous pressure data can be found in limbs with and without the stigmata of CVI. However, because venous pressure is so important, the sources of abnormal venous pressure must be understood.

Pathogenesis
Lower limb venous hypertension is derived from 2 sources. The first and most carefully studied is reflux of gravitational origin coursing down linear, axial, venous segments.[7] This is **hydrostatic pressure,** the weight of a blood column from the right atrium. Normally, the weight of this column is arrested by venous valves. However, if these valves fail to coapt, the weight of the blood presses inexorably distally. Ultimately, the highest pressures generated by this mechanism are expressed at ankle and foot level, where they are measured in centimeters of water or millimeters of mercury.

The second mechanism of venous hypertension is **dynamic.** This is the force of muscular contraction usually contained within compartments of the leg. However, superficial to deep perforating veins penetrate the deep crural fascia. Their anatomic angulation and their contained valves normally prevent compartmental pressure from being transmitted to subcutaneous tissues and skin. Failure of this check valve mechanism allows intracompartmental forces to be transmitted directly to unsupported subcutaneous veins and dermal capillaries.[2] There, the effective vessels elongate, dilate, and lose their valve competence. Thus, venous hypertension is both hydrostatic and hydrodynamic. The effects are additive and are amplified by the pulsatile nature of muscular forces generated by exercise.

A. Importance of Perforating Veins: At the level of the skin, the 2 abnormal hemodynamically forces meet and produce additive effects. Here, failed perforator check valves are believed to be of prime importance. Cockett's[11] influence on this subject led to the naming of leg/ankle perforating veins for him. Although 3 named perforators have been described, many more are actually of clinical importance. Figure 32–1 shows characteristic perforating veins, although many variable patterns exist.

Tremendous pressure exerted by large perforating veins in the lower leg during exercise has been described.[3] Also, bidirectional flow through the perforating veins during ambulation with inward flow during a foot-lifting phase (diastole) and outward flow in the

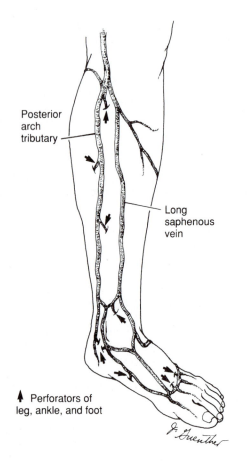

Posterior
arch
tributary

Long
saphenous
vein

↑ Perforators of
leg, ankle, and foot

J. Guenther

Figure 32–1. Schematic drawing of veins of lower leg. Note prominent posterior arch tributary, perforating veins, and veins of foot and distal plantar arch.

entering the capillary bed. This may produce a high degree of peripheral vascular resistance and tissue ischemia. According to Schmid-Schonbein,[44] "this phenomenon may be the basic physiologic mechanism in myocardial ischemia, stroke, shock, and many other diseases." This common pathway of tissue destruction may operate in CVI, the severe changes in the integrity of the skin and subcutaneous tissues being triggered by leukocyte activation, proteolytic enzyme release, and free radical activity.

In CVI, dependency and later limb elevation may result in a relative reperfusion phenomenon. Just as reperfusion effects as studied in limbs, mesentery, and myocardium are shown to be due to white cell trapping and activation, the same changes may be operative in CVI. Activated leukocytes release proteolytic enzymes, superoxide radicals, and other chemotactic substances.[46] A chain of tissue destructive events follows. Supporting these observations is a study of biopsies from skin of patients with a variety of venous dysfunction, including varicose veins, lipodermatosclerosis, and history of ulceration.[45] In this important study, white cell count increased from a median of 6 white blood cells per mm^2 in limbs with varicose veins to 45 white blood cells per mm^2 in limbs with lipodermatosclerosis to 217 in limbs with ulceration. The predominant infiltrating cells were seen to be T lymphocytes and macrophages.

An associated increase in number of capillaries was observed in the papillary dermis. It is uncertain whether accumulation of macrophages and T cells in areas of skin afflicted with CVI is the cause of CVI or an effect of it. An inflammatory response to tissue damage from any cause would lead to similar findings. Although far from complete, a unifying theory of causation of the skin changes of CVI can be based on these newly documented cellular changes.

Clinical Findings

In slender subjects, greater or lesser saphenous venous insufficiency and associated varicosities are seen in the physical examination. Examination is best performed by a seated examiner with the patient standing on a 46-cm platform as described by Ruckley.[42] A large, dilated, and tortuous saphenous vein is visible and palpable. Perforating veins can be defined by palpation of fascial defects. A physical sign of greater saphenous reflux is a downward groin impulse on coughing, which is thought to be transmission of blood distally through dilated, incompetent valves. This may be associated with a palpable thrill. Tapping the column of blood by percussion of the vein may demonstrate pressure transmission through the static column of blood in the incompetent vein.

Traditional, and in fact antique, physical tests have been described. These now have mainly tradition to recommend them as they are largely indirect. The Perthes' test was the first test used for deep venous occlusion and dates from 1895. In this test,[41] the entire

"foot-on-the-ground" phase (systole) has been documented.[8] Other calf perforating veins such as in the area of the gastrocnemius muscle also transmit pressure externally. One of the most important is the anteromedial calf perforator named for Boyd. In the thigh, perforators named in honor of several surgeons are recognized (Dodd and Hunter perforators).

A third factor that contributes to venous hypertension is proximal saphenous flow from the plantar veins and perforators in the foot into the saphenous and communicator veins at the ankle. This observation has been emphasized to be of importance in recurrent ulcerations by Negus.[38]

B. Cellular Changes: Fascinating cellular changes due to venous hypertension occurring in the skin have been uncovered. These suggest new theories of tissue damage and of ulceration. Elevated venous pressure has been observed in association with lower extremity white blood cell trapping.[37] When lipodermatosclerosis and ulceration are present, about 30% of circulating white blood cells are seen trapped after 1 hour of limb dependency.[51] Because white cells are larger than red cells, they deform very slowly on extremity is tightly wrapped with elastic bandages to compress varices. The patient then exercises. A complaint of severe pain with exercise suggests deep venous occlusion with superficial veins serving as collateral pathways of flow.

The most historically important traditional test is the Brodie-Trendelenburg test.[9,54] With the patient supine, the lower limb is elevated about 45 degrees above horizontal to ensure maximum venous drainage. Tourniquets of at least 1 inch in diameter are placed at the saphenofemoral junction in the groin, supplemented with other tourniquets occluding distal venous segments as needed. These are placed to allow sequential removal. The patient is then asked to stand. The pattern of superficial venous refill is noted, and the rate of refilling is timed. Filling of the superficial veins with tourniquet in place in under 30 seconds suggests incompetent valves in the distal perforating veins and deep venous incompetence.

Tourniquet removal in the sequence just explained may demonstrate patterns of refilling of superficial veins and varices due to leakage from the saphenofemoral junction or named perforators. This time-honored test has limitations, as shown in Figure 32–2 when a single tourniquet is used to evaluate the long saphenous vein. Rapid refilling can occur by means of Dodd or Hunterian perforators into a mainly distal incompetent saphenous system. The difficulty of accurately compressing the saphenofemoral junction high in the groin is also illustrated. Since physical examination has its limitations, more precise diagnostic evaluations are required to decide on the pattern and extent of venous surgery.

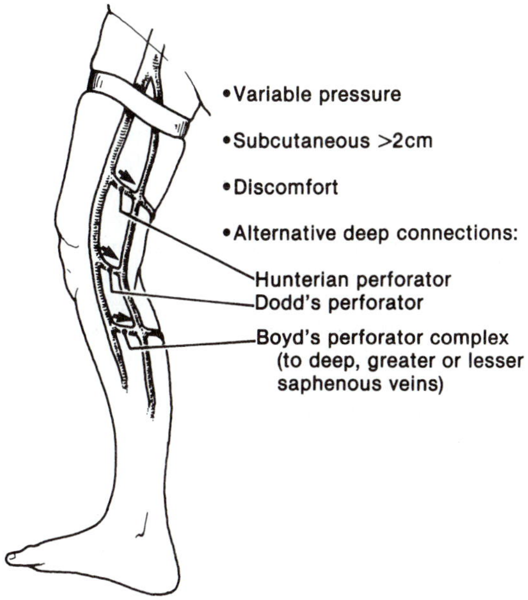

The continuous-wave Doppler instrument has an ability to identify long saphenous reflux of nonjunctional origin and limbs in which stasis symptoms and visible varicosities were of nonsaphenous origin. However, the continuous-wave Doppler device cannot clearly isolate reflux in individual veins. It detects velocity of blood flow from any vein lying in the path of the ultrasound beam. At the femoral level, detected reflux might have as its origin the femoral vein, the saphenous vein, a venous anomaly, or a duplicated long saphenous vein.

Duplex technology has markedly changed evaluation of venous function. The B-mode ultrasound component allows imaging of the superficial and deep veins. Venous flow can be assessed by observation of the intraluminal moving echoes produced by red blood cell microaggregates.[47] Flow toward and away from the heart can be color-coded to allow more rapid vessel identification as well as presence or absence of pathologic reflux flow. Venous valves can be identified, with their leaflets often seen as normal, shortened, thickened, nonfunctional, or functional.

Duplex examination of the supine patient is frequently done for detection of deep venous thrombosis. However, in the supine subject, the venous valves are open in a floating position. Even when there is no flow, the valves remain open. Valve closure requires a reversal of flow with a pressure gradient that is higher proximally than distally.[55] Manual compression proximally does not reliably produce the requisite pressure gradient and sufficient flow velocity (30 m/sec) in a distal direction to effect valve closure. Although a Valsalva maneuver can close proximal valves such as the iliofemoral valve, distal valve closure of the popliteal and crural levels is not accomplished. Thus, venous valve function cannot be assessed reliably in a person who is supine.

Use of the hand-held Doppler instrument and duplex technology complement each other. The former has become part of the office examination of venous insufficiency just as it is part of the examination of every patient with arterial disease. However, in patients with severe venous insufficiency, the most important diagnostic evaluation is color-flow duplex scanning. Valvular insufficiency at the saphenofemoral junction is determined precisely.[56,58]

As the examination begins with the Doppler, it is well to know sensitivity and specificity as well as the predicted values of physical examination compared with Doppler insonation using the hand-held instrument. These are shown in Tables 32–1 and 32–2.[17] High specificity and predictive valve for physical and Doppler examination are found when evaluating patients who are slender and in whom the subcutaneous tissue measures less than 2.5 cm. In these patients, the positive "tap-cough-thrill" tests[42] are accurate.

- Variable pressure
- Subcutaneous >2cm
- Discomfort
- Alternative deep connections:
  - Hunterian perforator
  - Dodd's perforator
  - Boyd's perforator complex (to deep, greater or lesser saphenous veins)

Figure 32–2. Limitations of tourniquet testing. (Reprinted, with permission, from DePalma RG, Rose S, Bergan JJ: Treatment of varicosities with saphenous origin: A dialogue. In: *Varicose Veins and Telangiectasias.* Bergan JJ, Goldman MP [editors]. Quality Medical Publishers, 1993.)

Table 32–1. Comparison of physical examination and Doppler ultrasonography with duplex scanning.

	Sensitivity	Specificity	Positive Predictive Value	Negative Predictive Value
Physical examination	48% (24/50)	73% (22/30)	75% (24/32)	46% (22/48)
Doppler ultrasound	48% (24/50)	83% (25/30)	83% (24/29)	49% (25/51)

n = 80 limbs with saphenofemoral junction incompetency.

If a patient has no history of deep thrombophlebitis and no signs of deep venous incompetence in the ankle skin, a duplex examination can be omitted before treatment of primary saphenofemoral incompetence. However, the duplex examination does reveal unexpected findings that affect surgical judgment. (For a more complete treatise on this subject, see the recent monograph, Quantitative Measurements in CVI.)

In the future, use of color-flow duplex scanning for mapping superficial venous insufficiency will become dominant. It will measure reflux duration[14] and reflux volume and velocity, as well as provide information on vein diameter and cross-sectional area.

A number of other tools to elucidate venous pathophysiology have been applied: photoplethysmography (PPG), light reflection rheography (LRR), mercury strain gauge plethysmography (MSG), and air plethysmography (APG). Among these, the PPG proved useful early because it allows variants of the classic Brodie-Trendelenburg test. First, PPG documented rapid venous refill in the foot. Then application of tourniquets was thought to show whether this rapid distal refill was of deep or superficial origin. However, this test proved nonspecific. van Bemmelen showed that an examination of the skin alone was as useful as the PPG. In this regard, duplex has proven that vein diameter is important to the existence of venous reflux and that this variable is reversible after appropriate surgical intervention.[62]

Although some extremities with chronic venous insufficiency and some with only varicose veins differ substantially hemodynamically from one another, there is considerable overlap in hemodynamic measurements.[6] Air plethysmography has shown this considerable hemodynamic overlap among limbs with early varicosities, normal limbs, and those with chronic venous insufficiency.[13] Air plethysmography has not been used widely by many practitioners because it has little impact on decisions for therapy of an individual limb. It remains a useful research device.

In deciding on therapy in a limb with severe CVI, it is important to know which pathologic process—obstruction or reflux—is dominant in each of the important vein segments. The PPG, LRR, MSG, and APG instruments do not provide this information.

Only imaging techniques such as magnetic resonance phlebography and contrast phlebography can define chronic obstruction. Also, only duplex evaluation and phlebography identify function of individual vein segments. When the patient is a possible surgical candidate for correction of deep venous insufficiency, ascending phlebography will demonstrate segmental venous occlusion. Certain patterns of disease such as unilateral iliac vein occlusion are suitable for direct intervention.[52] More important, descending phlebography will reveal sites of valvular incompetence, which may be correctable by valveplasty using modern techniques of venous reconstructive surgery.[28]

Differential Diagnosis

The differential diagnosis of CVI, with its accompanying characteristic skin changes of edema and liposclerosis, is usually straightforward. However, Kaposi's sarcoma mimics CVI (Fig 32–3). Kaposi's lesions are usually widespread and may be pigmented, which is exacerbated in areas of limb dependency. Also, the characteristic Kaposi's lesions can be sparse initially. In immunocompromised persons, the lesions can initially occur unilaterally. This can be deceptive.

Another manifestation of CVI may be a bursting calf pain on exercise, which is relieved by leg elevation. This pain is usually caused by severe iliofemoral or iliofemoral-caval occlusion. Differentiation of this type of pain from arterial insufficiency claudication may be difficult when edema and induration render the taking of the pedal pulse difficult. Measurement of ankle arterial pressure and recording of pulse waves using plethysmography separates venous from arterial claudication. Rarely, arteriography may be required.

Table 32–2. Comparison of physical examination and Doppler ultrasound with color-flow duplex.

	Sensitivity	Specificity	Positive Predictive Value	Negative Predictive Value
Physical examination	47% (8/17)	60% (3/5)	80% (8/10)	25% (3/12)
Doppler ultrasound	47% (8/17)	80% (4/5)	89% (8/9)	31% (4/13)

n = 22 limbs with history of prior stripping.

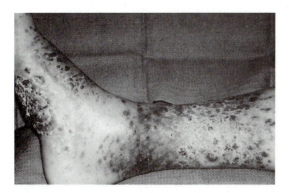

Figure 32–3. Kaposi's sarcoma. Note raised crusted lesions superimposed on general pigmentation. Lesion of arch of foot is atypical for venous stasis.

Unilateral lymphedema characteristically appears in young females during late adolescence or early adulthood. This process, lymphedema praecox, is completely painless, and its characteristic doughy consistency and slow pitting on finger pressure are clinically recognizable. Appearing later in life as lymphedema tarda may make it appear to be a swelling of venous origin. The best diagnostic differentiation of lymphedema from CVI is color-flow duplex scanning. This eliminates the need for lymphangiography, and phlebography is not required if duplex scanning reveals a normal deep venous system.

Options for Treatment

Effective options for treatment of CVI have increased remarkably. Many of these options are in the arena of venous reconstruction. However, new methods of detaching deep venous pathophysiology from the superficial venous system are also proving effective. A better understanding of cellular mechanisms in venous disease is also making pharmaceutical approaches more rational.

A. Medical Treatment: Conservative treatment of CVI always precedes consideration of surgical intervention. Nonoperative treatment relies on limb compression to counteract the effects of venous hypertension.[34] This is achieved by gradient elastic support, which compresses interstitial tissue. Limb compression devices in addition to fitted elastic support stockings include Unna's paste boot, short-stretch and long-stretch elastic bandages, and a semirigid Velcro support, the CircAid appliance.

Of the latter, the most time-honored treatment for ulceration is Unna's paste boot, which is applied continuously until healing is achieved. When the ulcer has healed, below-knee gradient stockings are fitted. These deliver 30–40 mmHg ankle pressure and are prescribed in a carefully fitted form. The stockings provide progressively decreasing pressure proximally.[5] Almost always, below-knee stockings suffice. In fact,

above-knee stockings or other compression devices crossing the knee are cumbersome and occlude the popliteal vein on knee flexion. Rarely do patients require devices delivering ankle pressure higher than 40 mmHg. In patients with concomitant arterial insufficiency, stockings delivering less pressure at the ankle are required to prevent skin necrosis. Support stockings are always removed at bedtime.

Treatment of stasis ulceration, complicated sepsis, and cellulitis demand bed rest and limb elevation. The initial period of bed rest may require hospital wound care.[34] Plain gauze dressing changes and ulcer cleansing with saline compresses are used initially. Tetracycline has been found to be an effective antibiotic for patients with CVI, but organism-specific antibiotics tailored for bacteria cultured from the ulcer bed should be used. Tetracycline is thought to have a nonspecific effect on the cytokine-activation phenomenon. If the patient develops a severe id reaction (derived from the term, *dermatophytid*) with a generalized rash remote from the stasis ulceration, energetic treatment with systemic corticosteroids or systemic antifungal agents may be necessary. The generalized reaction always disappears after ulcer healing.

B. New Drug Treatment Options: Several classes of drugs have been shown to have possible usefulness in CVI:[12] fibrinolytics, hydroxyrutosides, prostaglandins, methylxanthines, and antioxidants. Because one theory of venous ulceration invokes pericapillary fibrin cuff blockade of oxygen diffusion, fibrinolytic therapy has been proposed by Browse and Burnand. However, in a study comparing a fibrinolytic anabolic steroid with placebo in limbs receiving conventional compression therapy, no significant difference in healing was observed between the treatment groups. Another study revealed that patients reported subjective improvement. However, the patients were unable to differentiate treatments by anabolic steroids from placebo. Fibrinolytic treatment, of historic importance, has not been generally accepted.

Another class of drugs, the hydroxyrutosides, have been used for many years in Europe for symptomatic varices. These agents are thought to restore the barrier properties of the fiber matrix between the capillary and endothelial cells. The chief finding is decrease in leg edema and subjective reduction in the symptom of tired legs. The hydroxyrutosides have no proven role in the management of severe venous stasis, although they apparently relieve symptoms of CVI.

A treatment regimen using intravenous prostaglandin E$_1$ (PGE$_1$) compared with placebo has been tried as treatment for patients with venous ulceration. In a 6-week period, 8 of 20 patients treated with prostaglandin had complete ulcer healing compared with only 2 of 22 patients receiving placebo.

Of greater importance is the action of the methylxanthines, which improve red cell deformability. These agents also inhibit alterations in the microvasculature induced by interleukin 2 (IL-2). In a report of a placebo-controlled, double-blind study using the methylxanthine, pentoxifylline, Weitgasser[64] reported that 26 of 30 patients on active treatment showed improvement over the study period as contrasted with only 13 of 29 patients receiving placebo.

Another double-blind, placebo-controlled study[3] involved 12 patients with CVI and persistent leg ulcers. Pentoxifylline was administered both intravenously and orally for the first 7 days and orally for another 60 days. Four of 6 patients receiving the active agent experienced ulcer healing. In a multiclinic study, oxypentifylline, orally 400 mg 3 times daily, was compared with placebo.[7] Compression bandaging was applied to both groups of patients. Complete healing of the ulcers occurred in 28 of 30 limbs treated by the active agent compared with only 12 of 42 patients treated with placebo. Specific results were significant ($p < 0.01$).

In addition to compression bandaging, Salim[36] found the use of the free radical scavengers, allopurinol and dimethylsulfoxide, to significantly improve ulcer healing in the treated groups at endpoints of 4, 8, and 12 weeks. The object of this treatment is to block effects of toxic oxygen metabolites and proteolytic enzymes. Allopurinol is a potent scavenger of hydroxy radicals and also inhibits formation of the enzyme, xanthine oxidase, an important mediator of reperfusion effects. Although none of these drugs has been widely used in the USA, they introduce the possibility of pharmacotherapy for CVI.

C. Surgical Treatment: Surgical intervention in CVI is indicated when conservative measures have failed or are predicted to fail. Such surgical techniques are directed toward control of sources of venous hypertension. This may be achieved by axial (saphenous) stripping to abolish gravitational reflux, by removing varicose clusters to detach relevant sources of hydrodynamic pressure, or by reconstructing veins.

First, gravitational forces should be controlled. Superficial venous incompetence is a major contributor to CVI in most limbs and has been shown to be a logical first target in treating CVI. Saphenous stripping was a part of the treatment of 55% of DePalma's series of patients. In Bergan's duplex study of advanced CVI, 10 of 58 (17%) limbs had only superficial reflux. Superficial reflux was the major contributor to CVI in another 17 limbs.

Linton[33] emphasized the importance of interruption of incompetent communicating and perforating veins using a medial longitudinal incision to control CVI skin changes. Operations to alleviate these changes include a variety of techniques of subfascial and extrafascial interruption of perforating veins. These can be combined with removal of the long saphenous vein.

In 1974, DePalma[16] used a modification of Linton's principles to interrupt perforating and communicating veins to minimize transmission of venous hypertension to the skin and subcutaneous tissues. This procedure had as its goal complete interruption of incompetent perforating and communicating veins and grafting of ulcers in one operation. It differed from the traditional approach in that rather than creating a longitudinal incision that was notorious for its poor healing, a series of bipedicle flaps in natural skin lines were fashioned to provide access to offending veins in the lower leg. A follow-up report detailed experience in 68 extremities among 53 patients followed up for up to 12 years. There were 4 recurrences during that period. These related to failure to wear support stockings or to lateral recurrences related to development of short saphenous or lateral perforator incompetence.

More recently, a shearing operation[21,48] using a proximal skin line incision and skin grafting of ulcers greater than 3 cm in diameter has been found to be useful.[18] Removal of greater or lesser saphenous veins can be combined with femoral valveplasty based on preoperative duplex scanning and phlebography. However, valveplasty, as indicated by duplex scanning and descending phlebography, was needed in only 2 of 54 instances in a recent operative series. Figure 32–1 shows the anatomy of the long saphenous vein, the posterior arch tributary, and the perforating veins. Figure 32–4 shows use of the shearing phlebotome, which completely divides posterior arch perforators and communicating veins superficial to the fascial level. In the area of ulceration where subcutaneous tissue is effaced, subfascial dissection includes careful division of short communicating branches from the posterior tibial vein. Long-term appearance of the limb after the procedure is shown in Figure 32–5. In a 10-year follow-up of over 80 limbs, there have been 4 recurrences and 1 delayed healing lasting 21 days. This is in contrast to the many healing problems encountered with the longitudinal Linton incision.

Hospitalization time has been reduced from an average of 14 days to 3–4 days; when skin grafting is required, 7 or more days may be needed. Skin recurrences related to lateral recurrence after a medial procedure or severe proximal obstruction such as vena cava thrombosis have produced ulcer recurrences. Recurrence occurs when patients with obstruction fail to wear support stockings postoperatively.

1. Direct venous reconstruction–As previously mentioned, the logical approach to management of severe venous stasis includes outpatient care with graded elastic compression, careful attention to skin hygiene, and avoidance of allergenic medications. When this therapy fails, appropriate diagnostic studies, including noninvasive evaluation with duplex and Doppler scanning, as well as invasive evaluation by ascending and descending phlebography, can be done.

The first choice of surgical therapy would be removal of superficial varicosities. This should be combined with subfascial or superficial interruption of perforating veins as indicated by preoperative diagnostic studies. Whether this is done in the limb with intact skin or in the presence of ulceration becomes the surgeon's choice, but in any event, lifetime-graded elas-

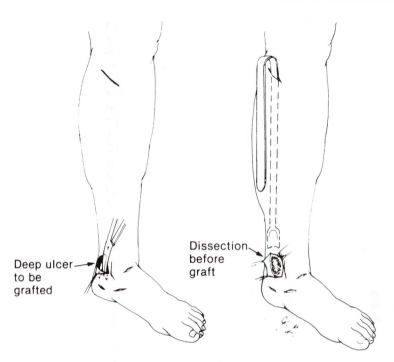

Deep ulcer to be grafted

Dissection before graft

Figure 32–4. Essentials of subcutaneous shearing operation. Subfascial dissection is done in the area of ulceration to divide branches from the posterior tibial vein. (Reprinted, with permission, from DePalma RG: Surgical treatment of chronic venous ulceration. In: *Venous Disorders.* Bergan JJ, Yao JST [editors]. WB Saunders, 1992.)

tic compression remains the keystone of therapy of venous stasis. The intractable patient is one who fails this first surgical event. The patient with a postoperative recurrent ulcer is then thought to be a candidate for direct venous reconstruction.

2. Venous reconstruction—Clinical reconstructive surgery of the venous system became feasible after 1960, chiefly through the work of Palma in Uruguay. His 1958 publication[39] was obscure, but his 1960 publication in the English language[40] has become a standard reference. Direct reconstruction of the femoropopliteal venous segment actually became feasible before Palma in the early 1950s. However, the description of this reconstruction by Warren and Thayer[63] went virtually unnoticed. The reason for this was probably the predominance of arterial reconstructive surgery in that era as well as the explosive subsequent growth of this specialty. Note that Warren's description of his results are similar to those given for all venous reconstructive surgery since that time. ". . . at the time of follow-up examination . . . those who had ulcers showed them still healed or, having recurred, had done so with less severity and often a longer period of freedom than had been the case preoperatively. In those who had not suffered from ulcers, the criteria for improvement was a diminution in dermatitis or edema. No patient was cured."

Experimental venous valve surgery began in the early 1950s[22] and continued with the work of McLaghlin[35] in the 1960s. The breakthrough in direct venous reconstruction was the invention of the valveplasty by Kistner in 1968, but his operation became generally known only after 1975.[31] At that time, surgeons could evaluate patients for direct reconstruction by selecting those who had failed conservative care and conventional subfascial perforator interruption. They could investigate such patients by ascending and descending venography with a view toward performing cross-pubic bypass, saphenopopliteal bypass, or valveplasty.

The additional contribution of Kistner is difficult to overestimate in which the venous stream could be redirected through a competent proximal valve: venous segment transfer. In the development of valveplasty for primary valvular insufficiency and of vein segment transfer, Kistner added a number of new procedures that might be applicable to patients who failed conventional therapy. He pointed out that use of direct venous reconstruction, combined with conventional therapy, produced good to excellent long-term results in over 80% of patients.[29] The role of perforator veins was summarized by Kistner's statement that, "when interruption of incompetent perforators was performed in addition to femoral vein reconstruction, an excellent result was achieved."

Kistner's teachings have been taken up over the world,[26] but a cautionary message has been sent: Primary valve repair alone is not sufficient in management of chronic venous stasis.[27] Furthermore, this last report emphasizes the need for objective evaluation of venous reconstructive surgery. Clinical results alone

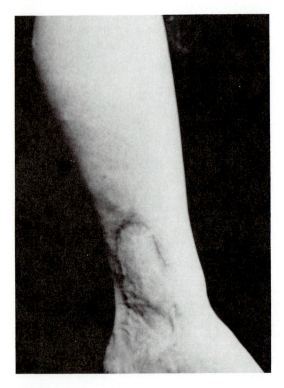

Figure 32–5. Long-term appearance 10 years after shearing procedure ulcer excision and skin graft in 50-year-old woman wearing 30-mm graded support stockings.

ciple of direct free venous reconstruction has found application in bypass of vena cava by spiral vein grafting.[20,49] Whether or not prosthetic reconstruction of the vena cava[53] will work remains a matter for further observation.

Experimental venous valve autotransplantation received some attention in the 1960s.[59,60] Further investigations using distal arteriovenous fistulae showed the feasibility of the procedure.[32] Surgical interest became concentrated on the procedure after the reports of Taheri[50] and associates.

The numerous reports on valve transplantation that followed stimulated interest in this field, but the unfortunate consequence has been that valve transplantation has been undertaken as a primary surgical procedure in treating some patients with venous stasis. Failures of such procedures have unnecessarily discredited the procedure.

Prognosis

Results of nonoperative treatment of venous stasis ulcer have been summarized recently.[34] An overall recurrence rate calculated by life-table method was 29% at 5 years. Compliant patients using consistent support fared better with only a 16% ulcer recurrence rate. The shearing operation and vein stripping have a recurrence rate of 10% over a 10 year period in 58 limbs. This is related mainly to severe hypertension resulting from proximal obstruction.

provide an unacceptable method of recording results. Only objective scientific data proves useful.

3. Advances in venous reconstruction–The ingenious principle of providing a venous bypass by performing a single venous anastomosis as described by Palma was an important forward step. Nevertheless, modifications of this bypass may make the procedure more applicable to an increasing number of patients. For example, the addition of a distal arteriovenous fistula may increase patency of a venous bypass. This was described by Gruss.[23,24] The addition of externally reinforced PTFE grafts, with or without arteriovenous fistulas, may be an important contribution as well. These modifications must be proved and objectively documented before they can be accepted as standard surgical procedures. Furthermore, free venous bypasses as described by Danza[15] and associates may find selected application, and the same prin-

Conclusions

As summarized above, the last few years have provided a considerable advance in understanding venous pathophysiology and the cellular mechanisms involved in CVI. Future research directions will include a better understanding of vein wall, venous valve, and perivenous tissue functions. More direct surgical approaches, including external valveplasty and reconstruction of major veins will be applied with predictable increasing success. At present, these are applied only after correction of superficial reflux has been accomplished, but in the future, venous reconstruction may be more liberally applied.

A better understanding of the molecular alterations in the skin of CVI will allow new medical approaches to be used for palliation of this condition. Thus, the future looks bright for research in venous insufficiency and for treatment of CVI patients.

REFERENCES

1. Andalon AA: La plastie valvulaire dans l'insuffisance veineuse profonde. J Malad Vasc 982;7:201.
2. Arnoldi CC: Venous prezssure in patients with valvular

incompetence of the veins of the lower limb. Acta Chir Scand 1966;132:628.
3. Arnoldi CC: In: *Controversies in the Management of*

Venous Disorders. Eklof B, Gjores JE, Thulesius O, Bergqvist D (editors). Butterworth Publishers, 1989:14.

4. Barbarino C: Pentoxyfylline in the treatment of venous ulcers of the leg. Am Med Res Opin 1992;12:547.

5. Bergan JJ: Conrad Jobst and the development of pressure gradient therapy for venous disease. In: *Surgery of the Veins.* Bergan JJ, Yao JST (editors). Grune & Stratton, 1985:529.

6. Bergan JJ: New developments in surgery of the venous system. Cardiovasc Surg 1993;1:624–631.

7. Bjordal RI: Haemodynamic studies of varicose veins and the post thrombotic syndrome. In: *The Treatment of Venous Disorders.* Hobbs JT (editor). MTP Press Ltd, 1977:37.

8. Bjordal RI: Simultaneous pressure flow recordings in varicose veins of the lower extremity. Acta Chir Scand 1970;136:309.

9. Brodie B: Lectures Illustrative of Various Subjects in Pathology and Surgery. Volume XII. Longmares, Green & Co., 1840.

10. Browse NL, Burnand KG: The postphlebitic syndrome: A new look. In: *Venous Problems.* Bergan JJ, Yao JST (editors). Year Book, 1979:395.

11. Cockett FB, Elgan-Jones DE: The ankle blow out syndrome. Lancet 1953;1:17.

12. Colgan MP, Moore DJ, Shanik DG: Drug therapy for venous ulcers: New methods of treatment. Phlebology 1992;(Suppl):41.

13. Cordts PR et al: Physiologic similarities between extremities with varicose veins and chronic venous insufficiency utilizing air plethysmography. Am J Surg 1992; 164:260.

14. Czeredarezuk M, Branas CC, Weinyarten MJ: Duplex imaging and distal cuff deflation to measure venous reflux time. J Vasc Technol 1992;16:284.

15. Danza R, Navarro T, Baldizan J, Olivera D: Injerto venovenoso libre: Indicaciones, tecnica y resultados (11 anos de experiencia). Cir Uruguay 1980;50:485.

16. DePalma RG: Surgical therapy for venous stasis. Surgery 1975;76:910.

17. DePalma RG, Hart MT, Zanin L, Massarin EH: Physical examination, Doppler ultrasound and colour flow duplex scanning: Guides to therapy for primary varicose veins. Phlebology 1993;8:7.

18. DePalma RG: Surgical therapy for venous stasis: Results of a modified Linton operation. Am J Surg 1979; 137:810.

19. DePalma RG: Surgical treatment of chronic venous ulceration. In: *Phlebologie 92.* Raymond-Martinbeau P, Prescott R, Zummo M. (editors). John Libbey Eurotext, 1992:1235.

20. Doty B: Bypass of superior vena cava. J Thorac Cardiovasc Surg 1982;83:326.

21. Edwards JM: Shearing operations for incompetent perforating veins. Br J Surg 1976;63:885.

22. Eiseman B, Balette W: An operative technique for the construction of venous valves. Surg Gynecol Obstet 1953;97:731.

23. Gruss JD et al: Anwendung von kunststoff bei der Palma operation. Angio 1979;1:51.

24. Gruss JD: Zur Modifikation des femoralis Bypass nach may. VASA 1975;4:59.

25. Homans J: The late results of femoral thrombophlebitis and their treatment. N Engl J Med 1946;235:249.

26. Huse JB et al: Direct venous surgery for venous valvular insufficiency of the lower extremity. Arch Surg 1983;118:719.

27. Johnson ND et al: Late objective assessment of venous valve surgery. Arch Surg 1981;116:1461.

28. Kamida CB, Kistner RL: Descending phebology: The Straub technique. In: *Atlas of Venous Surgery.* Bergan JJ, Kistner RL (editors). WB Saunders, 1992:105.

29. Kistner RL: Late results of venous valve repair. In: *Long-Term Results of Vascular Surgery.* Yao JST, Pearce WL (editor). WB Saunders, 1993:451.

30. Kistner RL: Surgical repair of a venous valve. Straub Clin Proc 1968;34:41.

31. Kistner RL: Surgical repair of the incompetent femoral vein valve. Arch Surg 1975;110:1336.

32. Kroener JM, Bernstein EF: Valve competence following experimental venous valve autotransplantation. Arch Surg 1981;116:1467.

33. Linton RR: The communicating veins of the lower leg and the operative technique for their ligation. Ann Surg 1938;107:582.

34. Mayberry JC, Moreta GL, Taylor LM, Porter JM: Nonoperative treatment of venous ulceration. In: *Atlas of Venous Surgery.* Bergan JJ, Kistner RL (editors). 1992:81.

35. McLaghlin AD et al: Valve replacement in the recanalized incompetent superficial femoral vein in dogs. Ann Surg 1965;162:446.

36. Moulton S et al: Gravitational reflux does not correlate with clinical status of venous stasis. Phlebology 1993;8:2.

37. Moyses C, Cederholm-Williams SA, Michel CC: Haemoconcentration and the accumulation of white cells in the feet during venous stasis. Int J Micro Circ Clin Exp 1987;5:311.

38. Negus D: The distal long saphenous vein in recurrent ven-ous ulceration. In: *Phlebologie.* Raymond-Martinbeau, Prescott R, Zummo M (editors). J Libbey Eurotext 1992;1291.

39. Palma EC et al: Tratamiento de los trastornos postflebiticos mediante anastomosis venosa safeno-femoral controlateral. Bull Soc Surg Uruguay 1958;29:135.

40. Palma EC, Esperon R: Vein transplants and grafts in the surgical treatment of the postphlebitic syndrome. J Cardiovasc Surg 1960;1:94.

41. Perthes G: Uber die operation der untershenkelvaricen nach Trendelenburg. Dtsch Med Wochenschr 1895; 21:253.

42. Ruckley CV: *A Color Atlas of Surgical Management of Venous Disease.* Wolfe Medical, 1992:91.

43. Salim AS: The role of oxygen-derived free radicals in the management of venous (varicose) ulcerations: A new approach. World J Surg 1991;15:264.

44. Schmid-Schonbein GW: Granulocyte: Friend or foe. Nips 1988;3:6.

45. Scott HJ, Coleridge-Smith PD, Scurr JH: Histological study of white blood cells and their association with lipdermatosclerosis and venous ulceration. Br J Surg 1991; 78:210.

46. Scurr JH, Coleridge-Smith PD: Pathogenesis of venous ulceration. Phlebology 1992;(Suppl)13.

47. Sigel B et al: Red cell aggregation as a cause of blood flow echogenicity. Radiology 1983;148:799.

48. Simpson CJ, Smellie GD: The phlebotome in the management of incompetent perforating veins and venous ulcerations. J Cardiovasc Surg 1987;28:274.

49. Smith ER, Brantigan CO: Bypass of superior vena cava obstruction using spiral vein graft. J Cardiovasc Surg 1983;24:259.

50. Taheri SA et al: Surgical treatment of postphlebitic syndrome with vein valve transplant. Am J Surg 1982;144:221.

51. Thomas PRS, Nash GP, Dormandy JA: White cell accumulation in the dependent legs of patients with venous hypertension: A possible mechanism for trophic changes in the skin. Br Med J 1988;296:1693.

52. Thomas ML: Ascending and descending phlebography. In: *Atlas of Venous Surgery.* Bergan JJ, Kistner RL (editors). WB Saunders, 1992:95.

53. Trainini JC et al: Superior vena cava bypass. Texas Heart Inst J 1983;10:201.

54. Trendelenburg J: Uber die Unterbinding der Vena saphena magna bei Unterschekelvaricen. Beitr Klin Chir 1890–1891;195.

55. van Bemmelen PS, Beach K, Bedford G, Strandness DE Jr: Quantitative segmental evaluation of venous valvular reflux with ultrasound scanning. J Vasc Surg 1989; 10:425.

56. van Bemmelen PS, Bergan JJ (editors): Photoplethysmography and light reflection rheography. In: *Quantitative Measurement of Venous Incompetence.* RG Landes Co, 1992;37.

57. van Bemmelen PS, Beach K, Bedford G, Strandness DE Jr: The mechanisms of venous valve closure. Arch Surg 1990;125:617.

58. Vasdekis SN, Clarke GH, Nicolaides AN: Quantification of venous reflux by means of duplex scanning. J Vasc Surg 1989;10:670.

59. Waddell WG et al: Venous valve transplantation in postphlebitic and postthrombotic veins. Arch Surg 1967; 95:826.

60. Waddell WG et al: Venous valve transplantation. Arch Surg 1964;88:27.

61. Walsh J, Bergan JJ, Beeman S, Moulton SL: Femoral vein reflux is abolished by saphenous vein stripping. Ann Vasc Surg (in press).

62. Walsh JC, Bergan JJ, Moulton SL, Beeman S: Proximal venous reflux adversely affects distal venous function. Surg 1994;8:566–570.

63. Warren R, Thayer TR: Transplantation of the saphenous vein for postphlebitic stasis. Surgery 1954;35:867.

64. Weitgasser H: The use of pentoxifylline (Trental 400) in the treatment of leg ulcers: Results of a double-blind trial. Pharmatherapeutica 1983;3:143.

Deep Venous Thrombosis & Pulmonary Embolism

33

John G. Adams, Jr., MD, & Donald Silver, MD

Although the incidence of deep venous thrombosis and pulmonary embolism in hospitalized patients remains uncertain, it is accepted that these disorders affect a substantial number of hospitalized patients and carry significant morbidity and mortality. In a recent study, the average annual incidence of deep venous thrombosis was 48 per 100,000 patients, whereas the incidence of pulmonary embolism with or without documented deep venous thrombosis was 23 per 100,000 patients. The in-hospital fatality rate from venous thromboembolism was 12%. Extrapolation from these data suggests that about 170,000 patients are treated for an initial episode of venous thromboembolism in short-stay hospitals in the USA each year and that an additional 90,000 patients are treated for recurrent disease. Studies using radiolabeled fibrinogen or venography have revealed an incidence of deep venous thrombosis of 20–30% in patients undergoing general surgical procedures and an incidence of 50% in patients undergoing orthopedic surgical procedures. Pulmonary embolism occurs in about 1% of these patients. Other investigators have estimated that about 630,000 symptomatic cases of pulmonary embolism occur in the USA each year and that pulmonary embolism is the primary cause of death in 100,000 patients annually.

DEEP VENOUS THROMBOSIS

Essentials of Diagnosis
- Stasis.
- Venous injury.
- Increased coagulability.

General Considerations
The pathogenesis of thrombosis, documented by Virchow in 1856, consists of interactions between an injured vessel and stasis and increased coagulability of blood. Stasis and local acceleration of the coagulation process are the most important factors in thrombus formation; the evolution and composition of thrombi differ according to the interactions of these factors.

Venous thrombi usually form under conditions of low or disturbed flow and are composed of erythrocytes and fibrin with relatively few platelets. Stasis predisposes to the thrombosis by allowing the activated clotting factors to become concentrated with reduced exposure to the natural anticoagulants. Venous thromboses usually begin in valve pockets where areas of maximum stasis occur or at sites of venous injury. Most venous thrombi probably begin as platelet aggregates in the depths of valve pockets. These small thrombi are usually rapidly lysed through the activity of the plasminogen activator of the venous endothelium. Activation of coagulation, due to release of tissue factor following surgery, trauma, or from other stimuli, results in increased thrombus formation, which may overwhelm the local fibrinolytic activity, especially in the presence of venous stasis.

Deep venous thrombosis occurs most often in the calf veins, especially the soleal veins. These are followed in decreasing order of frequency by the other calf veins, femoral veins, common iliac veins, and inferior vena cava. Thrombosis has been found to be more common in the left lower extremity and may be related to compression of the left common iliac vein by the right common iliac artery (May-Thurner syndrome). The thrombosis remains confined to the calf (distal deep venous thrombosis) without propagation or embolism about 80% of the time and usually undergoes spontaneous lysis or recanalization. The thrombosis propagates proximally (proximal deep venous thrombosis) into the popliteal, femoral, or iliac veins in the remaining 20% of patients. If not treated, 10–20% of patients with proximal deep venous thrombosis will manifest clinical pulmonary embolism.

Phlegmasia can be described as extensive iliofemoral venous thrombosis associated with marked edema of the lower extremity; the outflow obstruction may compromise arterial flow and produce ischemia of the distal leg and foot. The edema is caused by the impaired venous and lymphatic (related to compression of the perivascular lymphatics) return. In phlegmasia alba dolens, the less severe form of phlegmasia, the extremity is edematous and pale but not ischemic; neural function remains normal. In phlegmasia cerulea dolens, the extremity is blue and markedly edematous, and it often exhibits petechiae and bullae. The extremity is at risk for arterial insufficiency and neural compression with the development of sensory and motor deficits of the distal leg and foot. Both types of phlegmasia are associated with a large loss of fluid into the tissues of the lower extremity. The hypovolemia from this "third-spaced" fluid may cause a reduced cardiac output, which increases the risk of extension of the thrombotic process and pulmonary embolism. The mortality rate associated with phlegmasia cerulea dolens has been reported to be as high as 42%. Untreated phlegmasia cerulea dolens may result in venous gangrene of the foot and occasionally the leg.

Clinical Findings

A. Signs and Symptoms: Most patients with deep venous thrombosis do not have symptoms. When manifestations are present, pain is the predominant symptom and occurs in 50% of patients. Edema of the affected extremity may be present secondary to thrombotic obstruction of the veins, inflammation of the perivascular tissues, or lymphatic obstruction. Distention of the superficial veins and cutaneous erythema may be present. Homans' sign (pain in the calf with forced dorsiflexion of the foot) is nonspecific for the diagnosis of deep venous thrombosis.

The entire lower extremity with phlegmasia alba dolens is edematous and pale; arterial inflow and neurologic function remain normal. With progression of the obstructing thrombotic process (phlegmasia cerulea dolens), the extremity becomes markedly edematous and blue; petechiae and bullae are often present. Initially, arterial inflow and neurologic function may be normal, but later stages are characterized by arterial insufficiency and the development of motor and sensory deficits of the distal leg and foot. If the venous outflow obstruction persists, venous gangrene may develop (Fig 33–1).

B. Imaging Studies: Ascending venography remains the "gold standard" of diagnosis of deep venous thrombosis. However, noninvasive diagnostic procedures are being used more frequently. The noninvasive procedures have been categorized into direct and indirect methods. Impedance plethysmography is an indirect method of detecting deep venous thrombosis. It measures the effects of venous obstruction on normal physiologic fluctuations in leg volume and electrical impedance. Direct methods of detecting deep venous thrombosis such as Doppler ultrasonography and duplex scanning examine either hemodynamic (Doppler) or morphologic (B-mode) properties of the blood flow and the venous system.

1. Ascending venography–During ascending venography, an invasive diagnostic procedure, contrast is injected into the veins of the extremity. Classically, the examination is performed with the patient in the semi-upright position (40–60° from the horizontal) with no weight bearing on the extremity under examination. The contrast is injected into a vein on the dorsum of the foot, and examination of the veins of the extremity is performed with fluoroscopy and multiple

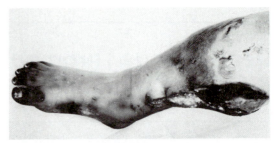

Figure 33–1. Extensive right iliofemoral venous thrombosis with edema, discoloration, and gangrenous changes of the toes and foot. Note the fasciotomy that was used to decompress the neurovascular compartments of the lower leg.

films. The venographic criteria for the diagnosis of deep venous thrombosis include one or more of the following: constant filling defects on more than one view; cut-off of the dye column with a nonopacified segment of vein; presence of collateral flow (especially in the pelvis); and presence of tortuous, "corkscrew" collaterals (Fig 33–2).

The complications associated with venography are pain, extravasation of contrast, and, on rare occasions, thrombosis. Because of the technical demands and complications associated with venography, it is being replaced by noninvasive methods of evaluating deep venous thrombosis.

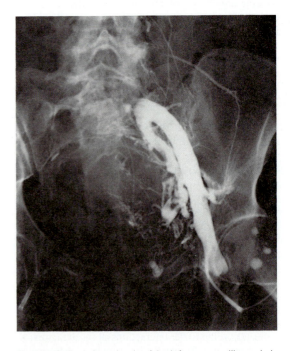

Figure 33–2. A thrombosis of the left common iliac vein is demonstrated by venography. Note pelvic and iliac collaterals.

2. Impedance plethysmography–Impedance plethysmography is an indirect, noninvasive method of detecting deep venous thrombosis, which assesses volume changes in a limb by measuring changes in electrical resistance between 2 pairs of circumferential electrodes placed on the extremity. With a change in the blood content of an extremity, a proportional change in the resistance to an electrical current occurs as measured by the voltage changes along the current path. In a compilation of 10 different studies in which impedance plethysmography was compared with venography in symptomatic patients, impedance plethysmography had a sensitivity of 92% and a specificity of 88% for the detection of thrombi involving the popliteal or more proximal veins. Impedance plethysmography is not considered accurate for the detection of calf vein or nonoccluding thrombi.

3. Doppler ultrasonography–Continuous-wave Doppler ultrasonography is the simplest and most rapid method of evaluation of the extremity for deep venous thrombosis. The common femoral, superficial femoral, popliteal, and tibioperoneal veins are evaluated for the presence or absence of spontaneous venous flow with or without phasic respiratory variations and the response to thigh or calf compression. Thrombosis is suggested by the absence of spontaneous flow and the absence of augmentation of flow with respiratory variation and compression. The results of 18 studies encompassing 1189 patients comparing Doppler ultrasonography with venography for occlusive thrombi proximal to the calf demonstrated a sensitivity of 83% and a specificity of 88%. Doppler ultrasound scanning frequently fails to detect thrombi that are distal to the calf or are only partially occlusive. In addition, Doppler ultrasonography is not good for evaluation of recurrent deep venous thrombosis in patients with the postthrombotic syndrome because the abnormal Doppler signals do not distinguish old from new thromboses.

4. Duplex scanning–B-mode ultrasonography allows one to image the venous system, visualize venous flow, evaluate valve cusp movement, visualize thrombus, and differentiate acute from chronic thrombus based on echogenicity and venous wall changes. The combination of real-time imaging and Doppler ultrasonography is referred to as duplex scanning. The common femoral, superficial femoral, popliteal, and calf veins are examined for their compressibility, movement of red cell aggregates, movement of valve cusps, flow variation with respiration, and flow variation with distal compression of the extremity. The addition of color-flow imaging provides the advantages of distinguishing veins from arteries, reducing the need for Doppler flow interrogation, and facilitating the identification of the calf veins (Fig 33–3). Recent studies indicate that duplex scanning detects deep venous thrombosis with a sensitivity of 88–98% and a specificity of 86–95%. Note that duplex scanning is operator-dependent; that is, several months of experi-

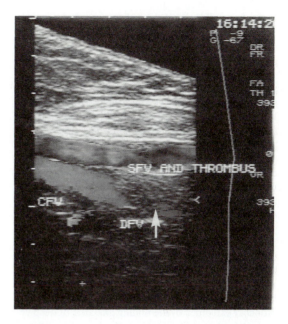

Figure 33–3. A thrombosis (*arrow*) of the superficial femoral vein (SFV) is demonstrated by duplex examination. (CFV, common femoral vein; DFV, deep femoral vein.)

ence are required to acquire proficiency in performing the study. The high degree of sensitivity and specificity in establishing the presence of deep venous thrombosis has allowed the noninvasive duplex scan to become the preferred initial test for the evaluation of deep venous thrombosis.

Risk Factors

The more common risk factors for venous thromboembolism are listed in Table 33–1. Identification and proper management of patients with increased risk for developing thromboembolic complications should help to decrease the morbidity and mortality associated with these disorders.

Table 33–1. Venous thromboembolism risk factors.

Age over 40	Other factors
Pregnancy/estrogens	Varicose veins
Obesity/immobility	Myeloproliferative disorders
Heart disease	Hyperlipidemia
Malignancy	Diabetes mellitus
Trauma	Hemolytic-uremic syndrome
Sepsis	Thrombotic thrombocytopenic
Hypercoagulable states	purpura
Previous DVT/PE	Lupus-like anticoagulants
Cryofibrinogenemia	Intravascular hemolysis
Behçet's syndrome	Homocystinuria
	Cushing's syndrome
	Ulcerative colitis

DVT, deep vein thrombosis; PE, pulmonary embolism.

A. Age: The incidence of venous thromboembolism increases linearly with increasing age. A higher incidence of deep venous thrombosis has been reported in postoperative patients over 40 years of age compared with that found in patients under 40 years of age. Three causal factors have been proposed to explain this increase. (1) As the soleal veins age, they lose their elasticity, and the resulting dilatation and tortuosity contributes to an increase in the stasis of blood. (2) The decrease in muscle mass of the "venous pump" results in decreased pump effectiveness and additional venous stasis. (3) Last, there is an increased incidence of associated conditions and diseases (eg, malignancy, heart disease), which predispose older patients to thromboembolic complications.

B. Gender: Females are generally at increased risk for the development of thromboembolic disease. Although the incidence of deep venous thrombosis is higher in female outpatients, the incidence of deep venous thrombosis in hospitalized patients appears to be equal in males and females. This discrepancy is probably explained by the finding that 50% of deep venous thromboses in females occur in young women and are related to pregnancy. If pregnant patients are deleted from the study population, the incidence of deep venous thrombosis appears to be equal in males and females. This concept is further supported by autopsy studies in which the incidence of detectable pulmonary emboli was found to be the same in males and females.

C. Pregnancy/Estrogen Therapy: An increased risk of thromboembolism exists in women using exogenous estrogens and in pregnant women (particularly during the puerperium). These women are said to be in a hypercoagulable state. The hypercoagulable state of pregnancy has been described as a state of compensated disseminated intravascular thrombosis. By the third trimester, factors II, VII, VIII, IX, X, and fibrinogen are elevated, and antithrombin III (AT III) and protein S levels are decreased. In addition, the plasminogen activating system may be either inhibited by increased levels of plasminogen activator inhibitors (PAI-1 and PAI-2) produced by the placenta or by suppression of the plasminogen activators at the endothelial cell level. Exogenous estrogens decrease AT III levels, increase levels of factor VII and X, decrease venous tone, and increase blood viscosity. Platelet aggregation in response to thrombin is also enhanced by the increased estrogens.

The incidence of venous thrombosis in women using estrogens has been shown to be increased 2–11 times that which occurs in women not using estrogens. Also, a positive correlation exists between estrogen dosage and the risk of venous thrombosis. The relative risk of venous thrombosis is 1.0 in women receiving oral contraceptives containing 50 μg estrogen, 3.2 at a dose of 100 μg, and 5.9 at a dose of 150 μg. No correlation has been found between postmenopausal estrogen use and thrombosis. On the other hand, estrogen

therapy for prostate carcinoma increases the risk of deep venous thrombosis in males.

D. Obesity/Immobility: Immobility due to obesity, hospitalization, trauma, or surgery is associated with an increased risk of thromboembolism. The incidence of deep venous thrombosis and pulmonary embolism in obese patients is about twice that in nonobese patients. In addition to stasis, evidence exists that the impaired fibrinolytic system in obese patients may result in a hypercoagulable state. Prolonged immobility associated with paraplegia, cerebrovascular accident, Guillain-Barré syndrome, catatonia, tetanus, and respiratory insufficiency have been found to result in an increased risk of thromboembolic disease. Immobility results in stasis of blood in the venous sinuses of the calf.

The risk of thromboembolic complications associated with surgery is difficult to differentiate from the risk contributed by other associated conditions (eg, immobility, age). However, it is agreed that surgery contributes to an increased risk of deep venous thrombosis and pulmonary embolism; the magnitude and duration of the operation appear to have a greater effect on the incidence of both thrombosis and embolism than does the site of the operation (except orthopedic procedures).

E. Heart Disease: Patients over the age of 30 years with any form of heart disease have a 3.5-fold increased risk of deep venous thrombosis and pulmonary embolism. The more severe the heart disease, the greater the risk of thromboembolic complications. Autopsy studies have shown that pulmonary emboli principally arise from the leg veins in patients with heart disease, although right heart mural thrombi have been found in 10–20% of cardiac patients with autopsy-proven pulmonary emboli. The severity of the heart disease and the disturbances of cardiac rhythm directly influence the occurrence of thromboembolism in cardiac patients. Cardiac disturbances may influence cardiac output, venous return, or the extent of immobilization of the patient. No evidence has been found that alterations in blood coagulation or endothelial injury contribute to thrombus formation in patients with cardiac disorders.

F. Malignancy: Malignancy and thrombosis have been associated since the description by Trousseau (1861) of recurrent thrombosis in cancer patients. The incidence of thrombotic events in patients with malignancy is estimated to be between 5% and 15%. The risk of pulmonary embolism is increased 2- to 3-fold in patients with cancer. Deep venous thrombosis occurs in up to 50% of patients with pancreatic cancer. Some malignancies such as mucin-secreting adenocarcinomas, multiple myeloma, and promyelocytic leukemia are known to secrete tissue thromboplastin. Proteases that activate factor X are secreted by breast, vaginal, and colonic cancers. Cancer patients frequently have elevated levels of factors V, VIII, IX, X, and fibrinogen and decreased levels of AT III. The tenuous balance between coagulation and fibrinolysis in cancer patients is easily disturbed leading to thrombosis or, rarely, hemorrhage.

G. Trauma: Any patient subjected to major trauma is at risk for developing deep venous thrombosis and pulmonary embolism, regardless of the site of injury or his or her age. Deep venous thrombi have been documented in 35–86% of patients hospitalized for trauma. The estimated occurrence of pulmonary embolism in patients hospitalized for trauma is 2%, with 1% resulting in death. Pulmonary embolism has been described as being the leading cause of death in the injured elderly. The risk of pulmonary embolism can be classified according to injury, with the risk being 2–5% for head and chest trauma, 5–8% for burns, 14% for spinal fractures, 27% for pelvic fractures, and 45–60% for tibial and femoral fractures. Activation of the extrinsic coagulation pathway by trauma leads to release of tissue thromboplastin, which, together with the induced venous stasis, predisposes the patient to damaging venous thrombosis.

H. Sepsis: There is a 2-fold increased risk for the development of deep venous thrombosis in patients who develop postoperative infection. Sepsis predisposes to thrombosis via multiple mechanisms. Gram-positive bacteria may directly cause platelet aggregation. Gram-negative bacterial endotoxin may stimulate platelet aggregation but may also, through interaction with leukocytes and endothelial cells, cause tissue factor-like activation of the coagulation system. Endotoxin is also known to be one of the major causative stimuli for the development of disseminated intravascular coagulation.

I. Hypercoagulable States: Congenital and acquired hypercoagulable syndromes (Table 33–2) are associated with a predisposition to thrombosis. AT III and protein C are the plasma proteins primarily responsible for the prevention of thrombosis. Congenital deficiencies of these proteins are inherited as autosomal dominant traits. Patients with heterozygotic traits demonstrate an increased tendency to develop thrombosis; the homozygote condition is frequently incompatible with life.

Table 33–2. Hypercoagulable syndromes.

Congenital	Acquired
Antithrombin III deficiency	Antiphospholipid syndrome
Protein C deficiency	Malignancy
Protein S deficiency	Sepsis
Heparin cofactor II deficiency	Pregnancy/estrogens
Plasminogen abnormalities	Diabetes
Fibrinogen abnormalities	Vasculitides
Homocystinuria	Myeloproliferative disorders
Hyperlipidemia	Heparin-induced thrombocytopenia
	Protein C,S deficiencies
	Antithrombin III deficiency
	Trauma/thermal injury
	Major operative procedures

The incidence of congenital AT III deficiency is about 1 in 2000. Acquired AT III deficiencies occur in patients with disseminated intravascular coagulation, hepatic insufficiency, nephrotic syndrome, pregnancy, administration of exogenous estrogens, and L-asparaginase chemotherapy. AT III is the major plasma inhibitor of thrombin and also inhibits factors IXa, Xa, XIa, and XIIa. Patients with levels of AT III lower than 60% of normal are predisposed to venous thrombosis. The level of AT III in heterozygotes is typically 40–60% of normal. Thromboembolic events usually begin during the second decade of life in patients with AT III deficiency. Although spontaneous thrombotic episodes may occur, inciting events such as operative procedures, trauma, pregnancy, oral contraceptive or estrogen use, and infection are frequently related events. Arterial thrombosis is uncommon. Recurrent thrombosis occurs in 60% of untreated patients.

The initial treatment for patients with thromboembolic disorders diagnosed with AT III deficiency is anticoagulation with heparin. Prior to anticoagulation, the plasma AT III concentration must be corrected to a functional activity of at least 80% of normal. Transfusions of AT III concentrate, fresh frozen plasma, or cryoprecipitate can correct the deficiency. Frequent monitoring of AT III levels during replacement is necessary because of the shortened half-life of AT III during the administration of heparin. Heparin can be administered simultaneously with the AT III replacement. The prolongation of the activated partial thromboplastin time (aPTT) indicates adequate AT III replacement. Following initial anticoagulation with heparin, the management of the AT III-deficient patient with deep venous thrombosis and pulmonary embolism is oral anticoagulation with warfarin for 3–6 months. Long-term anticoagulation with warfarin is recommended for patients with AT III deficiencies who experience recurrent thrombotic events.

Protein C deficiency is among the more prevalent congenital hypercoagulable disorders with the incidence of the heterozygous deficiency being as high as 1 in 200–300 persons in the general population. Protein C is a vitamin K-dependent plasma protein which, when activated by the thrombin-thrombomodulin complex, inhibits clot formation and enhances fibrinolytic activity. There is a striking disparity between the prevalence of protein C deficiency and the expression of symptoms. Fifty percent of persons expressing the heterozygotic form of the disease develop thromboses before the age of 30 years. Thromboses are usually venous (superficial thrombophlebitis, deep venous thrombosis, mesenteric venous thrombosis, and pulmonary embolism). However, arterial thrombotic episodes may occur.

Protein C deficiency has been associated with warfarin-induced skin necrosis. Because of the short half-life of protein C (6–7 hours), the administration of warfarin rapidly results in decreased levels of protein C in all patients. The reduction of the concentration of protein C before reductions of factors II, IX, and X (factor VII also has a 6–7-hour half-life) can contribute to cutaneous microvascular thrombosis, especially in patients with preexisting protein C deficiency. Purpura fulminans neonatalis, an almost universally fatal condition involving thrombosis of the cutaneous capillaries and veins, may occur in some infants with homozygous protein C deficiency.

The diagnosis of protein C deficiency is established by the results of functional and immunologic assays. Heterozygous patients typically have protein C levels that are 50–60% of normal. Patients with protein C deficiency and thrombosis are treated with anticoagulation or fibrinolytic therapy or both. Warfarin is used for long-term anticoagulation, but heparin must be administered with the warfarin for the first few days to avoid increasing the hypercoagulable state. Warfarin therapy is continued indefinitely. In asymptomatic patients with protein C deficiency, prophylactic anticoagulant therapy does not appear warranted; however, prophylaxis should be initiated to prevent complications during situations in which the risk of thrombosis is increased.

Protein S is a vitamin K-dependent plasma protein, which functions as a cofactor for the anticoagulant and fibrinolytic actions of activated protein C. Similar to the other inheritable hypercoagulable disorders, the onset of symptoms in patients with low or abnormal proteins occurs at a young age (average 25 years), and patients typically present with superficial thrombophlebitis, deep venous thrombosis, mesenteric thrombosis, or pulmonary embolism. Arterial thrombosis is unusual.

The diagnosis of protein S deficiency is established by functional and immunologic assays that determine the free and total protein S activities. Patients with plasma levels of protein S antigen of about one-third to one-half of normal or with levels of protein S functional activity of less than 70% of normal have an increased tendency to develop recurrent venous thrombotic disease. The management of patients who present with complications of protein S deficiency is the same as that for patients with protein C deficiency.

J. Previous Deep Venous Thrombosis/ Pulmonary Embolism: Patients with previous deep venous thrombosis or pulmonary embolism have an increased risk for developing thromboembolic complications. Studies have documented that patients with previous thromboembolic disease undergoing surgery have a 60–70% incidence of deep venous thrombosis. Patients with a history of thromboembolic disease have a 3-fold increase of thromboembolic complications in the postoperative period.

K. Other Risk Factors: Patients with varicose veins have a 2-fold increased risk for developing venous thromboembolic disease. An increased risk of thromboembolism accompanies several of the myeloproliferative disorders including primary thrombocythemia, polycythemia rubra vera, and agnogenic myeloid metaplasia. Hyperlipidemia, diabetes mellitus, hemolytic-uremic syndrome, and thrombotic thrombocytopenic purpura predispose to thrombosis because of their effects on platelets. Hyperlipidemia may activate platelets by modulating adenylate cyclase activity or increasing thromboxane A_2, leading to increased aggregation. Diabetes mellitus affects platelets and the vessel wall by increasing thromboxane A_2, factor VIII:vWF and fibrinogen while decreasing platelet sensitivity to prostacyclin. Both thrombotic thrombocytopenic purpura and hemolytic-uremic syndrome are characterized by the deposition of platelet-fibrin thrombi in the microcirculation.

The lupus-like anticoagulants are IgG or IgM immunoglobulins to platelet and endothelial cell membrane phospholipids. These immunoglobulins have been found to be associated with systemic lupus erythematosus, connective tissue disorders, some malignancies, peripheral vascular disease, and certain drugs (procainamide and hydralazine). The lupus-like anticoagulants have been associated with a high incidence of thromboembolic events (as high as 50%) in patients undergoing vascular reconstructions. The mechanism responsible for the thrombosis is not well defined. The proposed mechanisms include inhibition of the conversion of plasminogen to plasmin, inhibition of AT III, inhibition of prostacyclin synthesis by the endothelial cell, alteration of platelets resulting in increased adhesiveness, and inhibition of thrombomodulin resulting in a decrease in the anticoagulant effects of protein C.

Intravascular hemolysis resulting from transfusion of incompatible blood, hemolytic anemia, paroxysmal nocturnal hemoglobinuria, and cardiopulmonary bypass may promote thrombosis by making available phospholipids that accelerate the intrinsic coagulation pathway. Homocystinuria, an inborn error of metabolism, leads to an increase of homocysteine in the plasma and tissues; the increase of homocysteine has been associated with increased platelet consumption and a high incidence of thromboembolism. An increased incidence of thromboembolic disease has also been noted in patients with Cushing's syndrome, ulcerative colitis, cryofibrinogenemia, and Behçet's syndrome.

Treatment

The incidence of venous thrombosis and pulmonary embolism may be reduced by limiting venous stasis or administering drugs to inhibit coagulation. Ambulation increases venous return and reduces thrombosis. The efficacy of early mobilization and leg exercises in preventing thrombosis is most beneficial in elderly patients undergoing major operations. Anticoagulant drugs effectively prevent venous thrombosis when properly administered. Since platelets play an ancillary role in venous thrombosis, antiplatelet drugs are generally not effective in preventing venous thrombosis.

A. Preventive Measures:

1. Compression devices–Elastic stockings and pneumatic compression devices increase venous return. Data from 4 randomized trials evaluating the use of elastic stockings for the prevention of deep venous thrombosis revealed a 9.3% incidence of deep venous thrombosis in patients wearing stockings and an incidence of 24.5% in control patients. Pneumatic compression devices also lower the rates of lower extremity venous thrombosis. The pneumatic pumps rhythmically compress the leg compartments and increase venous return and fibrinolytic activity. The external pneumatic compression appears to be as effective as low-dose subcutaneous heparin in preventing venous thrombosis in surgical patients. A combination of low-dose heparin and pneumatic compression stockings may be more effective in preventing venous thrombosis than either alone.

2. Subcutaneous heparin–Heparin acts as a catalyst for inactivation of thrombin, factor Xa, and the other serine proteases by AT III. It is a glycosaminoglycan with a molecular weight between 5000–40,000 daltons. Commercial heparin preparations are derived from pork and beef, lung, or intestine. The AT III binding site has been identified as a pentasaccharide that is present in only one-third of the molecule's saccharide chains.

Small amounts of heparin administered subcutaneously prevent thrombosis by enhancing antithrombin activity. Low-dose heparin prophylaxis is effective for low- to moderate-risk patients with normal levels of AT III and thrombin. Low-dose heparin is less effective in high-risk patients with highly activated coagulation systems and, consequently, low levels of AT III. Pooled data from randomized clinical trials evaluating deep venous thrombosis prophylaxis in general surgical patients revealed a reduction in the incidence of deep venous thrombosis from 19.1% (288 of 1507) in control patients to 6% (50 of 831) in patients receiving low-dose subcutaneous heparin. Low-dose heparin prophylaxis has not proved to be as effective in patients with excessive activation of their coagulation systems (as in malignancies, femur and hip fractures, hip surgery, and so on).

Low-dose subcutaneous heparin effectively prevents fatal pulmonary embolism in general surgical patients. In a large multicenter trial in which 4121 patients were randomized to receive either low-dose subcutaneous heparin or placebo, only 2.5% (2 of 80) of the deaths in the heparin group were directly attributed to pulmonary embolism, compared with 16% (16 of 100) of the deaths among the control group. This significantly lower incidence of fatal pulmonary embolism has been confirmed in other studies.

The low-dose subcutaneous heparin regimen consists of administering 5000 units (U) subcutaneously 2 hours preoperatively, followed by 5000 U every 8–12 hours postoperatively. Laboratory monitoring of the aPTT is usually not needed. Patients may develop the heparin-induced thrombocytopenia syndrome from low doses of heparin; therefore, patients receiving heparin should initially have daily platelet counts. The incidence of serious hemorrhagic complications with low-dose subcutaneous heparin is low. The risk of fatal hemorrhage is about 0.2%.

3. Low molecular weight heparin–Fractionation of heparin produces low molecular weight heparin fragments that have high anti-factor Xa activity, but whose anticoagulant effects measured by aPTT are not as great as unfractionated heparin. Theoretically, low molecular weight heparin should prevent thrombosis and have a lower incidence of hemorrhagic side effects and may be less antigenic.

Several investigators have advocated the use of low molecular weight heparin for prophylaxis of venous thrombosis. In a study in which patients undergoing abdominal surgery were randomized to receive either low molecular weight heparin or unfractionated heparin, the patients in the low molecular weight heparin group had a significantly lower incidence of venous thrombosis (2.5%) than patients receiving unfractionated heparin (7.5%). There was no difference in the incidence of wound hematomas or serious bleeding episodes between the 2 groups. Although these results appear promising, other investigators have questioned the efficacy and safety of low molecular weight heparin, suggesting that the incidence of bleeding complications associated with its administration may actually be higher than those observed with unfractionated heparin.

4. Warfarin–Warfarin is an effective and proven agent for preventing venous thromboembolism. Warfarin inhibits the liver's synthesis of active vitamin K-dependent coagulation factors II, VII, IX, and X. It also decreases the production of vitamin K-dependent protein C and protein S. Decreases in factor activity are dependent on the circulating half-lives of the factors; factor VII reaches a steady state after 1–2 days, whereas prothrombin (factor II) takes up to 10 days.

Numerous studies have established the efficacy of prophylactic warfarin administration in preventing venous thrombosis and pulmonary embolism. In a study of patients with hip fractures, the incidence of clinical venous thrombosis decreased from 28.7% in the control group to 2.7% in the treated group. At autopsy, the incidence of thrombosis decreased from 83% to 14%, respectively. The incidence of pulmonary embolism in several studies of patients on warfarin therapy averaged 1.2% compared with 8.4% in untreated patients. The risk of serious hemorrhage ranged between 3% and 7%, whereas fatal hemorrhages occurred in 0.3% of the patients receiving warfarin.

Prophylactic use of warfarin seems justified in groups in whom low-dose subcutaneous heparin has not proved effective. The high-risk categories include patients with recent femur or hip fractures, patients undergoing hip surgery, and patients with malignancies capable of inducing a prethrombotic state. Warfarin prophylaxis should be used cautiously with careful monitoring of prothrombin times. Patients with liver disease or vitamin K deficiency (malnourished condition or receiving long-term intravenous alimentation without vitamin K supplementation) or the elderly should receive reduced initial doses of warfarin. Numerous drugs may affect the actions of warfarin (Table 33–3). The maintenance dose of warfarin should keep the prothrombin time 1.5–1.7 times the control.

The most common complication of warfarin therapy is hemorrhage. The incidence of clinically significant hemorrhage in patients on well-controlled warfarin therapy is about 4.3% per treatment year. Warfarin's anticoagulant effect is reversed with subcutaneous, oral, or intravenous administration of vitamin K or the administration of intravenous fresh frozen plasma. Other complications of warfarin therapy include dermatitis, alopecia, hypersensitivity reactions, nausea, emesis, and diarrhea. Warfarin is not used during pregnancy because it crosses the placenta and has teratogenic effects. Skin necrosis is a rare but dramatic complication of warfarin therapy, which occurs most commonly in women within the first few days of administration. Anticoagulation with heparin during initial administration of warfarin is recommended to avoid this complication. Avoidance of "loading doses" of warfarin may also decrease the risk of warfarin-induced skin necrosis.

5. Dextran–Dextran is a partially hydrolysed glucose polymer available in 2 preparations: dextran 70 (average molecular weight 70,000 daltons) and dextran 40 (average molecular weight 40,000 daltons; "low molecular weight dextran"). Dextran decreases platelet adhesiveness and alters the release reaction

Table 33–3. Warfarin interactions.

Potentiates Effect (Prolongs PT)	Inhibits Effect (Shortens PT)
Medications	**Medications**
Alcohol	Barbiturates
Allopurinol	Cholestyramine
Amiodarone	Corticosteroids
Anabolic steroids	Diuretics
Aspirin	Glutethimide
Cimetidine	Griseofulvin
Clofibrate	OCPs
Disulfiram	Rifampin
Erythromycin	
Metronidazole	**Disease States**
NSAIDs	Uremia
Phenylbutazone	High vitamin K diet
Phenytoin	High vitamin C diet
Quinidine	Hypermetabolic states
Thyroxine	Low vitamin K diet
Trimethoprim-sulfamethoxazole	Hepatic insufficiency

PT, prothrombin time; OCPs, oral contraceptives; NSAIDs, nonsteroidal anti-inflammatory agents.
The effect of warfarin may be potentiated or retarded by interaction with numerous medications and disease states.

causing decreased aggregation. Dextran also decreases plasma concentrations of factor VIII:vWF. The adsorption of dextran on platelet surfaces in combination with low levels of factor VIII:vWF may account for the decreased platelet function. Dextran, at high concentrations, also interferes with the polymerization of fibrin, causing clots that form to be more susceptible to lysis by plasmin. Dextran acts additionally as a plasma volume expander, increasing blood flow and reducing venous stasis.

Dextran has been used prophylactically to prevent both venous and arterial thrombosis. When the results of several studies were combined, venous thrombosis was found in 15.6% (115 of 738) of patients receiving dextran prophylactically compared with 24.2% (193 of 799) of control patients. Dextran has been reported to reduce the incidence of venous thrombosis following femur fractures or hip surgery by 50%. However, a prospective study that examined the use of dextran 70 in high-risk surgical patients revealed no reduction of the incidence of pulmonary embolism or mortality compared with control patients. In a multicenter prospective study, the incidence of fatal pulmonary embolism was about the same for patients who received dextran 70 as for patients treated with low-dose subcutaneous heparin.

Doses of dextran between 500 mL of 6% solution and 1000 mL of 10% solution per 24 hours, used for a period of 72 hours, have proved effective. Dextran infusion can be associated with serious complications including pulmonary edema secondary to plasma volume expansion, hemorrhage, renal failure, and rare anaphylactoid reactions. Fewer side effects have been reported with dextran 40 than with dextran 70. Because of questions regarding dextran's effectiveness and the potential complications associated with its use, it is a second-line agent in the prevention of thromboembolic disease.

B. Medical Treatment: Multiple options including heparin anticoagulation, thrombolytic therapy, and surgery are available for the management of deep venous thrombosis.

1. Heparin– Clinical trials have established the efficacy of intravenous heparin in preventing the progression of thromboembolic complications in patients with deep venous thrombosis. Therapeutic heparin anticoagulation is the first line of treatment for deep venous thrombosis of the popliteal or proximal veins of the leg. Anticoagulation is accomplished by administering a 5000–20,000-U (100–200 U/kg) intravenous heparin bolus, followed by a continuous maintenance infusion. Clinical trials have shown that the heparin dosage must be adjusted to keep the aPTT at least 1.5 times control values to ensure a low incidence of recurrent thromboembolism. The maintenance dosage usually varies 600–2000 U heparin per hour. Intravenous heparin therapy is continued for 4–6 days. Oral anticoagulation with warfarin is begun on the second to third day of heparin therapy. The heparin is discontinued after the prothrombin time is at least 1.5 times control values.

Heparin should be continued in patients with continued active thrombosis and restarted in patients with recurrences of the thrombosis. Long-term oral anticoagulation with warfarin is continued for 3–6 months. Self-administered subcutaneous heparin, 5000 U twice a day for 3–6 months, is a satisfactory alternative to oral anticoagulation.

It is uncertain whether patients with calf vein thrombosis should receive anticoagulation therapy, since only about 20% of these thrombi propagate proximally. It has been suggested that these patients should be followed by venography, ^{125}I-fibrinogen scanning, impedance plethysmography, or ultrasonography, and should receive anticoagulation when proximal propagation of the thrombus occurs. However, many treat deep calf vein thrombosis with heparin followed by warfarin.

If deep venous thrombosis is treated as outlined, the risk of recurrent thromboembolism is less than 5%. However, long-term follow-up studies of patients have shown that they are at risk for developing the postphlebitic syndrome. Several studies have indicated that more than 80% of deep venous thrombosis patients who are treated with heparin develop stasis ulcerations in their malleolar area after being followed up for 4–7 years. These studies emphasize that although heparin markedly reduces the risk of recurrent thromboembolism in patients with deep venous thrombosis, it does not prevent the venous, especially the valvular, damage that contributes to the long-term morbidity.

The major complications of heparin therapy are hemorrhage and thrombocytopenia. Bleeding is the most common complication, occurring in 10–20% of patients during continuous intravenous infusion. Bleeding rarely occurs unless the aPTT is prolonged more than 2–3 times the control for several hours. The incidence of bleeding may approach 50% in patients with underlying bleeding diatheses such as uremia and thrombocytopenia. The elderly, especially females, are at greater risk for bleeding while receiving heparin.

The heparin-induced thrombocytopenia syndrome is an idiosyncratic drug reaction to heparin, which can result in thrombosis or, rarely, bleeding. Two types of heparin-induced thrombocytopenia occur. An acute form has few clinical sequelae; however, the delayed form can lead to devastating thrombohemorrhagic complications and even death. The delayed form of the syndrome is seen in about 4–5% of patients receiving heparin and generally occurs within 2–15 days of therapy during the initial exposure to heparin. It may occur on the first day of re-exposure to heparin. This form of heparin-induced thrombocytopenia syndrome has been associated with a morbidity rate of 61% and a mortality rate of 23% if detected late and rates of 22.5% and 12%, respectively, if detected and treated early. The incidence and severity of the delayed form

of heparin-induced thrombocytopenia syndrome are independent of the dose, type, or route of administration of heparin. The pathophysiology of the syndrome is thought to be an IgG-heparin immune complex disorder involving both the Fab and Fc portions of the IgG molecule.

The heparin-induced thrombocytopenia syndrome should be suspected when a patient receiving heparin has a falling platelet count or a platelet count of less than 100,000/cm³, increased resistance to anticoagulation with heparin, or new thrombohemorrhagic complications. If heparin-induced thrombocytopenia is suspected, all sources of heparin should be eliminated, platelet function inhibitors should be administered, and, if needed, an alternate form of anticoagulation (warfarin or dextran) should be used. Confirmation of the diagnosis is made by platelet aggregometry or ^{14}C-serotonin release studies. In patients with known heparin-induced thrombocytopenia syndrome who require heparin reexposure, platelet function inhibiting agents appear to exert a protective effect from the thrombohemorrhagic complications but not the thrombocytopenia. Preliminary studies also suggest that ancrod may be an acceptable alternative to heparin.

Contraindications to heparin therapy include serious active bleeding, recent neurosurgical procedures, malignant hypertension, and cerebral or subarachnoid hemorrhage. Relative contraindications are recent surgery, gastrointestinal bleeding, hemorrhagic diathesis, and recent stroke.

2. Thrombolytic therapy–The fibrinolytic system maintains vascular patency by lysing fibrin accumulations. Plasminogen, the precursor of the active fibrinolytic enzyme plasmin, is closely bound to fibrinogen and remains bound to fibrin. Therefore, if sufficient plasminogen activator could be generated in or on the thrombus, the plasminogen in or on the thrombus could be converted to plasmin and thus induce thrombolysis. The obvious advantage of using thrombolytic agents to treat deep venous thrombosis is lysis of the thrombus with, theoretically, preservation of venous valvular function.

Thrombolytic agents that have been evaluated in the treatment of deep venous thrombosis are streptokinase, urokinase, and recombinant human tissue type plasminogen activator. Streptokinase is a nonenzymatic protein that is produced by group C β-hemolytic streptococci. It combines with plasminogen to form an activator complex, which then converts plasminogen to plasmin. Thus, the quantity of streptokinase administered must be sufficient to result in plasmin production, but an excessive quantity could cause all the plasminogen to be incorporated into the activator complex and be unavailable for conversion to plasmin. Urokinase and tissue plasminogen activator directly convert plasminogen to plasmin (Fig 33–4). Urokinase is isolated from human urine or cultured from human embryonic kidney cells and is nonantigenic. Recombinant human tissue type plasminogen activator is biologi-

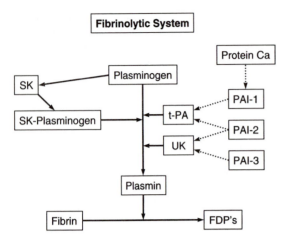

Fibrinolytic System

Figure 33–4. The fibrinolytic process is regulated by plasminogen activators and inhibitors. Plasminogen is activated to plasmin, the active fibrinolytic enzyme, by urokinase and tissue plasminogen activator. Streptokinase forms a complex with plasminogen, which converts additional plasminogen to plasmin.

cally identical with the tissue plasminogen activator that is present in most cells of the body. Because streptokinase and urokinase have no specific affinity for plasminogen attached to fibrin, they activate both fibrin-bound and circulating plasminogen. Conversely, tissue plasminogen activator has a higher affinity for plasminogen in the presence of fibrin. This specificity results in activation of plasmin on the fibrin clot, with limited activation of circulating plasminogen.

Urokinase and streptokinase have reduced the size and have completely lysed thromboemboli in experimental and clinical studies. Both agents are most effective when given to patients with thromboemboli that are less than 5–7 days of age. The best results have been obtained in patients who have had symptoms for less than 48 hours. Streptokinase and urokinase have been noted to accelerate lysis of thromboemboli with restoration of venous patency and the preservation of valvular function in 26–57% of treated patients. In a recent summary of studies comparing anticoagulation and thrombolysis in the treatment of deep venous thrombosis, 82% of the patients in the anticoagulation group demonstrated no clearing of thrombus, whereas 4% demonstrated complete lysis. In the group of patients receiving thrombolytic therapy, 45% had significant or complete resolution of the thrombus with an additional 18% exhibiting partial lysis. These data demonstrate an advantage of thrombolytic therapy in the management of deep venous thrombosis.

A significantly lower incidence of postphlebitic sequelae has been observed in patients with deep venous thrombosis who were treated with thrombolytic therapy than in those treated with anticoagulation. However, others have demonstrated no difference in the incidence of postphlebitic syndrome in patients treated

with thrombolytic therapy and those treated with anticoagulant therapy in long-term follow-up. Patients in whom complete lysis of the deep venous thrombosis was achieved with thrombolytic therapy demonstrate markedly reduced valvular reflux at long-term follow-up when compared with patients in whom lysis of the deep venous thrombosis was incomplete.

Catheter-directed thrombolysis of thromboses of the iliofemoral system has been introduced as a new technique. Local delivery of the thrombolytic agent to the thrombus has many theoretical advantages over systemic administration including local delivery of a greater concentration of the thrombolytic agent to the thrombus and decreased systemic activation of the thrombolytic system. Preliminary experience with this technique has shown promising results; however, further investigation is needed to evaluate this mode of therapy.

The major complication encountered during the administration of thrombolytic agents is hemorrhage, which occurs 2–5 times more frequently than in patients receiving heparin. The increased incidence of hemorrhagic complications has led to the development of contraindications to the administration of thrombolytic agents (Table 33–4). In addition, vascular invasive procedures should be reduced to a minimum and should include only those procedures in which bleeding can be controlled by direct pressure in patients receiving thrombolytic therapy. Sensitivity reactions are rarely encountered during urokinase infusions; however, they occur in 10–25% of patients receiving streptokinase.

Thrombolytic agents with a greater affinity for fibrin are being developed. The newer agents should generate less systemic lysis and less complications. Pro-urokinase, one of the new agents, is an inactive zymogen of urokinase that also has a high affinity for fibrin-bound plasminogen. Clinical trials evaluating pro-urokinase are underway.

Although thrombolytic agents appear to be able to lyse fresh (less than 5 days old) thromboemboli and to preserve valve function, further controlled clinical trials are needed to substantiate their effectiveness before they are accepted for general use. Heparin re-

Table 33–4. Contraindications to systemic thrombolytic therapy.

Absolute
  Active internal bleeding
  Recent CVA
  Intracranial pathology
  Recent eye surgery
Relative
  Recent major surgery/trauma/CPR
  Active peptic ulcer disease
  Uncontrolled hypertension
  Pregnancy
  Diabetic hemorrhagic retinopathy

CVA, cerebral vascular accident; CPR, cardiopulmonary resuscitation.

mains the agent of choice for the management of thromboembolism.

C. Surgery: Patients with deep venous thrombosis who have a contraindication to anticoagulant therapy and those who have recurrent pulmonary embolism while properly anticoagulated are candidates for interruption of the inferior vena cava, either directly or by intraluminal device, to prevent fatal pulmonary embolism. Transvenous insertion of a Greenfield vena caval filter protects 96% of patients from pulmonary embolism while maintaining patency of the inferior vena cava in over 95% of the patients.

Iliofemoral thrombectomy has not been used extensively in the USA for the treatment of iliofemoral thrombosis because the risk/benefit ratio has been high. However, acceptable results of iliofemoral thrombectomy have been documented. In a multicenter, prospective, randomized trial, patients with iliofemoral thrombosis treated by thrombectomy demonstrated a higher patency of the iliofemoral system (76%) compared with patients treated with anticoagulation (35%) at 6 month follow-up. In addition, patent femoropopliteal segments with competent valves were observed in 52% of the thrombectomy group compared with 26% of the anticoagulation group. In another study, good results were reported in 86% of patients followed up for 4 years after iliofemoral thrombectomy. Although controversial, iliofemoral thrombectomy is being advocated more frequently for the treatment of major iliofemoral thrombosis of recent duration in young healthy patients and those in whom the thrombosis propagates despite treatment with anticoagulation or thrombolytic therapy.

PULMONARY EMBOLISM

Essentials of Diagnosis
- Dyspnea.
- Hemoptysis.
- Pleuritic pain.
- Tachycardia.
- Clinical thrombophlebitis.
- Atypical asthma.

General Considerations
Pulmonary emboli occur when portions of thrombi break off and travel to the lungs. Pulmonary emboli arise most commonly from thrombi in the iliofemoral system, but may arise from calf, pelvic, and much less often upper extremity venous thrombi. Pulmonary embolism occurs in 10–20% of patients with confirmed proximal deep venous thrombosis and much less frequently in patients with calf vein thrombosis.

Clinical Findings
A. Signs and Symptoms: Pulmonary embolism mimics many of the disorders that occur in the chest, mediastinum, and epigastrium. The classic triad of symptoms—dyspnea, hemoptysis, and pleuritic pain—occurred in only 28% of the 160 patients in the Urokinase Pulmonary Embolism Trial (UPET) and in only 20% of patients with massive embolization. However, 2 of the 3 symptoms occurred in 65% of the patients. Dyspnea occurred in 81%, pleuritic pain in 72%, and hemoptysis in 34% of the 160 patients. Tachypnea, the most common finding associated with pulmonary embolism, was present in 88%. Tachycardia was present in 43% and clinical thrombophlebitis in 30% of the patients in the trial.

B. Imaging Studies: Although the chest radiograph is frequently obtained, it is rarely diagnostic of pulmonary embolism. The Westermark sign (hyperlucency in an area of oligemia) is an infrequent finding on the radiograph. Pulmonary infarction, frequently accompanied by pleural effusion, occurs in about one-third of patients with pulmonary embolism. The infarctions usually occur in patients with preexisting cardiac or pulmonary disorders, which compromise the pathways of oxygenation (bronchial arterial circulation, pulmonary arterial circulation, and the airways). Conversely, patients without preexisting cardiopulmonary disease who develop pulmonary embolism rarely suffer pulmonary infarction. The electrocardiogram, like the chest film, may suggest pulmonary embolism but usually is not diagnostic. Electrocardiographic changes occur in up to 87% of patients with pulmonary embolism and are more pronounced in those with previous cardiopulmonary disease.

Pulmonary perfusion scanning has become the most used diagnostic procedure for determining the presence of pulmonary embolism. It can be performed rapidly with minimal risk to the patient. The initial scan is useful in establishing the diagnosis of pulmonary embolism; subsequent scans are of value in monitoring embolus resolution and in detecting new emboli. Scans should be performed as soon as pulmonary embolism is suspected. A diagnostic scan should include anterior, posterior, and right and left lateral views. The perfusion scan should be compared with a current chest radiograph and a ventilation scan. Parenchymal lesions detected with the chest radiograph (eg, atelectasis, bullae, pneumonia, tumor, effusion) are frequently associated with hypoperfusion. Therefore, when altered perfusion exists in radiographically abnormal areas of the lung, the perfusion scan is nondiagnostic.

Reduced perfusion in areas that appear normal on the chest radiograph is suggestive of pulmonary embolism. The ventilation scan also detects regions of altered ventilation. A scan that demonstrates a decrease in ventilation and perfusion in the same lung area indicates airway or parenchymal disease, whereas a normal ventilation scan and an abnormal perfusion scan in the proper clinical setting are highly suggestive of pulmonary embolism (Fig 33–5).

Pulmonary angiography remains the most reliable modality for establishing the diagnosis of pulmonary embolism. Like the perfusion scan, the pulmonary angiogram is most reliable if performed immediately after embolization and becomes less reliable with the passage of time because thrombolysis occurs rapidly in the pulmonary circulation. Although pulmonary angiograms have been performed by injecting contrast material into the right heart or even into the central veins, the best definition of the pulmonary vascular tree is obtained by injecting contrast into the main, right, and left pulmonary arteries with additional selective pulmonary artery injections as indicated (Fig 33–6). In addition to angiographic evaluation of the pulmonary arterial tree, the right ventricular and pulmonary arterial pressures should be determined because they are almost always elevated with clinically significant pulmonary embolism. In addition, mixed venous blood samples should be obtained for blood gas determinations.

C. Laboratory Tests: The triad of elevated lactic dehydrogenase, bilirubin, and normal serum glutamic oxalic transaminase occurred in only 4% of the patients in the UPET and has not been found reliable in establishing the diagnosis of pulmonary embolism. Blood gas studies indicate the degree of hypoxemia accompanying the embolization; the carbon dioxide pressures are usually low because of the associated hyperventilation. In addition, the difference between alveolar PCO_2 and arterial PCO_2 may be widened because of the increased alveolar dead space.

Treatment

A. Medical: The goals of management of pulmonary embolism are to support and maintain life during the acute episode, to stop the propagation of the thromboembolus, to augment spontaneous or induced fibrinolytic removal of the thromboembolus, and to prevent recurrences. With early diagnosis and prompt and aggressive therapy, most patients will survive the embolization and have a low rate of recurrence.

The response to pulmonary embolization is determined by the size of the embolus and the patient's cardiopulmonary status. Some patients tolerate massive embolization well, but those with cardiopulmonary compromise may tolerate small emboli poorly. Although the administration of oxygen by mask or nasal prongs helps most patients, tracheal intubation and respiratory assistance may be necessary when the hypoxia is profound. Hypotension or a failing heart usually dictates the need for inotropic agents and vasopressors. In addition, some clinicians recommend aggressive fluid administration to increase the filling of the left atrium and thus improve cardiac output. The fluid must be given cautiously with constant monitoring of the pulmonary artery and right ventricular pressures. If significant hypoxia or hypotension occurs, the patient will require cardiopulmonary support. Intensive nursing care and adequate monitoring of vital functions are essential components of the care provided for these patients. The management of pul-

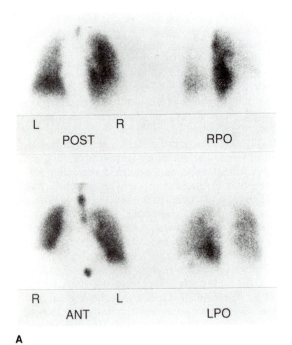

A

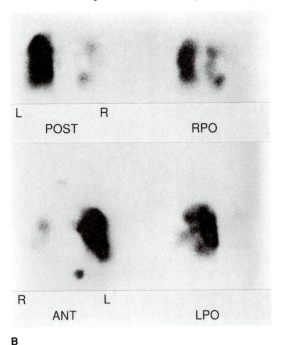

B

Figure 33–5. *A:* Views of a ventilation scan demonstrating normal ventilation. *B:* Views of the perfusion phase of the study demonstrating multiple segmental and subsegmental defects of perfusion involving most of the right lung and, to a lesser extent, the left lung. These perfusion defects do not have similar changes on the ventilation scan and therefore have a high probability of representing pulmonary embolism. (POST, posterior; ANT, anterior; RPO, right posterior oblique; LPO, left posterior oblique.)

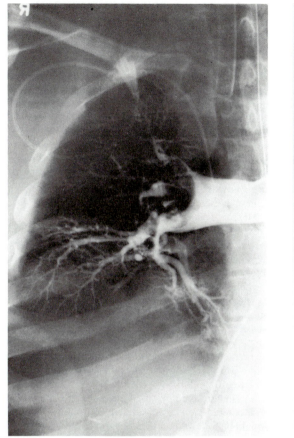
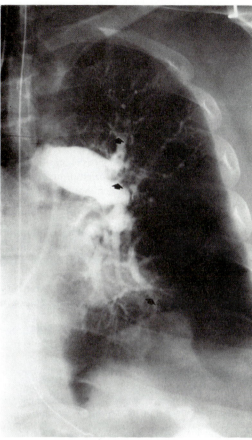

A B

Figure 33–6. Pulmonary angiograms of a multitrauma victim who developed deep venous thrombosis and pulmonary embolism. Pulmonary artery pressure was 50/25 mmHg. *A:* Selective right pulmonary angiogram demonstrates a large embolus at the bifurcation of the right pulmonary artery with almost total occlusion of the right, middle, and upper lobe arteries. There is partial occlusion of the right lower lobe artery. *B:* Selective right pulmonary angiogram reveals multiple emboli (*arrows*) in the branches of the left pulmonary artery. A large portion of the left lateral lower lobe is not perfused.

monary embolism also includes anticoagulation, thrombolytic therapy, and embolectomy.

1. Anticoagulation–Heparin remains the principal agent for treating pulmonary embolism. The first controlled trial of the use of heparin in patients with pulmonary embolism was reported in 1960. Although it was not well designed, the study clearly demonstrated the therapeutic advantage of heparin. If the patient has no contraindications, intravenous heparin should be administered as soon as the diagnosis of pulmonary embolism is suspected and continued during the diagnostic procedures. The average adult patient usually receives 10,000–20,000 U heparin as the initial dose and 800–1000 U per hour during the diagnostic evaluation. If pulmonary embolism is confirmed, additional heparin is administered to increase the total dose to that described earlier for the management of deep venous thrombosis. When sufficient amounts of heparin are given to stop the clotting process, the aPTT becomes about twice that of the control. Larger amounts of heparin are required initially; as the coagulation process slows, smaller amounts of heparin are required. After 24–48 hours, the aPTT is maintained at 1.6–1.8 times that of the control.

Intravenous administration of heparin is continued for 5–10 days or longer if recurrent embolization or continued active thrombosis is present in the legs or pelvis. After the acute episode, the patient is administered less intense anticoagulation, usually warfarin, which is continued for a minimum of 3 months. Elastic stockings and avoidance of positions of stasis are prescribed to reduce the incidence of recurrent embolization. Proper, prompt management of the pulmonary embolism is usually adequate management for the residual thrombosis at the source of the embolus.

Heparin is tolerated well by most patients. Overt bleeding, which occurred in 27% of the 78 patients treated with heparin in the UPET, is almost always related to the use of excessive amounts of heparin or to an invasive diagnostic procedure. Twelve of the 78 patients had recurrent embolism, as demonstrated by ventilation-perfusion scans, whereas 6 others had clinical evidence of recurrent embolism, yielding a possible recurrence rate of 23%. The percentages of recurrent embolism were 18% with adequate heparin therapy and 44% with inadequate heparin therapy. Recurrent embolization during the early days of heparin treatment should be interpreted not as a failure of management but as a result of management. The heparin has stopped the clotting process, lysis is occurring, and thrombus at the source of the original embolus undergo lysis, fragmentation, and embolization. The recurrent emboli are generally not clinically significant because they usually undergo lysis in a few days.

Most patients, treated promptly, survive pulmonary embolism, with the in-hospital mortality rate ranging from 5% to 9%. Death occurring during pulmonary embolism usually results from cardiac failure.

2. Thrombolysis—Many patients die from massive pulmonary embolism because of right ventricular failure secondary to the sudden increase in pulmonary vascular resistance caused by the embolism. Thrombolytic therapy offers a theoretical advantage over heparin, which acts to arrest the thrombotic process and allow spontaneous lysis to occur, because it is capable of rapidly lysing the thrombus and thereby lowering the pulmonary hypertension and increasing the cardiac output. The UPET and the Urokinase-Streptokinase Pulmonary Embolism Trial (USPET) compared the therapeutic effects of heparin with thrombolytic therapy in patients with pulmonary embolism. In the UPET, patients who received urokinase had significantly accelerated resolution (as demonstrated by angiography and lung scans) of thrombus and improved pulmonary hemodynamics compared with patients who received heparin. Although no significant differences were demonstrated for in-hospital morbidity and mortality rates between the 2 groups, patients with massive pulmonary emboli appeared to gain the greatest improvement with 24 hours of urokinase infusion. Hemorrhagic complications were high in both the thrombolytic and heparin groups—45% and 27%, respectively—and were partly attributed to the number of invasive procedures required under the experimental protocol. In the USPET, urokinase treatment for 12 hours proved to be as effective with respect to early resolution of the thrombus as either streptokinase or

urokinase administered for 24 hours. The incidences of recurrent embolism in the 3 groups were not significantly different, nor were the 2-week or 6-month mortality rates.

One-year follow-up of pulmonary embolism patients in the UPET revealed no difference in mortality between the patients treated with heparin and those treated with urokinase. The pulmonary hemodynamics of 40 patients who participated in the UPET were studied at 1 year; patients initially treated with thrombolytic therapy demonstrated significantly improved pulmonary hemodynamics (capillary blood volume and pulmonary diffusing capacity) compared with patients initially treated with heparin.

In another study in which 23 patients with angiographically proven pulmonary embolism were randomized to receive either heparin or urokinase, follow-up at 7 years showed improved pulmonary hemodynamics both at rest and during exercise (pulmonary artery pressure and pulmonary vascular resistance) in the patients who received thrombolytic therapy.

The data indicate that thrombolytic agents accelerate the lysis of pulmonary emboli and may be more beneficial than heparin in patients with massive pulmonary embolism. Therefore, thrombolytic therapy is recommended for patients with massive pulmonary embolism involving one or more lobes and for those with cardiopulmonary insufficiency and shock. Thrombolytic therapy should be used in conjunction with compression devices to reduce venous stasis and should be followed up with heparin and warfarin anticoagulation. Heparin remains the treatment of choice for most patients, especially those with pulmonary embolism without hemodynamic compromise.

B. Surgical: Operative embolectomy has traditionally been reserved for the patient with massive pulmonary embolism and cardiac collapse. The diagnosis of pulmonary embolism must be confirmed by angiography before operative intervention. The operative mortality rate for embolectomy is about 50%. Retrospective analysis has led many investigators to propose thrombolytic therapy as the initial treatment for such patients, reserving embolectomy for nonresponders. An alternative to operative embolectomy has been the use of catheter-directed suction embolectomy; investigators report a 32% operative mortality rate and a 56% overall survival rate using this technique, which may be performed in the radiology suite.

REFERENCES

Ahn SS: The hypercoagulable states: A comprehensive review for the vascular surgeon. Semin Vasc Surg 1990;3:6.

Ahn SS et al: Postoperative thrombotic complications in patients with the lupus anticoagulant: Increased risk after vascular surgical procedures. J Vasc Surg 1988;7:749.

Anderson FA et al: A population-based perspective of the hospital incidence and case-fatality rates of deep vein thrombosis and pulmonary embolism: The Worcester DVT study. Arch Intern Med 1991;151:933.

Anonymous: Prevention of fatal postoperative pulmonary

embolism by low doses of heparin: An international multicentre trial. Lancet 1975;2:45.

Anonymous: The urokinase pulmonary embolism trial: A national cooperative study. Circulation 1973;47(Suppl 2):1.

Anonymous: Urokinase-streptokinase embolism trial: Phase 2 results: A cooperative study. JAMA 1974;229:1606.

Arnesen H, Hoiseth A, Ly B: Streptokinase or heparin in the treatment of deep vein thrombosis: Follow-up results of a prospective study. Acta Med Scand 1982;211:65.

Barritt DW, Jordon SC: Anticoagulant drugs in the treatment of pulmonary embolism: A controlled trial. Lancet 1960; 1:1309.

Bergqvist D et al: Low molecular weight heparin once daily compared with conventional low-dose heparin twice daily: A prospective double-blind multicentre trial on prevention of postoperative thrombosis. Br J Surg 1986;73: 204.

Bonnar J, Daly L, Sheppard BL: Changes in the fibrinolytic system during pregnancy. Semin Thromb Hemost 1990; 16:221.

Clagett GP, Reisch JS: Prevention of venous thromboembolism in general surgical patients: Results of meta-analysis. Ann Surg 1988;208:227.

Cole CW, Bormanis J: Ancrod: A practical alternative to heparin. J Vasc Surg 1988;8:59.

Coller BS et al: Deficiency of plasma protein S, Protein C, or antithrombin III and arterial thrombosis. Arteriosclerosis 1987;7:456.

Comerota AJ, Aldridge SC: Thrombolytic therapy for acute deep vein thrombosis. Can J Surg 1992;36:359.

Comerota AJ et al: Venous duplex imaging: Should it replace hemodynamic tests for deep venous thrombosis? J Vasc Surg 1990;11:53.

Comp PC: Hereditary disorders predisposing to thrombosis. Prog Hemost Thromb 1986;8:71.

Comp PC, Esmon CT: Recurrent venous thromboembolism in patients with a partial deficiency of protein S. N Engl J Med 1984;311:1525.

Coon WW: Epidemiology of venous thromboembolism. Ann Surg 1977;186:149.

Coon WW: Risk factors in pulmonary embolism. Surg Gynecol Obstet 1976;143:385.

Coon WW: The spectrum of pulmonary embolism: Twenty years later. Arch Surg 1976;111:398.

Coon WW, Coller FA: Clinicopathologic correlation in thromboembolism. Surg Gynecol Obstet 1959;109:259.

Elliot MS et al: A comparative randomized trial of heparin versus streptokinase in the treatment of acute proximal venous thrombosis: An interim report of a prospective trial. Br J Surg 1979;66:838.

Haimovici H: Ischemic forms of venous thrombosis: Phlegmasia cerulea dolens and venous gangrene. Heart Bull 1967;16:101.

Hirsh J et al: Evolution of thrombosis. Ann N Y Acad Sci 1987;516:586.

Kakkar VV, Lawrence D: Hemodynamic and clinical assessment after therapy for acute deep vein thrombosis. Am J Surg 1985;150:54.

Kakkar VV, Murray WJ: Efficacy and safety of low-molecular-weight heparin (CY216) in preventing postoperative venous thromboembolism: A co-operative study. Br J Surg 1985;72:786.

Kakkar VV et al: Natural history of postoperative deep-vein thrombosis. Lancet 1969;2:230.

Kelton JG et al: Heparin-induced thrombocytopenia: Laboratory studies. Blood 1988;72:925.

Laster J, Elfrink R, Silver D: Reexposure to heparin of patients with heparin-associated antibodies. J Vasc Surg 1989;9:677.

Laster J et al: The heparin-induced thrombocytopenia syndrome: An update. Surgery 1987;102:763.

Lindner DJ et al: Long-term hemodynamic and clinical sequelae of lower extremity deep vein thrombosis. J Vasc Surg 1986;4:436.

Lohr JM et al: Lower extremity calf thrombosis: To treat or not to treat? J Vasc Surg 1991;14:618.

Manabe S, Matsuda M: Homozygous protein C deficiency combined with heterozygous dysplasminogenemia found in a 21-year-old thrombophilic male. Thromb Res 1985; 39:333.

Marciniak E, Wilson HD, Marlar RA: Neonatal purpura fulminans as expression of homozygosity for protein C deficiency. (Abstract). Blood 1983;62(Suppl 1):303a.

Marlar RA, Neumann A: Neonatal purpura fulminans due to homozygous protein C or protein S deficiencies. Semin Thromb Hemost 1990;16:299.

Miletich J, Sherman L, Broze G Jr: Absence of thrombosis in subjects with heterozygous protein C deficiency. N Engl J Med 1987;317:991.

Molina JE, Hunter DW, Yedlicka JW: Thrombolytic therapy for iliofemoral venous thrombosis. Vasc Surg 1992;26: 630.

Moser KM, LeMoine JR: Is embolic risk conditioned by location of deep venous thrombosis? Ann Intern Med 1981;94:439.

Nicolaides AN, Sumner DS (editors): Impedance plethysmography. In: *Investigation of patients with deep vein thrombosis and chronic venous insufficiency.* Med-Orion, 1991.

Okrent D, Messersmith R, Buckman J: Transcatheter fibrinolytic therapy for left iliofemoral venous thrombosis. J Vasc Intervent Radiol 1991;2:195.

Oliver MA: Duplex scanning in venous disease. Bruit 1985;9:206.

Philbrick JT, Becker DM: Calf deep venous thrombosis: A wolf in sheep's clothing? Arch Intern Med 1988;148: 2131.

Plate G et al: Thrombectomy with temporary arteriovenous fistula: The treatment of choice in acute iliofemoral venous thrombosis. J Vasc Surg 1984;1:867.

Rabinov K, Paulin S: Roentgen diagnosis of venous thrombosis in the leg. Arch Surg 1972;104:134.

Robinson DL, Teitelbaum GP: Phlegmasia cerulea dolens: Treatment by pulse-spray and infusion thrombolysis. AJR 1993;160:1288.

Schwartz HP et al: Plasma protein S deficiency in familial thrombotic disease. Blood 1984;64:1297.

Semba CP et al: Iliofemoral venous thrombosis: Treatment with regional thrombolysis. (Abstract). J Vasc Intervent Radiol 1993;4:54.

Sharma GV, Burleson VA, Sasahara AA. Effect of thrombolytic therapy on pulmonary-capillary blood volume in patients with pulmonary embolism. N Engl J Med 1980; 303:842.

Sharma GVRK et al: Long-term hemodynamic benefit of thrombolytic therapy in pulmonary embolic disease. (Abstract). J Am Coll Cardiol 1990;15:65A.

Silver D, Kapsch DN, Tsoi EK: Heparin induced thrombocytopenia, thrombosis and hemorrhage. Ann Surg 1983;198:301.

Sipes SL, Weiner CP: Venous thromboembolic disease in pregnancy. Semin Perinatol 1990;14:103.

Stewart JR, Greenfield LJ: Transvenous vena caval filtration and pulmonary embolectomy. Surg Clin North Am 1982;62:411.

Strandness DE Jr et al: Long-term sequelae of acute venous thrombosis. JAMA 1983;250:1289.

Tolleffsen DM: Laboratory diagnosis of antithrombin and heparin cofactor II deficiency. Semin Thromb Hemost 1990;16:162.

Trousseau A: *Clinique Medicale de l'Hotel-Dieu de Paris.* Bailliere, 1861.

Van Ramshorst B et al: Duplex scanning in the diagnosis and follow-up of DVT. In: *Angiologie.* Boccalon H (editor). John Libbey Eurotext, 1988.

Welch WH: *Papers and Addresses.* Johns Hopkins University Press, 1920.

White RH et al: Diagnosis of deep-vein thrombosis using duplex ultrasound (see comments). Ann Intern Med 1989; 111:297.

Lymphatic Disease

34

Robert Y. Rhee, MD, & Peter Gloviczki, MD

The primary function of the lymphatic system is to transport extracellular fluid from the interstitial space back into the blood circulation. The lymphatic system, in coordination with the immune system, also functions as a protective filter against foreign body invasion. The formation of interstitial fluid is regulated by Starling forces of hydrostatic and osmotic pressure across the walls of capillaries. The hydrostatic pressure forces an ultrafiltrate of the blood plasma into the interstitial space, most of which is reabsorbed at the venous capillaries. However, about 2–4 L of protein-rich (75–150 g) fluid is not reabsorbed during a 24-hour period and must be carried back into the intravascular space by the lymphatic system. Hence, lymphatic vessel dysfunction, occlusion, or trauma can interfere with fluid dynamics and immunologic function. Failure to return lymph fluid from the interstitial space to the venous circulation results in stasis and abnormal lymph accumulation in the distal compartments. Lymphedema develops when there is insufficient collateral circulation and all compensatory mechanisms have been exhausted. In addition, because transport of excess tissue fluid containing lymphocytes, different plasma proteins, immunoglobulins, and cytokines is impaired, chronic inflammatory changes in the subcutaneous tissue and skin occur.

ANATOMY OF THE LYMPHATICS

The adult lymphatic system consists of peripheral lymph vessels, lymph nodes, and major lymphatic trunks. The lymphatic capillaries, which are composed of a single layer of attenuated endothelial cells, absorb the excess interstitial fluid. Although these capillaries lack a basal membrane, they are nonetheless anatomically similar to the arterial and venous counterparts. However, larger lymphatic vessels are anatomically and functionally very different from those in the venous system. The venous system is filled with a liquid column, which responds immediately to changes in pressure or resistance. On the other hand, the lymphatic system is rarely filled entirely with fluid. The lymph column completely fills the lymphatic channels only in longstanding stasis.

Unidirectional flow is maintained by bicuspid lymphatic valves and, in the initial lymphatics, by supporting microfibrils that extend from the endothelial cell to the interstitial tissue. The large gap junctions between the endothelial cells allow for absorption of large molecules. The smaller lymph components are actively phagocytosed through the endothelial cells. The lymph is then collected by the afferent lymph vessels and transported to the lymph-conducting elements of the lymph nodes that filter and further conduct the lymph fluid to efferent lymphatic channels.

The superficial medial lymphatic system is responsible for at least 80% of lymph transport in the lower extremities (Fig 34–1). The lateral superficial bundle, which is located near the lesser saphenous vein, also functions to transport lymph back from the distal compartments of the lower leg. Also, a deep lymphatic network runs in close proximity to the tibial and peroneal vessels and transports lymph through the popliteal lymph nodes into the deep femoral lymphatics. The superficial and deep systems join in the inguinal lymph nodes and drain toward the aortoiliac lymphatic system. The cisterna chyli is located between the aorta and the inferior vena cava, usually at the level of L1–L2. Mesenteric lymphatics merge with the pelvic and lower extremity lymphatics at this level. The thoracic duct collects and transports the lower body's lymph from the cisterna chyli and drains into the left subclavian vein (Fig 34–2).

The anatomy of the upper extremity lymphatics parallels that of the artery and vein. The medial arm bundle is the most significant pathway for lymph drainage (Fig 34–3). However, after trauma to this major lymphatic vessel during axillary node dissection, the drainage of lymph is secondarily channeled through the lateral lymphatic bundle to the deltoideopectoral and supraclavicular nodes. The lymphatic channels from the right upper extremity and upper thorax drain into the subclavian trunk, which in turn drains into the venous system at the junction of the right jugular and subclavian veins.

LYMPHEDEMA

Essentials of Diagnosis

- Progressive, painless swelling of the extremity.
- Nonpitting edema with a distal to proximal distribution.
- Hyperkeratosis, fissuring of the skin, onychomycosis.

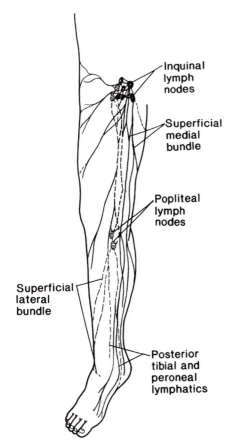

Figure 34–1. Anatomy of the lower extremity lymphatic system. (Reproduced, with permission, from Gloviczki P: Microsurgical treatment for chronic lymphedema: An unfulfilled promise? In: *Venous Disorders.* Bergan JJ, Yao JST [editors]. WB Saunders, 1990.)

Labels in figure:
- Inquinal lymph nodes
- Superficial medial bundle
- Popliteal lymph nodes
- Superficial lateral bundle
- Posterior tibial and peroneal lymphatics

- "Buffalo hump" edema at metatarsal head of the foot.
- "Stemmer's sign" or squared toes.

General Considerations

Lymphedema develops when the transport capacity of the lymphatic system is exceeded by lymph production in the affected area of the body. The disorder is characterized by the complications of excessive accumulation of interstitial fluid with a high protein content. In patients with lymphatic obstruction, numerous compensatory mechanisms develop. These include collateral lymphatic circulation, spontaneous lymphovenous fistulas, and increased activity of tissue macrophages. If the lymphatic transport is impaired because of injury or obstruction to the lymph vessels or lymph nodes, the compensatory mechanisms can function effectively for extended periods. Indeed, lymphedema of the limbs may not develop for several months or years following inguinal or axillary node dissection.

The high protein lymph accumulation results in a chronic, nonpitting edema. The high protein content also produces a fibrotic reaction in the subcutaneous tissue, leading to a relentless scarring process, which can further damage the lymphatic vessels. Fibrosis of the lymph vessels leads to loss of permeability and intrinsic contractility. Dilatation of the lymph vessels causes valvular incompetence, and the inflammatory and fibrotic changes destroy the valve leaflets, further decreasing the transport capacity of the lymphatic system. Further progression of lymphedema results in fibrotic obstruction of the lymph nodes and the major lymph vessels. The larger collaterals, which function effectively during the initial period of obstruction, also occlude with time. Dermal lymphatics are often the only outlet for lymphatic drainage during the chronic phase of lymphedema.

The filtering function of the lymphatics is dysfunctional in lymphedema. The removal of particulate matter, infectious agents, and macromolecules is impaired, predisposing the edematous extremities to soft tissue infections. Obstructive lymphangitis further destroys the lymphatic system and results in progression of the disease.

Lymphedema can be classified according to its etiology (primary or secondary), genetics (familial or sporadic) and time of onset of edema (congenital, praecox, tarda). Primary lymphedema is presumed to be a developmental abnormality and may be present at birth (congenital), may manifest during the second or third decade of life (praecox), or may develop after age 35 years (tarda). Secondary lymphedema is an acquired disorder, resulting from a known underlying disease process such as infection, trauma, radiation injury, tumor, or lymphoproliferative disease. Although the latter classifications are useful in delineating cause, the treatment strategies are not based on these distinctions. Instead, the stage or the nature of the anatomic abnormality is important in planning effective therapy.

Clinical Findings

A. Signs and Symptoms: A careful history and physical examination frequently reveal the cause of a swollen extremity and suggest the diagnosis of lymphedema. The most common form of primary lymphedema (80%), lymphedema praecox, occurs more frequently in females, usually in the second or third decades. The onset of swelling often coincides with puberty or pregnancy. The natural history is one of slowly progressive swelling of the ankle and lower legs with proximal involvement during the more recent months. A family history of chronic leg swelling may indicate familial lymphedema. Secondary lymphedema is more common than the primary form and can develop after regional node dissection, radiation treatment, infection, trauma, or malignant obstruction of lymph vessels or nodes. Filariasis is the most com-

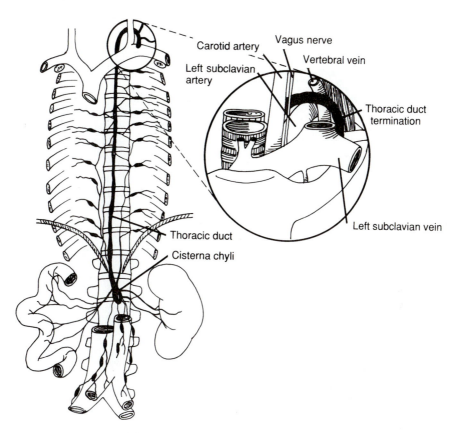

Figure 34–2. Anatomy of the mesenteric and thoracic lymphatic system. (Reproduced, with permission, from Gloviczki P: Lymphatic reconstructions. In: *Vascular Surgery,* 4th ed. Rutherford RB [editor]. WB Saunders, in press.)

mon cause of secondary lymphedema in Third World countries. In the USA, malignancy and the surgical or radiologic treatment for malignant diseases account for most cases.

The edema from lymphatic dysfunction may be partially pitting during the earlier stages when the compensatory mechanisms have not been depleted. During the later stages, the edema becomes nonpitting and intractable and does not regress completely, even with prolonged elevation. The distribution of the edema is diagnostic of a lymphatic cause (Fig 34–4). Edema usually starts distally in the perimalleolar area with obliteration of the contours of the ankle in advanced cases. The dorsum of the forefoot above the metatarsal head is usually involved, creating the typical "buffalo hump" deformity. In the early stages, pinkish discoloration with a mildly elevated temperature caused by increased vascularity may be seen. In the later stages, the skin is usually thick and shows areas of hyperkeratosis and lichenification. The leather-like skin with *peau d'orange* appearance is a reflection of longstanding disease, and squaring of the toes reflects the high protein content of the edema (Stemmer's sign).

Although eczematous dermatitis may occur, ulceration of the skin is rare. Yellow discoloration or club-

bing of the nails secondary to impaired lymphatic drainage of the nailbed may also be seen. Secondary fungal infections of the skin are common, and small vesicles filled with lymph may be present. Although a feeling of heaviness is common, pain is an unusual complaint in a patient with lymphedema. If pain does occur, another diagnosis such as venous disease or infection should be considered. During the initial evaluation, sequential limb girth measurements should be obtained, and venous pathology should be ruled out with noninvasive evaluations.

B. Imaging Studies:

1. Lymphoscintigraphy–Lymphoscintigraphy is now the diagnostic test of choice in evaluating lymphedema. The technique is noninvasive and generally comfortable for the patient. The study involves interstitial injections of small amounts of a radiolabeled antimony trisulfide (technetium-99m [^{99m}Tc]-labeled Sb_2S_3) or human serum albumin (HSA) colloid into the interdigital space and subsequent imaging of the extremity with a dual-headed gamma counter. The resulting anatomic distribution of the radiolabeled colloid is then assessed for evidence of lymphatic dysfunction or obstruction. The study is performed with the patient in the supine position. A foot dynamometer is used in the lower extremity and a

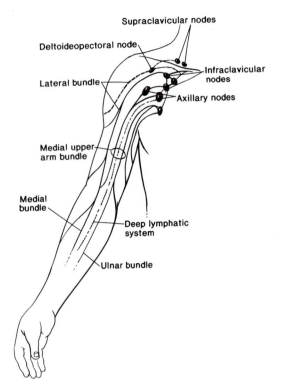

Figure 34–3. Anatomy of the upper extremity lymphatic system. (Reproduced, with permission, from Gloviczki P: Microsurgical treatment for chronic lymphedema: An unfulfilled promise? In: *Venous Disorders*. Bergan JJ, Yao JST [editors]. WB Saunders, 1990.)

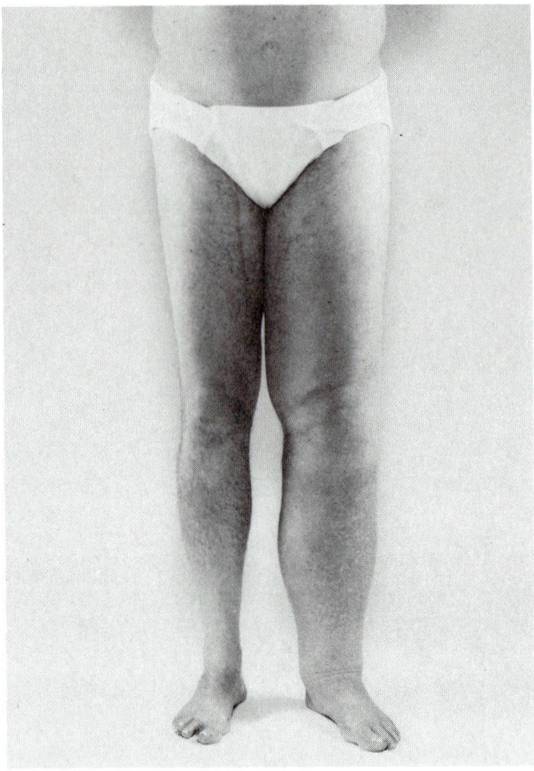

Figure 34–4. Patient with chronic secondary lymphedema of the left lower extremity.

squeezable rubber ball in the upper extremity to initiate exercise during the test. The ^{99m}Tc-labeled colloid (350–450 µCi) is injected into the web space between the second and third toes (or fingers) bilaterally with a tuberculin syringe and a 27-gauge needle. The injection may be associated with a transient (5–10 seconds) burning sensation in some of the patients. The number of injected particles with this dose may range from 10^9 to 10^{13}. This radiopharmaceutical is regulated as an investigational drug in the USA by the Food and Drug Administration.

After the injection, patients are exercised for 1 minute every 5 minutes during the first hour. The measured exercise is crucial in obtaining reproducible images in the groins. A large-field gamma camera is positioned to include the groin region and the extremity, and a total of 12 images is obtained in 1 hour. At the end of the first hour and after 3 hours, 20-minute images of the whole body are obtained. The patient is encouraged to ambulate between takes of the total body images. Direct injection into the deep lymphatic system (posterior to the lateral malleolus) does not offer improved images of the deep system. Upper extremity studies can be obtained in a similar fashion, using a squeezable plastic ball for exercise.

The lymphoscintigram is reviewed for evidence of proper injection, the time of visualization of the regional lymph nodes, distribution pattern of the tracer, transport kinetics, and appearance of lymph vessels and nodes. The activity of regional nodes should maximize between 15 and 60 minutes. Any delay in activity of longer than 60 minutes suggests dysfunction of the lymphatic transport system. The data are collected and graded from 0 to 45 (higher numbers represent more abnormal results) and entered into a standardized report format (Table 34–1). This semiquantitative transport index (TI) is used to document the severity of the edema.

Patients with edema due to chronic venous insufficiency have normal or enhanced lymph transport. A normal lymphoscintigram, however, may not always have predictable uptake of the tracer by the regional lymph nodes. Therefore, evidence of asymmetry of the patterns of lymphatic drainage is an important criterion for evaluation. Following injection of the tracer, the activity normally ascends the anteromedial aspect of the leg into the thigh (Fig 34–5). Usually, multiple channels can be identified in the calf, but in the thigh, because the lymph vessels run close together, differentiation may be difficult. After 60 minutes, activity

Table 34–1. Lymphoscintigraphy in lymphedema.

Components*	Score†			
	0	3	5	9
Transport kinetics	no delay	mild delay	extreme delay	no flow
Distribution pattern	normal	partial dermal	diffuse dermal	no flow
Time index	Time in minutes for appearance of regional lymph nodes, multiplied by 0.04			
Lymph nodes	normal	visible, diminished	barely visible	not seen
Lymph vessels	normal	visible, diminished	barely visible	not seen

* Components of lymphatic transport index (TI).
† Normal score < 5.

should be localized to the regional nodes with faint hepatic, gallbladder, and para-aortic node uptake.

A lymphoscintigram is considered abnormal with evidence of any one of the following: (1) delayed or absent clearance of the tracer from the injection site, (2) dermal backflow (cutaneous pattern) or collaterals, (3) reduced, faint, or no uptake in the regional lymph nodes, and (4) abnormal tracer accumulation suggestive of extravasation, lymphocele, or lymphangiectasia (Figs 34–6 and 34–7). Primary lymphedema may be differentiated from the secondary type by demonstration of aplasia or hypoplasia of the ducts. However, because chronic secondary lymphedema can also result in such changes, clinical differentiation based on history and physical examination is more valuable than the subtle findings on lymphoscintigraphy.

Lymphoscintigraphy is a semiquantitative study. A clear, reproducible qualitative interpretation by an expert nuclear radiologist is essential. In our institution, the sensitivity of the qualitative interpretation is excellent (92%) with a specificity of close to 100% for the diagnosis of lymphedema. It remains the test of choice in differentiating lymphedema from edemas of other origin.

2. Computed tomography (CT)–CT is used to rule out any obstructing mass or tumor that may result in decrease of the transport capacity of the lymphatic system. Consistent with the presence of lymphedema is the finding of coarse, nonenhancing, tubular reticular structures in the subcutaneous tissue with a honeycombed appearance.

3. Magnetic resonance imaging (MRI)–MRI is also valuable for verifying the presence of obstructing masses in secondary lymphedema. It is particularly sensitive in identifying vascular malformations and soft tissue tumors. MRI can be used to differentiate lipedema and chronic venous edema from lymphedema. Typically, lipedema has increased amounts of subcutaneous fat without increased vascularity or signal changes consistent with excess fluid. The ratio of the superficial to the deep compartment is increased in lipedema compared with a normal ratio in venous edema and lymphedema. MRI can also delineate nodal and large lymphatic trunk anatomy proximal to the lymphatic obstruction, which cannot be visualized with lymphoscintigraphy.

4. Lymphangiography–When vital dye is injected into the subcutaneous tissue, it is rapidly collected by the subdermal or superficial dermal lymphatics. The dye is easily seen and is used to identify

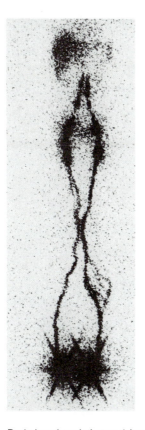

Figure 34–5. Body lymphoscintigram 1 hour after injection of tracer. The patient had bilateral lower extremity swelling but no evidence of abnormal lymphatic kinetics or anatomy. There are several collateral lymph channels at the left popliteal region. (Reproduced, with permission, from Cambria A et al: Noninvasive evaluation of the lymphatic system with lymphoscintigraphy: A prospective, semiquantitative analysis in 386 extremities. J Vasc Surg 1993;18:773.)

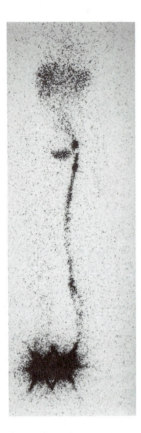

Figure 34–6. Body lymphoscintigram in a patient with right lower extremity swelling. Note absence of uptake in the right groin lymph nodes with no identifiable distal lymph channels.

tients who are candidates for microvascular lymphatic reconstruction. It is also useful in patients with lymphangiectasia, chylous reflux, chylous ascites, and chylothorax to image the anatomy of pelvic and abdominal lymph ducts and the thoracic duct. The complications of lymphangiography are rare and include allergic reaction to iodine, obstructive lymphangitis, pulmonary embolization due to the oily contrast (via spontaneous lymphovenous anastomoses), and pain during the procedure.

Differential Diagnosis

Systemic causes of extremity edema include cardiac, hepatic, renal, and endocrine dysfunction (Table 34–2). Underlying cardiac diseases such as congestive heart failure, chronic constrictive pericarditis, and severe tricuspid regurgitation are some of the most common cardiac causes. Liver or kidney failure, hypoproteinemia, Cushing's syndrome, and myxedema may also be associated with extremity swelling. The edema from these causes manifest as bilateral, soft, pitting edema, which improves with medical control of the systemic pathology. However, the most com-

larger lymphatic vessels, which are then cannulated to obtain direct contrast lymphangiograms. The technique is usually performed with the patient under local anesthesia (1% lidocaine). After 1 ml of isosulfan blue dye (Lymphazurine) has been injected subcutaneously into the first and second interdigital spaces, a small transverse incision is made in the dorsum of the forefoot. The lymphatic vessels are then dissected and cannulated under direct vision with a 30-gauge intracatheter. Then, a constant infusion of lipid-soluble contrast medium (usually ethiodized oil) is started at 1 mL over 8 minutes (maximum dose 7 mL for each limb). If the infusion is done too quickly, the dye will extravasate through the vessel wall or the vessel may rupture, making interpretation difficult. The limb is then imaged radiographically during the course of the injection and serially thereafter. In patients with severe lymphatic obstruction, the contrast may remain in the lymph nodes for several weeks to months after the initial injection.

Direct-contrast lymphangiography is now rarely used for diagnosis of lymphedema. It can be used to define detailed anatomy of the lymph vessels in pa-

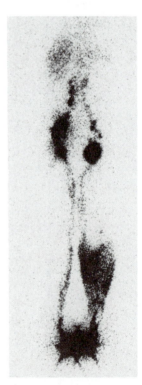

Figure 34–7. Body lymphoscintigram in a patient with Hodgkin's disease. A lymphocele is noted in the left groin at the site of a previous lymph node biopsy. There is a dermal pattern in the left calf. (Reproduced, with permission, from Cambria RA et al: Noninvasive evaluation of the lymphatic system with lymphoscintigraphy: A prospective, semiquantitative analysis in 386 extremities. J Vasc Surg 1993;18:773.)

Table 34–2. Differential diagnosis of chronic leg swelling.

Systemic Causes	Local or Regional Causes
Cardiac failure	Chronic venous insufficiency
Hepatic failure	
Renal failure	Lymphedema
Hypoproteinemia	Lipedema
Hyperthyroidism (myxedema)	Congenital vascular malformation
Allergic disorders	
Idiopathic cyclic edema	Arteriovenous fistula
Hereditary angioedema	Trauma
Drugs	Snake or insect bite
Antihypertensives	Infection, inflammation
Methyldopa	Hematoma
Nifedipine	Dependency
Hydralazine	Rheumatoid arthritis
Hormones	Postrevascularization edema
Estrogen	
Progesterone	Soft tissue tumor
Anti-inflammatory drugs	Hemihypertrophy
Phenylbutazone	
Monoamine oxidase inhibitors	

mon cause of unilateral extremity swelling is venous disease.

Chronic venous insufficiency is the most difficult to differentiate from lymphedema. A history of deep venous thrombosis or stasis ulcers at the ankle level supports venous insufficiency. Venous edema from venous hypertension also tends to be painful and pitting, and is associated with dermatitis and superficial varicosities. Noninvasive venous studies such as impedance plethysmography and duplex ultrasonography may further help to differentiate the 2 disease processes.

Congenital vascular malformations of the extremities may also be difficult to differentiate from lymphedema. Klippel-Trénaunay syndrome can mimic lymphedema. Characteristic changes of this syndrome are port-wine stains, increase in the length of the affected extremity, atypical lateral varicosities, and abnormality of the deep venous system. In patients with large-shunt arteriovenous fistulas (Parkes Weber syndrome), a bruit or thrill is present with a pulsatile, dilated superficial venous system. Other conditions producing symptoms of unexplained limb swelling are lipedema, trauma-induced reflex sympathetic dystrophy, obesity, hematoma, Baker's cyst, and osteoarthritis.

Nonoperative Treatment

Most patients with chronic lymphedema can be managed with conservative, nonoperative treatment. The goals of treatment are to decrease the volume of the extremity, to limit the progression of the disease, and to prevent repeated episodes of lymphangitis and cellulitis. Before initiating treatment, every attempt should be made to define the cause of the edema. Chronic venous insufficiency and systemic causes should always be ruled out.

A. Preventive Treatment: Lymphedema is generally easier to treat in the earlier stages before irre-

versible fibrosis of the lymphatic vessels occurs. Secondary lymphedema can be prevented in certain situations when the proper treatment is started early or when preventive measures are instituted. In filarial infections, prompt therapy with antiparasitic agents (diethylcarbonate or ivermectin) appears to limit the extent of lymphatic damage. Lymph node dissections for treatment of malignancies should be limited in patients in whom survival or tumor recurrence does not depend on the extent of the dissection. Judicious use of adjuvant radiation therapy is also important. Secondary infections should be aggressively treated and measures to prevent new infection such as meticulous hygiene, topical fungal infection control, and the use of protective clothing to prevent trauma to the skin should be initiated early. In patients with recurrent infections, daily antibiotic prophylaxis may be necessary.

B. Medical Treatment: The use of diuretics for fluid reduction is controversial. The effect is usually temporary, and secondary hemoconcentration is a serious side effect. Diuretics may be used judiciously in patients with symptomatic acute lymphedema after the diagnosis is confirmed. Short-term treatment may also be useful for alleviation of symptoms in patients in the terminal phase of a malignant disease or in those whose lymphedema is related to their menstrual cycle. Dietary sodium restriction should also be part of the initial treatment regimen.

Direct treatment with pharmacologic agents has only a limited role in the treatment of chronic lymphedema. However, benzopyrones have been shown to reduce lymphedema by increasing proteolysis by tissue macrophages. They enhance an alternate pathway for the removal of excess protein from the interstitial space. Theoretically, if the intercellular protein concentration is reduced, the retained lymphatic fluid will also diminish. A recent prospective, randomized trial in Australia showed that this treatment with 5,6-benzo-α-pyrone was efficacious, but slow in reducing edema fluid in patients with chronic lymphedema.

C. Mechanical Reduction: Reducing the size of the extremity is the mainstay of nonoperative therapy for lymphedema. Occasionally, maintaining the reduction at the extremity's pre-edema size is possible if proper treatment is instituted early. In patients with chronic lymphedema in whom fibrosis has developed, the brawny tissues typically do not become normal following reduction techniques.

Elevation of the extremity to 45 degrees is a simple and effective method of reducing lymphedema. The limitation to this therapy is the bedrest required for effective treatment. Although hospitalized patients do well with this approach, outpatient therapy is limited by patient compliance.

Simple, regularly scheduled massage of the affected limb (manual lymphatic drainage [MLD]) can enhance lymphatic drainage and keep the tissues soft and decompressed. This technique originates from Germany, but is gaining slow acceptance in the USA. Massage is performed sequentially in 4 quadrants (upper, lower, right, left). The contralateral compartment is massaged. This massage of the more normal regions helps to drain cutaneous lymph fluid from the massaged area, allowing it to receive fluid from the adjacent involved area. The process is repeated in stages along the length of the limb in a proximal to distal direction, but massaging each segment in a distal to proximal fashion. These sessions should be performed 2–3 times per week. The patient is fitted with an elastic stocking between and after the sessions.

External compression with custom-fitted, heavy-duty elastic stockings should be an integral part of any treatment plan. Limbs affected with lymphedema generally require at least 40–50-mmHg rated stockings. The length of the stockings should be sufficient to cover all of the edematous portions of the limb. If compression of the thigh is required, the stocking should be supported by a leotard-type waist extension. These stockings should be worn at all times when the patient is not supine and should ideally be fitted after a period of immobilization with leg elevation.

Sequential air compression devices may be used to aid in "milking" the edema fluid out from the extremity. The affected limb is placed in a pneumatic boot with several compartment that are intermittently inflated. The created pressure gradient forces lymph fluid out of the involved limb and into the trunk where the lymphatic system functions normally. An average cuff pressure of 90–100 mmHg and a ratio of 1:3 for compression and decompression are used. Typically, patients are hospitalized 2–3 days with daily 6–8-hour treatments. A reduction of limb size of about 20% can be expected during a 3–6-month treatment period. Outpatient therapy with comparable devices (Lymphapress) have also been successful in achieving similar reductions. The most important predictor of poor outcome in lymphedema patients is the degree of subcutaneous fibrosis. In one series, 80% of patients with poor response to the treatment had lymphedema for more than 10 years. These devices are contraindicated in the presence of active infection, deep venous thrombosis, or congestive heart failure.

Surgical Treatment

Only 5–10% of all patients with lymphedema ultimately require surgical treatment. The indications for surgical intervention are (1) impaired function and movement of the involved extremity because of its size and weight, (2) recurrent episodes of cellulitis and lymphangitis, (3) intractable pain, (4) lymphangiosarcoma, and (5) cosmesis. Operations for lymphedema are divided into 2 major groups: excisional procedures and lymphatic reconstruction.

A. Excisional Operations: Excisional procedures remove a portion of lymphedematous subcutaneous tissue, with varying portions of the skin. The following operations can be performed.

1. Charles' procedure–Total skin and subcutaneous tissue excision of the lower extremity from the tibial tuberosity to the malleoli is the most radical of the excisional operations. The deep fascia is also removed if there is extensive fibrosis. The proximal and distal aspects of the excision are tapered to prevent a step deformity. The wound is then covered with a split-thickness or full-thickness skin graft, usually from an uninvolved donor site. These grafts are difficult to manage with frequent localized sloughing (especially in areas of recurrent cellulitis), excessive scarring, hyperkeratosis, and dermatitis. The Charles' procedure is reserved for the few patients who are not candidates for reconstruction or flap procedures. The long-term results are fair.

2. Modified Homans' procedure–The modified Homans' procedure involves localized excision of the fibrosed subcutaneous tissue with preservation of the overlying skin. A proximal pneumatic tourniquet is used for hemostatic control during the procedure. A medial incision extending longitudinally 1 cm posterior to the tibial border is used to excise the affected subcutaneous tissue. Moderately thick flaps (1–1.5 cm) are elevated anteriorly and posteriorly to the mid-sagittal plane in the calf. The redundant skin is excised and the wound carefully closed to allow uninterrupted apposition of the flaps to the underlying fascia. No subcutaneous or dermal sutures are used. Suction catheters are then placed after hemostasis and tourniquet deflation. The results are directly related to the amount of subcutaneous tissue excised. The patients are susceptible to recurrences and should be maintained on a salt-restricted diet and elastic compression stockings. The results of this procedure in Miller's experience are promising with 65–80% obtaining significant reduction in the size of the affected extremity and a noticeable improvement in their level of function.

3. Thompson's procedure–The transfer of normal lymphatic tissue to a diseased segment is the primary goal of this subcutaneous flap procedure. The Thompson procedure also involves resecting a portion of the diseased tissue, creating a longitudinal "dermis-flap." After the subcutaneous excision, a flap edge is then deepithelialized and buried (sutured) in the deep muscular compartment. In theory, the buried dermis flap enhances the formation of new lymphatic connections between the subdermal lymphatic plexus of the flap and the deep lymphatic channels. However, new channels of lymphatic drainage could not be demonstrated in patients who have undergone this procedure. Therefore, the benefit is believed to be the result of subcutaneous edematous tissue excision, rather than the dermal flaps. Consequently, Thompson's procedure does not offer any better functional outcome than the previously described Homans' operation.

B. Lymphatic Reconstructions: Improvement in the flow of the lymphatic transport system is ideally the most direct and physiologic method of treating lymphatic obstruction. Efforts to increase lymph transport by implanting a piece of omentum or a segment of ileum (mesenteric bridge operations) to the affected areas to promote the formation of new lymphatic communications have had only marginal success. Recent developments in microvascular techniques have allowed direct reconstructions of the lymphatic channels. However, physiologic lymphatic reconstructions are indicated in only a small subset of patients who have obstruction at the root of the involved extremity, with preserved lymphatics distally. Unfortunately, patients with primary lymphedema usually have diffuse disease and are poor candidates for reconstruction.

1. Lymphovenous anastomoses–Direct lymphovenous anastomoses have had varying degrees of success. The rationale for the operation is based on the observation that in patients with chronic lymphedema, spontaneous lymphovenous anastomosis can occasionally be demonstrated by lymphangiography. These communications between the lymphatic and venous systems are considered natural compensatory mechanisms for lymphatic hypertension that occurs early in the course of the disease. Thus, direct reconstructions on the lymphatic system must be initiated before the development of subcutaneous fibrosis and lymphatic vessel sclerosis. Microvascular surgical techniques have enabled surgeons to anastomose blood vessels less than 2 mm in diameter with excellent patency.

The indications for lymphovenous anastomoses are limited. Patients must have had recent-onset secondary lymphedema without previous episodes of cellulitis or lymphangitis. They must also have first undergone a trial of conservative, nonoperative treatment. Venous hypertension is also a contraindication to this type of reconstruction because of its reliance on forward flow through the anastomoses. Preoperative evaluation should include lymphoscintigraphy and, in selected patients, direct-contrast lymphangiography. An ideal candidate is a patient with a proximal pelvic lymphatic obstruction with dilated infrainguinal lymph vessels. CT is obtained to rule out any underlying mass or malignancy.

If the patient meets all of the latter criteria, he or she is hospitalized 24–48 hours before surgery for preoperative extremity lymph reduction using elevation and intermittent compression methods. With the patient with leg edema under general anesthesia, a transverse incision at the midthigh level or a longitudinal incision in the groin is made. Lymph vessels of the superficial medial lymphatic bundle are dissected under an operating microscope with 5–40 × magnification. An attempt is made to visualize the lymph vessels with isosulfan blue dye, which is injected subcutaneously distal to the incision. The lymphatic vessels appear as whitish, fluid-filled channels, which can sometimes be difficult to differentiate from fibrous bands and small nerves. If contrast lymphangiography was performed within 24 hours of the operation, the contrast-filled lymphatics can be identified using an image intensifier

and a C arm. After the lymphatic vessels and the veins are identified, a standard microsurgical anastomosis is performed using 6–8 interrupted 11-0 monofilament, nonabsorbable sutures (Fig 34–8). An average of 2–4 anastomoses per patient is constructed (Fig 34–9). The postoperative limb is wrapped with elastic bandage and elevated 30 degrees using pillows. Measurement of limb circumference and volume in conjunction with lymphoscintigraphy is used to assess results.

Experimental anastomoses using normal femoral lymph vessels and a tributary of the femoral vein in dogs yielded a patency rate of 50% at 3–8 months after surgery by cinelymphangiography. The results in humans were more difficult to document. For example, in 14 patients who underwent lymphovenous anastomoses, only 5 limbs maintained the initial improvement 46 months after surgery. This improvement occurred in 4 of 7 patients with secondary lymphedema and in only 1 of 7 patients with primary lymphedema. Indirect evidence of patency (lymphoscintigraphy) and clinical findings were used to assess outcome. Postoperative lymphangiography has been avoided because of the risk of further progression of the disease along the major lymphatic channels secondary to chemical lymphangitis. In a series of 90 patients with lymphovenous anastomoses, 73% had subjective improvement and 42% experienced long-term improvement. This technique can be considered in a select group of patients with secondary lymphedema. However, direct confirmation of its long-term patency is unavailable.

2. Lymphatic grafting–The concept of lympholymphatic grafting is attractive, since some of the problems inherent in lymphovenous anastomoses (such as venous hypertension causing reversal of flow into the lymphatic circuit) can be avoided. Also, since no platelets and only low levels of procoagulant factors are in the lymph fluid, patency should be better than anastomoses with a blood-filled system. Preoperative evaluation should be conducted in a fashion similar to that for lymphovenous reconstructions. This technique is used primarily for unilateral secondary lymphedema such as postmastectomy lymphedema and proximal lower extremity obstruction. It is important to document normal lymphatics in the donor leg with lymphoscintigraphy before considering surgery.

In postmastectomy lymphedema, autotransplantation of a major lymphatic bundle from the medial aspect of the thigh to the arm can be performed. The distal anastomosis is performed on the proximal arm with epifascial and subfascial lymph vessels in an end-to-end fashion. The proximal anastomosis is best performed in the neck to one of the larger descending lymphatic vessels of the thoracic duct (Fig 34–10). The procedure for lower extremity reconstruction is a transposition of a normal lymphatic trunk in the thigh to the diseased limb with a lympholymphatic anastomosis in the groin (cross-femoral grafting). A longitudinal thigh incision is used to harvest 2–3 lymphatic

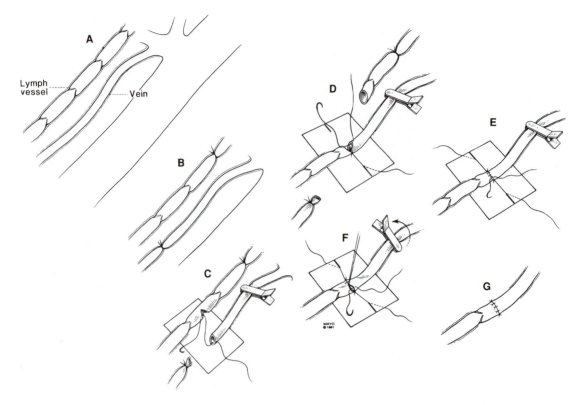

Figure 34–8. The technique of microsurgical end-to-end lymphovenous anastomosis. (Reproduced, with permission, from Gloviczki P et al: The natural history of microsurgical lymphovenous anastomoses: An experimental study. J Vasc Surg 1986;4:148.)

vessels. They are transected distally after ligation and tunneled subcutaneously above the pubis to the contralateral side. An end-to-end anastomosis is performed under an operating microscope using 11-0 interrupted absorbable sutures (Fig 34–11). In a report of Baumeister and Siuda (1990) on 55 patients undergoing such procedures, 80% of the patients were noted to have improvement (volume reduction) after a mean follow-up of 3 years. Long-term patency rate of the lymphatic grafts is unknown.

Complications

A. Infection: Lymphatic dysfunction can predispose the limb to cellulitis and lymphangitis. The infections occur because of decreased clearance of infectious agents and foreign bodies from the subcutaneous space. In addition, accumulation of the protein-rich lymph fluid within a confined space allows unimpeded proliferation of bacteria. Obstructive lymphangitis may also complicate and further aggravate lymphedema. Most frequently caused by β-hemolytic streptococci or staphylococci, lymphangitis can ascend quickly to the more proximal regions causing damage to larger lymphatic vessels and result in systemic sepsis secondary to proliferation within the venous system.

B. Lymphangiosarcoma: Longstanding lymphatic stasis, chronic inflammation, and a locally depressed immune state predispose the lymphatic circulation in the affected limb to malignant degeneration. Lymphangiosarcoma arising from chronic lymphedema is rare. Persistent nonhealing bruises or purple-red nodules should be evaluated to rule out associated malignancy. If a sarcoma does develop, it is usually extremely aggressive, and early amputation of the affected limb should be considered. The chances for long-term survival of these patients are poor.

Prognosis

Chronic untreated lymphedema may progress to irreversible, diffuse, subcutaneous fibrosis with a steady increase in the size and weight of the involved limb. In some patients, an elephantiasis-type extremity may result in huge lower legs or arms requiring special clothing. Fortunately, most patients with lymphedema improve with conservative therapy. However, most patients never regain their normal appearance despite optimal medical and surgical treatment. Only 5–10% of all patients require surgical treatment. The clinical course of secondary lymphedema is more favorable when early treatment is initiated.

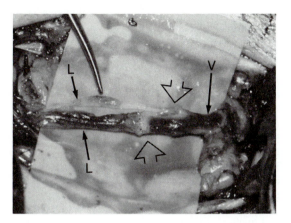

Figure 34–9. Two lymphovenous anastomoses (*arrows*) after microsurgical reconstruction. V, vein; L, lymphatic vessel. (Reproduced, with permission, from Gloviczki P: Treatment of acquired lymphedema: Medical and surgical. In: *Current Therapy in Vascular Surgery.* Ernst CB, Stanley JC [editors]. BC Decker, 1991.)

PRIMARY CHYLOUS DISORDERS

Essentials of Diagnosis

- Protein-rich, fatty lymph (chyle) accumulation in a body cavity.
- Chylous fluid with specific gravity greater than 1.012 g/dL, protein greater than 3 g/dL, and fat content 0.4–4 g/dL.
- Incompetent lymphatic valves.
- Dilatation of lymphatics (lymphangiectasia).
- Chylorrhea from lymph-filled vesicles in the lower extremity or perineum.

General Considerations

Chyle is a sterile, odorless, alkaline fluid that is milky in appearance. Its protein concentration is around 4 g/dL with a fat content of 0.4–4 g/dL.

The abnormal accumulation of lymph fluid or chyle in a compartment of the body outside the lymphatic system is the key feature of chylous disorders. **Primary chylous disorders** are usually caused by congenital lymphangiectasia or megalymphatics, with or without obstruction of the thoracic duct or a main lymphatic trunk. The spectrum of primary chylous disorders includes chylous reflux, chylous ascites, and chylothorax. In these patients, the lymphatic valves may be incompetent with resulting reflux of chyle into the lower extremities, perineum, or genitalia. This reflux of lymph fluid leads to accumulation of chyle in the distal compartments that are drained by the diseased lymphatic channel. Chylorrhea or oozing from vesicles in the skin of the limb, scrotum, or labia can cause extreme patient distress, not only physiologically but psychologically as well.

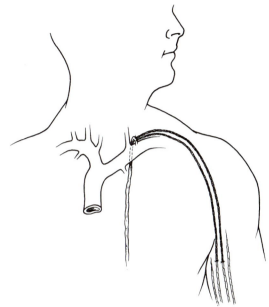

Figure 34–10. Lymph vessel transplantation for chronic postmastectomy upper extremity edema. The lower extremity lymph vessels are transplanted and anastomosed distally to the arm lymph ducts and proximally to the thoracic duct. (Reproduced, with permission, from Gloviczki P et al: Treatment of acquired lymphedema: Medical and surgical. In: *Current Therapy in Vascular Surgery. II,* Ernst CB, Stanley JC [editors]. BC Decker, 1991.)

Reflux into the kidney may cause chyluria whereas rupture or transudation of lymph into the abdominal or thoracic cavity can cause chyloperitoneum or chylothorax, respectively. Other areas that have been shown to accumulate chyle are the pericardium, lungs, and tracheobronchial tree. Rupture of lymphatic vessels into the lumen of the gut may result in a protein-losing enteropathy. **Secondary chylous disorders** are usually caused by trauma or malignancy. Lymphoma is the tumor most commonly associated with causing secondary obstruction of the lymphatic system, whereas iatrogenic operative trauma is the most common cause of chylous ascites and chylothorax.

Clinical Findings

The loss of chyle from the lymphatic system into body cavities such as the abdomen and thorax may result in severe metabolic and nutritional derangements. The continuing loss of fat and protein is responsible for chronic malnutrition in these patients. Hypocalcemia, hypocholesterolemia, lymphopenia, and anemia have also been reported. The immune function of patients with chylous disorders is often depressed, with a history of urinary and respiratory infections. In patients with chylous reflux into the lower extremities or genitalia, there is usually unilateral involvement

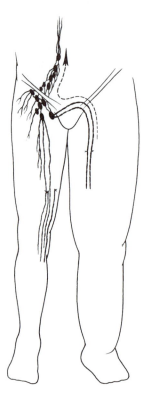

Figure 34–11. Lymph vessel transposition for chronic lower extremity secondary lymphedema. The normal right lymph vessels are transposed and anastomosed to the distal left lymphatic system. (Reproduced, with permission, from Gloviczki P: Treatment of acquired lymphedema: Medical and surgical. In: *Current Therapy in Vascular Surgery. II,* Ernst CB, Stanley JC [editors]. BC Decker, 1991.)

with ipsilateral cutaneous vesicles. Chylous ascites can almost always be detected by physical examination and diagnostic sampling of the ascitic fluid. Chylothorax may occur as a result of direct thoracic duct injury as discussed later, or secondary to chylous ascites. The diagnosis is confirmed by sampling the fluid in the chest.

The Sudan fat stain is diagnostic of fat content in the chylous fluid. Contrast lymphangiography is the test of choice in localizing the area of obstruction or trauma. In primary chylous ascites, a thorough search for malignancy with either CT or MRI should be carried out before therapeutic intervention.

Differential Diagnosis

Chylous vesicles from lymphatic valvular incompetency must be differentiated from primary infections and allergic reactions by aspiration and Gram staining. Chylous ascites and chylothorax should be sampled and analyzed for protein and lipid content as well as for cytology. Other causes of ascites or pleural effu-

sion such as congestive heart failure, malignancy, and infection should be ruled out.

Treatment

A. Medical: The goal of medical treatment for chylous disorders is to decrease the body's production of chyle. This can be best accomplished by diet restriction of cholesterol and fat. A medium-chain triglyceride oral diet or total parenteral nutrition should be used to control the production and influx of new chyle. Repletion of proteins and calcium lost in chyle is also important. In chylous ascites and chylothorax, drainage in the early stages may be therapeutic, but recurrence of the fluid accumulation is inevitable.

B. Surgical: Surgical intervention with excision and ligation of the diseased lymphatic vessel or thoracic duct is the treatment of choice in most patients with this disorder. Four hours before the operation, the patient is given a fatty meal to delineate the chylous leak or obstruction. Radical excision or ligation of the incompetent retroperitoneal lymph vessel is the most effective technique for controlling chylous reflux. A retroperitoneal approach through a flank incision is preferred. Ligation of the retroperitoneal lymph vessels should be done under direct vision, taking extreme care to avoid avulsing or tearing the delicate lymphatics. Lymphovenous anastomoses may be attempted if the ducts are dilated.

Intractable, recurring primary chylous ascites is an indication for exploration. The prognosis for these patients is good if a clearly definable area of rupture is identified preoperatively or during the exploration. The involved area is then oversewn or excised. However, if the mesenteric lymphatic trunks are fibrosed or hypoplastic with diffuse transudation of chyle, direct ligation cannot be performed and a peritoneal venous shunt (LeVeen) may be of benefit. In a patient with a persistent chylothorax, the leaking thoracic duct or the ruptured diaphragmatic or chest wall lymphatics should be identified and ligated, if possible. Mechanical pleurodesis is performed if ligation is unsuccessful. An anastomosis between the thoracic duct and the azygos vein may also be considered if the anatomy is favorable.

LYMPHATIC COMPLICATIONS OF VASCULAR SURGERY

General Considerations

Because of its close proximity to the arterial and venous systems, the lymphatic system is frequently injured during vascular procedures. The lymph vessels run parallel with arteries and veins, and some are inevitably transected during dissection. Lymph nodes adjacent to major arteries and veins may also be injured during the operation. Fortunately, the normal lymphatic system can regenerate and reestablish flow after minor trauma in most instances. However, injury to major lymphatic vessels during arterial reconstructions, such as postbypass edema, lymphocele (groin, retroperitoneum), or lymphatic fistula are not uncommon complications. Chylous ascites and chylothorax may also occur in some patients after operations in the abdomen and chest.

A. Postbypass Edema:

1. Clinical findings and diagnosis–Lower extremity edema can be a complication in 50–100% of patients following infrainguinal bypass procedures. The edema usually becomes evident after the patient begins ambulation. Physical examination is frequently diagnostic; the edema is typically nonpitting and painless. Duplex scanning should be used in patients with marked swelling to rule out deep venous thrombosis.

2. Treatment–After the diagnosis of postbypass lymphedema has been confirmed, the treatment of choice is nonoperative. Frequent elevation of the extremity and, selectively, compression stockings (30–40 mmHg at the ankle level) are suggested. Care must be taken not to compress below-knee vein grafts that are placed immediately under the skin. We avoid the use of stockings in patients following pedal bypasses because of the possibility of compression to the graft at the ankle. Medical treatment with diuretics, mannitol, or corticosteroids have not proved very useful in this setting.

B. Lymphatic Fistula:

1. Clinical findings and diagnosis–Persistent leakage of clear, yellowish fluid from a groin incision soon after the operation is diagnostic. If lymphocutaneous fistulas develop several months after surgery, infection of an implanted prosthetic graft should be suspected. The workup of these patients should include CT, white cell scan, or lymphoscintigraphy.

2. Treatment–Lymphatic fistulas should be managed initially with conservative treatment. Local wound care, systemic antibiotics, bedrest, and leg elevation should be started as soon as the diagnosis is made. If the output of the fistula does not decrease after several days of conservative treatment, operative repair of the traumatized lymphatic vessel is indicated. Injection of isosulfan blue dye into the subcutaneous tissue of the first and third interdigital spaces of the foot is often helpful in identifying the affected lymphatic channels in the operating room. The groin incision is reopened with meticulous sterile technique and the site of the lymphatic injury identified by observing the blue-stained lymphatic fluid leaking from the damaged vessel. The ends of the vessels are then oversewn, and the wound is closed in multiple layers to prevent further extravasation into a potential space.

C. Lymphocele:

1. Clinical findings and diagnosis–A lymphocele is a localized lymph collection with a pseudocapsule. A typical lymphocele is a soft, nontender swelling in the postbypass groin, with intermittent drainage of clear lymph fluid if there is an associated fistula. Large lymphoceles can cause localized discomfort, pain, and extremity edema (from compression effects on the remaining lymph vessels and the venous system). In contrast to seromas, lymphoceles by definition communicate with one or more lymphatic channels. Lymphoscintigraphy is the test of choice for demonstration of such connections (see Fig 34–7). The groin is the most common site of lymphocele formation. Ultrasonography is useful in differentiating lymphoceles from a hematoma or soft tissue infection. Retroperitoneal lymphoceles are rare; their reported incidence is less than 0.1% following aortic reconstruction. Patients may present with unexplained abdominal pain, nausea, or distention. CT is the diagnostic test of choice. If the lymphocele is noted many months or years after the operation, graft infection must be ruled out.

2. Treatment–Enlarging groin lymphoceles that recur after aspiration are treated surgically. The goal of surgery is to identify and ligate the connection with the lymph vessels and to resect the lymphocele. In patients with retroperitoneal lymphoceles, serial ultrasonography or CT is needed to assess the progression. If the lymphocele is increasing or causes local compression to adjacent structures, needle aspiration under radiographic guidance is performed for diagnostic and therapeutic reasons. After ruling out a graft infection with Gram's stains and cultures, the patient is observed for signs of recurrence. If the lymphocele recurs, operative repair should be considered. Again, isosulfan dye may be helpful in delineating connecting lymphatics and identifying the extent of the lymphocele. The lymphocele can be simply unroofed and the site of lymphatic leak oversewn. If a prosthetic graft is exposed, it should be covered by retroperitoneal tissue or a piece of omentum.

D. Chylous Ascites:

1. Clinical findings and diagnosis–Chylous ascites from injury to intra-abdominal and mesenteric lymphatic channels following aortic reconstruction is an uncommon but significant complication. Progressive abdominal pain, distention, and nausea are the most common symptoms. The workup of this postoperative complication is similar to that of primary chylous ascites and should include CT and paracentesis.

2. Treatment–Most patients with chylous ascites after abdominal vascular surgery can be managed nonoperatively with diet control and serial, therapeutic paracentesis. If the conservative treatment fails to control the ascites, operative intervention with direct ligation or oversewing of the injured lymphatic vessel is indicated.

E. Chylothorax:

1. Clinical findings and diagnosis–Injury to the lymphatic channels in the thoracic cavity during aortic reconstruction is rare. Chylothorax following other thoracic procedures such as esophageal resection is more common. It can also occur after translumbar aortography or after repair of congenital vascular anomalies, most frequent following surgery for aortic coarctation in children. The diagnostic test of choice is the chest radiograph. As with chylous ascites, sampling of the effusion fluid confirms the diagnosis.

2. Treatment–Initial treatment for chylothorax is tube thoracostomy with closed-suction drainage. If the chest tube and diet modification fail to control the chylous effusion or if severe metabolic complications occur from loss of essential electrolytes in the chyle, operation is indicated. Direct surgical closure of the thoracic duct may not be possible, especially when evidence of inflammation is in the region of the duct. Therefore, oversewing the thoracic duct at the level of the diaphragm is usually the safest and most effective method. In some patients, mechanical pleurodesis may be required to control the chylous effusion. Chemical pleurodesis is not effective for intractable chylothorax.

Preventive Measures

To prevent postbypass lymphedema, groin lymphoceles, and fistulas, meticulous care must be taken to preserve the lymphatics around the femoral sheath. The vertical groin incision should be placed lateral to the femoral artery, and the inguinal lymphatics should be retracted medially. The vascular sheath of the femoral and popliteal arteries should be opened through a vertical incision. Minimal dissection in the lymphoadipose tissue around the vessels should be performed. If the lymphatic vessels are severed, the ends should be ligated or cauterized to avoid a leak. It is recommended to leave a skin bridge between the groin incision and the incision in the thigh for dissection of the more distal saphenous vein. Short multiple skin incisions for dissection of the saphenous vein may result in less injury to the superficial lymphatics of the thigh.

The principles of lymphatic preservation should also be applied to intra-abdominal and thoracic dissections. In the abdomen, care must be taken not to injure the cisterna chyli, which is located in about 50% of patients at the level of the second lumbar vertebra between the inferior vena cava and the abdominal aorta. If the cisterna chyli or the thoracic duct are injured, lateral closure with 7-0 monofilament sutures should be attempted. Injured large lymphatic vessels in the lumbar, para-aortic, or mesenteric regions should always be ligated or clipped during the operation.

REFERENCES

AbuRahma AF, Woodruff BA, Lucente FC: Edema after femoropopliteal bypass surgery: Lymphatic and venous theories of causation. J Vasc Surg 1990;11:461.

Asby ER, Abdou S, Miller TA: Lymphedema and tumors of the lymphatics. In: *Vascular Surgery: A Comprehensive Review,* 4th ed. Moore WS (editor). WB Saunders, 1993.

Baumeister RG, Siuda S: Treatment of lymphedemas by microsurgical lymphatic grafting: What is proved? Plast Reconstr Surg 1990;85:64.

Browse NL: The diagnosis and management of primary lymphedema. J Vasc Surg 1986;3:181.

Cambria RC et al: Noninvasive evaluation of the lymphatic system with lymphoscintigraphy: A prospective, semiquantitative analysis in 386 extremities. J Vasc Surg 1993;18:773.

Casley-Smith JR, Morgan RG, Piller NB: Treatment of lymphedema of the arms and legs with 5,6-benzo-alpha-pyrone. N Engl J Med 1993;329:1158.

Földi E, Földi M, Clodius L: The lymphedema chaos: A lancet. Ann Plast Surg 1989;22:505.

Garrett HE Jr et al: Retroperitoneal lymphocele after abdominal aortic surgery. J Vasc Surg 1989;10:245.

Gloviczki P: Microsurgical treatment for chronic lymphedema: An unfulfilled promise? In: *Venous Disorders.* Bergan JJ, Yao JST (editors). WB Saunders, 1991.

Gloviczki P: Section 18: Management of lymphatic disorders. In: *Rutherford's Vascular Surgery,* 4th ed. Rutherford RB (editor). WB Saunders (in press).

Gloviczki P: Treatment of secondary lymphedema: Medical and surgical. In: *Current Therapy in Vascular Surgery. II.* Ernst CB, Stanley JC (editors). BC Decker, 1991.

Gloviczki P, Bergman RT: Lymphatic problems and revascularization edema. In: *Complications in Vascular Surgery,* 2nd ed. Bernhard VM, Towne JB (editors). Quality Medical Publishing, 1991.

Gloviczki P et al: Microsurgical lymphovenous anastomosis for treatment of lymphedema: A critical review. J Vasc Surg 1988;7:647.

Gloviczki P et al: The natural history of microsurgical lymphovenous anastomoses: An experimental study. J Vasc Surg 1986;4:148.

Kalman PG, Walker PM, Johnston KW: Consequences of groin lymphatic fistulae after vascular reconstruction. J Vasc Surg 1991;25:210.

Kinmonth JB: *The Lymphatics: Surgery, Lymphography and Diseases of the Chyle and Lymph Systems,* 2nd ed. Edward Arnold Publishers, 1982.

Kleinhans E et al: Evaluation of transport kinetics in lymphoscintigraphy: Follow-up study in patients with transplanted lymphatic vessels. Eur J Nucl Med 1985;10:349.

O'Brien BMC et al: Long-term results after microlymphaticovenous anastomoses for the treatment of obstructive lymphedema. Plast Reconstr Surg 1990;85:562.

O'Donnell TF Jr: Management of primary lymphedema. In: *Current Therapy in Vascular Surgery. II.* Ernst CB, Stanley JC (editors). BC Decker, 1991.

Pappas CJ, O'Donnell TF Jr: Long-term results of compression treatment for lymphedema. J Vasc Surg 1992;16:555.

Persson NH, Takolander R, Bergqvist D: Edema after lower limb arterial reconstruction: Influence of background factors, surgical technique and potentially prophylactic methods. VASA 1991;20:57.

Servelle M: Surgical treatment of lymphedema: A report on 652 cases. Surgery 1987;101:483.

Weissleder R, Thrall JH: The lymphatic system: Diagnostic imaging studies. Radiology 1989;172:315.

Weissleder H, Weissleder R: Lymphedema: Evaluation of qualitative and quantitative lymphoscintigraphy in 238 patients. Radiology 1988;167:729.

Vascular Trauma

35

Douglas B. Hood, MD, Albert E. Yellin, MD, FACS, & Fred A. Weaver, MD

General Considerations

Trauma has become a critical public health problem in the USA, and vascular trauma is an important component of this problem. In 1986, an estimated 450,000 vascular injuries occurred in the USA, of which roughly 41,000 were fatal. The direct cost of treating these injuries amounted to $1.1 billion. Because vascular injuries tend to occur in young males, the indirect cost, including lost productivity and wages resulting from death and disability, was $13.4 billion. The total cost of $14.5 billion represents 0.37% of the United States Gross National Product.

A. Incidence: The incidence of vascular trauma is increasing. A 30-year review of the incidence of vascular trauma in Houston from 1958 to 1988 revealed an average number of 27 patients per year with vascular injury during the initial years, which grew to 213 patients per year during the final year of the review. This increase exceeded the population growth during the same time period. The authors attribute the increase in vascular trauma to an increase in violent crimes, increased use of guns, and faster ambulance transport times, which enables more of these injured patients to arrive at the hospital alive. These trends are evident in all major urban areas.

B. Causes: Approximately 90% of arterial injuries are due to penetrating trauma. Much of our knowledge regarding the management of penetrating injuries comes from experience gained during the major armed conflicts of the 20th century. However, there are important differences between vascular injuries caused by military weapons and those seen in the civilian setting. Military injuries are typically caused by weapons that produce very high muzzle velocity (>2500 ft/sec). The energy of a projectile is proportional to the square of its velocity ($E = 1/2mv^2$), and as the energy of these high-velocity missiles is transferred to the body, massive tissue destruction occurs. In addition to injury produced directly from the bullet, injury is produced remote from the bullet tract from concussive forces and from secondary missiles such as fragments of bone and bullet casing. Also, a temporary cavity is created as a result of the radial forces of the bullet; this produces a suction effect, drawing dirt and clothing into the wound.

In contrast, civilian wounds are generally caused by lower-velocity weapons, which produce less destruction of the surrounding tissues. Typical low-velocity weapons are knives, ice picks, other handheld instruments, and handguns. The injury from these weapons is generally confined to the missile tract itself. Recently, however, an increase in the use of military weapons (eg, AK-47s) has occurred in the civilian population, and more extensive wounds are being seen. Shotguns also cause extensive wounds when fired at close range because of the distribution pattern of the multiple pellets and embedded wadding.

Blunt trauma accounts for the remaining 10% of vascular injuries. Blunt vascular injuries tend to occur in areas where there are strong attachments of vessels to adjacent bone, tendon, and soft tissue. An injury such as a bony fracture or dislocation produces traction on nearby vessels with subsequent intimal stretch and disruption, which may lead to dissection of the vessel wall, thrombosis, or both. In addition, fracture fragments may directly lacerate or transect adjacent vessels. A direct blow may also lead to intimal injury and thrombosis.

The surgeon who will be caring for trauma victims must understand not only the pathophysiology of vascular trauma, but also the evolving diagnostic modalities and current treatment protocols.

Classification of Arterial Injuries

Most of the attention in treating vascular trauma is directed at the management of arterial, rather than venous, injuries. This is because most major morbidity (tissue ischemia and resulting amputation) arises after arterial injuries, whereas major venous injuries may be undetected. Symptoms of chronic venous insufficiency that may result from long-term sequelae of venous injury do not arise for years, if at all. Just as several different mechanisms may produce arterial injury, several different types of arterial injury of varying severity occur.

A. Contusion: Contusion of the arterial wall with intramural hematoma formation may result from a direct blow or the concussive effect of a bullet. The hematoma may produce a mass effect, which can critically narrow or occlude the vessel lumen, or may weaken the wall of the artery and result in delayed pseudoaneurysm formation. Arteriographically, this injury is seen as a concentric or eccentric narrowing of the contrast column (Fig 35–1).

B. Intimal Disruption: Traction on the vessel after blunt injury, a direct blow from a blunt instru-

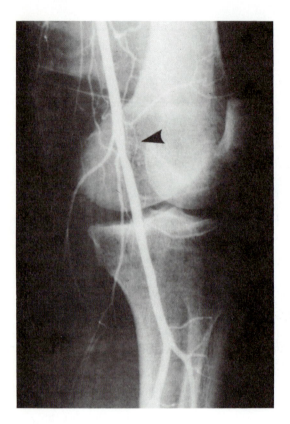

Figure 35–1. Intramural hematoma of the popliteal artery.

ment, or the concussive effect of a bullet may cause intimal disruption. Frequently, no overt clinical signs of trauma are found on inspection of the external surface of the artery. Arteriographically, intimal disruption is characterized by loss of the normal smooth contour of the vessel lumen or it appears as a linear defect (Fig 35–2).

C. Puncture: Arterial puncture injuries may result from ice picks, knives, shotgun pellets, or percutaneous vascular procedures. Many of these injuries heal uneventfully, but a few may persist and become expanding pseudoaneurysms. Puncture injuries are seen as an eccentric irregularity or outpouching of the contrast column on arteriography.

D. Lateral Disruption: A tangential injury in which the circumference of the vessel wall is only partially destroyed can result in a lateral disruption. The portion of the vessel wall that remains intact prevents retraction and thrombosis of the injured ends. This injury commonly presents with active bleeding or as a large pulsatile hematoma. When this type of injury results in a contained area of hemorrhage, it is called a *pseudoaneurysm.* Pseudoaneurysms may enlarge to several centimeters in size over time. Large pseudoaneurysms may produce pressure on adjacent structures, and there is a risk of rupture with continued expansion. The arteriographic appearances of lateral

disruption and pseudoaneurysm are similar. They are seen as an eccentric pooling of contrast medium (Figs 35–3 and 35–4).

E. Arteriovenous (AV) Fistulae: AV fistulae result as a direct effect of concomitant injuries to adjacent arteries and veins, or may develop in a delayed fashion when necrosis of adjacent injuries occurs. Early venous filling on arteriography is pathognomonic of an AV fistula (see Fig 35–4), but it is frequently not possible to definitively localize the precise orifice of the fistulous connection.

F. Transection: Arterial injury may result in complete disruption of the vessel wall. The transected ends usually retract, constrict, and thrombose. Thus, rather than presenting with hemorrhage, patients with these injuries typically present with signs of end-organ ischemia. The arteriographic appearance is of an occlusion, in which the actual site of injury cannot be seen, or of active extravasation of contrast if complete thrombosis has not occurred.

Principles of Treatment

A. Clinical Evaluation: The diagnosis of arterial injury is obvious in the patient who presents with exsanguinating external hemorrhage, an expanding or pulsatile hematoma, an absent pulse, or signs of ischemia. However, physical signs of most arterial injuries are more subtle, and the diagnosis less obvious. A high degree of suspicion and an active search for major arterial injuries are needed to prevent the delayed complications that are likely to occur if a major injury is missed. These complications include intimal dissection and thrombosis, distal embolization of thrombus that may form at the site of injury, continued expansion with delayed rupture of a pseudoaneurysm, and late development of ischemic symptoms such as claudication.

The patient who presents with signs of obvious ischemia or with massive bleeding, either externally or into one of the body cavities, should be taken directly to the operating room for exploration without delay. If arteriography is deemed necessary for an extremity injury, it can be done on the operating table prior to exploration. Active external bleeding is controlled by direct pressure during transport to the operating room. A member of the surgical team may need to continue to apply this pressure with a gloved hand while the operative field is prepared and draped around him. The use of tourniquets to control bleeding should be avoided because they occlude flow through collaterals which are important in preserving distal perfusion. The blind placement of clamps or other instruments into a bleeding wound should also be condemned, because this often results in irreparable injury to arteries, veins, nerves, or other vital structures. Embedded weapons should not be removed prior to arrival in the operating room because this may precipitate major bleeding. Similarly, probing the depths of a wound should be done only in an operating room.

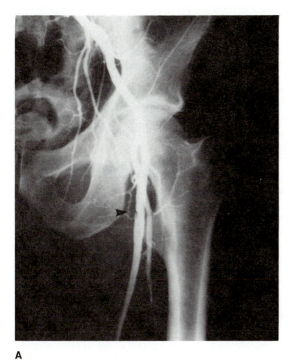

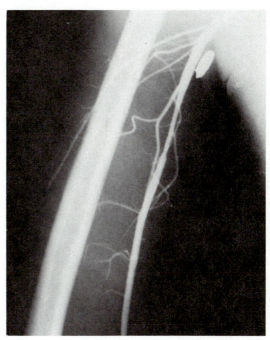

A

B

Figure 35–2. Arterial intimal disruption. **A:** Intimal flap. **B:** Diffuse intimal injury.

For the patient who has stable vital signs without signs of active bleeding or acute limb-threatening ischemia, time is available to more precisely define the anatomy of any potential vascular injury and to assess and prioritize associated injuries. For potential cervical, thoracic, and extremity vascular injuries, the evaluation generally includes diagnostic arteriography in the stable patient. Abdominal vascular injuries are accompanied by a high incidence of injury to other organs which invariably require operative intervention, and an extensive diagnostic workup is seldom necessary prior to celiotomy. Since the principles of diagnosis of vascular injuries vary according to the region injured, diagnostic algorithms for each of these regions are discussed under the corresponding heading later in the chapter. Some common, universal principles of treatment of arterial injuries, regardless of the specific location of injury, are presented here.

B. Nonsurgical Treatment: Not all arterial injuries need to be surgically repaired. Occlusive injuries to minor branch vessels may be safely observed, as may occlusive injuries of a single tibial or distal forearm vessel. In addition, a number of nonocclusive injuries heal without specific intervention. The healing power of these minimal, nonocclusive injuries has been likened to that of the puncture site for percutaneous vascular catheterization and to the extensive intimal disruption that occurs with balloon angioplasty. In the experience of many, the following injuries may be safely observed, provided that the wounding agent

is of low velocity, the distal circulation is intact, and no active hemorrhage is present: intimal defects, pseudoaneurysms of less than 5 mm diameter, and intimal flaps that are adherent or protrude downstream. If a nonoperative management strategy is adopted, the patient must be followed closely and should have healing or nonprogression of the injury documented by repeat duplex scanning or arteriography. The safety of

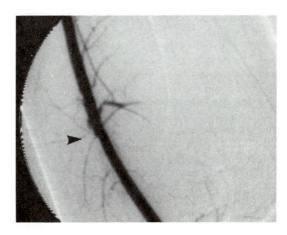

Figure 35–3. Small pseudoaneurysm (*arrow*). Note the presence of contrast outside of the normal confines of the arterial wall.

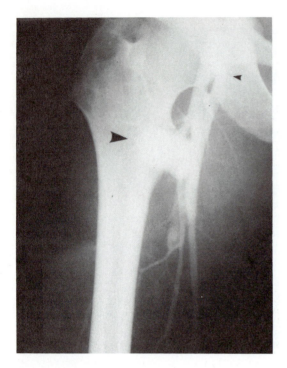

Figure 35–4. Large pseudoaneurysm of the superficial femoral artery (*large arrow*) with associated arteriovenous fistula to the superficial femoral vein (*small arrow*).

this approach has been documented in our published series of 61 such injuries (including injuries of the cerebral and extremity arteries) in which no complications occurred. Only 1 patient in this series subsequently required operation, which was done for a pseudoaneurysm that enlarged on serial arteriography. The concept of conservative or nonoperative treatment of minimal injuries is controversial and considered radical by some who advocate operative repair of all identified arterial injuries.

Some arterial injuries may be managed by transluminal embolization at the time of diagnostic arteriography. Appropriate injuries include low-flow AV fistulas, pseudoaneurysms, and even active bleeding from noncritical arteries. Noncritical arteries include the distal profunda femoris artery, branches of the hypogastric arteries, and muscular branches of major arteries. Arteriographic embolization may be preferable for injuries in locations that are difficult to expose surgically or for those in which exposure would produce a disfiguring scar, such as branches of the external carotid artery. Some arteries, such as the vertebral and some branches of the hypogastric, are actually hazardous to expose surgically because of their anatomic location and the potential for major hemorrhage or postoperative functional deficit. Injuries to these vessels are better treated by transluminal embolization, if at all possible. Embolization can also be of value in conjunction with operative repair. Even if an injury

cannot be completely occluded, flow across the lesion may be diminished, thus decreasing the risk and magnitude of hemorrhage at operation. Temporary, transluminal placement of an inflatable balloon catheter may also be of value to occlude a bleeding artery while the patient is prepared for surgical intervention.

C. Surgical Treatment: Once identified, all other arterial injuries should be repaired in the operating room. Several technical principles guide surgery for arterial trauma, regardless of the location of the specific injury. The patient should be volume resuscitated with crystalloid and blood, if necessary, before the operation. This is often best done in the operating room. Dissection and exposure of the area of injury may precipitate a prodigious amount of bleeding that will not be tolerated by the hypovolemic patient. Every effort to prevent hypothermia should be undertaken, including the use of warmed intravenous fluids, blood, and anesthetic gases, and placement of a heating blanket on the operating table. Broad-spectrum antibiotic coverage is begun as soon as possible, preferably prior to the start of the operation, to obtain therapeutic tissue levels at the time of incision.

The entire affected extremity or body cavity must be prepared, draped, and included in the operative field. This is particularly important for extremity injuries so that appropriate proximal vascular control can be achieved and the condition of the distal part can be constantly assessed. Also, an uninjured leg is included in the operative field for harvest of a segment of saphenous vein if a graft is needed. Depending on the site of injury and the expected size of the graft that may be needed, the saphenous vein can be harvested from the ankle or thigh. With lower extremity arterial injuries, the saphenous vein should be harvested from the contralateral uninjured extremity to preserve the superficial venous system of the injured extremity in case a concomitant ipsilateral deep venous injury is present. If both lower extremities are injured, a segment of cephalic vein harvested from an arm may serve as a graft.

On the extremities, incisions are placed longitudinally over the injured artery so that they may be extended proximally or distally if additional exposure is needed. For abdominal injuries, a vertical midline incision is usually sufficient to expose any injury that may be found, although a thoracic extension of the incision may be required for suprarenal aortic or caval injuries. Thoracic vascular injuries require median sternotomy or lateral thoracotomy, depending on the site of injury.

Vascular control should be obtained proximal and distal to the site of injury prior to its unroofing to prevent uncontrolled blood loss when the lesion is exposed. If proximal or distal control cannot be rapidly obtained in the face of ongoing hemorrhage, a finger or sponge stick can compress and tamponade the area of injury. Alternatively, a Foley or Fogarty catheter, depending on the vessel size, can be inserted through the injury into the lumen and the balloon inflated. These maneuvers arrest hemorrhage until more definitive exposure and control of the vessel are obtained. Collateral arteries should be preserved when possible to protect against distal ischemia or thrombosis during repair. However, some collaterals may have to be sacrificed for adequate exposure and mobilization of the vessel.

All injured arteries must be débrided to normal-appearing intima prior to repair. This is particularly true with high-velocity gunshot wounds, shotgun wounds, and blunt injuries in which the intima may be damaged for a considerable distance from the obvious site of injury. Balloon thrombectomy catheters should be carefully passed proximally and distally if there is any question of the presence of intraluminal thrombus remote from the site of injury. Distal thrombosis seen on preoperative arteriography may alternatively be treated with direct intra-arterial infusion of a thrombolytic agent such as urokinase. The risk of provoking distant bleeding after limited local infusion of a thrombolytic agent is very small. Anticoagulation with heparin is of value in limiting thrombus propagation during the time of repair. Heparin may be administered systemically or, if a contraindication exists such as a head or intra-abdominal injury, it may be administered directly into the injured vessel. Note that in the latter instance, collateral circulation gradually disperses the heparin, and it may need to be administered more than once.

Depending on the extent and location of injury, repair can be accomplished by lateral arteriorrhaphy, excision of the area of injury with end-to-end anastomosis or placement of an interposition graft, or bypass grafting. Primary repair is preferable, but may not be possible if excessive tension is placed on the anastomosis. If a graft is required, autogenous material is preferred for small-caliber (4–6 mm) arteries. Prosthetic grafts are used exclusively for aortic and large-caliber arterial injuries not amenable to primary repair. Grafts made of polytetrafluoroethylene (PTFE) may be preferable to those made of Dacron because of the alleged ability of PTFE to better resist infection in a contaminated field.

Routine completion arteriography is useful to document a technically precise repair. If a technical defect such as anastomotic narrowing is present, the anastomosis should be revised. Distal arterial spasm seen on completion arteriography may be treated with the direct intra-arterial infusion of vasodilators such as papaverine or tolazoline. However, be aware that arterial spasm seen on arteriography can be a sign of an occult compartment syndrome, as will be discussed later.

Postoperative Complications

A. Early: The early postoperative complications of vascular repair after trauma are bleeding and thrombosis. Bleeding may occur from the site of repair as a result of inadequate suture technique or may be from a site of missed injury. Thrombosis of the site of repair may result from a myriad of causes. These include inadequate débridement of the injured ends of the vessel with intimal irregularity remaining in the sutured end, faulty technique in suture placement, and failure to clear the proximal or distal circulation of thrombus prior to completion of repair. A missed proximal or distal injury may also result in thrombosis. Most such problems can be avoided by insisting on restoration of normal pulses at the initial operation or by using completion arteriography to examine the site of repair and distal run-off. Postoperatively, the patient must be monitored for these complications by frequent assessment of vital signs and pulses. If either bleeding or thrombosis is suspected, the patient should be returned to the operating room for exploration.

Wound infection can be a devastating complication of vascular repair. Patients with infection may present early with erythema, warmth, and drainage from the wound or may present late with an infected pseudoaneurysm or chronic osteomyelitis. Infection is the most common reason for amputation following a successful vascular repair. A policy of aggressive débridement of all devitalized tissue minimizes the risk of infection, even if this requires several trips to the operating room.

B. Late: Late complications of vascular repair include pseudoaneurysm formation at the suture line, AV fistula formation, and delayed thrombosis.

Causalgia is a particularly dreaded complication following vascular injury. It is caused by injury to associated nerves rather than the vascular injury itself. Nerve injury may be a result of direct trauma from the wounding agent itself or from operative dissection, or it may be a result of nerve ischemia from delayed repair of the vascular injury. Causalgia is a difficult diagnosis to make with certainty. It classically presents as a triad of symptoms in the affected limb: burning pain, sympathetic dysfunction, and limb atrophy. Causalgia may be treated by sympathetic blockade, and if the response is good, by surgical sympathectomy.

CEREBROVASCULAR INJURIES

Essentials of Diagnosis

- History of penetrating or blunt cervical trauma.
- Neck hematoma, pulse deficit, or bruit.
- Possible neurologic deficit.
- Arteriography.

Carotid Arteries

Ninety percent of carotid artery injuries are due to penetrating trauma, and 10% are due to blunt trauma. The mortality rate associated with penetrating injury is 10–30% and up to 40% after blunt injury.

A. Clinical Findings: The index of suspicion of a carotid artery injury is raised by the physical findings of a pulse deficit, bruit, or cervical hematoma. Neurologic deficits contralateral to the side of injury, and ipsilateral Horner's syndrome or dysfunction of cranial nerves IX–XII may or may not be present. Neurologic deficits may be difficult to identify because of associated head injury, systemic hypotension, or the patient's use of psychoactive substances prior to the time of injury. Injuries of the esophagus and trachea are frequently associated with those of the carotid arteries because of their close proximity in the neck.

B. Penetrating Injuries: For purposes of diagnosis and treatment of penetrating wounds, the anterior neck may be divided into 3 anatomic zones. Zone I extends from the sternal notch to the head of the clavicle, zone II from the clavicle to the angle of the mandible, and zone III from the angle of the mandible to the base of the skull. In the evaluation of penetrating trauma to zones I and III of the neck, arteriography is mandatory. Injuries to zone I may involve the great vessels, and if an arterial injury is present, arteriographic localization is necessary to plan the proper incision for exposure. Carotid artery injuries in zone III at the base of the skull can be extremely difficult to expose surgically, and arteriography is indispensable in formulating an operative plan.

Carotid artery injuries in zone II are relatively easy to expose surgically. Some surgeons advocate operative exploration of all zone II neck wounds that penetrate the platysma, with repair of any injuries that are found. Others pursue a more selective approach to operation and prefer to evaluate such patients with arteriography to rule out injury to the cervical vessels (Fig 35–5). The role of duplex scanning is also currently being evaluated in the management of these patients and may replace invasive arteriography for zone II injuries. If a selective approach to surgical exploration of zone II neck injuries is followed, evaluation of the aerodigestive tract with bronchoscopy and either esophagoscopy or contrast radiography of the esophagus is essential in addition to arteriography.

Note that active external hemorrhage or an expanding cervical hematoma causing potential airway compromise requires immediate surgical exploration without preoperative diagnostic studies, regardless of the zone of injury.

C. Treatment: Operative repair should be considered for almost all penetrating injuries of the carotid arteries. The few exceptions include those injuries in patients with a dense neurologic deficit and a large infarct on CT scan or patients with a normal neurologic examination and an occlusive injury that would require a complex repair. In the asymptomatic patient with an occlusive injury, there is a small risk of thrombus propagation with extension into the middle cerebral artery. If there is no contraindication, our policy has been to anticoagulate these patients immediately and continue anticoagulation for 3–6 months. Also, care must be taken to avoid systemic hypotension for at least 72 hours after injury to inhibit thrombus prop-

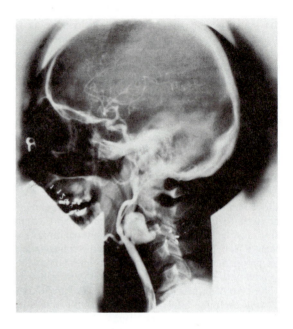

Figure 35–5. Pseudoaneurysm arising from the proximal portion of the internal carotid artery.

agation and to aid in the development of collateral perfusion to the brain. Minimal injuries, as described earlier, may be safely observed with expected healing of the injury site. These injuries include small (less than 5 mm) pseudoaneurysms and intimal defects. Patients with minimal injuries who are treated nonoperatively must undergo repeat evaluation in 1–2 weeks with either arteriography or duplex scanning to rule out progression of the lesion.

Most carotid artery injuries are best managed surgically. The carotid artery is exposed in the neck through an incision overlying and parallel to the anterior border of the sternocleidomastoid muscle. Median sternotomy may be necessary to expose the most proximal portion of the common carotid artery in the chest. Exposure of the distal internal carotid artery is difficult, but a few extra centimeters of exposure may be gained by division of the digastric muscle, removal of the angle of the mandible, or by anterior subluxation or division of the mandible. The latter maneuvers often require the assistance of an oral surgeon.

Injuries of the common and internal carotid arteries are repaired by the usual techniques of lateral arteriorrhaphy or excision of the area of injury with either primary re-anastomosis or graft replacement for more complex wounds. An injury that destroys the first portion of the internal carotid artery may be reconstructed by oversewing the origin of the artery at the common carotid bifurcation. The external carotid artery is then ligated and divided a few centimeters distal to its origin, and its proximal stump transposed and anastomosed to the distal segment of the internal carotid artery (Fig 35–6). For distal internal carotid artery injuries that are actively bleeding and cannot be exposed and controlled rapidly, a balloon catheter can be placed into the distal lumen of the artery either through the injury or through a proximal arteriotomy. After the balloon is inflated and hemorrhage is controlled, the area of injury can be dissected and definitively treated, or, if that is still not possible, the balloon may be left in place and the artery allowed to thrombose. External carotid artery injuries are repaired if simple, but complex repair or grafting is generally not undertaken and the vessel is ligated.

During repair of internal carotid artery injuries, an intraluminal shunt may be used to maintain prograde flow. A shunt is especially important to maintain cerebral perfusion if back-bleeding from the distal internal carotid artery is sluggish or if the measured stump pressure is less than 50 mmHg. The use of a shunt in this situation allows the operation to proceed without undue haste or concern regarding cerebral ischemia. If a shunt is used, the patient should be systemically anticoagulated with heparin. The shunt should first be passed through the lumen of any graft that will be used prior to its placement into the native artery. The repair or anastomosis is then performed and the shunt removed just prior to placement of the last few sutures. Shunting is generally not necessary during repair of proximal common carotid artery injuries in which the carotid bifurcation is intact because antegrade flow in the internal carotid artery can usually be maintained via collaterals of the external carotid artery.

Ligation of the common or internal carotid artery after penetrating injury is almost never required because repair is possible in almost all cases. Ligation is necessary only for very distal, unreconstructible injuries of the internal carotid artery. Embolization with detachable balloons at the time of diagnostic arteriography may be performed in lieu of operative ligation for such lesions. Following ligation or embolization of the internal carotid artery, patients should be anticoagulated for 3 to 6 months to inhibit thrombus propagation into the cerebral arteries. Carotid artery ligation may be followed by extracranial-intracranial bypass (superficial temporal to middle cerebral artery bypass) if preservation of ipsilateral cerebral perfusion is considered essential, but this is a formidable procedure and is rarely indicated.

Injuries to other cervical structures are commonly associated with carotid artery injuries. Injuries of the internal jugular vein may be repaired by lateral suture, or the vein may be ligated without sequelae. Soft tissue (fascia and muscle) should be interposed between the repair of an associated injury to the aerodigestive tract and any vascular repair. The sternocleidomastoid muscle is an excellent choice for this. The muscle may be detached from its insertion on the mastoid process and the muscle belly rotated to protect the vascular repair in case dehiscence of the pharyngeal repair occurs. Endotracheal intubation should be undertaken early in the course of management of these patients, so that tracheostomy may be avoided as a source of contamination of the vascular repair.

D. Blunt Injuries: Blunt injuries of the carotid arteries may result from direct blows, stretch of the vessels over the transverse process of the second cervical vertebra in hyperextension injuries, and basilar skull fractures. Blunt injury produces vessel contusion or intimal damage, which frequently progresses to dissection of the arterial wall and complete thrombosis of the lumen. These injuries usually involve the distal internal carotid artery rather than the common carotid artery, which is more commonly injured with penetrating trauma. There is often a characteristic lucid interval lasting from hours to days between the time of injury and the appearance of neurologic symptoms. However, the common association of a closed head injury in many of these patients may make it difficult to recognize a change in neurologic status. The patient may complain of hearing a "buzzing" sound, or a carotid bruit may be present on physical examination. Diagnosis of blunt carotid artery injury requires a high index of suspicion, especially in patients with neurologic deficits unexplained by computed tomography (CT) scanning of the brain. The diagnosis is confirmed by arteriography.

Because many blunt carotid artery injuries are extensive and involve the distal internal carotid artery, they are frequently not suitable for operative repair. Although controversial, data suggest that patients with

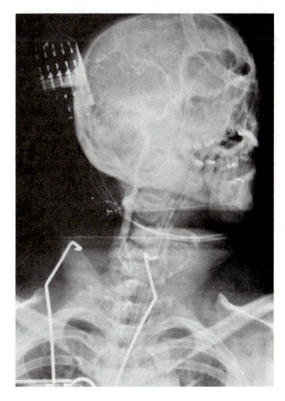

Figure 35–6. Completion arteriogram after external carotid-internal carotid transposition for the injury seen in Figure 35–5.

blunt injuries should be treated nonoperatively with systemic anticoagulation to limit distal thrombus propagation and embolization.

Vertebral Arteries

A. Clinical Evaluation: Before the routine use of arteriography to evaluate trauma victims, vertebral artery injuries were infrequently discovered. More recently, the liberal use of diagnostic arteriography has uncovered a significant number of these injuries. In the absence of an AV fistula, the diagnosis of vertebral artery injury on clinical grounds alone is highly unusual. There are generally no signs of injury on physical examination, and symptoms of vertebrobasilar ischemia are rarely present. In fact, when a neurologic deficit is present, it is usually due to associated injury of the central nervous system or carotid arteries.

The vertebral artery is the first branch of the subclavian artery (Fig 35–7). It courses through the posterior triangle of the neck to enter the foramen in the transverse process of the 6th cervical vertebra. Surgical exposure of this first portion of the subclavian artery is relatively simple through a supraclavicular incision. The second portion courses within the vertebral foramina to exit the first cervical vertebra, and its exposure may be exceedingly difficult. Exposure requires re-

moval of the anterior arch of the bony transverse processes. In addition, this portion of the artery is surrounded by an extensive venous network, which may be a source of major hemorrhage during dissection. The 3rd and 4th portions of the vertebral artery require craniotomy for exposure.

B. Treatment: Because of the rare incidence of adverse sequelae after ligation and the difficult and sometimes hazardous surgical exposure, an injured vertebral artery is rarely repaired. Angiographic embolization is the treatment of choice for most injuries. Embolization proximal and distal to the area of injury is not always necessary, since proximal interruption of flow alone may be sufficient to cause distal thrombosis. Even if an injury such as a pseudoaneurysm or AV fistula cannot be completely occluded by embolization, partial interruption of its blood supply may diminish flow through the lesion and decrease the risk and magnitude of hemorrhage at operation. Occlusive injuries to the vertebral arteries need only be observed; no intervention is necessary. Primary operative repair of a vertebral artery injury should be undertaken only when arteriographic evidence of a hypoplastic or absent contralateral vessel is found, which occurs in less than 5% of patients. In that case, occlusion of the normal vessel by embolization may cause posterior cerebral ischemia.

THORACIC INJURIES

Essentials of Diagnosis

- Penetrating trauma in which a missile has traversed the mediastinum.
- Major blunt trauma with abnormal chest x-ray (usually showing widened mediastinum).
- Aortography.

General Considerations

Major arterial injuries of the thorax and abdomen are often rapidly fatal. Patients who present with unstable vital signs and penetrating thoracic or abdominal wounds should undergo operative exploration without delay. For the patient presenting in extremis in whom a missile has traversed the mediastinum, emergency thoracotomy with cross-clamping of the aorta may be lifesaving. However, many patients with major vascular injuries of the trunk have remarkably few physical signs. Patients who are stable are invariably found to have a hematoma at the site of arterial injury, which has been contained by the surrounding soft tissues and has tamponaded the injury.

Clinical Evaluation

A. Signs and Symptoms: The pulse examination is frequently entirely normal in patients with arterial injuries of the torso because of the large caliber of these vessels and the fact that these injuries are rarely completely occlusive. However, an abnormal pulse

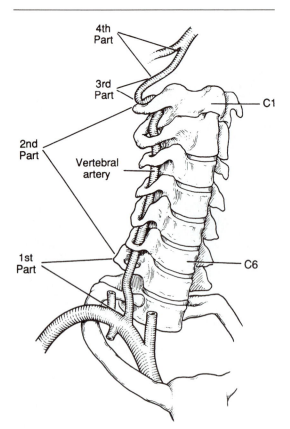

Figure 35–7. Anatomic divisions of the vertebral artery.

examination is a strong predictor of the presence of a major vascular injury. The clinician should search for asymmetry of pulses between the 2 upper extremities and between the upper and lower extremities.

Injuries of the thoracic aorta and great vessels most frequently follow penetrating trauma of the thorax or base of the neck. Any patient seen with penetrating trauma to the base of the neck or in which a missile has traversed the mediastinum should undergo arteriography to exclude great vessel injury.

The thoracic aorta is particularly susceptible to blunt injury. Ninety percent of blunt injuries of the thoracic aorta occur in the descending portion, typically just distal to the ligamentum arteriosum where the relatively mobile aortic arch meets the fixed descending thoracic aorta. Major decelerative force applied at this area produces disruption of the inner layers of the aortic wall, resulting in pseudoaneurysm formation or complete disruption of the aortic wall and free, usually fatal, hemorrhage.

Eighty to 90% of patients with aortic transection die at the scene of injury, and this is the cause of death in about 15% of all fatalities from motor vehicle accidents. Of those patients who reach the hospital alive, one-third die within 24 hours if untreated. Diagnosis requires a high index of suspicion and an aggressive approach to evaluation.

Clues to the presence of blunt aortic transection on physical examination include systemic hypotension and pulse asymmetry between the upper or upper and lower extremities. Breath sounds may be decreased on the left due to a hemothorax. Associated sternal and rib fractures are common, a reflection of the magnitude of the force sustained by the thoracic cavity.

Blunt injuries of the branches of the aortic arch, such as avulsion of the origin of the innominate artery from the aortic arch, also occur, but are uncommon. Fractures of the 1st and 2nd ribs may be associated with blunt injuries of the great vessels. Some have advocated arteriography in all patients with these fractures to rule out vascular injury. However, in the absence of a displaced posterior 1st rib fracture or a pulse deficit on physical examination, a vascular injury is unlikely.

B. Imaging Studies: Findings on chest radiography that are associated with aortic transection include a superior mediastinum that is widened to greater than 9 cm, an obscured or indistinct aortic knob, left apical capping, a left pleural effusion, deviation of the trachea to the right, depression of the left mainstem bronchus, deviation of the nasogastric tube (esophagus) to the right, and associated fractures of the ribs and sternum. Several of these signs are also associated with fractures of the thoracic spine with surrounding hematoma; therefore, these patients should be maintained in spinal immobilization until such a fracture is ruled out. Also, the superior mediastinum may erroneously appear widened on the supine anteroposterior chest film obtained in the emergency room on many patients without aortic injury. An upright film may clarify the findings and provide a more accurate assessment of the mediastinum (Fig 35–8).

Aortography is the definitive diagnostic test and should be performed in all patients with a history of major decelerative trauma and a suspicious chest x-ray or physical findings. When injury is present, the aortogram usually demonstrates the tear just distal to the takeoff of the left subclavian artery (Fig 35–9). Diagnosis is also possible with a contrast-enhanced CT scan or transesophageal echo, but the aortogram is most sensitive and more precisely defines the location of the injury, which is important in planning operative repair.

Treatment

A. Proximal Aorta: Patients with injuries to the ascending aorta and aortic arch are rarely treated because few make it to the hospital alive. Proximal, ascending aortic injuries may result from major blunt trauma, such as a motor vehicle accident with steering wheel injury that produces rapid deceleration, sternal fracture, and secondary aortic laceration. Exposure is accomplished by median sternotomy. Small injuries may be directly repaired with mattress sutures after control with a fingertip or partially occluding aortic clamp. Larger injuries, in the rare patient who survives, may require cardiopulmonary bypass and prosthetic graft repair.

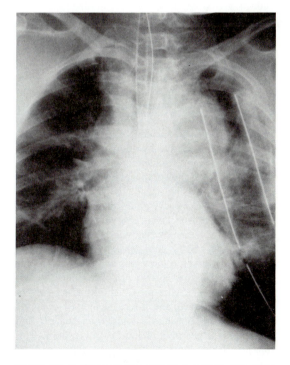

Figure 35–8. Chest radiograph in a patient with blunt transection of the thoracic aorta. Note the widened mediastinum, loss of contour of the aortic knob, shift of the trachea to the right, and depression of the left mainstem bronchus.

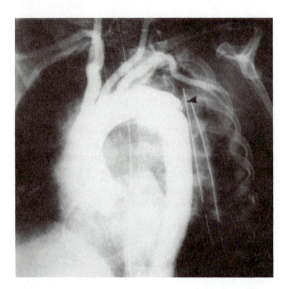

Figure 35–9. Aortogram of the patient seen in Figure 35–8. There is a contained disruption of the proximal descending thoracic aorta (arrow) distal to the takeoff of the left subclavian artery.

B. Descending Aorta: The treatment of descending thoracic aortic transection is surgical, but it may include a period of preoperative stabilization in the intensive care unit or operating room to optimize hemodynamic parameters, including prevention or control of arterial hypertension, while other life-threatening injuries to the head or abdomen are attended to and while the necessary resources required in the operating room are mobilized. However, operation should be delayed for no more than a few hours.

Exposure is accomplished by left posterolateral thoracotomy. The use of a double-lumen endotracheal tube facilitates exposure by allowing selective deflation of the left lung. The site of aortic injury is often surrounded by a subpleural hematoma. Distal control is obtained by passing a tape around the aorta below the hematoma. The injury typically lies just below the takeoff of the left subclavian artery, and proximal control must be obtained by encircling the aorta between the subclavian and left common carotid arteries with a tape passed medial to the vagus and recurrent laryngeal nerves. A tape is also placed around the left subclavian artery. After proximal and distal control have been achieved, the pleura is incised over the hematoma, the hematoma rapidly evacuated, and clamps placed just proximal and distal to the laceration. The clamps should be placed close together to exclude a minimal number of intercostal arteries. The intercostals are important collateral channels to preserve spinal cord perfusion and prevent cord ischemia and paraplegia during aortic cross-clamping.

A transverse incision is made in the aorta at the site of the laceration, the aorta completely transected, and the area of injury débrided. Dacron graft interposition is generally preferable to and more rapid than primary repair. A 2–3-cm length of graft is usually all that is needed. The injured aorta is very friable and may not hold sutures well; Dacron pledgets can be used to buttress the sutures. It has been stated that cord ischemia is unlikely if aortic cross-clamp time is 30 minutes or less, and graft interposition can usually be accomplished within that time. An even more rapid repair can be achieved by inserting a sutureless graft, consisting of a tubular woven Dacron graft with a grooved polypropylene ring at each end. The graft is inserted through the aortotomy. Umbilical tapes are then passed around the aorta and graft proximally and distally, pulled tight in the appropriate grooves, and tied. Several anchoring mattress sutures are also placed in the Dacron cuff and aortic wall to help secure this type of graft.

Complex repairs that require longer periods of cross-clamp time may require left-heart (atriofemoral) or complete cardiopulmonary bypass to provide aortic perfusion distal to the clamps. Alternatively, an aortoaortic heparin-bonded shunt (Gott shunt) can be used.

Penetrating injuries of the thoracic aorta may be repaired by lateral suture, patch aortoplasty, or graft insertion, depending on the extent of the injury.

C. Great Vessel Injuries: Injuries to the innominate and proximal left common carotid arteries are best approached through a median sternotomy. The incision may be extended vertically into the neck or along the superior border of the clavicle if more distal control is necessary. The proximal left subclavian artery arises from the posterior aspect of the aortic arch, and its origin is best approached through a left anterolateral thoracotomy. More distal exposure of the left subclavian artery may be accomplished by dividing the sternum superiorly and incising along the superior border of the left clavicle, thus creating a "trap door," which exposes the vessel in its entirety.

Great vessel injuries are repaired primarily whenever possible, but usually require graft insertion. Very proximal innominate or left common carotid artery injuries that cannot be primarily repaired may be treated by oversewing the proximal stump at the aorta. A graft is then placed at a different site on the aorta, and vessel continuity is restored. If the distal innominate artery is injured, a bifurcated graft may be used and sutured to the ends of the right subclavian and common carotid arteries. Very proximal left subclavian artery injuries may be treated by oversewing the proximal stump and transposing the distal end to the side of the left common carotid artery. Associated injuries to the brachiocephalic veins are repaired, if feasible, but may be ligated without serious sequelae.

ABDOMINAL INJURIES

Essentials of Diagnosis
- Penetrating or blunt abdominal trauma with persistent hypotension and distending abdomen.
- Active hemorrhage or retroperitoneal hematoma found at time of abdominal exploration.

General Considerations
Major abdominal vascular injuries are most often due to penetrating trauma and are fatal in 20–40% of cases. A major abdominal vascular injury may result in rapid, exsanguinating hemorrhage into the peritoneal cavity or a retroperitoneal, mesenteric, retrohepatic, or portal hematoma. Many patients with abdominal vascular injuries present in shock and there is little time for preoperative diagnostic evaluation. Abdominal vascular injuries are generally diagnosed at the time of celiotomy. Major abdominal vascular injury should be suspected in any patient presenting with a penetrating wound between the nipples above and the inguinal crease below, especially in the presence of a distended abdomen. Penetrating injuries may involve any vessel, but most frequently involve the inferior vena cava. Abdominal vascular injury after blunt trauma is not common, but, if present, usually involves the renal arteries, the retrohepatic vena cava, or the iliac vessels in association with fractures of the bony pelvis. Abdominal vascular injuries are generally found in combination with injuries to the hollow and solid abdominal viscera; only rarely are they found as isolated injuries.

When exploring the abdomen with suspected major vascular injury, the importance of adequate volume resuscitation prior to celiotomy is paramount. Release of the tamponading effect of the abdominal wall after incision may cause a rapid fall in blood pressure and even cardiac arrest in the incompletely resuscitated patient. The entire thorax and abdomen should be prepared and draped into the operative field. On opening an abdomen which is filled with blood and in which massive hemorrhage is on-going, rapid proximal control of the aorta can be obtained by placing an aortic occluder at the diaphragmatic hiatus to compress the supraceliac aorta against the vertebral bodies. This device may be left in place and compressed by an assistant; or, the gastrohepatic ligament can be opened, the aorta exposed at the diaphragmatic hiatus, and a large vascular clamp applied. Alternatively, proximal control may be gained by performing a left thoracotomy and cross-clamping the thoracic aorta. This may even be done prior to celiotomy for suspected major abdominal vascular injuries and, when performed in the emergency room, may permit salvage of 2–3% of patients with penetrating abdominal trauma who arrive at the hospital in a moribund state. After proximal control of the aorta is obtained, more definitive localization and control of the source of abdominal bleeding then follows.

Aortic Injuries
Abdominal aortic injuries usually present as a central retroperitoneal hematoma but may present with active intraperitoneal hemorrhage. The route of exposure and control of the aorta depends on the suspected site of injury. Pararenal and suprarenal aortic injuries are best exposed by means of a medial visceral rotation maneuver, with medial mobilization of the left colon, spleen, and pancreas, with or without the left kidney. This is performed by incising the lateral peritoneal reflection of the colon and the ligamentous attachments of the spleen and sweeping the viscera medially, staying in the avascular, retroperitoneal plane. This maneuver provides wide exposure, especially of the upper abdominal aorta. Extension of a vertical midline incision across the costal margin into the left 7th or 8th intercostal space as a thoracoabdominal incision, in addition to the medial visceral rotation, provides even more generous exposure of the suprarenal or supraceliac aorta. Exposure of the supraceliac aorta is impossible without such a thoracic extension of the incision. Exposure of an infrarenal aortic injury is best obtained by a direct anterior approach, elevating the transverse colon cephalad, incising the ligament of Treitz, retracting the small bowel to the right, and incising the peritoneum directly over the aorta.

Smaller injuries of the aorta are frequently amenable to simple primary repair with a monofilament, nonabsorbable suture. Larger injuries may require patch aortoplasty, and more extensive injuries require prosthetic grafting. In the presence of extensive contamination from associated enteric injuries, there is a potential risk of infection of prosthetic materials. In this case, a graft may be placed in situ, but the retroperitoneum must be irrigated copiously with antibiotics and débrided of all devitalized tissue. The peritoneum should be closed securely over the graft; if that is not possible, the omentum should be wrapped around the graft. Alternatively, in the presence of gross contamination of the retroperitoneum by enteric contents, the infrarenal aorta may be oversewn and ligated and an extra-anatomic axillary-bifemoral bypass performed through clean tissue planes after the abdomen is closed.

Iliac Vessel Injury
Most major iliac artery injuries are due to penetrating trauma. Physical signs of this injury include an absent or diminished femoral pulse and the presence of a bruit in the groin. Intraoperatively, patients with iliac artery injuries present with active pelvic bleeding or

with a retroperitoneal hematoma in the lateral aspect of the pelvis.

A. Surgical Treatment: Exposure of the iliac arteries begins with exposure of the distal aorta. On the right, the peritoneal incision extends around the base of the cecum, and the cecum is elevated. Dissection is then carried caudally on top of the common iliac artery. The ureter crosses anterior to the distal common iliac artery and should be retracted laterally. Exposure of the left common iliac artery is achieved by continuing the peritoneal incision over the distal aorta caudad and angled to the left. Again, the ureter should be retracted laterally. Often, this longitudinal incision does not provide adequate exposure of the left external and internal iliac arteries. If needed, the lateral peritoneal attachments of the sigmoid colon can be incised and the colon retracted medially, thus exposing these distal vessels.

Repair of common or external iliac artery injuries is achieved by lateral repair, excision of the area of injury and end-to-end anastomosis, or graft replacement. In the presence of severe enteric contamination, the common or external iliac artery may be ligated and an extra-anatomic femorofemoral bypass graft performed. The internal iliac artery, if injured, may be ligated with impunity because of the rich network of collaterals across the pelvis.

B. Associated Injuries: The iliac veins are closely adherent to the arteries and are often injured concurrently. Hasty dissection of the arteries may result in iatrogenic laceration of an iliac vein. Venous bleeding can be torrential and difficult to localize, particularly when it is from the hypogastric vein. Repair is difficult because of the thin, friable vein wall. Iliac vein injuries are repaired when possible, but usually are ligated. The lower extremities should be wrapped with elastic bandages and kept elevated after repair or ligation of the iliac veins to minimize postoperative edema, promote venous flow, and minimize the potential for postoperative thrombosis.

Pelvic fractures associated with severe blunt trauma may cause disruption of multiple branches of the internal iliac arteries and veins. This may result in fatal hemorrhage and must always be kept in mind as a source of occult major bleeding. Patients with hemorrhage respond to stabilization of the pelvic fracture with an external fixator in almost all cases; those that do not should undergo pelvic angiography with embolization of arterial bleeding sites. If discovered at operation, a nonexpanding pelvic hematoma due to blunt trauma should not be explored. The injury should be left to tamponade. Management of an expanding pelvic hematoma is more complex. The injured branch vessels can be extremely difficult to localize, and to attempt this in the operating room may provoke rapidly fatal hemorrhage. In this situation, the best course of action is to pack the pelvis, close the abdomen, and transport the patient to the angiography suite for embolization.

Mesenteric Arteries

Injuries of the visceral branches of the abdominal aorta can be quite complex and are generally associated with extensive injuries to the viscera themselves, most frequently to the liver and small bowel.

The celiac trunk is approached through the gastrohepatic ligament, through the gastrocolic ligament with superior retraction of the stomach, or by the left-sided medial visceral rotation maneuver previously described. Celiac artery injuries are repaired, if possible. If necessary, ligation of the celiac artery may be performed and is usually well-tolerated because of the rich collateral network from the superior mesenteric artery (SMA) through the gastroduodenal artery.

Injuries of the proximal SMA are exposed by medial visceral rotation or by direct dissection at the mesenteric root. Exposure of the retropancreatic portion of the SMA may require division of the body of the pancreas followed by distal pancreatectomy. SMA repair is accomplished by lateral suture or interposition grafting, preferably with autogenous graft material. The proximal SMA may also be ligated, but ligation without revascularization results in an unacceptably high incidence of subsequent bowel necrosis. Aorta to SMA bypass should be performed in cases of very proximal SMA injury not amenable to primary repair. The injured inferior mesenteric artery can usually be ligated without sequelae in the young trauma patient.

Renal Vessels

Renal artery injuries may be caused by penetrating or blunt trauma. Thrombosis of the renal artery from blunt trauma may result when rapid deceleration moves the relatively mobile kidney in the retroperitoneum, stretching the vessels and producing intimal fractures and flaps or complete arterial disruption. A direct blow can also cause contusion of the artery with resultant thrombosis.

A. Diagnostic Evaluation: Diagnostic clues to the presence of a renal artery injury include pain and tenderness in the epigastrium or flank and microscopic or gross hematuria. However, hematuria is absent in roughly 20% of patients with significant renal artery injury. Oliguria or anuria may represent bilateral injury or injury to the renal artery supplying a solitary kidney. Intraoperative findings suggestive of a renal vascular injury include a lateral or central retroperitoneal hematoma and a cyanotic-appearing kidney.

Renal vascular injuries frequently result in nephrectomy; therefore, evaluation of the function of both kidneys is critical to avoid removal of the only functioning kidney. Do not assume that an opposite kidney that is palpated intraoperatively is functional. For the unstable patient suspected of harboring a potential renal injury, a 1-shot intravenous pyelogram (IVP) in the emergency room prior to exploration takes very little time and should be done to document function of the contralateral uninjured kidney. Alternatively, an IVP may be done in the operating room at the time of exploration in patients found to have a significant renal injury. For the stable patient suspected of having a renal vascular injury, a CT scan is the optimal diagnostic tool. A delay or absence of contrast enhancement of the kidney may indicate injury to the renal vasculature and should be followed by renal arteriography.

B. Treatment: For bilateral renal artery injuries, revascularization of at least one kidney should be attempted in the hemodynamically stable patient, even if this requires ex vivo operative techniques or autotransplantation. For unilateral injuries, major destruction of the main renal vein, collecting system, or renal parenchyma should dissuade attempts at repair. Also, extensive associated injuries to other organs that render the patient unable to tolerate additional operating time or blood loss are an indication for nephrectomy rather than repair of the vascular injury.

An occasional renal artery injury is amenable to lateral suture or resection of the area of injury with end-to-end anastomosis, but most require aortorenal grafting with saphenous vein. Hypogastric artery is the preferred graft in younger patients because of the tendency toward aneurysmal degeneration of vein grafts in this position followed over many years. Complex injuries to the renal branch vessels require ex vivo techniques to repair, but should be attempted only in the most stable patients. Renovascular hypertension may occur after arterial repair in some patients followed long term. Such patients may later be candidates for remedial revascularization or nephrectomy.

Injuries to the main renal veins should be repaired by lateral suture, if possible. Ligation of segmental venous branches can be performed without untoward sequelae because of the extensive intraparenchymal communications with other venous tributaries. This is in contrast to the segmental arterial branches, which are end-arteries and cannot be ligated without sacrificing renal parenchyma. The left renal vein may be ligated proximally, provided that the gonadal and adrenal collaterals are preserved. The right kidney does not tolerate ligation of its main venous outflow, and in the case of a major right renal vein injury not amenable to repair, nephrectomy should be performed. The internal jugular vein is a suitably sized replacement for a renal vein should a graft be necessary.

C. Special Considerations: The kidney is able to tolerate 2–4 hours of warm ischemia, although loss of excretory function begins after 30 minutes. Although little function is retrievable after 6 hours of total ischemia, there have been occasional reports of successful repair as long as 24 hours after injury, with some return of excretory function. The probability of retrieving significant renal function after prolonged periods of total occlusion of the main renal vessels depends on the amount of flow to the kidney through collaterals. Extensive mobilization of the kidney or ureter will disrupt these collaterals.

Inferior Vena Cava

Because they occur in a low pressure system, most abdominal venous injuries are quickly tamponaded by the resulting hematoma or adjacent organs and do not typically result in rapid hemorrhage. Hemorrhage occurs during abdominal exploration when the hematoma is dislodged. Localization of the injury in the depths of the hematoma can be difficult.

Injuries to the inferior vena cava (IVC) may produce a retroperitoneal hematoma that is located either centrally or in the right lateral region. Exposure is best obtained by reflecting the right colon and duodenum medially. Control of the injury site can be obtained by compressing the cava above and below the injury with sponge sticks, by encircling the IVC above and below the injury with tapes, or by placing a side-biting clamp around the injury. Care must be taken to avoid lacerating the lumbar branches of the IVC, which would lead to additional hemorrhage. Lateral suture repair can be accomplished for most injuries, and up to a 50% narrowing is acceptable.

Do not overlook injuries of the posterior wall of the IVC. These injuries may be approached by longitudinal extension of a concomitant anterior injury, if present. The posterior hole can be repaired with sutures placed from within the lumen. An alternative approach is to mobilize the IVC by dividing several lumbar veins. The IVC is then rotated to expose the posterior injury site. The infrarenal IVC may be ligated if necessary after an extensive injury, and there have been reports of survival after ligation of the suprarenal IVC. However, repair of the suprarenal IVC is preferred. Internal jugular vein, spiral saphenous vein, and externally supported PTFE grafts have been used successfully in this position. After repair or ligation of the vena cava, the lower extremities should be wrapped in elastic bandages and elevated to minimize postoperative edema and promote venous flow. These patients should be observed closely to detect postoperative venous thrombosis.

Injuries to the retrohepatic vena cava and hepatic veins are among the most challenging vascular injuries to treat successfully. Injudicious attempts to mobilize the liver and directly expose the area of injury are frequently met with massive hemorrhage or fatal air embolism. These injuries are often best treated by hepatic packing with return to the operating room for pack removal after the patient has been stabilized and the injury tamponaded. Occasionally, packing fails to arrest hemorrhage; when this occurs, the injury must be exposed and repair performed. Invariably, successful repair requires wide exposure of the liver, with extension of the abdominal incision into either a median sternotomy or right thoracotomy, and incision of the diaphragm down to the cava. Extension of the incision should be performed sooner rather than later in the course of the operation.

Vascular inflow to the liver is controlled by compressing or cross-clamping the aorta at the level of the diaphragmatic hiatus and by placing a vascular clamp across the hepatoduodenal ligament to compress the hepatic artery and portal vein (Pringle maneuver). Tourniquets or clamps to control the IVC are placed below the liver but above the renal veins in the abdomen and within the pericardium above the liver. Alternatively, an intracaval shunt (chest tube or endotracheal tube) can be placed through the right atrial appendage of the heart, across the injury, and encircled with tapes above and below the liver to isolate the injury and decrease bleeding during exposure and repair. The ligamentous attachments of the right lobe of the liver are then incised, and the liver is rotated medially, exposing the retrohepatic vena cava and hepatic veins. The vena cava usually can be repaired by direct suture, but the hepatic veins must frequently be oversewn.

Portal and Mesenteric Veins

Injuries to the portal and superior mesenteric veins should be repaired if at all possible. The supraduodenal portal vein is exposed by a Kocher maneuver, rotating the duodenum and the head of the pancreas medially. The vein is carefully dissected away from the common bile duct within the hepatoduodenal ligament. Division of the pancreas and distal pancreatectomy may be necessary for exposure of the retropancreatic portion of the portal vein. Ligation of the portal and superior mesenteric veins is compatible with survival, but acute ligation carries a high incidence of intestinal ischemia and infarction due to venous hypertension, congestion, and thrombosis. If these veins are ligated, a second-look celiotomy with resection of infarcted bowel (if present) should be undertaken after 24–48 hours. After ligation, massive fluid sequestration occurs in the intestines and requires aggressive replacement in the postoperative period to prevent systemic hypovolemia.

INJURIES TO THE EXTREMITIES

Essentials of Diagnosis

- Penetrating or blunt extremity trauma.
- Active hemorrhage, expanding hematoma, or signs of acute limb ischemia.
- Abnormal pulse examination or ankle-brachial index (ABI) <1.00.
- Arteriography.

Diagnostic Consideration

Physical signs associated with peripheral arterial trauma may include the 5 Ps of acute arterial occlusion (pain, pallor, pulselessness, paresthesias, and paresis), coolness, and mottling of the affected part. In addition, a hematoma may be present over the site of injury, which may or may not be expansile. A palpable thrill or audible bruit at the site of or distal to an area of injury are uncommon, but when present are virtually diagnostic of arterial injury. Neurologic deficits frequently accompany vascular injuries, either as a result of direct injury to nerves running in close proximity to the injured vessels or as a result of ischemia of these same nerves.

In the extremities, pulses are often present but diminished distal to an arterial injury. An abnormal pulse examination is a very sensitive indicator of arterial injury. Nevertheless, distal pulses are normal in more than 50% of patients with documented major arterial injuries. The pulse wave may be transmitted through clot, intimal flaps, and collateral networks. Thus, reliance on the pulse examination alone is inadequate for the diagnosis of occult arterial injury.

Many arterial injuries of the extremities are clinically occult and represent a significant diagnostic challenge. Because of the severity of soft tissue destruction seen in military wounds, routine exploration of all penetrating wounds in proximity to a neurovascular bundle was standard practice during the Korean War. When applied to civilian injuries, this practice resulted in an extremely high number of negative explorations, up to 84% in one series. Refinement and ready availability of arteriography allowed this modality to replace wound exploration in the patient with a proximity injury. However, as in wound exploration, mandatory arteriography for proximity injury resulted in a large number of normal arteriograms, at a significant cost. In the absence of objective clinical findings (eg, pulse deficit, hematoma, nerve injury), arteriograms performed for proximity alone demonstrate arterial injury in only 6–9% of patients.

Recent studies have shown that Doppler-derived ankle or wrist brachial indices may be used to stratify patients according to risk of major arterial injury and may be useful in selecting patients for further study with arteriography. These results are valid only for injuries distal to the axillary fold or inguinal crease. The index is calculated by determining the ratio of the lower of the 2 ankle or wrist systolic opening pressures in the injured extremity to the brachial artery opening pressure in an uninjured extremity.

A prospective analysis of 514 consecutive patients with penetrating extremity trauma revealed that a pulse deficit by physical examination and an index of less than 1.00 were the only significant independent predictors of a major arterial injury. The sensitivity of an index of less than 1.00 in predicting major arterial injury was 96%. The negative predictive value was 99%; that is, in patients with an ABI equal to or greater than 1.00, there was a 99% certainty that no major arterial injury existed. These patients can thus be safely observed without subjecting them to the potential risks and costs of arteriography.

The diagnosis of vascular injury associated with blunt extremity trauma is more difficult. Vascular damage should be suspected with crush injuries, displaced fractures, and joint dislocations (especially

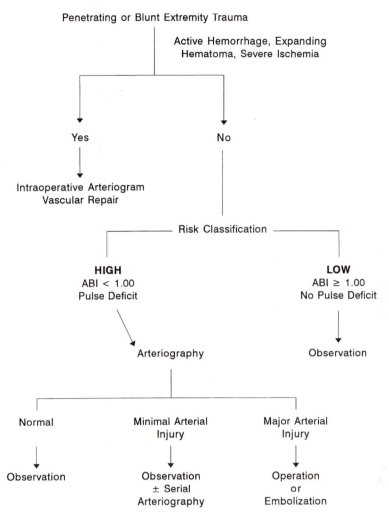

Figure 35–10. Algorithm for the assessment and management of penetrating or blunt extremity trauma. Note the indications for arteriography (pulse deficit or ABI <1.00). Minimal injuries are as defined in the text.

those of the knee). The importance of a careful physical examination in identifying arterial injuries cannot be overemphasized, and diagnostic arteriography should be used liberally when any abnormality of the examination is present. If the physical examination is normal, pulses are intact, and the ABI is 1.00 or greater, our experience indicates that screening arteriography is not warranted, even in the presence of a knee dislocation (Fig 35–10).

Much interest exists in the use of noninvasive technologies such as duplex or color-flow duplex scanning in the assessment of peripheral vascular trauma. These techniques prevent the potential complications of arteriography and are less expensive to perform. Early reports show a 95% or greater sensitivity in predicting major arterial injury. However, these studies are technically demanding, and are heavily reliant on the skill of the technologist and the ability of the surgeon to interpret the findings.

Upper Extremity

A. Subclavian Artery: Extrathoracic subclavian artery injuries most commonly result from penetrating trauma, but may occur after blunt trauma, particularly in association with posterior displaced 1st rib fractures or clavicle fractures. Clinical signs include a pulse deficit in the upper extremity, a hematoma at the base of the neck, and associated brachial plexus injuries. Because of the rich collateral network around the shoulder, physical signs of injury to the subclavian and axillary arteries, such as upper extremity pulse deficits or ischemia, are frequently absent or ambiguous. Therefore, a high index of suspicion must be maintained to avoid overlooking these critical injuries. Arteriography should be used liberally in the evaluation of wounds to this area.

The surgical approach to proximal subclavian artery injuries is median sternotomy for right-sided injuries or anterolateral thoracotomy for left-sided injuries. More distal injuries may be exposed through a supraclavicular incision alone, with or without resection of a portion of the clavicle. The most distal injuries may necessitate an additional infraclavicular incision with division or partial resection of the clavicle to achieve complete exposure.

Several important structures lie in proximity to the subclavian artery, which must be avoided during dissection. The subclavian vein is situated anterior and inferior to the artery and has many delicate branches that are easily avulsed, causing significant bleeding. The phrenic nerve lies on the anterior surface of the anterior scalene muscle. This muscle may require division for exposure of the middle third of the subclavian artery and, if so, the nerve must be protected. The vagus nerve crosses anterior to the first portion of the subclavian artery. The recurrent laryngeal nerve courses around the origin of the subclavian artery, the aorta, and the ligamentum arteriosum on the left and around the origin of the subclavian from the innominate artery on the right. On the left side, the thoracic duct enters the venous system at the confluence of the subclavian and jugular veins.

The subclavian artery is a somewhat delicate vessel in its midportion, and sutures have a tendency to tear through the wall. Rather than perform a primary repair under tension, graft interposition or an end-to-side subclavian-carotid anastomosis should be undertaken without hesitation. There seems to be no disadvantage in terms of long-term patency to the use of prosthetic graft material in this location. The use of prosthetic graft also eliminates the possibility of size mismatch, which may be a problem if vein is used.

B. Axillary Artery: The axillary artery extends from the lateral border of the first rib to the inferior edge of the teres major muscle. Axillary artery injuries can be associated with blunt anterior dislocation of the shoulder and fractures of the humeral neck, but are more commonly due to penetrating trauma. The axillary artery is surrounded by the cords of the brachial plexus, and a very high incidence of neurologic injury is associated with injury of the axillary artery.

The best approach to the axillary artery is through a horizontal infraclavicular incision, which may be extended onto the arm if necessary. The axillary artery is made up of 3 portions. The first portion, medial to the pectoralis minor muscle, is exposed by separating the fibers of the pectoralis major muscle. The second and third portions, beneath and lateral to the pectoralis minor, are better approached beneath and lateral to the pectoralis major muscle by dividing the insertion of the pectoralis minor. One must be careful in dissection of this region not to injure the nerves of the brachial plexus. Primary repair can usually be accomplished for axillary artery injuries, but saphenous vein or prosthetic interposition grafting should be used when necessary.

C. Brachial Artery: Brachial artery injuries are commonly iatrogenic, resulting from cardiac catheterization and diagnostic or therapeutic radiologic procedures. Blunt injuries of the brachial artery are associated with supracondylar fractures of the humerus, but again, most injuries are a result of penetrating trauma. Diagnosis is usually obvious if the injury is above the takeoff of the profunda brachii artery, but because of the rich collateral flow that this vessel provides, injuries to the brachial artery below its takeoff can be more difficult to discern clinically.

The surgical approach to a brachial artery injury is through a longitudinal incision directly over the area of injury. Lateral repair of this vessel is rarely possible because of its small size, but usually enough artery can be mobilized to perform a tension-free end-to-end primary repair. When primary repair is impossible, saphenous or cephalic vein is ideal for use as an interposition graft.

D. Radial and Ulnar Arteries: Isolated injury to either the radial or the ulnar artery in the forearm rarely causes ischemic problems, because of collateral filling from the uninjured vessel through the palmar arches. Occlusive injuries of a single vessel do not require therapeutic intervention in the absence of ischemic signs or symptoms. However, actively bleeding injuries require treatment. Nonocclusive injuries such as large pseudoaneurysms or AV fistulas may enlarge over time and necessitate intervention. A single vessel may be ligated or embolized with little morbidity. Repair may be undertaken in the absence of other major bodily injuries requiring attention. Repair is mandatory if a previous injury to the other vessel has occurred, if the palmar arch is not complete by Allen's test or angiography, if any sign of distal ischemia is present, or if both vessels are injured. In general, because the ulnar artery is the larger of the 2, it should be the preferential vessel reconstructed.

Lower Extremity

A. Femoral Arteries: Injuries to the common and profunda femoral arteries are uncommon because of their short length and proximal location. Superficial femoral artery injuries are very common. Exposure of the femoral vessels is obtained through a vertical or oblique incision in the groin, which may be extended down the anteromedial aspect of the thigh for more distal injuries. If more proximal control is necessary, the external iliac artery can be exposed by dividing the inguinal ligament vertically or by making a separate transverse incision above the ligament for retroperitoneal exposure and control. Femoral injuries are repaired by the previously described techniques, namely, lateral suture, resection with primary reanastomosis, or graft interposition. The profunda femoral artery may be ligated in an emergency situation as long as the superficial femoral artery is patent, but it is generally preferable to repair injuries to the proximal profunda femoral artery because of its key role as a collateral.

B. Popliteal Artery: Popliteal artery injuries resulting in acute occlusion are associated with the highest rates of amputation for any site of vascular injury. For example, ligation of the popliteal artery resulted in a 73% amputation rate during World War II. This high amputation rate is due to the lack of preformed collaterals around the knee; it also reflects the magnitude of associated venous, soft tissue, skeletal, and neurologic injuries. Associated trifurcation and popliteal vein injuries occur in about 30% of patients with popliteal artery injuries.

The popliteal artery is particularly susceptible to blunt injury because of its tight attachments to the adductor magnus tendon above and to the fibrous arch of the soleus muscle and interosseous membrane below the knee (Fig 35–11). Knee dislocation (posterior or anterior) or fracture of the supracondylar femur or tibial plateau causes stretch of the vessel, which may produce intimal tears. One-third of patients with knee dislocation have a popliteal artery injury that can be documented by arteriography. Routine arteriography

has been recommended for all knee dislocations, but it has been demonstrated that a careful pulse examination by an experienced physician and the use of ABIs can detect all significant injuries that require operative repair. Experienced trauma surgeons can be more selective in their use of arteriograms.

The injured popliteal artery is best exposed through a medial incision, which allows extension proximally or distally as needed. In a minority of cases in which the location of the injury is precisely known by preoperative arteriography, the posterior approach may be used. Early systemic anticoagulation in the absence of any contraindication is essential to arrest thrombus formation in the small vessels of the leg distally. Associated popliteal vein injuries should be repaired whenever possible in an attempt to minimize postoperative venous hypertension and the likelihood of a compartment syndrome. Concurrent use of mannitol, an oxygen free radical scavenger, has been reported to markedly decrease the incidence of compartment syndrome and its sequelae.

In a recent series from our institution, 100 popliteal artery injuries were identified. Successful repair and limb salvage were accomplished in 89 extremities. One patient underwent primary amputation because of

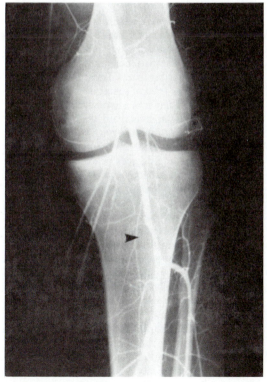

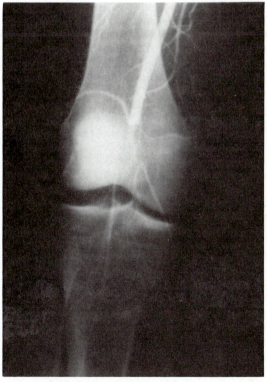

A
B

Figure 35–11. Arteriograms demonstrating nonocclusive (**A**) and completely occlusive (**B**) injuries of the popliteal artery after blunt trauma.

severe associated orthopedic, neurologic, and soft tissue injuries rendering any attempt at repair futile. Ten repairs were unsuccessful. In five, extensive thrombosis of the tibial vessels precluded successful revision, and the other 5 were associated with invasive sepsis and no attempt at revision of the vascular repair was made.

C. Infrapopliteal Arteries: Injuries to the tibial vessels are managed in a similar manner to that already described for forearm vascular injuries. Preferably, perfusion to at least 2 of the 3 tibial vessels should be maintained. This means that if the tibioperoneal trunk is injured, it should be repaired, usually with a saphenous vein graft. Displaced fractures of the tibia and fibula often compress and occlude a tibial artery or cause an area of spasm seen on arteriography. Frequently, pulsatile flow is restored after reduction and fixation of the fracture.

D. Venous Injuries: About 50% of all extremity arterial injuries are associated with concomitant venous injuries. Simple venous injuries amenable to lateral suture should be repaired. The treatment of more complex venous injuries that require end-to-end anastomosis or graft replacement is controversial. Whether repair provides any advantage over ligation of these complex injuries is unclear. Those who advocate repair refer to experimental studies that demonstrate a reduction in limb arterial flow following acute ligation of the major venous outflow of the limb. It has been hypothesized that venous ligation may thus lead to a higher rate of failure of arterial repairs. Also, repair of major lower extremity venous injuries theoretically lessens the potential incidence of chronic venous insufficiency. Those who are less enthusiastic about venous repair refer to the high incidence of thrombosis of these repairs and the risk of pulmonary embolization.

Meyer and associates, in a series employing routine venography 7 days after venous repair, showed that 14 of 36 repairs (39%) had thrombosed. Of those repairs requiring interposition vein grafting, 59% had failed at 1 week. Clearly, this study demonstrates a high incidence of thrombosis of complex venous repairs. Limb salvage in this series was 100% and was unaffected by the high rate of thrombosis of venous repairs. Clinical studies have been inconsistent in their findings regarding arterial patency, compartment syndrome, venous thromboembolism, and chronic venous insufficiency, and the issue remains unsettled.

When injured veins are repaired, meticulous attention to technique is essential. Thrombosis will occur if there is the slightest anastomotic imperfection. Prosthetic graft material should not be used in the venous system of the extremities because the rate of thrombosis in this position is prohibitive. The seriously injured patient may not be able to tolerate the additional operating time and potential additional blood loss that venous repair may entail, and in these situations the injured veins are best treated by ligation.

Whether the venous injury is repaired or ligated, the affected extremity should be kept elevated and wrapped with elastic bandages in the postoperative period to minimize edema. Also, the use of heparin, dextran, or other antiplatelet agents may be useful to inhibit thrombosis of the repair.

E. Associated Injuries:

1. Orthopedic–In most instances of combined orthopedic and vascular trauma to the limbs, the arterial repair should be completed and distal perfusion restored prior to orthopedic stabilization. However, when there is severe instability of the limb, an external fixator may be initially placed to provide stabilization. Alternatively, an intraluminal shunt can be placed in the artery across the injury after gentle proximal and distal thrombectomy has been performed and perfusion restored to the distal limb. Definitive repair of the vascular injury is then deferred until orthopedic stabilization has been obtained. A fractured limb should be brought out to length prior to repair of a vascular injury to avoid subsequent tension on the repair at the time of orthopedic stabilization.

2. Neurologic–Neurologic injury occurs in about 50% of upper extremity vascular injuries and 25% of those of the lower extremity. Invariably, the nerve injury, not the vascular injury, determines the long-term functional status of the traumatized extremity. The vascular injury can almost always be repaired and perfusion restored.

Repair of neurologic injuries is generally performed 2–3 months after the acute injury occurs. This delay allows physiologic nerve regrowth and repair to occur. Injured nerve ends seen at the initial operation should be tagged with nonabsorbable suture to permit easier identification at the time of subsequent repair. An exception to delayed repair is a nerve cleanly transected by a sharp instrument; in this case, the nerve should be repaired at the time of initial exploration.

3. Soft tissue–Peripheral vascular injuries are associated with varying degrees of damage to the surrounding soft tissues. More severe soft tissue injury occurs with blunt trauma, high-velocity gunshot wounds, and shotgun blasts. Soft tissue injuries are treated at the time of initial operation by débridement of all grossly nonviable tissue, removal of foreign bodies, and copious irrigation. The wounds are inspected frequently during the postoperative period, and the patient is taken back to the operating room for repeat débridement as often as necessary.

An unexplained, persistent postoperative fever is often the only sign of hidden devitalized tissue. Débridement of devitalized tissue is essential to reduce the incidence of wound sepsis, which is a major cause of delayed amputation following vascular repair. Occasionally, extensive débridement of devitalized soft tissue must be performed, leaving a segment of vessel exposed. Blood vessels, especially at an anastomotic suture line, must be covered by soft tissue to prevent desiccation and disruption. Coverage may be accomplished by local mobilization and rotation of muscles, such as the sartorius or gastrocnemius muscle. However, if the soft tissue defect is large, another approach is required. Extra-anatomic bypass may be performed by ligating the exposed vessel proximally and distally and routing a graft through clean tissue planes around the area of exposure. Alternatively, a free flap of muscle, such as the rectus abdominus or latissimus dorsi muscle, may be required to provide coverage of the vessels and soft tissue defect.

Compartment Syndrome

The muscle groups, blood vessels, and nerves of the extremities are contained within fascial sheaths. Small increases in the volume of tissue within one of these noncompliant sheaths result in a large increase in pressure. A **compartment syndrome** occurs when the pressure within one or more of these osteofascial compartments rises and causes compromise of the blood flow to the muscles and nerves within that compartment. If the compartment pressure rises high enough, blood flow to that compartment may actually cease, and the structures within become ischemic.

A. Causes: An elevated compartment pressure may result from 3 causes: soft tissue trauma, reperfusion injury following limb ischemia, and venous outflow obstruction. Compartment syndrome most commonly occurs after blunt trauma resulting in muscle and soft tissue injury and edema, along with hemorrhage into the compartment from associated fractures. Reperfusion of a severely ischemic limb may result in compartment syndrome by triggering the production of oxygen-derived free radicals. These free radicals damage cell membranes, causing further cell injury and death, which is manifested as muscle edema and necrosis. Venous thrombosis causes venous outflow obstruction and venous hypertension, which may be severe enough to cause consequent compartmental hypertension. One, 2, or all 3 of these mechanisms may occur in the traumatized limb and result in a clinically manifest compartment syndrome.

B. Clinical Findings: Clinical signs of compartment syndrome include pain at rest or especially with passive range of motion of the distal part (hand or foot), diminished distal sensation, and tenseness or tenderness on palpation of the affected compartment. A diminution of the distal pulse does not occur until late in the course of the syndrome. Also, since skin perfusion is extrafascial, ischemic changes in the skin are not seen until late. The development of a motor deficit indicates irreversible ischemic damage to muscles and nerves. Spasm noted on arteriography may be a sign of an unrecognized compartment syndrome. The systemic consequences that may result from a compartment syndrome and muscle necrosis include shock, myoglobinuria, acute renal failure, acidosis, and hyperkalemia.

Measured compartment pressures of more than 30–40 mmHg are useful adjuncts to diagnosis, especially for those in whom the clinical examination is unreliable (small children and patients with an altered sensorium or those under general anesthesia). However, it should be stressed that the diagnosis of compartment syndrome is clinical and that compartment pressure measurement is not required, especially if this delays initiation of therapy. Reliance on measured compartment pressures alone to the exclusion of the clinical picture is to be discouraged, since there are many potential sources of measurement error.

C. Treatment: The treatment of a patient with an incipient or established compartment syndrome is immediate decompressive fasciotomy. This procedure should not be delayed for preoperative arteriography to assess potential vascular injury. If necessary, arteriography can be done on the operating table after fasciotomy is completed. Prophylactic fasciotomy should be considered in the absence of clinical findings in the following circumstances: when a significant time delay occurs between an injury that causes clinical ischemia and the restoration of arterial flow (greater than about 6 hours); when there is massive swelling of the extremity, which would make early detection of a developing compartment syndrome by physical examination difficult; when there is combined arterial and venous injury, especially if the vein is ligated; or when massive soft tissue injury is present.

Fasciotomy entails incision of the fascial envelope of the compartment, thus allowing the tissues to expand unrestricted and allowing the tissue pressure to fall. In performing fasciotomy, not only must the fascial envelope of the compartment be opened widely, but the overlying skin must be opened as well (dermotomy). The skin can also act as a tourniquet, resisting expansion of the tissues. Thus, if the skin is not opened, the compartments may not be adequately decompressed.

The lower extremity has 4 discrete compartments that must be decompressed individually (Fig 35–12). The most effective method to ensure complete decompression is by a double incision technique. A medial longitudinal incision is placed 2 cm posterior to the margin of the tibia, through which the superficial and deep posterior compartments are decompressed. Be careful not to injure the saphenous vein and nerve that lie in the subcutaneous tissue in this area. After the skin and subcutaneous tissue are divided, the fascia overlying the superficial posterior compartment is opened widely. The origin of the soleus muscle from the tibia is then divided, the soleus retracted posteriorly, the deep posterior compartment exposed, and its fascia incised. A second incision is placed on the lateral aspect of the leg between the tibia and fibula. The fascia overlying the anterior compartment is opened, decompressing this compartment. The intermuscular septum is then incised to decompress the lateral compartment. Care must be taken here to avoid injury to the superficial peroneal nerve, which lies just deep to this septum. An alternate method of lower extremity 4-

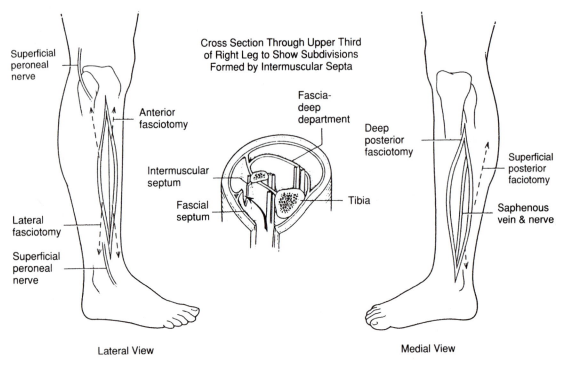

Superficial peroneal nerve

Anterior fasciotomy

Intermuscular septum

Fascial septum

Lateral fasciotomy

Superficial peroneal nerve

Cross Section Through Upper Third of Right Leg to Show Subdivisions Formed by Intermuscular Septa

Fascia-deep department

Deep posterior fasciotomy

Tibia

Superficial posterior faciotomy

Saphenous vein & nerve

Lateral View

Medial View

Figure 35–12. Technique of lower extremity fasciotomy.

compartment fasciotomy is through a single lateral incision, with or without resection of the fibula, but we believe this provides less complete decompression and do not advocate this approach.

Two compartments are found in the forearm: volar and dorsal. These compartments are interconnected and may be decompressed through a single volar incision (Fig 35–13). The incision is begun just proximal to the medial epicondyle of the humerus and carried obliquely across the antecubital crease. It then courses down the ulnar aspect of the forearm and across the wrist crease, again obliquely. After the muscular fascia is incised, the flexor retinaculum overlying the carpal tunnel is opened to decompress the median nerve. If the dorsal compartment still feels tense, it, too, is decompressed through a dorsal incision that begins distal to the lateral epicondyle and proceeds to the distal forearm.

Compartment syndrome may also develop in the foot, thigh, hand, or upper arm, each of which may require surgical decompression. However, these situations are uncommon and are beyond the scope of this discussion.

Fasciotomy wounds should be closed as soon as possible to prevent septic complications. If there is no muscle of questionable viability that may require repeated débridement, wound closure should be accomplished at the initial operation. If at exploration, no edema of the muscles is found and the skin edges can be brought together without tension, this should be

done, even if it can be done only on one side. A split-thickness skin graft may be used to cover any wound that cannot be closed without tension. Wounds that contain tissue of questionable viability are best left open, and the patient is returned to the operating room for reinspection and débridement at a later date. Delayed primary skin closure can be performed after it is certain that all nonviable tissue has been débrided, but these wounds more frequently require skin grafting to achieve closure.

To avoid or ameliorate the systemic effects of compartment syndrome and muscle necrosis, namely, acute renal failure, the patient must be well hydrated with a brisk urine output. This may require massive volume infusion and the use of loop diuretics such as furosemide or mannitol. There is evidence that mannitol also acts as a free radical scavenger, making it especially useful in the treatment of reperfusion injury. Alkalinization of the urine with the use of systemic bicarbonate has also been recommended to prevent the deleterious effects of myoglobin on the kidneys.

INTRAVASCULAR DRUG INJECTION

Vascular trauma may result from the intravascular injection of drugs into either the arterial or the venous system. Blood vessel injury from drug injection is most commonly seen in drug abusers, but may also be iatrogenic.

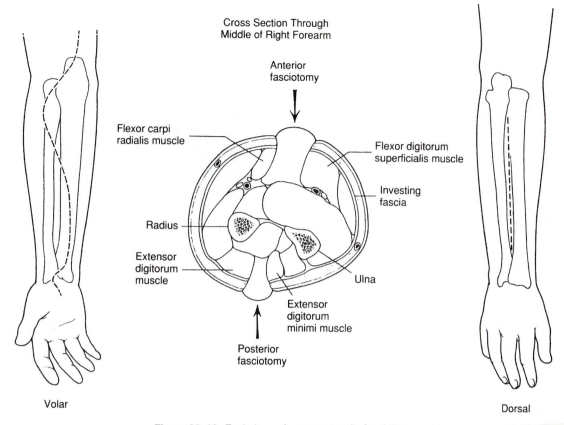

Cross Section Through
Middle of Right Forearm

Anterior
fasciotomy

Flexor carpi
radialis muscle

Flexor digitorum
superficialis muscle

Investing
fascia

Radius

Extensor
digitorum
muscle

Ulna

Extensor
digitorum
minimi muscle

Posterior
fasciotomy

Volar

Dorsal

Figure 35–13. Technique of upper extremity fasciotomy.

Venous injection

Venous damage associated with drug injection is the result of chronic or repetitive trauma, producing local irritation of the venous endothelium, which results in sclerosis and subsequent thrombosis. This process most frequently involves the superficial extremity veins but may extend into the deep venous system. Occasionally, injections are given directly into the femoral veins. Deep venous thrombosis (DVT) resulting from repetitive intravenous drug injection is treated by anticoagulation, just as with DVT resulting from any other cause. If septic thrombophlebitis is suspected, antibiotics are added to the regimen. *Staphylococcus aureus* is the most common organism isolated in these cases. Septic thrombophlebitis that does not respond to anticoagulation and antibiotic therapy requires surgical thrombectomy or vein excision. The common femoral vein may become pseudoaneurysmal after repeated injection, similar to an arterial mycotic aneurysm. Treatment entails complete excision of the affected vein, followed by proximal and distal ligation.

Mycotic aneurysms

Arterial mycotic aneurysms associated with drug injection result from repetitive needle trauma of the artery along with bacterial inoculation of the area surrounding the vessel. The arterial wall may become aneurysmal without direct needle trauma if infection extends from an adjacent site or if bacterial emboli from a distant site lodge in the vasa vasorum of the vessel wall and cause destruction. Arterial mycotic aneurysms are pulsatile in only 50% of cases and are inconsistently associated with bruits or loss of distal pulses. Unsuspected AV fistulas are encountered in about 5% of patients with arterial mycotic aneurysms. Complications of mycotic aneurysms include rupture, thrombosis, and distal embolization. Treatment entails the administration of parenteral antibiotics, wide débridement of all infected tissue, proximal and distal ligation of the aneurysmal vessel and removal of the entire infected arterial segment. Immediate revascularization for acute ischemia is not necessary in most patients. When revascularization is required, autogenous graft material is most often not available in these patients. The use of prosthetic material is complicated by a high incidence of septic complications. If revascularization must be done immediately, the grafts should be routed through extra-anatomic, noninfected tissue planes. If the patient does not require immediate revascularization, the tissues are allowed to heal and the infection to be cleared; if ischemic symptoms develop at a later date, a graft may be placed.

Arterial injection

Intra-arterial drug injection may result in a fulminant syndrome of acute limb ischemia involving small vessels and can progress to distal gangrene and tissue loss. The most common sites of intra-arterial injection, accounting for more than 80% of cases, are the radial and brachial arteries. Intra-arterial drug injection produces arterial and venous endothelial injury, leading to vessel spasm and thrombosis. The initial injury, even with intra-arterial injection, seems to be to the small veins. Venous thrombosis results in an increase in capillary hydrostatic pressure and transudation of fluid into the tissues. Elevated pressure in the soft tissues then ensues, impairing soft tissue perfusion and resulting in tissue ischemia and ultimately in gangrene. Thrombosis extends proximally into the arterioles but rarely extends into the larger named arteries.

Patients with intra-arterial drug injection present complaining of intense pain, which begins immediately after injection. Edema develops rapidly and can be severe, followed by stagnation of blood flow with cyanosis. Secondary arterial insufficiency and tissue hypoxia result in a cool extremity with progressive neurologic deterioration, ultimately resulting in gangrene of the digits. The distal pulse of the affected extremity is often normal or accentuated because of the degree of outflow obstruction. Arteriography generally demonstrates thrombosis of the digital arteries, but is rarely required to make the diagnosis and may actually aggravate the ischemic injury (Fig 35–14).

The treatment protocol followed in 48 patients with intra-arterial drug injury seen at the Los Angeles County University of Southern California Medical Center over a recent 16-year period involved the following: (1) heparin, 10,000 U intravenously given immediately, followed by a constant infusion to maintain the partial thromboplastin time 1.5–2.5 times the control; (2) dexamethasone, 4 mg intravenously every 6 hours; (3) low molecular weight dextran (Dextran 40) intravenous infusion at 20 mL/hr; (4) opiates or other analgesics for pain control; (5) extremity elevation; and (6) early use of passive and active range of motion.

Our treatment protocol was designed to minimize the various pathologic events that lead to tissue hypoxia and gangrene, namely, stasis, thrombosis, inflammation, and edema. Heparin is used to prevent thrombosis or propagation of clot in small veins and the capillary microcirculation, thereby preventing outflow obstruction, stasis, and occlusion of the arteries. Dexamethasone is used to protect cellular integrity, limit edema, and control the release of inflammatory mediators in response to tissue ischemia. Dextran minimizes platelet aggregation and sludging in small vessels. Elevation serves to reduce edema and alleviate stasis. Early mobilization with active and passive range of motion minimizes contracture development and residual motor deficit.

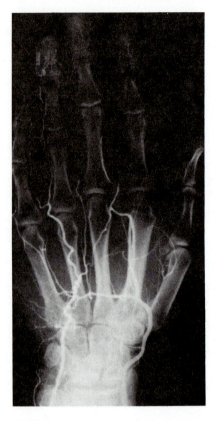

Figure 35–14. Typical digital arterial occlusion, here seen in the second and fourth digits, after intra-arterial drug injection.

Treatment was continued until all acute symptoms resolved or functional deficits stabilized, generally 3–8 days. After treatment of these 48 patients, 32 were found to have a normal extremity, 13 had limited tissue necrosis with dry gangrene, and 3 had neurologic dysfunction with an intact extremity.

IATROGENIC INJURIES

Vascular injury may occur as a result of the many invasive diagnostic, therapeutic, and monitoring procedures that have become routine in the management of many patients. Iatrogenic injury is the cause of 30% or more of the vascular trauma seen in many institutions. The brachial and femoral arteries are most commonly used to gain access to the vascular system and thus are most frequently injured. These injuries may manifest as bleeding and hematoma formation, thrombosis, dissection, embolization, or pseudoaneurysms and AV fistulas. An occasionally fatal but often occult complication is the unrecognized retroperitoneal perforation of an iliac artery by a guidewire or angioplasty catheter. Considerable hemorrhage into the retroperitoneal space can occur before obvious signs of hypovolemia are evident. When such complications occur in an elderly patient with coronary artery disease, a fatal myocardial infarction might occur.

General Considerations

A. Incidence and Risk Factors: The incidence of these complications is estimated to be between 1% and 2% of attempts at catheterization for cardiac and peripheral vascular procedures. A number of risk factors have been identified. Females generally have an increased risk because of the smaller size of their vessels. Atherosclerotic vessels are more likely than normal vessels to develop complications because of several reasons. A catheter introduced into a stenotic vessel may act as an obturator and produce vessel thrombosis. Atherosclerotic vessels are more likely to develop intimal flaps that may lead to dissection and thrombosis. Also, they are less elastic, which may prevent sealing of the catheter insertion site after the catheter is removed. Multiple punctures, a longer duration of catheterization, and multiple catheter exchanges result in a higher incidence of thrombotic complications. These factors relate to the experience of the angiographer as well as the complexity of the examination. The rate of complications is higher after therapeutic than after diagnostic procedures, a reflection of the larger sheaths required for the passage of balloons and stents. The use of aspirin, heparin, or thrombolytic agents increases the incidence of bleeding complications, but without heparin, thrombotic complications increase. In the femoral vessels, placement of the catheters into the superficial or profunda femoral arteries results in a higher complication rate than high entry into the common femoral artery. Finally, inadequate compression after the catheter is removed, especially if the puncture site is on the lateral aspect of the vessel after oblique vessel entry, results in a higher incidence of postprocedure complications.

B. Mechanism of Injury: The pathogenesis of brachial artery occlusive injuries due to catheterization has been described in detail and may apply to catheter-related occlusive injuries at all sites. Mechanisms of injury include, first, intimal disruption or dissection at the site of catheter entry or frank perforation of the arterial wall, which may lead to thrombus formation and vessel occlusion. Second, as the catheter lies inside the vessel, its shaft tends to rest against the posterior wall and may cause intimal ulceration or disruption proximal to the site of catheter entry. Third, thrombus may form on the outside of the catheter while it is residing in the intravascular space; as the catheter is removed at the conclusion of the procedure, the thrombus may be wiped off, leaving a plug inside the vessel and producing total occlusion. Another possible mechanism

of occlusion, after open catheterization, is narrowing at the site of suture closure of the arteriotomy. The arteriotomy should be closed transversely, not with a purse-string suture.

Diagnosis

Diagnosis of catheter-related trauma can usually be made clinically, and arteriography is rarely necessary. A hematoma is usually not difficult to discern, but differentiation from a pseudoaneurysm may be difficult. A pseudoaneurysm is frequently pulsatile or associated with a bruit, but these findings are inconsistent. Color-flow duplex scanning aids in this differentiation. AV fistulas following catheterization may be delayed in their presentation; duplex scanning is useful here also. Occlusive lesions may cause symptoms of acute ischemia or may be completely asymptomatic and noted only by a change in the pulse examination from prior to the procedure.

Treatment

Hematomas cause problems by compressing the surrounding structures, such as nerves. This is especially true after axillary puncture; a hematoma can track up into the axillary sheath, which is relatively noncompliant, and produce a brachial plexus palsy. A hematoma causing nerve compression should be evacuated as soon as possible because delay results in permanent disability. A hematoma may also put pressure on the overlying skin and cause blistering, ulceration, and frank necrosis. Débridement of skin may be necessary, along with evacuation of the hematoma, to permit adequate wound healing.

Small pseudoaneurysms may thrombose and heal and are safe to observe for a period of time. Ultrasound-guided compression of the neck of a small pseudoaneurysm may facilitate thrombosis in some patients. However, if pseudoaneurysms expand or are associated with an AV fistula, they should be surgically repaired.

Injuries that cause vessel occlusion or dissection and acute ischemic symptoms should be repaired as soon as possible. Injuries that do not produce acute ischemia should also be repaired. It has been documented that after iatrogenic brachial artery occlusive injuries, at least one-third of patients later develop ischemic symptoms requiring more complex bypass procedures if the injury is not immediately repaired.

Repair is optimally performed in the operating room, but may be done in the catheterization suite or even in the intensive care unit. Most repairs can be performed under local anesthesia. Depending on the extent of injury, repair may be accomplished by thrombectomy alone, débridement of the arteriotomy site and suture closure, patch angioplasty, local resection with reanastomosis, or graft interposition.

REFERENCES

Applebaum R et al: Role of routine arteriography in blunt lower-extremity trauma. Am J Surg 1990;160:221.

Blickenstaff KL et al: Trends in the management of traumatic vertebral artery injuries. Am J Surg 1989;158:101.

Dennis JW et al: Reassessing the role of arteriograms in the management of posterior knee dislocations. J Trauma 1993;35:692.

Fabian TC et al: Carotid artery trauma: Management based on mechanism of injury. J Trauma 1990;30:953.

Feld R et al: Treatment of iatrogenic femoral artery injuries with ultrasound-guided compression. J Vasc Surg 1992; 16:832.

Feliciano DV: Management of traumatic retroperitoneal hematoma. Ann Surg 1990;211:109.

Feliciano DV et al: Abdominal gunshot wounds: An urban trauma center's experience with 300 consecutive patients. Ann Surg 1990;208:362.

Fry WR et al: The success of duplex ultrasonographic scanning in diagnosis of extremity vascular proximity trauma. Arch Surg 1993;128:1368.

Frykberg ER, Vines FS, Alexander RH: The natural history of clinically occult arterial injuries: A prospective evaluation. J Trauma 1989;29:577.

Jackson MR et al: Abdominal vascular trauma: A review of 106 injuries. Am Surg 1992;58:622.

Johansen K et al: Non-invasive vascular tests reliably exclude occult arterial trauma in injured extremities. J Trauma 1991;31:515.

Johnson SB et al: Clinical results of decompressive dermotomy-fasciotomy. Am J Surg 1992;164:286.

Lynch K, Johansen K: Can Doppler pressure measurement replace "exclusion" arteriography in the diagnosis of occult extremity arterial trauma? Ann Surg 1991;214:737.

Mattox KL et al: Five thousand seven hundred sixty cardiovascular injuries in 4459 patients. Ann Surg 1989;209:698.

McAninch JW et al: Renal gunshot wounds: Methods of salvage and reconstruction. J Trauma 1993;35:279.

Meyer J et al: The early fate of venous repair after civilian vascular trauma: A clinical, hemodynamic, and venographic assessment. Ann Surg 1987;206:458.

Modrall JG, Weaver FA, Yellin AE: Vascular considerations in extremity trauma. Orthop Clin North Am 1993;24:57.

Munoz E, Cohen J: Epidemiology and the economics of vascular trauma. In: *Civilian Vascular Trauma.* Flanigan DP, Schuler JJ, Meyers JP (editors). Lea & Febiger, 1992.

Poole GV: Fracture of the upper ribs and injury to the great vessels. SGO 1989;169:275.

Schwartz MR et al: Refining the indications for arteriography in penetrating extremity trauma: A prospective analysis. J Vasc Surg 1993;17:116.

Skillman JJ, Kim D, Baim DS: Vascular complications of percutaneous femoral cardiac interventions: Incidence and operative repair. Arch Surg 1988;123:1207.

Stain SC et al: Selective management of nonocclusive arterial injuries. Arch Surg 1989;124:1136.

Stiles QR et al: Management of injuries of the thoracic and abdominal aorta. Am J Surg 1985;150:132.

Treiman GS et al: An effective treatment protocol for intraarterial drug injection. J Vasc Surg 1990;12:456.

Treiman GS et al: Examination of the patient with a knee dislocation: The case for selective arteriography. Arch Surg 1992;127:1056.

Wagner WH et al: Blunt popliteal artery trauma: One hundred consecutive injuries. J Vasc Surg 1988;7:736.

Weaver FA et al: Injuries to the ascending aorta, aortic arch and great vessels. SGO 1989;169:27.

Weaver FA et al: Is arterial proximity a valid indication for arteriography in penetrating extremity trauma? Arch Surg 1990;125:1256.

Weaver FA et al: The role of arterial reconstruction in penetrating carotid injuries. Arch Surg 1988;123:1106.

Index

NOTE: A *t* following a page number indicates tabular material and an *f* following a page number indicates a figure. Drugs are listed under their generic names. When a drug trade name is listed, the reader is referred to the generic name.

signs and symptoms, 182–183
treatment, 183
types, 112, 182
upper-extremity ischemia and, 157
Fibromyositis, differential diagnosis, 137
Fibronectin, 56, 57
Filariasis, lymphedema in, 392–393
5 Ps, of arterial occlusion, 418
Flow void principle, 28
Fluid balance, 80
effects of surgery, 81–83
Fluid replacement
intraoperative, 82–83
postoperative, 82–83
Fluid shift(s), associated with surgery, 81–83
Fluid volume, effects of trauma, 82
Foot. *See also* Diabetic foot
ulcers, in diabetic, 298–299
Foot drop, with acute limb ischemia, 285
Forefoot amputation, 347, 348*f*
Framingham study, 88–89
Fresh frozen plasma, for disseminated intravascular
coagulation, 69
Fungal infection, mycotic aneurysm and, 253

Gangrene, 2
amputation for, 346
in aortoiliac occlusive disease, 194, 195*f*
with deep venous thrombosis, 376, 376*f*
in diabetic patient, 346
dry, 2, 4*f*
in femoropopliteal occlusive disease, 333, 336
intestinal, 267, 269
with phlegmasia cerulea dolens, 376
wet, 2
Gastric artery aneurysms, 244*t*, 245*t*, 248
Gastroduodenal artery aneurysms, 244*t*, 245*t*,
248–249, 249*f*
Gastroepiploic artery aneurysms, 244*t*, 245*t*, 248
Giant cell arteritis, 111, 112–113
aortitis with, 127–128
clinical features, 128
treatment, 128
causes, 175
clinical features, 175–176
diagnostic criteria for, 173
epidemiology, 174
imaging studies, 175–176, 176*f*
incidence, 175
laboratory findings in, 175
pathophysiology, 175, 175*f*
patterns of vessel involvement in, 174–175
prognosis for, 176
signs and symptoms, 175
treatment, 176
upper-extremity ischemia and, 156
Glanzmann's thrombasthenia, 65
Glomerular capillary, 80, 81*f*
Glomerulus, renal, constituent parts, 80, 81*f*
Glycoprotein(s)
histidine-rich, elevation, 76

Ia, 57
Ib, 56*f*, 56–57
IIb:IIIa, 57
platelet, 56
Gradient elastic stockings, 369
Graft(s). *See also* Aortic grafts; Aortofemoral bypass
grafts; Extra-anatomic grafts;
Femoropopliteal bypass
aortoiliac, thrombosis, 232
aortomesenteric, antegrade, 271, 272*f*
aortovisceral bypass, 274
arterial emboli with, 283
basilic vein, for femoropopliteal bypass, 338
cephalic vein, for femoropopliteal bypass, 338
Dacron, 325, 328, 331, 409
endovascular, 39, 39*f*
iliofemoral, 204, 204*f*
lymphatic, for lymphedema, 399–400, 401*f*, 402*f*
polytetrafluorethylene, 325, 328, 331, 409
for femoropopliteal bypass, 338–339, 339*f*,
340–341
saphenous vein, for femoropopliteal bypass, 338,
339*f*
Great artery injuries, repair, 414
Greater saphenous vein
anatomy, 352, 352*f*
in chronic venous insufficiency, 366–368
superficial thrombophlebitis in, 362–363
varicosities, 355, 355*f*, 356, 366
high ligation and stripping with stab avulsion,
359–361, 360*f*
high ligation with stab avulsion, 359, 359*f*
Greenfield filter, 77, 385
Guidewires, angiographic, 13–14

Hageman factor. *See* **Factor XII**
Hand ischemia, 19, 153–159. *See also* Raynaud's phenomenon
causes, 153, 154*t*
clinical features, 153–156
diagnosis, 156–158
history-taking with, 153
imaging studies, 154–155
laboratory findings in, 155–156
physical findings in, 154
prognosis for, 159
signs and symptoms, 153–154
treatment, 158–159
Head and neck, vascular supply for, 89–91, 90*f*
collateralization of, 90–91
Heart disease. *See also* Coronary artery disease
atherosclerotic, arterial emboli with, 282
deep venous thrombosis and, 378
perioperative evaluation and management, 45–54
Heart valve(s), prosthetic, arterial emboli with, 282
Hemangioma(s), 309, 310*t*, 310–312
alarming, 312
biologic behavior, 310
cavernous, 314
clinical presentation, 310
coagulopathy with, 312